# Atlas of Nuclear Medicine Imaging


**Sheldon Baum, M.D.**

Director of Nuclear Medicine, Pennsylvania State University College of Medicine, Hershey, Pennsylvania

**Norman R. Vincent, M.D.**

Director of Nuclear Medicine, St. Vincent's Medical Center, Bridgeport, Connecticut

**Kenneth P. Lyons, M.D.**

Director of Nuclear Medicine, Veterans Administration Hospital, Long Beach, California

**Sing-yung Wu, M.D.**

Division of Nuclear Medicine, Veterans Administration Hospital, Long Beach, California

**Steven C. Gurkin, M.D.**

Director of Radiology, Colima Medical Group, Whittier, California



ACC APPLETON-CENTURY-CROFTS/New York

To Our Wives

Maureen Baum, Beverly Vincent,
Joanna Lyons and Adrienne Gurkin

---



81 82 83 84 85 / 10 9 8 7 6 5 4 3 2 1

Prentice-Hall International, Inc., London
Prentice-Hall of Australia, Pty. Ltd., Sydney
Prentice-Hall of India Private Limited, New Delhi
Prentice-Hall of Japan, Inc., Tokyo
Prentice-Hall of Southeast Asia (Pte.) Ltd., Singapore
Whitehall Books Ltd., Wellington, New Zealand

Library of Congress Cataloging in Publication Data
Main entry under title:

Atlas of nuclear medicine imaging.

Bibliography: p.
Includes index.
1. Radioisotope scanning—Atlases. 2. Nuclear medicine—Atlases. I. Baum, Sheldon. [DNLM:
1. Radionuclide imaging—Atlases. WN17 A8855]
RC78.7.R4A83 616.07′757′0222 80-10321
ISBN 0-8385-0447-7

Cover design: Dany Vincent
Text design: Jacquelyn Munn
Production: Matthew Collins, Bob Greiner, Jean Sabato

# Table of Contents

# Preface

This book is a comprehensive, detailed atlas of radionuclide imaging. It is an exhaustive compendium of normal and abnormal imaging and contains over 2800 illustrations.

For each procedure or organ system presented, detailed elaboration is made of the features that characterize a normal or abnormal imaging study. This is done with a dual approach: to illustrate the behavior and distribution of the particular radiopharmaceutical employed; and to emphasize the anatomic and functional characteristics of the scan or image itself. Labels and arrows have been used generously to identify anatomic structures that are seen on both normal and abnormal imaging.

The authors have attempted to present most major types of imaging abnormalities in this book. In a field such as nuclear medicine in which scientific progress and significant advances occur so rapidly, it is virtually impossible to assemble a collection of every abnormal imaging entity. Some areas of nuclear medicine, such as adrenal imaging, have not yet achieved widespread use and are not included in this edition. Also not included is emission computed tomography, which has not yet been accorded the preeminence for which it is ultimately destined in clinical nuclear medicine.

Although this is a multi-authored book, there was close collaboration between each of the five individual authors in order to avoid any sense of discontinuity or repetition.

Thanks are extended to Catherine Donahue and Nancy Bricker for their work in the preparation and organization of the manuscript.

Sheldon Baum
Norman R. Vincent
Kenneth P. Lyons
Sing-yung Wu
Steven C. Gurkin

# Acknowledgments

The assistance of the following people in the preparation of this Atlas is gratefully acknowledged: Sergio Alba, Susan Bott, Nancy Bricker, Mary Campbell, Judy Chronister, Nancy Cipkala, Vincent Czajkowski, James Dalzell, Maria Dell'Olio, Catherine Donahue, Christine Dunn, Nancy Elterich, Barbara Ann Eye, Mary Ann Gallo, Theresa Golazeski, Jean Hickey, Ken Irwin, William Koch, Cecelia A. Korchnak, Barbara Linderman, Elizabeth Meyer, Sally Nell, Cynthia Nielsen, Dorothy Potts, Michael Sheetz, Nancy Skultety, JoEllen Slabonik, Irene Tehan, Victoria Walker, Marianna Wright.

# 1/Liver, Spleen, and Hepatobiliary Imaging

Almost all liver–spleen imaging is performed following the intravenous administration of a radioactive colloid. The most commonly employed radionuclide for such imaging is Tc-99m sulfur colloid (SC), with a particle size of less than 0.1$\mu$ in diameter. The usual dose is 3 to 4 mCi.

Following the injection of Tc-99m SC, the radioactive particles become engulfed in the phagocytic cells of the reticuloendothelial system (RES), principally in the endothelial lining Kupffer cells of the liver and in the splenic macrophages. There is also some phagocytosis of the radiocolloid in the RES cells of the bone marrow, but to a far lesser degree than in the liver and spleen. In the normal subject there is almost total incorporation of the Tc-99m SC in the Kupffer cells and splenic macrophages within 5 minutes of intravenous administration.

Most liver and spleen imaging now includes both blood flow studies and static imaging. The blood flow studies are not usually helpful in assessing the presence or absence of a liver abnormality. However, great vessel abnormalities (superior vena cava obstruction, aneurysm of the abdominal aorta) may sometimes first be detected by this portion of the study.

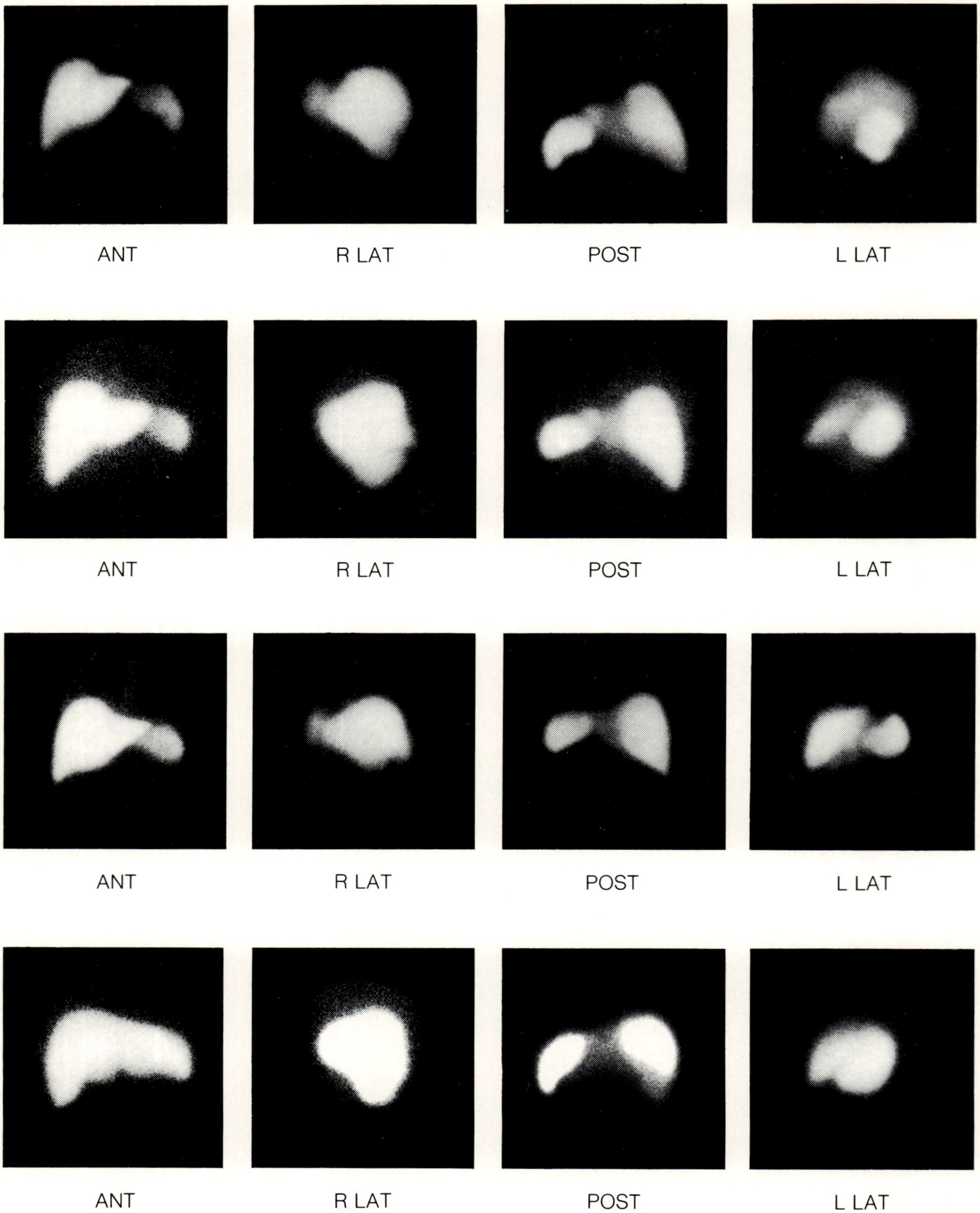


**FIG. 1.** (See legend next page)

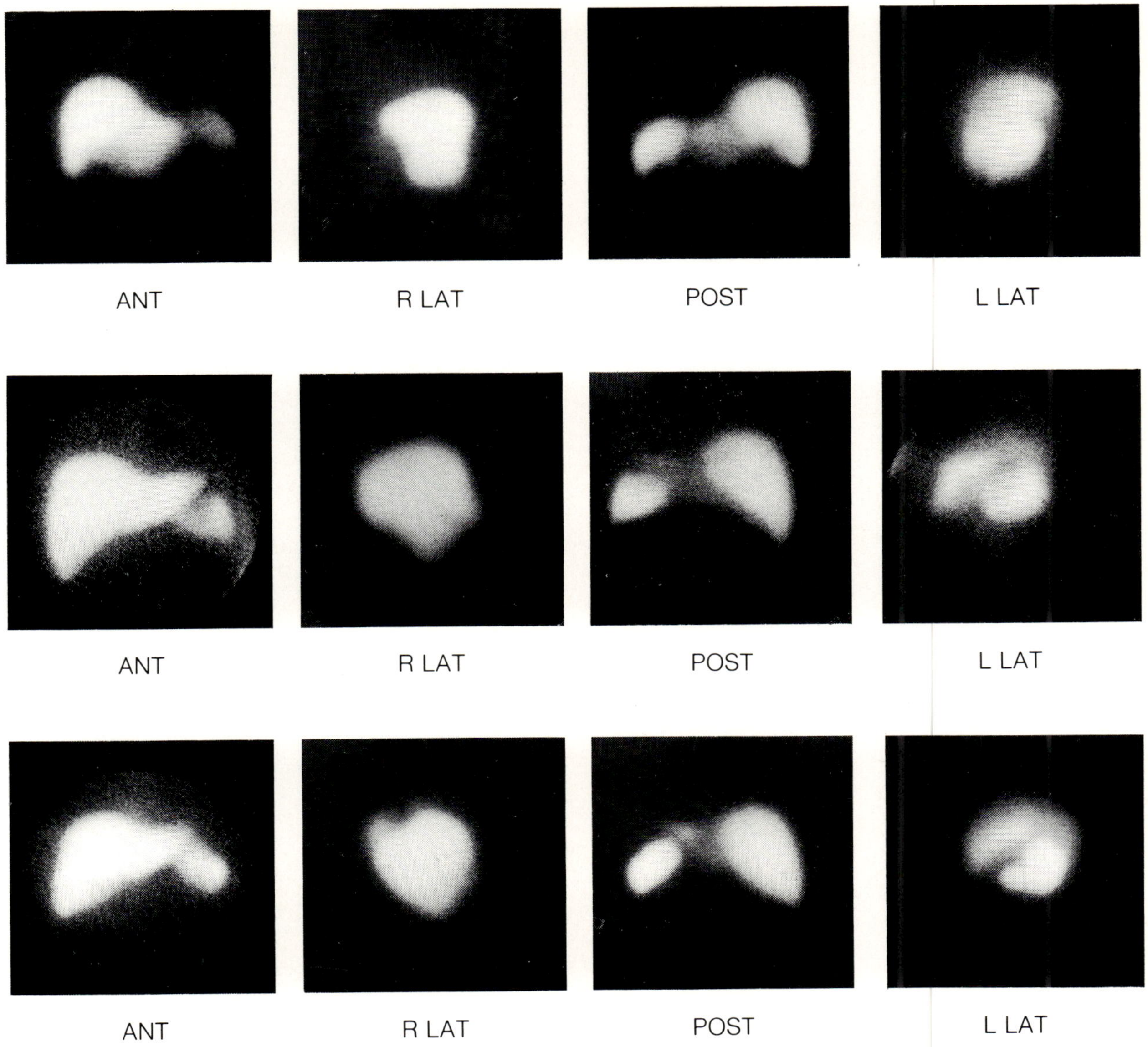


**FIG. 1. NORMAL LIVER–SPLEEN IMAGING. Positions.** Imaging is usually performed in the anterior, right lateral, posterior, and left lateral positions. Note the variability in hepatic configuration. Oblique positions may sometimes be helpful (see Fig. 45).

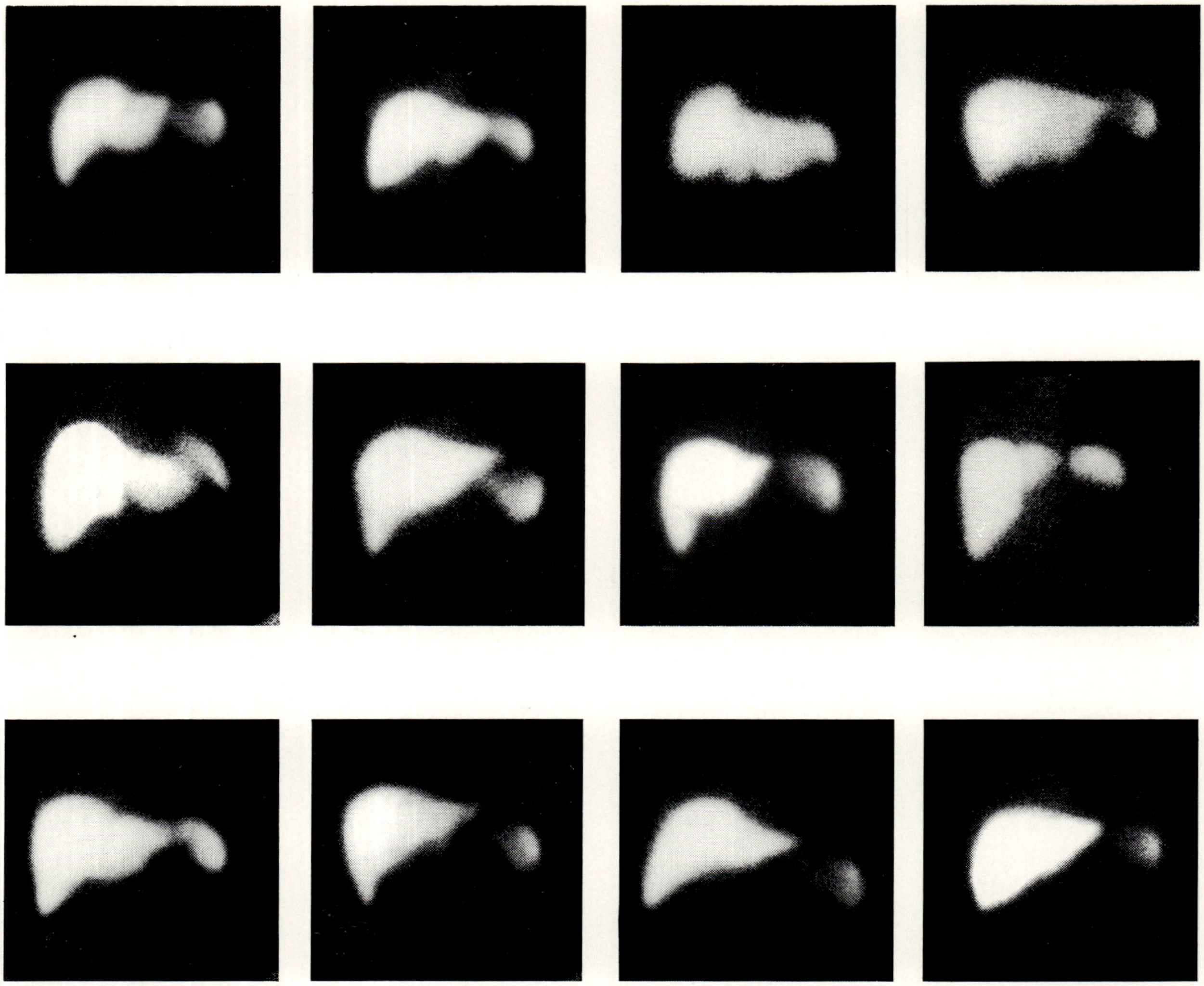

**FIG. 2.** NORMAL LIVER–SPLEEN IMAGING. **Anterior Position.** Both the liver and spleen are usually readily identified in the anterior position. The mass of the right lobe is usually four to five times greater than the left, and this is reflected in the relative radioactivity in each lobe. The normal reductions in radioactivity in the left lobe, especially in its lower half, may sometimes be mistakenly interpreted as a space-occupying lesion. The subdiaphragmatic portion of the right lobe is nicely rounded as it fits snugly underneath the right diaphragm. The medial portion of the right lobe and superior portion of the left lobe abut closely on the heart; this is the region of the cardiac impression. The lobar separation is not always easily recognized. The spleen is seen in the anterior position and, when of normal size, shows less radioactivity than is seen in the right hepatic lobe.

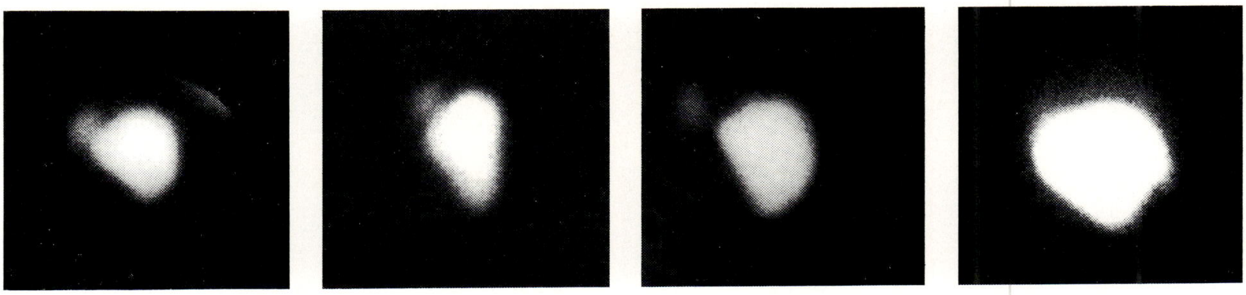

**FIG. 3.** NORMAL LIVER–SPLEEN IMAGING. **Right lateral position.** Anterior is to the viewer's right, posterior to his left. Unless there is unusual anterior extension of the left or right lobes, the anterior border is somewhat straightened with a relatively vertical appearance. The posterior border is also straightened but is somewhat diagonal. The lobes cannot be identified in this position. The subdiaphragmatic portion of the right lobe is smooth and rounded. The spleen, which is commonly located posteriorly, is usually identified in the right lateral position, a further demonstration of its posterior location. Its low radioactivity is a function of its distance from the collimator in this position.

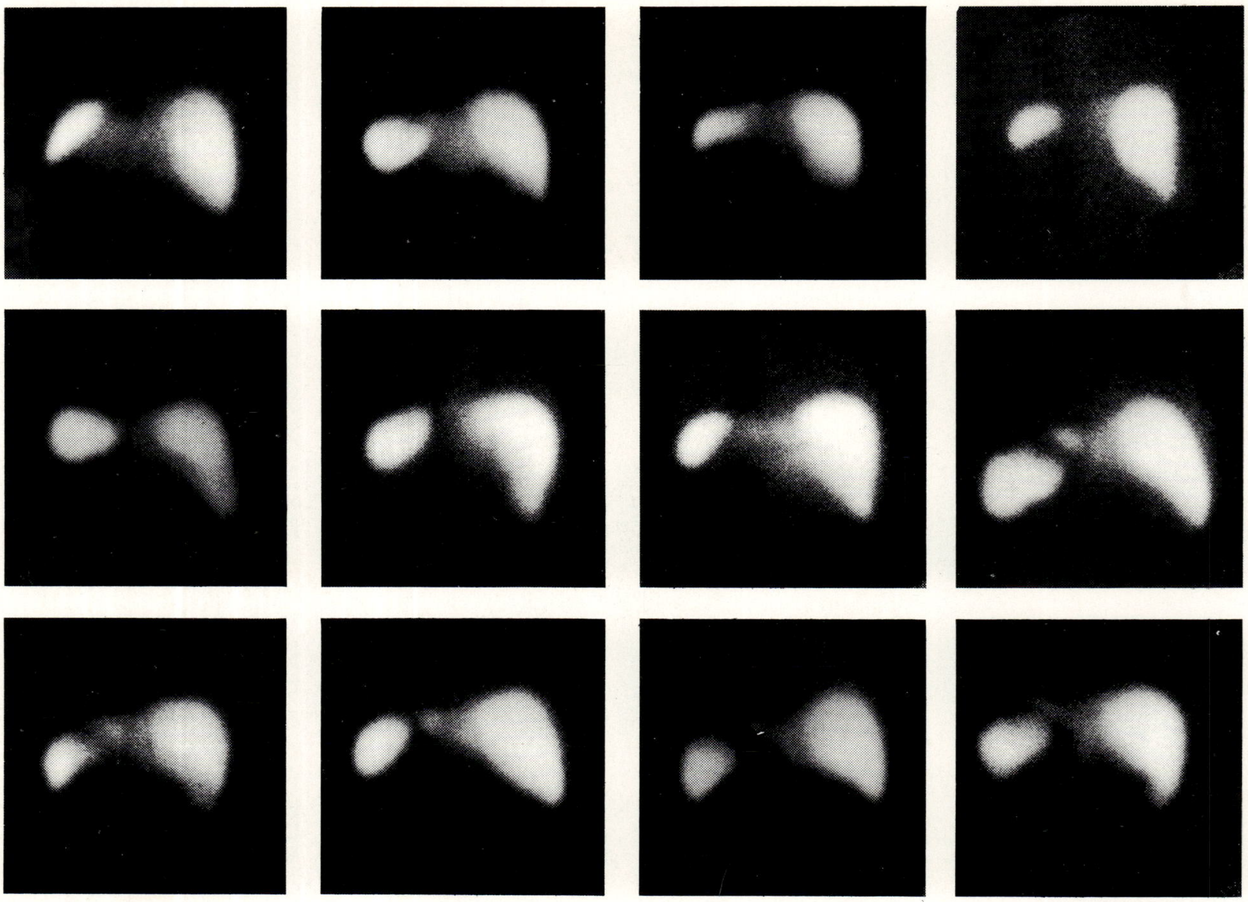

**FIG. 4.** NORMAL LIVER–SPLEEN IMAGING. **Posterior Position.** Although the right lobe of the liver may be readily seen in the posterior position, nonvisualization of the left lobe is common. Factors contributing to the failure to image the left lobe in this position include both its small mass and its far anterior position in relation to the detector. There may be a somewhat rounded reduction in radioactivity medially in the right lobe associated with the renal impression. The spleen is usually excellently visualized in the posterior position, and it is normal for the radioactivity in the spleen to be greater than in the liver, even in the absence of splenic enlargement.

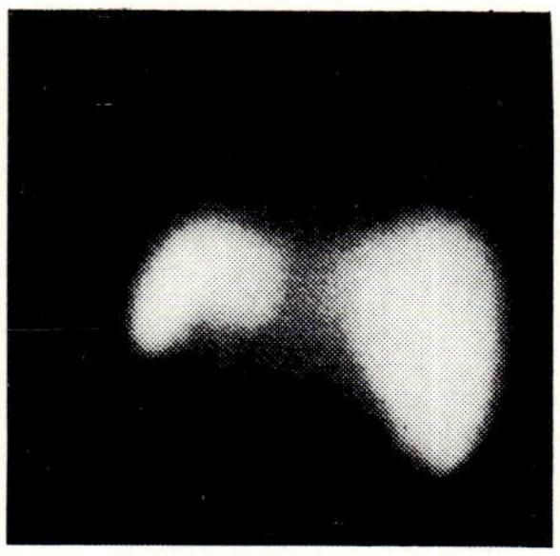

**FIG. 5.** NORMAL LIVER–SPLEEN IMAGING FOLLOWING RIGHT NEPHRECTOMY. **Posterior Position.** The area of reduced radioactivity commonly seen in association with the renal impression is no longer visualized.

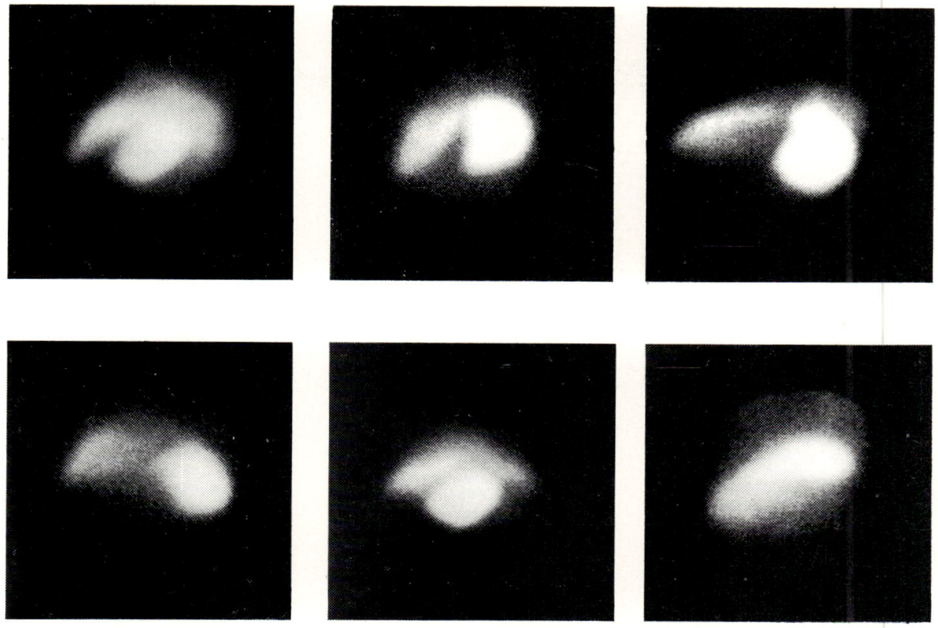

**FIG. 6.** NORMAL LIVER–SPLEEN IMAGING. **Left Lateral Position.** The spleen may be well outlined in its characteristic posterior location. Imaging in this view is especially helpful when information is needed concerning displacement or injury to the spleen. Although portions of the hepatic image normally can be identified in this position, there is no easily recognized delineation of the lobes of the liver.

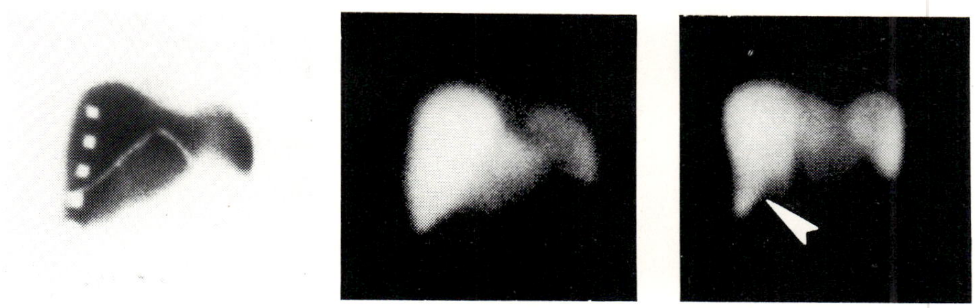

A ANT B ANT C ANT

**FIG. 7. REDUCTION IN LEFT LOBE RADIOACTIVITY.** Because of its greatly reduced mass compared to that of the right lobe, the left lobe of the liver commonly evidences reduced radioactivity. The reduction in radioactivity may be so prominent that a space-occupying lesion is sometimes suspected. In **A** the reduced uptake in the left lobe is readily appreciated. However, the reduced left lobe activity in **B** can be highly suggestive of a focal lesion. **C.** In this patient with an enlarged liver and spleen and a Riedel's lobe (large arrow), the reduced radioactivity in the left lobe, especially in its lower half, is a more pronounced reflection of the reduced mass of the left lobe compared to that of the right lobe. Note the accentuation of the lobar separation.

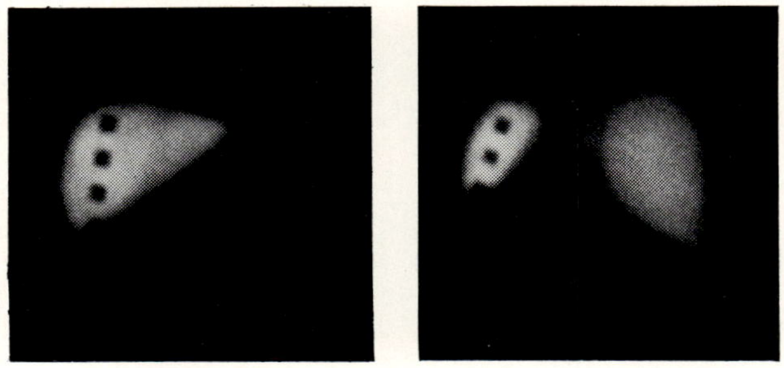

ANT Liver POST Spleen

**FIG. 8. NORMAL LIVER–SPLEEN IMAGING. Measurements.** Organ size can be determined with a scintillation camera through the use of a lead marker or similar device. In the method illustrated here, a ruler made up of 2 cm lengths of lead alternating with 2 cm blank areas is placed on the skin over the patient's liver to help determine its size. The longitudinal measurement from the subdiaphragmatic portion to the inferior portion of the right lobe is no greater than 19 cm. The spleen's longitudinal measurements are usually determined in both the anterior and posterior positions and, in the adult, should not exceed 10 cm.

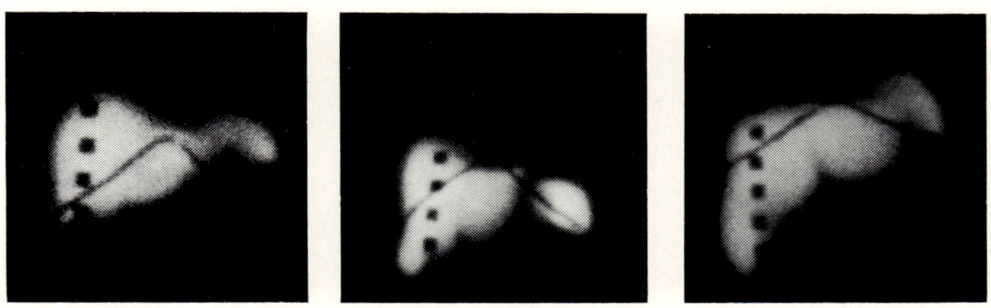

A ANT B C

**FIG. 9. NORMAL LIVER–SPLEEN IMAGING. Relation of Liver to Right Costal Margin. A.** For assistance to the clinician, the position of the liver in its relation to the right costal margin can be easily determined by the placing of a lead marker over the lowermost rib. Thus the amount the liver extends below the right costal margin can be calculated, and this should correspond roughly to the size of hepatic palpation. The palpable liver may sometimes not be enlarged, as is seen in **B** and **C,** in which the liver is of normal size but is relatively low-lying in its relation to the right costal margin. Similar determination can be made for the spleen by the outlining of the left costal margin. However, this is somewhat more difficult to identify in the healthy subject since the spleen rarely extends below the left costal margin.

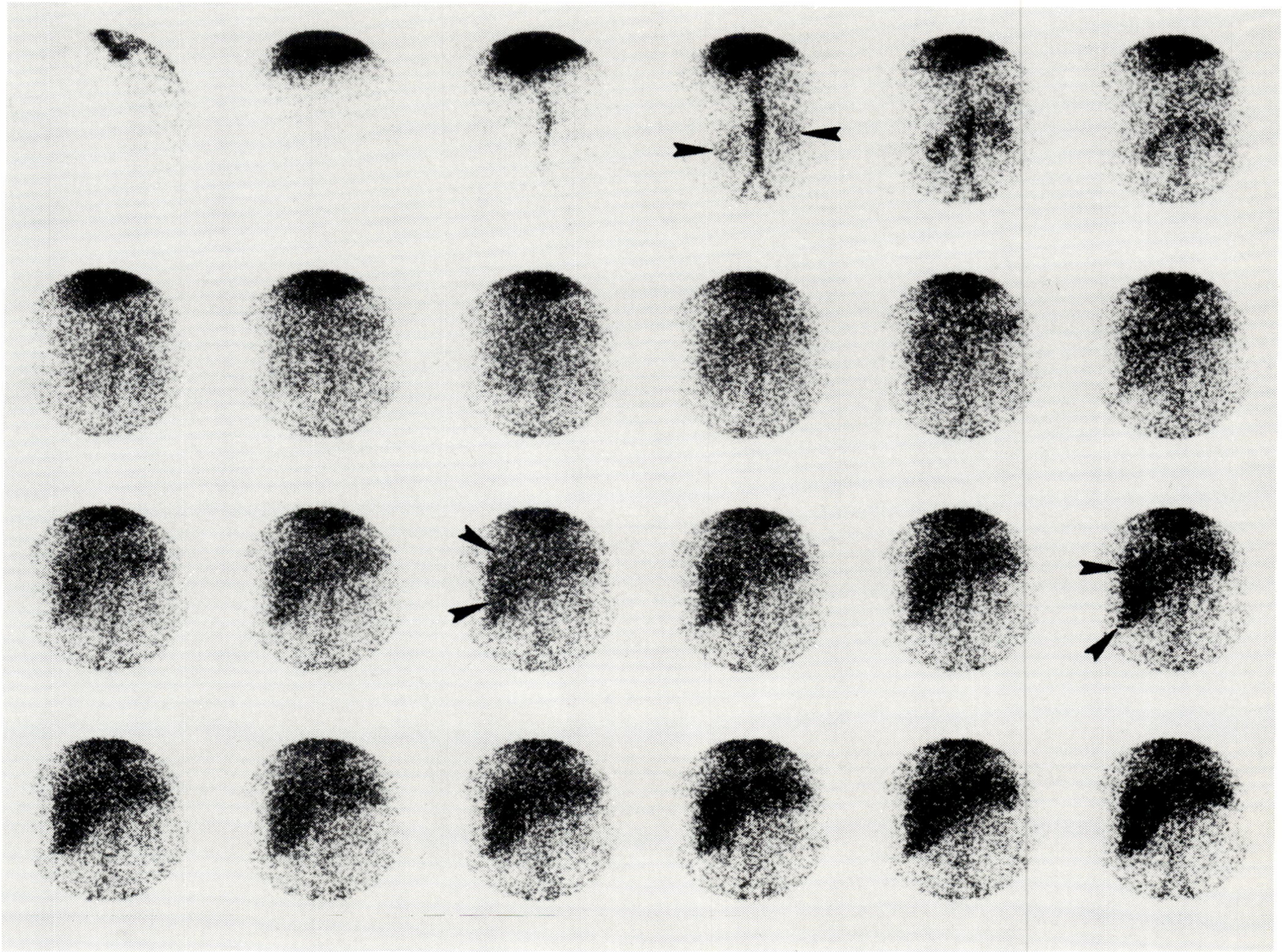

Blood Flow Study

**FIG. 10. BLOOD FLOW STUDIES PERFORMED IN CONJUNCTION WITH LIVER–SPLEEN IMAGING.** Following the IV administration of Tc-99m SC in an upper-extremity vein, imaging is performed as the radioactive material starts to become visualized in the abdominal aorta. Images in these studies were obtained at intervals of 3 seconds. There is little or no hepatic visualization during the arterial phase. Note the renal visualization during the arterial phase (arrows) in frames 4 and 5. The liver image starts to become well defined during the venous phase (arrows) as the Tc-99m-SC is delivered to the liver via the portal system (frames 14 and 15).

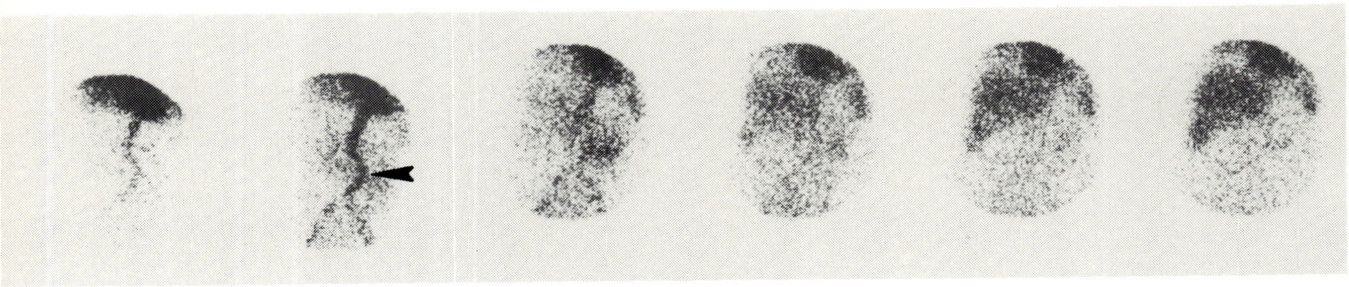

A

Blood Flow Study

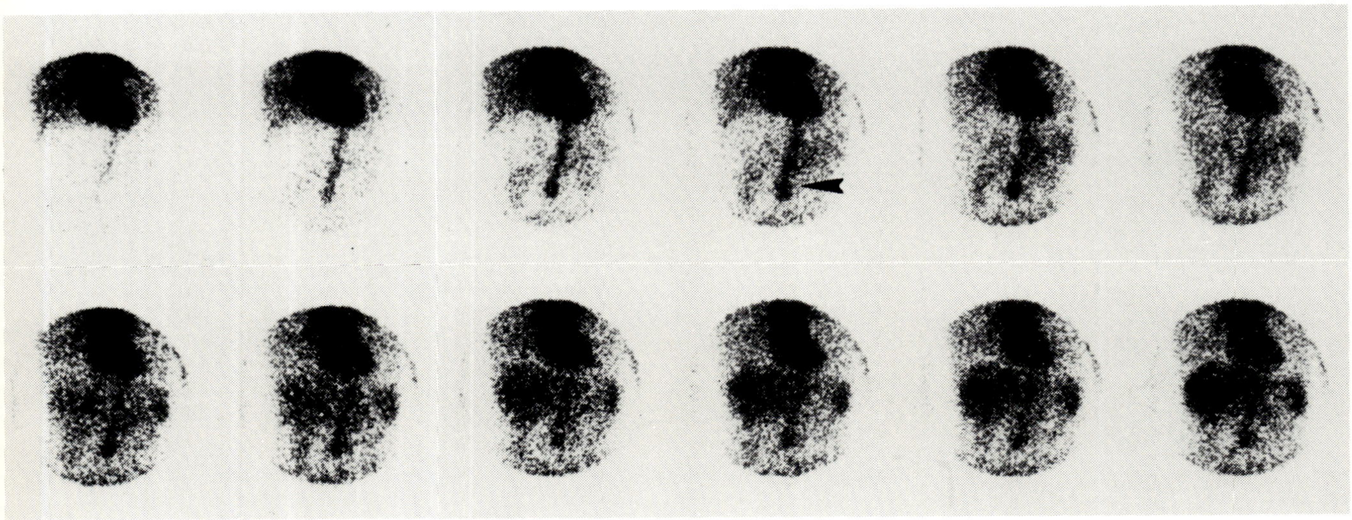

B

Blood Flow Study

**FIG. 11. UNSUSPECTED ABNORMALITIES DETECTED ON BLOOD FLOW STUDIES PERFORMED WITH LIVER–SPLEEN IMAGING.** Since the dose of the radiocolloid employed is relatively small (3 mCi), the images lack the clarity and definition of those produced by radionuclide venography and angiography, in which such radionuclides as Tc-99m pertechnetate or DTPA, administered in much larger doses, are used (see Chapter 8). **A.** Tortuosity of the abdominal aorta (arrow) is seen during the initial arterial phase. **B.** Aneurysm of distal abdominal aorta (arrow).

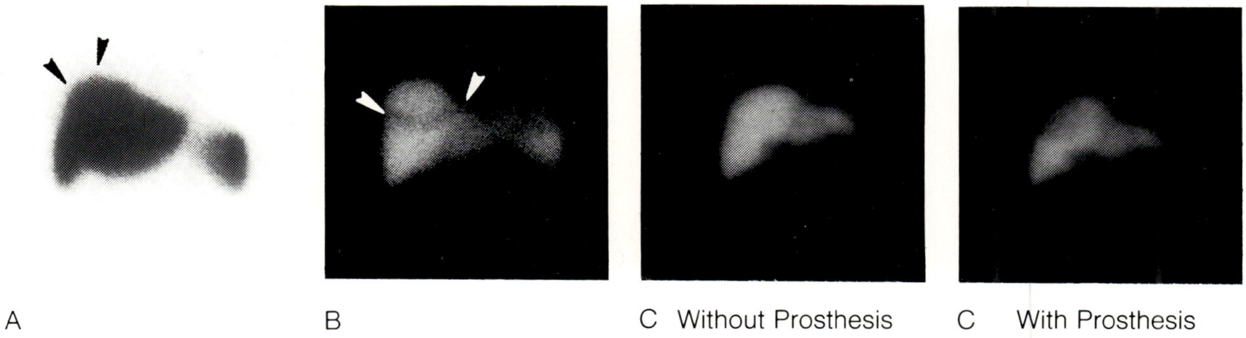


**FIG. 12. BREAST ARTIFACT. A.** Reduced radioactivity (arrows) due to overlying breast tissue recognized in the anterior position. **B.** Reduced radioactivity due to breast prosthesis. **C.** Imaging with and without prosthesis.

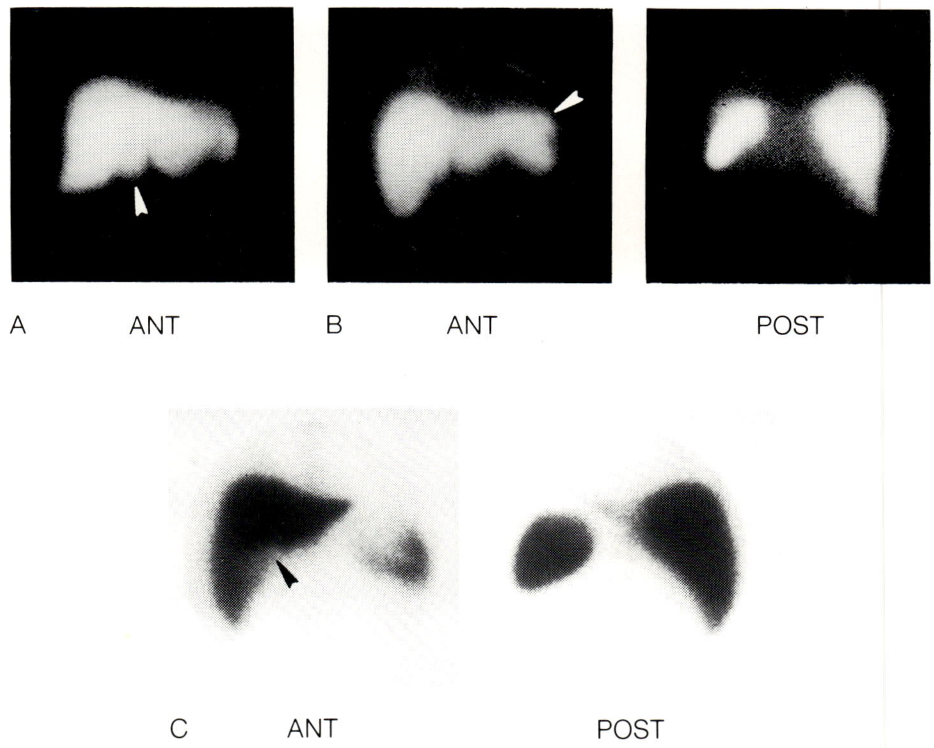


**FIG. 13. UNUSUAL LOBAR CONFIGURATION. A.** A quadrate lobe (arrow) may be identified in the anterior position. **B.** Extension of the left lobe (arrow) toward the left body wall is seen and appears to overlie the spleen. **C.** The posterior position of the inferior portion of the right lobe and the fossa in the region of the porta hepatis (arrow) almost suggests the presence of a lesion in the anterior position.

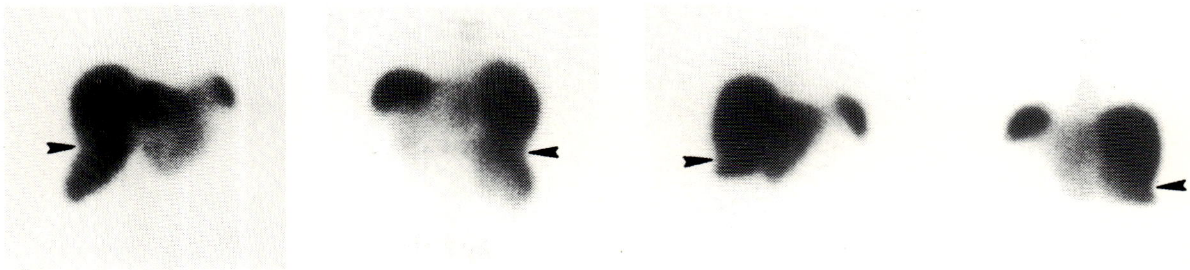

A ANT POST B ANT POST

**FIG. 14. GIRDLING EFFECT.** Marked lateral extension of the inferior portion of the right lobe is seen wherever the liver is not rigidly bound by the thoracic cage. There is usually no suggestion of a space-occupying lesion in the right lateral position. It is most frequently encountered in obese patients, usually females. **A.** Marked girdling effect as the right lobe extends below the limits of the thoracic cage (arrow). **B.** Girdling effect is more subtle as the right lobe extends below the limits of the thoracic cage (arrow).

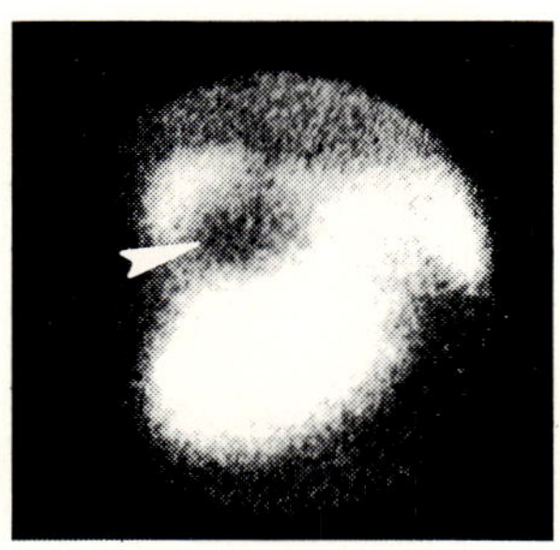

ANT

**FIG. 15. INTRAHEPATIC GALLBLADDER.** The gallbladder area is rarely identified in liver–spleen imaging. In this case, the intrahepatic gallbladder is responsible for the localized area of absent radioactivity (arrow). Its imaging appearance is identical to that of a tumor or other space-occupying lesion.

Variants of Normal

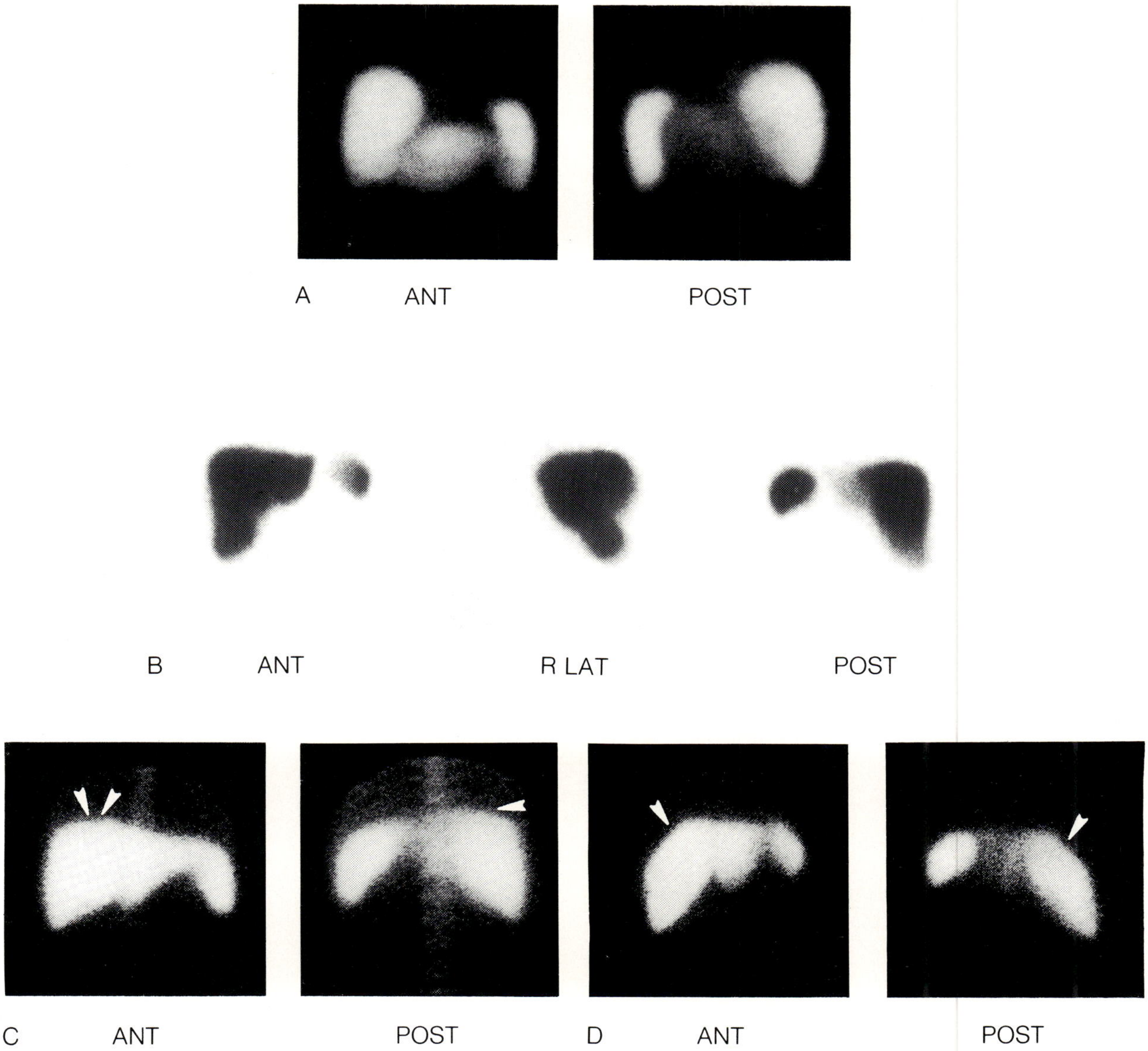



**FIG. 16. DIAPHRAGMATIC CHANGES. A.** Eventration of the right diaphragm results in the relatively elevated position of the subdiaphragmatic portion of the right lobe; findings are clearly visible in the anterior portion. **B.** Flattening of the subdiaphragmatic portion of the right lobe of the liver secondary to changes of pulmonary emphysema are visualized in the anterior, right lateral, and posterior positions. **C.** Flattening (arrows) associated with a right-sided pleural effusion seen in both the anterior and posterior positions. **D.** Straightening secondary to fibrothorax and pleural reaction. The sharply defined hepatic border hints that the changes may be pulmonary in origin.

## RIEDEL'S LOBE

Riedel's lobe of the liver is an additional lobe that is usually associated with, though sharply demarcated from, the inferior aspect of the right lobe. These lobes vary in size and are commonly responsible for a clinical impression of hepatomegaly or a right upper quadrant mass. The Riedel's lobe usually may be recognized in the anterior position alone, but in some cases delineation in right lateral and posterior positions is helpful. The direction of extension is best determined in the right lateral position. Rarely, the mass of the Riedel's lobe may be so small that identification through imaging may be difficult. This accessory lobe is encountered much more frequently in females than in males.

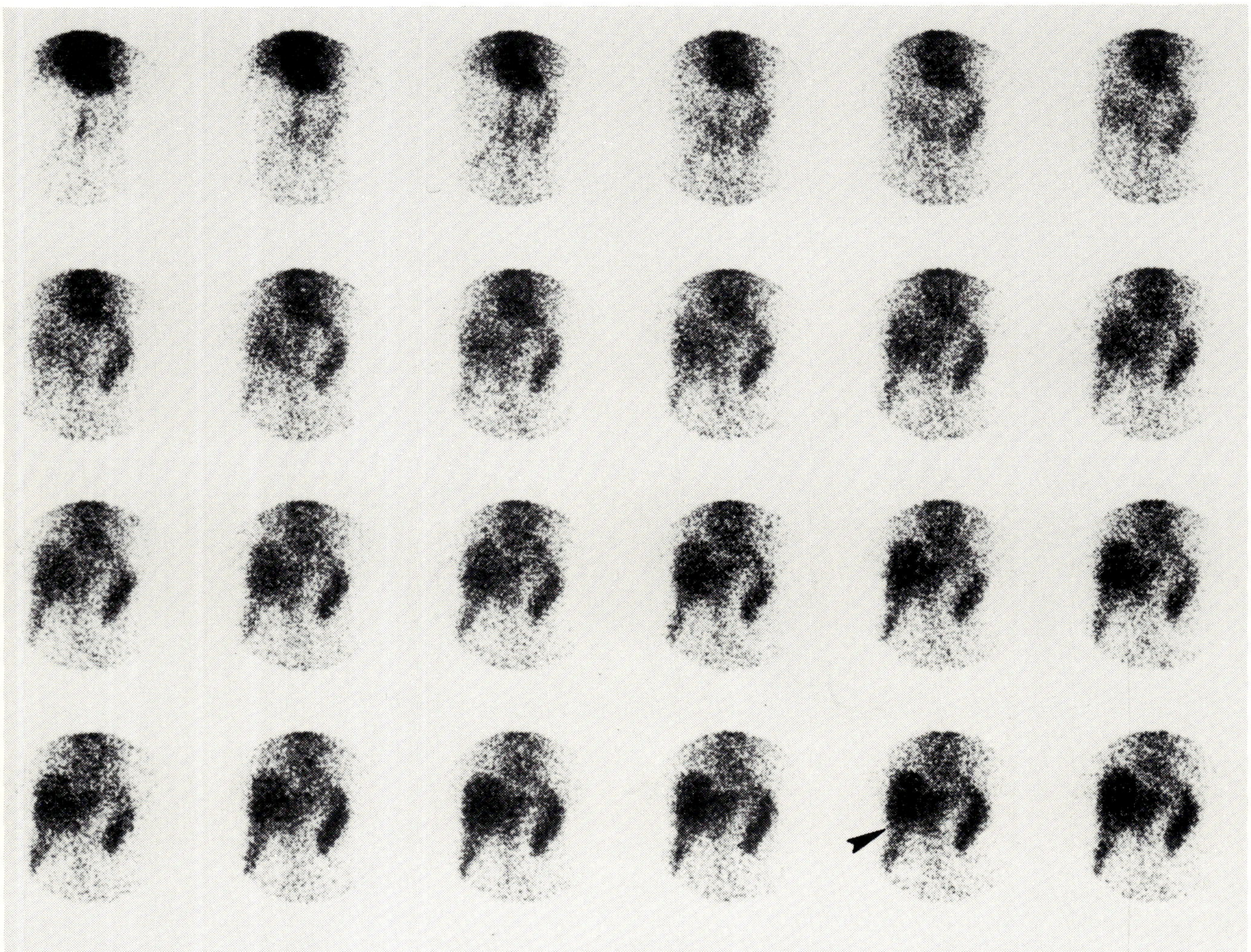

A

Anterior Blood Flow

**FIG. 17. A.** (See legend next page)

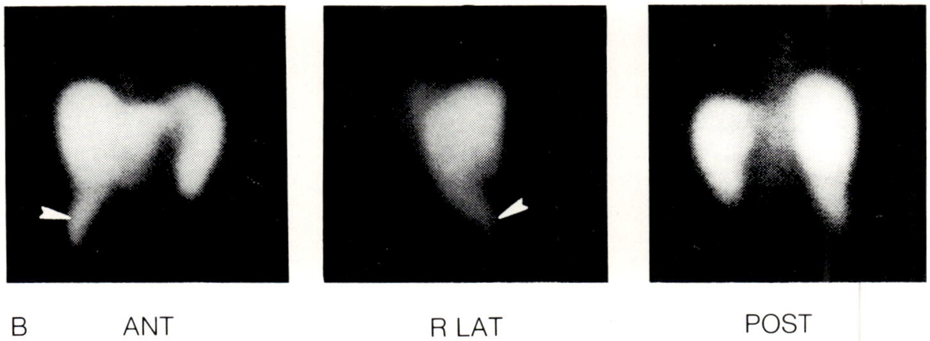


**FIG. 17.** ELONGATED RIEDEL'S LOBE. A. The blood flow study performed in the anterior position initially shows absent radioactivity at the site of the lobar separation (arrow) between the Riedel's lobe and right hepatic lobe. B. Static imaging shows the elongated tonguelike Riedel's lobe (arrow) extending anteriorly and inferiorly. The site of the lobar separation in the right lateral position may be confused with a space-occupying lesion.

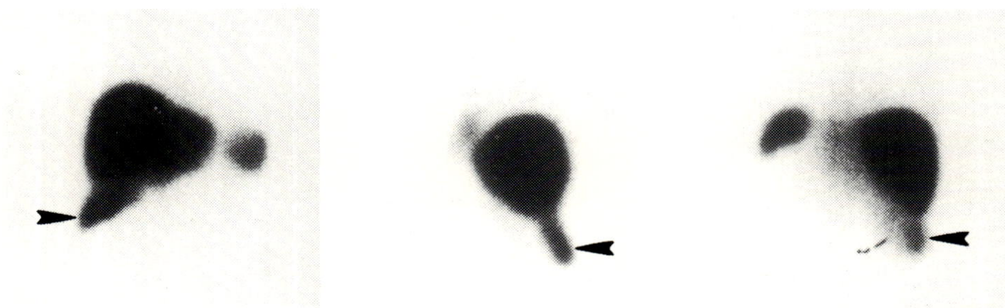

A ANT R LAT POST

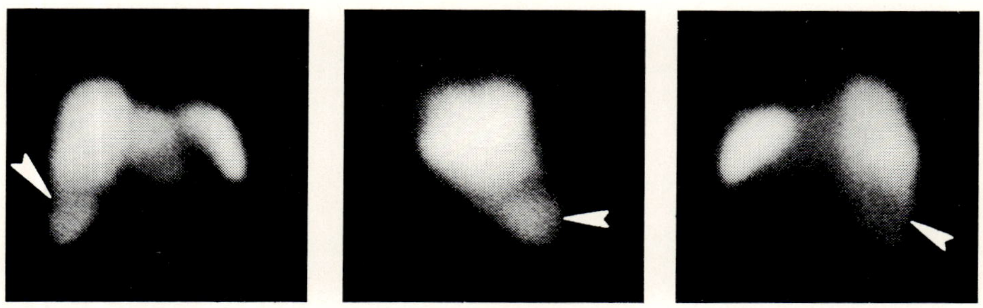

B ANT R LAT POST

**FIG. 18. RIEDEL'S LOBE WITH ANTERIOR EXTENSION.** The Riedel's lobe (small arrow) is readily recognized in the anterior position as the somewhat pedunculated portion of hepatic tissue extending inferiorly. The lobar separation (larger arrow) between the two lobes is easily identified. Note the anterior extension of the Riedel's lobe in the right lateral position. These accessory lobes are quite variable in size. In **A** the Riedel's lobe is sharply defined in the anterior, right lateral, and posterior positions. In **B** the pedunculated Riedel's lobe is somewhat ovoid, has a greatly reduced mass compared to the adjacent portion of the right lobe, and can be barely identified in the posterior position.

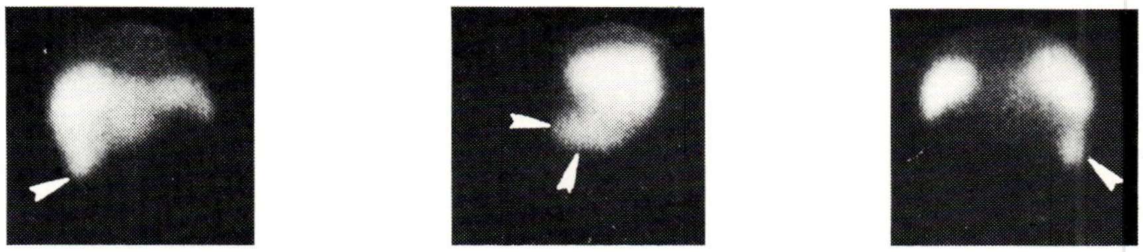

**FIG. 19. RIEDEL'S LOBE WITH POSTERIOR EXTENSION.** Although the Riedel's lobe (arrows) is easily visualized in the anterior and posterior positions, its marked posterior extension can be best appreciated in the right lateral position. Such posterior extension is uncommon.

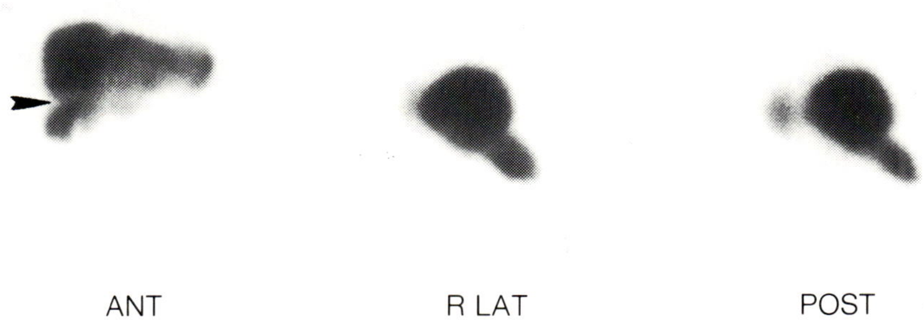


**FIG. 20. GLOBULAR RIEDEL'S LOBE.** The small, globular Riedel's lobe is easily palpated, and on physical examination it was thought that a subhepatic mass was present. Note the isolated position of the Riedel's lobe and the prominent lobar separation (arrow) in the anterior position. The marked anterior extension of the Riedel's lobe, as seen in the right lateral position, helps explain its prominence on palpation.

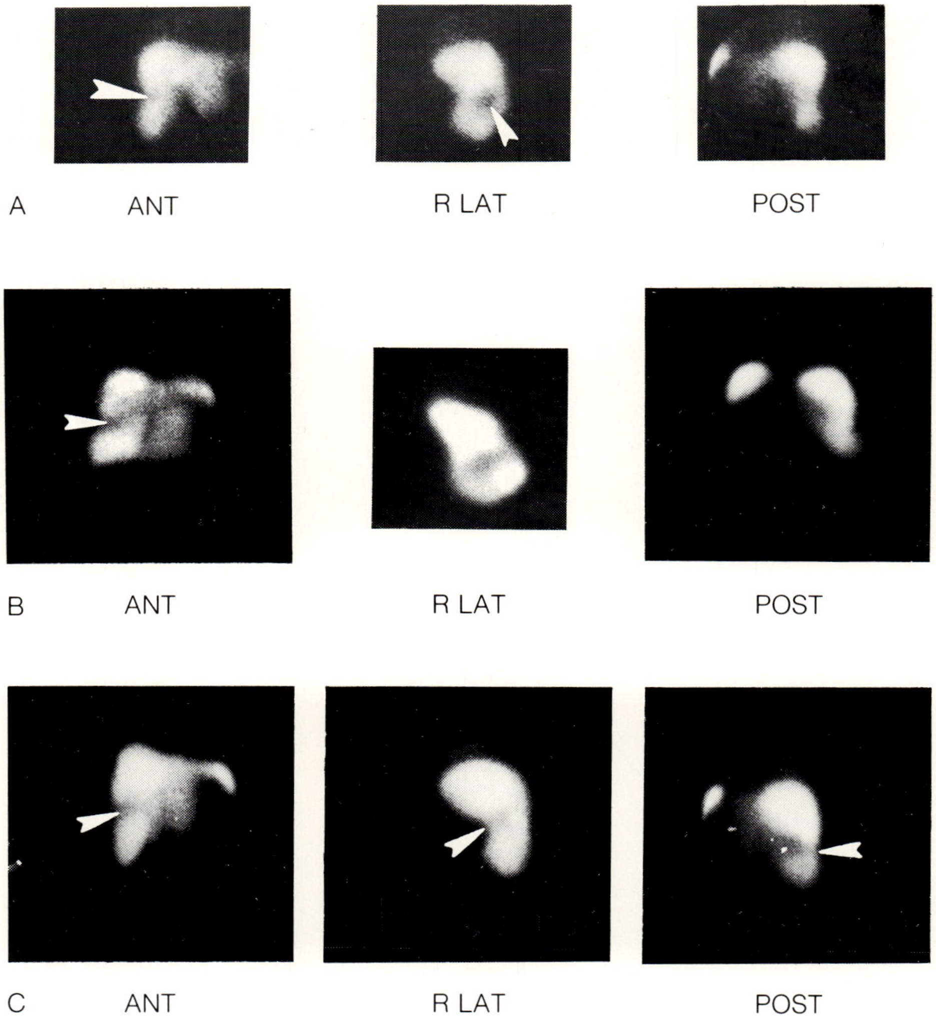


**FIG. 21. RIEDEL'S LOBE RESEMBLING A SPACE-OCCUPYING LESION.** The area of the lobar separation between the Riedel's lobe and the superior portion of the right lobe to which it is related may resemble a space-occupying lesion. **A.** In the anterior position, the area of separation between the right lobe of the liver and Riedel's lobe (larger arrow) is somewhat triangular. In the right lateral position, this separation appears as an area of absent radioactivity since the junctional region is farther from the collimator than the area of liver tissue either superior to it (right lobe) or inferior to it (Riedel's lobe). Thus the findings in the right lateral position may be mistakenly thought to be related to a space-occupying lesion. An extrahepatic mass was responsible for accentuation of the separation between the right and left lobes. **B.** In this liver with an unusual configuration, the lobar separation (arrow) is easily identified in the anterior position. However, in the right lateral position it is somewhat ovoid and has the appearance of a focal defect. **C.** Although the lobar separation is easily recognized in the anterior and posterior positions (arrows) it appears as a small, somewhat rounded area of absent radioactivity in the right lateral position (arrow).

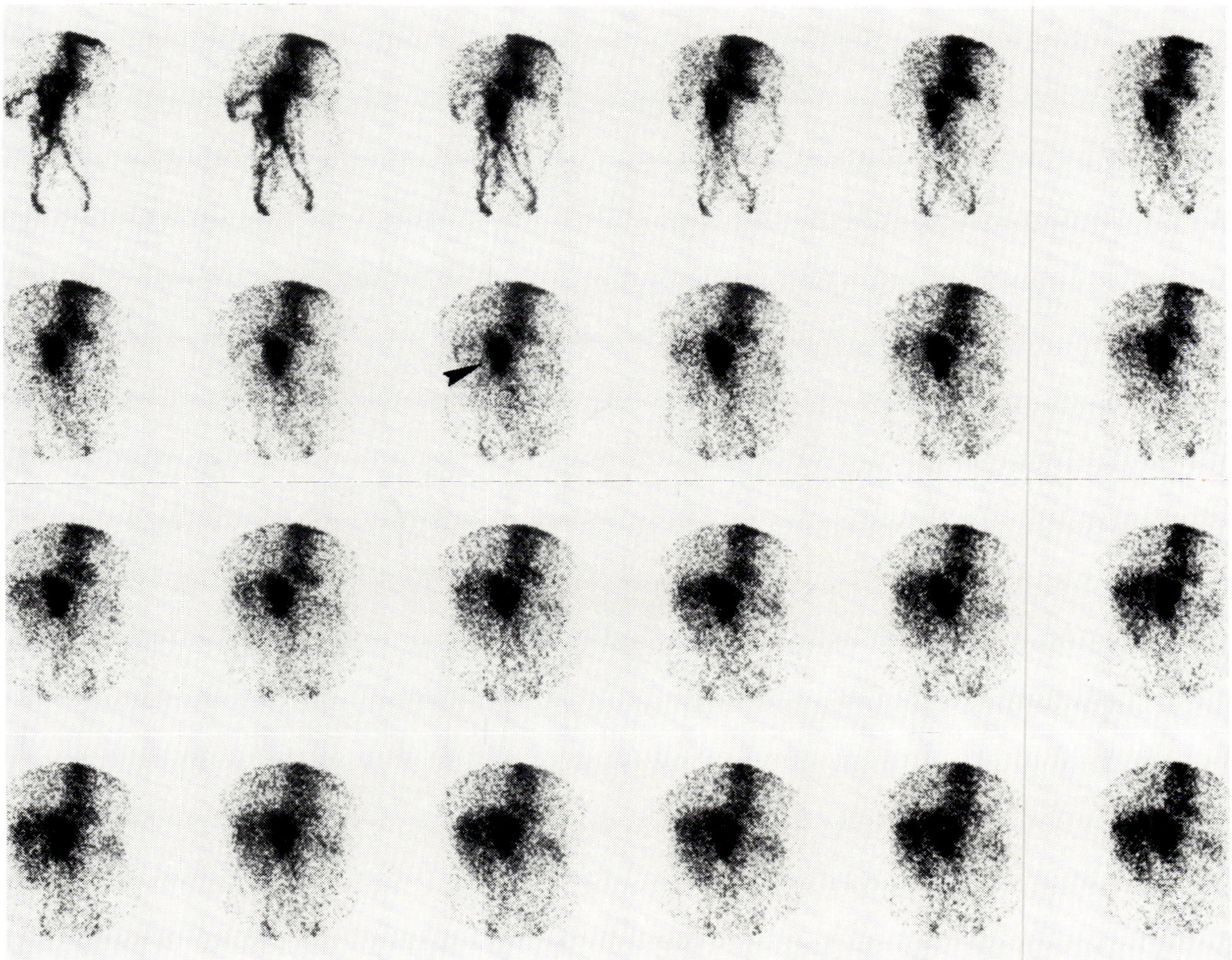

A Anterior Blood Flow

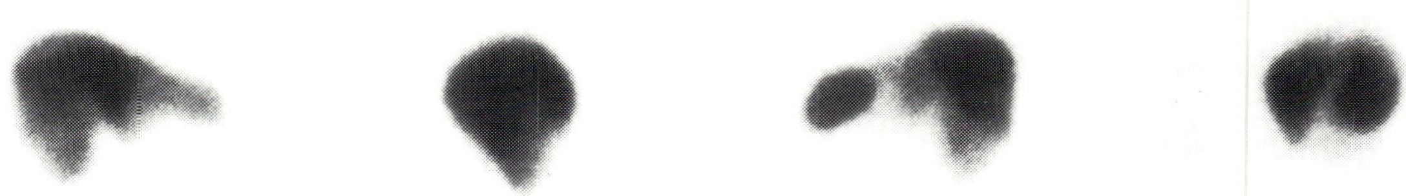

B ANT R LAT POST L LAT

**FIG. 22. SUPERIOR VENA CAVA OBSTRUCTION AND AREA OF INCREASED RADIOACTIVITY ON HEPATIC IMAGE. A.** Blood flow studies performed in conjunction with hepatic imaging, with frames obtained at intervals of 3 seconds. Numerous venous collaterals are almost immediately identified following IV administration of the Tc-99m SC in an upper extremity vein. The venous collaterals are numerous and extend down to the iliac veins. Note the appearance of the area of persistently increased radioactivity in frame 9 (arrow). This is probably due to increased portal flow in the left portal vein from collateral return through the internal mammary vein. **B.** Static imaging in the anterior position shows continuing increased activity in the area initially identified on the blood flow study.

## SPACE-OCCUPYING LESIONS

If there has been destruction or replacement of hepatic tissue with its accompanying Kupffer cells, a radioactive colloid cannot enter the involved region to be phagocytized; this is represented on the scan as an area of absent radioactivity. This is the basis for visualization of space-occupying lesions with hepatic imaging. The etiology of the space-occupying lesion cannot be determined from the radionuclide image alone. Thus tumor, cyst, abscess, and other focal lesions may have similar imaging appearances. In each of these types of abnormality, the remaining, uninvolved hepatic tissue usually demonstrates normal uptake of radioactive material. This is in contrast to diffuse liver diseases, such as Laennec's cirrhosis. In these cases, there is fairly uniform and widespread reduction in hepatic radioactivity, which is a manifestation, in part, of the extensive involvement of the entire liver in the disease process.

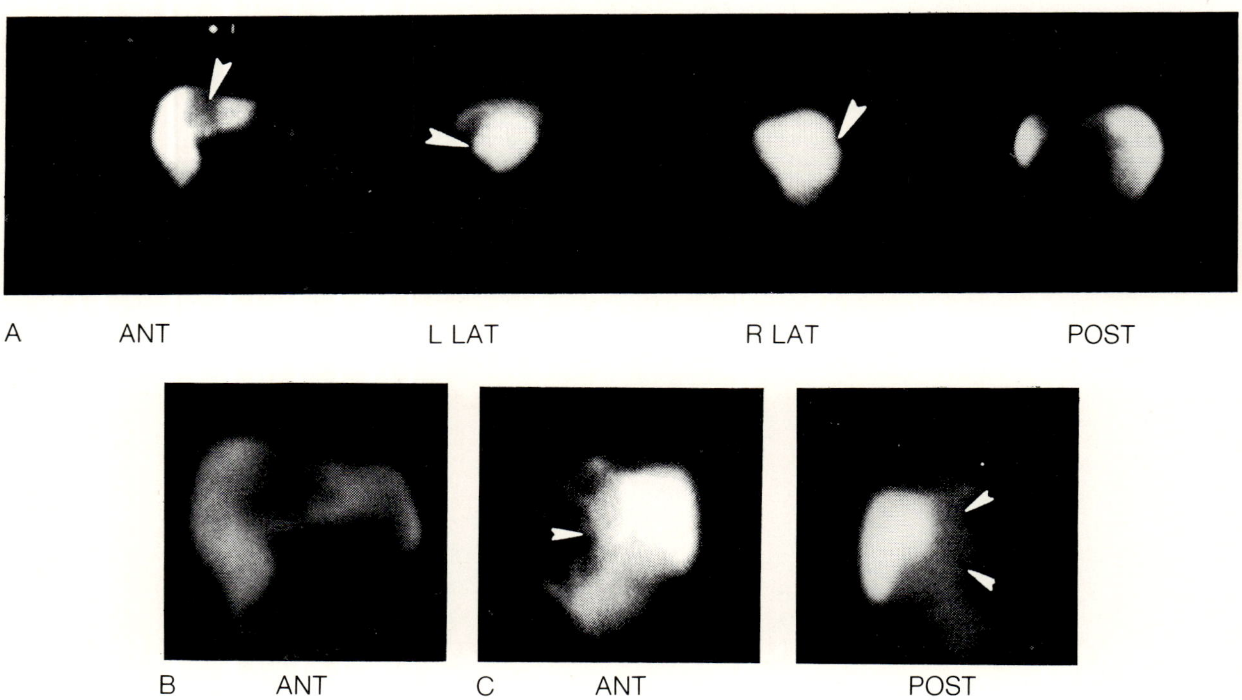


**FIG. 23. PRIMARY LIVER NEOPLASM: HEPATOCELLULAR CARCINOMA. A.** Note the somewhat irregular area of absent radioactivity (arrow) seen in the anterior position. This does not have the characteristic rounded appearance so commonly seen with metastases and hepatoma. Its far anterior location can be identified in both the right and left lateral positions ( large arrows ). **B.** Same patient one year later shows irregular extension of the tumor. **C.** Another patient with a malignant hepatoma and metastases elsewhere in the liver. The extensive right lobe replacement is seen in both the anterior and posterior positions (arrows). There are no specific imaging characteristics that distinguish hepatoma from other malignancies involving the liver.

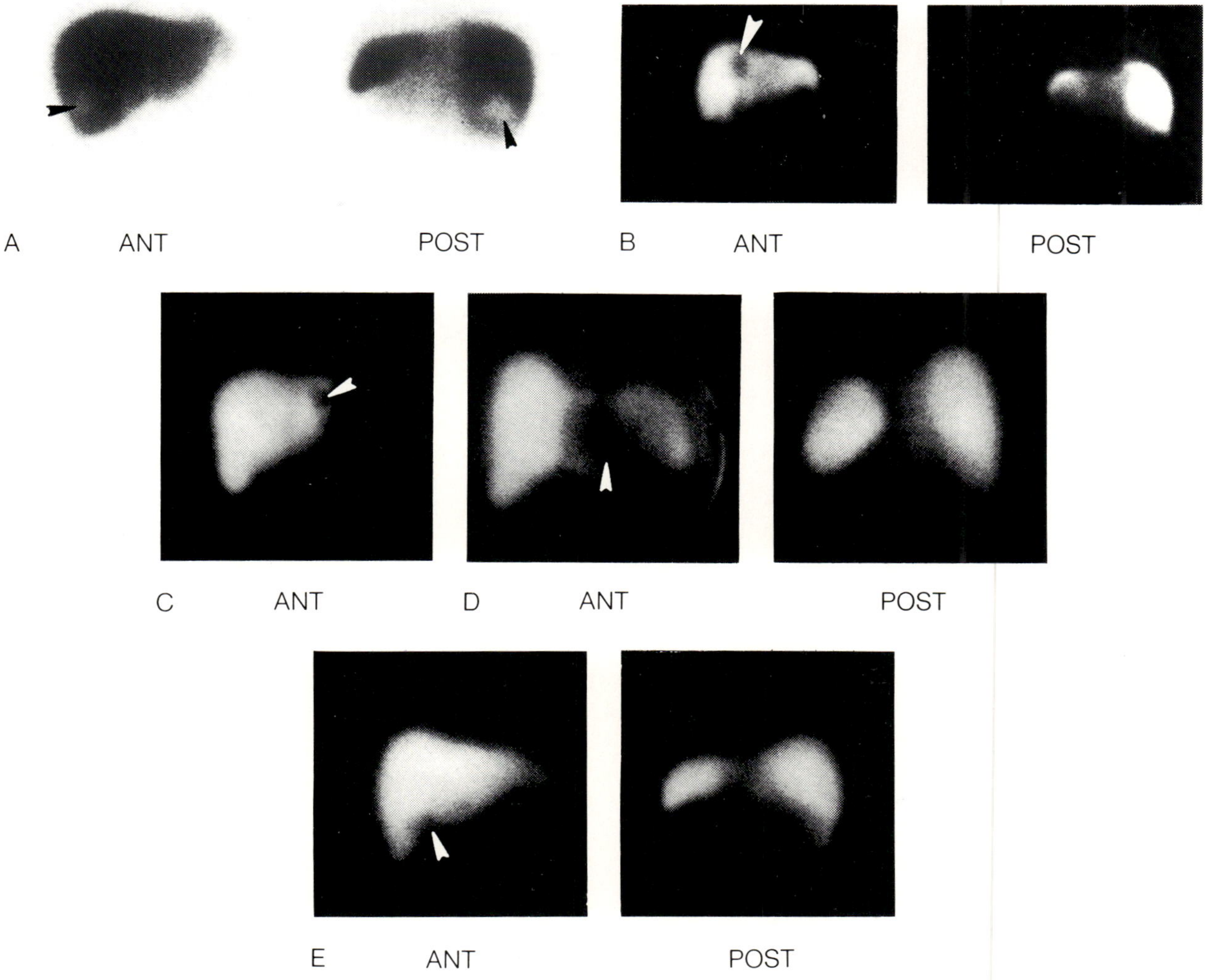


**FIG. 24. SOLITARY METASTASIS.** The solitary metastatic lesion has no hallmarks that distinguish it as a metastatic tumor rather than a primary neoplasm, cyst, or abscess. Developmental anomalies are sometimes misinterpreted as showing a solitary metastasis. **A.** Solitary metastasis in right lobe. The lesion (arrow) is clearly identified in the anterior and posterior positions. From its appearance in the anterior position, note its similarity to a Riedel's lobe (primary: bronchogenic carcinoma). **B**. Solitary metastasis in junctional region between right and left lobes (arrow). Accentuation of the lobar separation is usually seen as a semivertical area of reduced radioactivity. In this case, the metastasis is sharply defined and somewhat rounded (primary: carcinoma of breast). **C.** Small metastasis in left lobe (arrow). Solitary left lobe lesions may be difficult to identify because of the usual reduced radioactivity compared to that of the larger right lobe (primary: carcinoma of stomach). **D.** Large metastasis almost entirely replacing left lobe (arrow). The imaging characteristics are similar to those that might be seen with a large cystic lesion (primary: carcinoma of endometrium). **E.** Small metastatic lesion (arrow) along the inferior aspect of the left lobe (primary: carcinoma of breast).

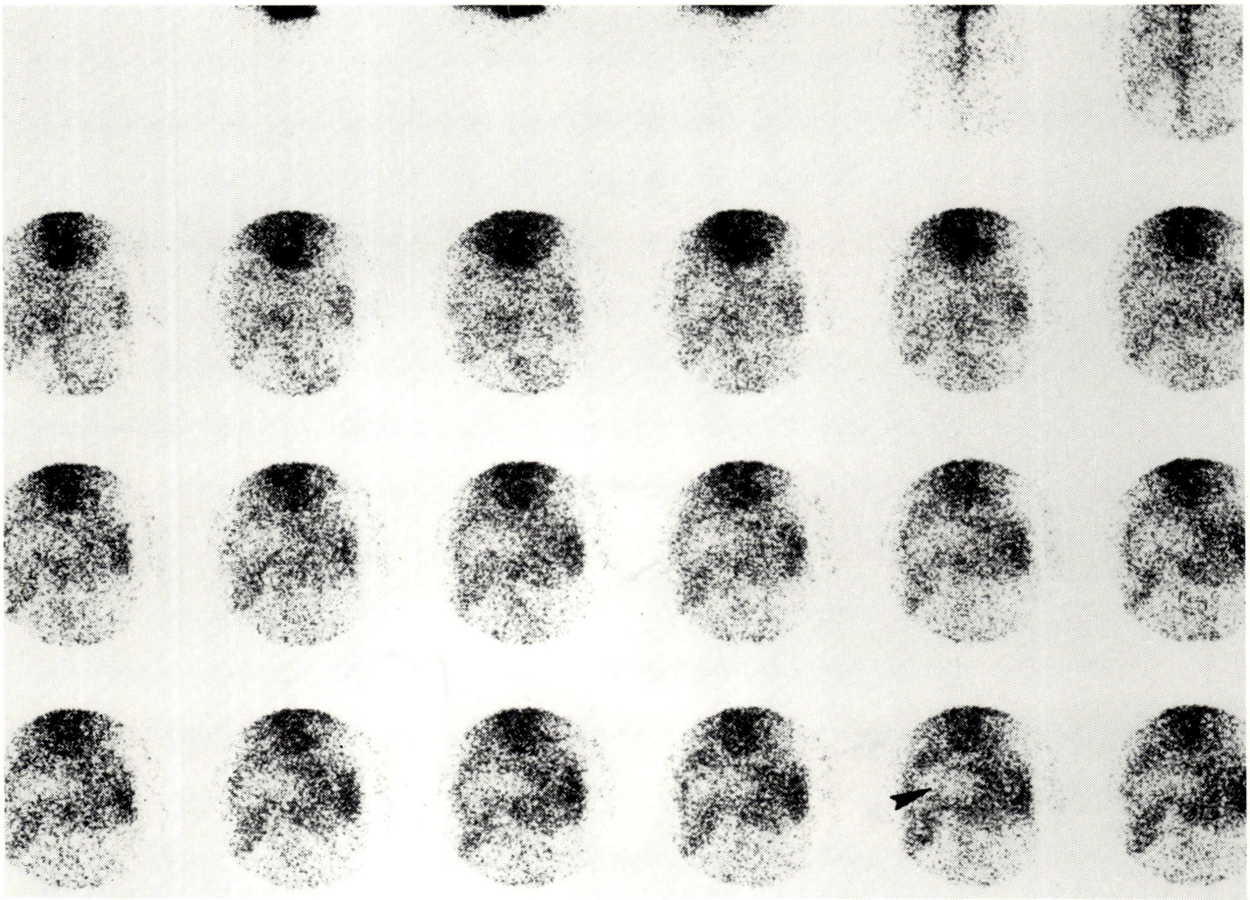

A Anterior Blood Flow

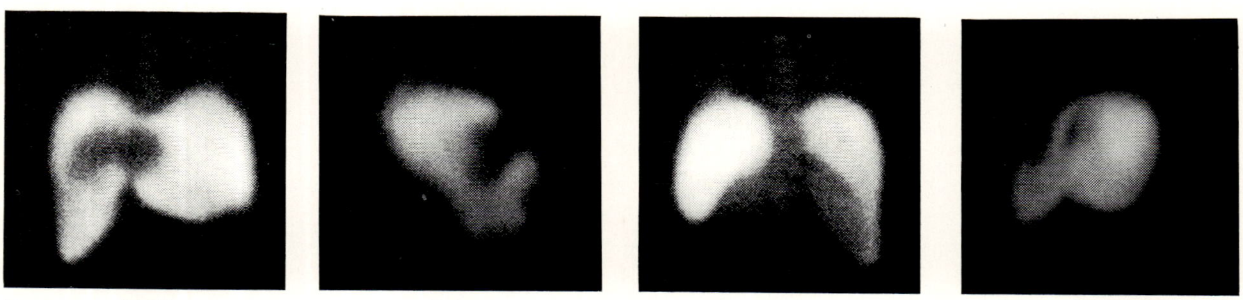

B ANT R LAT POST L LAT

**FIG. 25. SOLITARY AREA OF ABSENT RADIOACTIVITY DUE TO COALESCENCE OF SEVERAL METASTATIC LESIONS.** The visualization of what appears to be a solitary space-occupying lesion is often associated with the coalescence of several metastases. From the hepatic image alone it is sometimes difficult to determine whether the abnormality is due to a single metastatic lesion or the coalescence of several lesions. **A.** The blood flow study identifies what appears to be a solitary area of absent radioactivity, most clearly visible during the venous phase. **B.** Static imaging again clearly identifies the abnormal area in the anterior position, which appears at first to be a solitary metastasis. However, in the right lateral position, at least two contiguous lesions may be demonstrated.

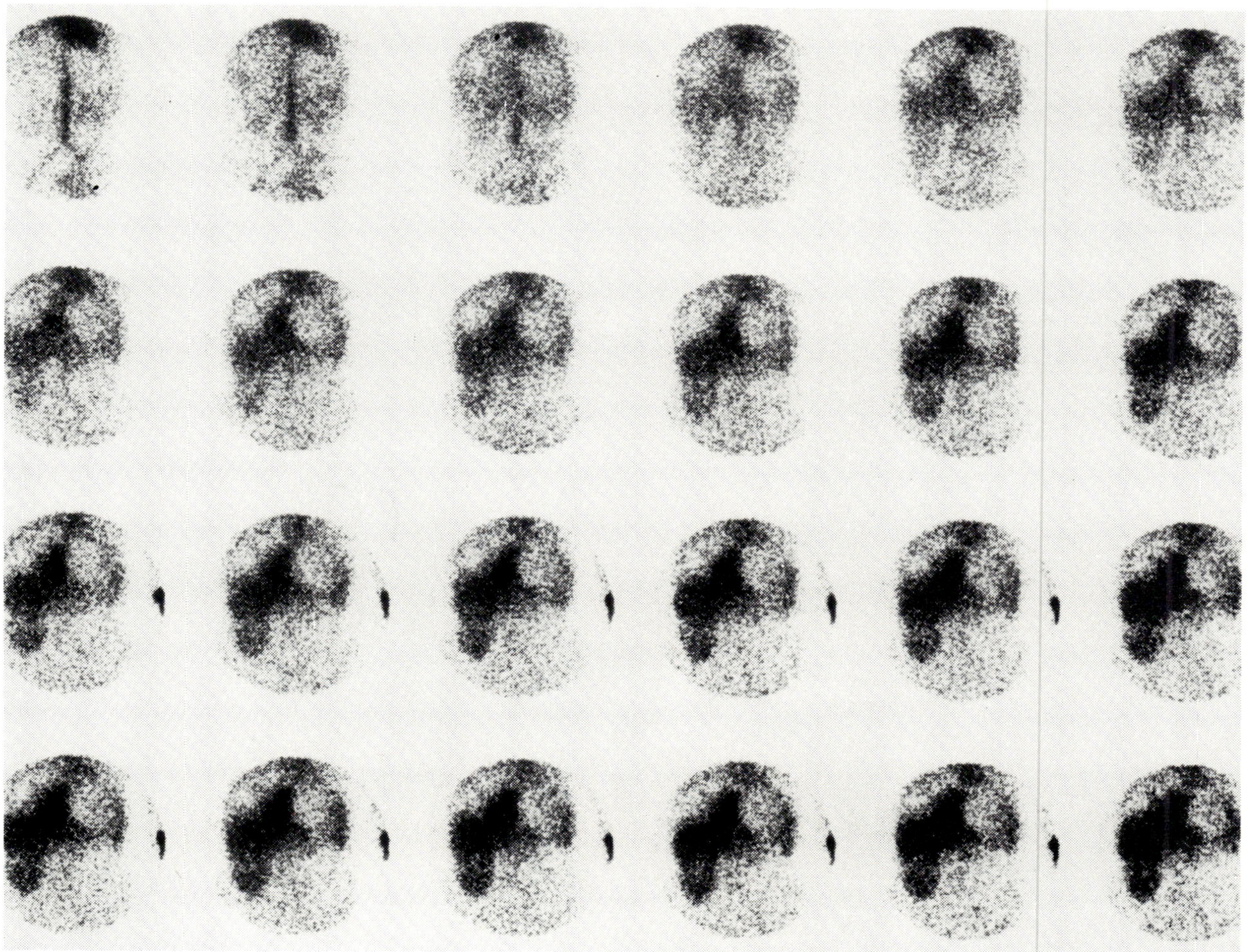

A Anterior Blood Flow

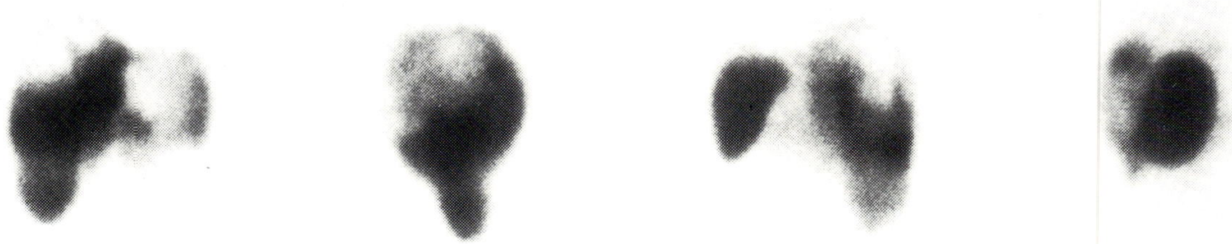

B ANT R LAT POST L LAT

**FIG. 26. MULTIPLE METASTASES AND HEPATOMEGALY. A. Blood Flow Study.** There is barely any identification of the liver during the arterial phase. Areas of radioactivity seen during the early phase grossly identify the uninvolved portions. **B. Static Imaging.** There is extensive neoplastic replacement of the subdiaphragmatic portion of the right lobe, with only a rim of functioning tissue surrounding the lesions. This is clearly visible in both anterior and posterior positions. Note the Riedel's lobe (primary: carcinoma of breast).

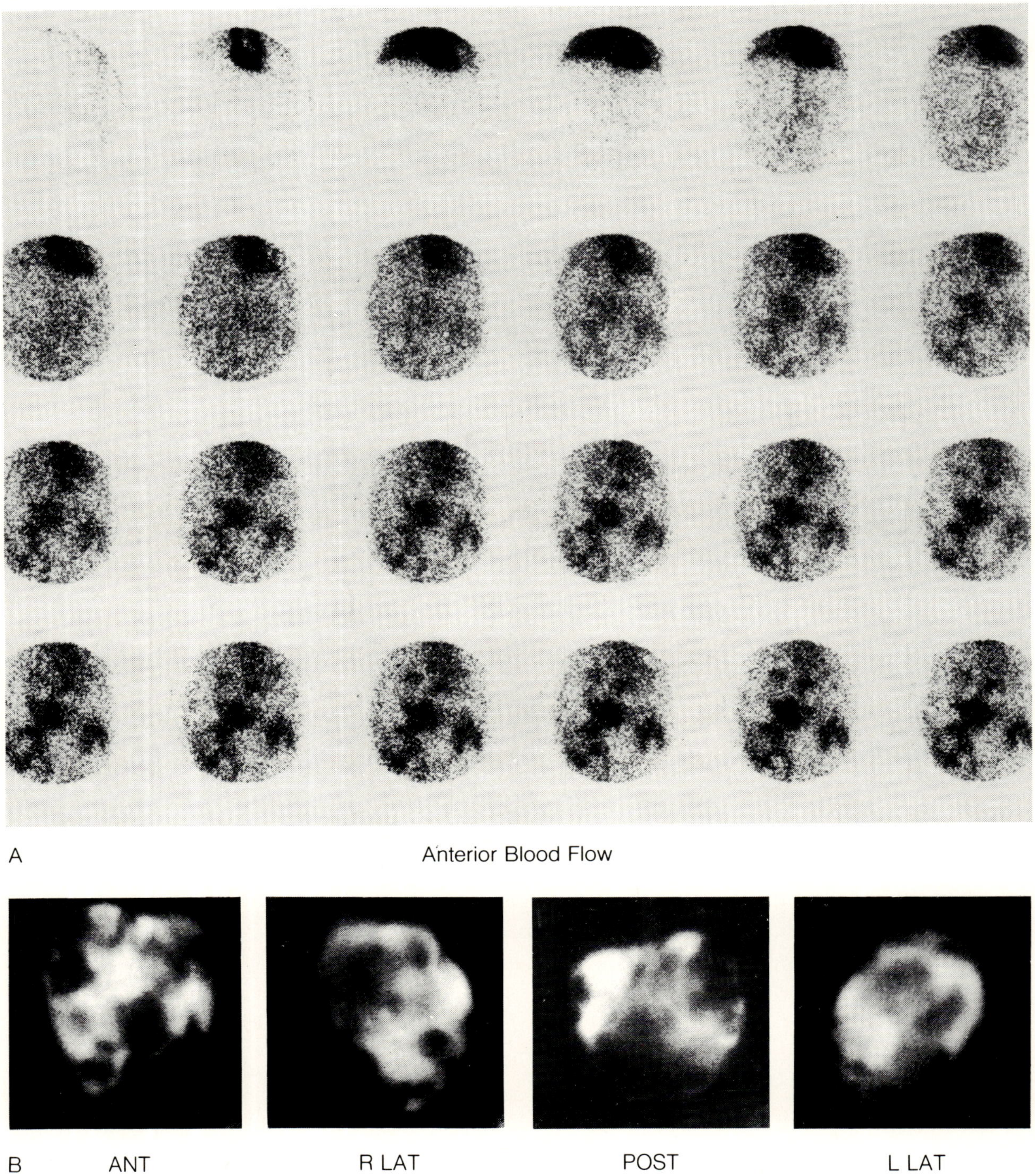


**FIG. 27.** MULTIPLE METASTASES AND HEPATOMEGALY. **A. Blood Flow Study.** During the venous phase, the remaining portions of uninvolved liver became visualized and appear as isolated areas of Tc-99m-SC uptake. **B. Static Imaging.** The multiple, somewhat rounded areas of absent radioactivity situated throughout the liver represent the extensive metastatic involvement of the organ. The lesions are clearly visible in all positions (primary: carcinoma of breast).

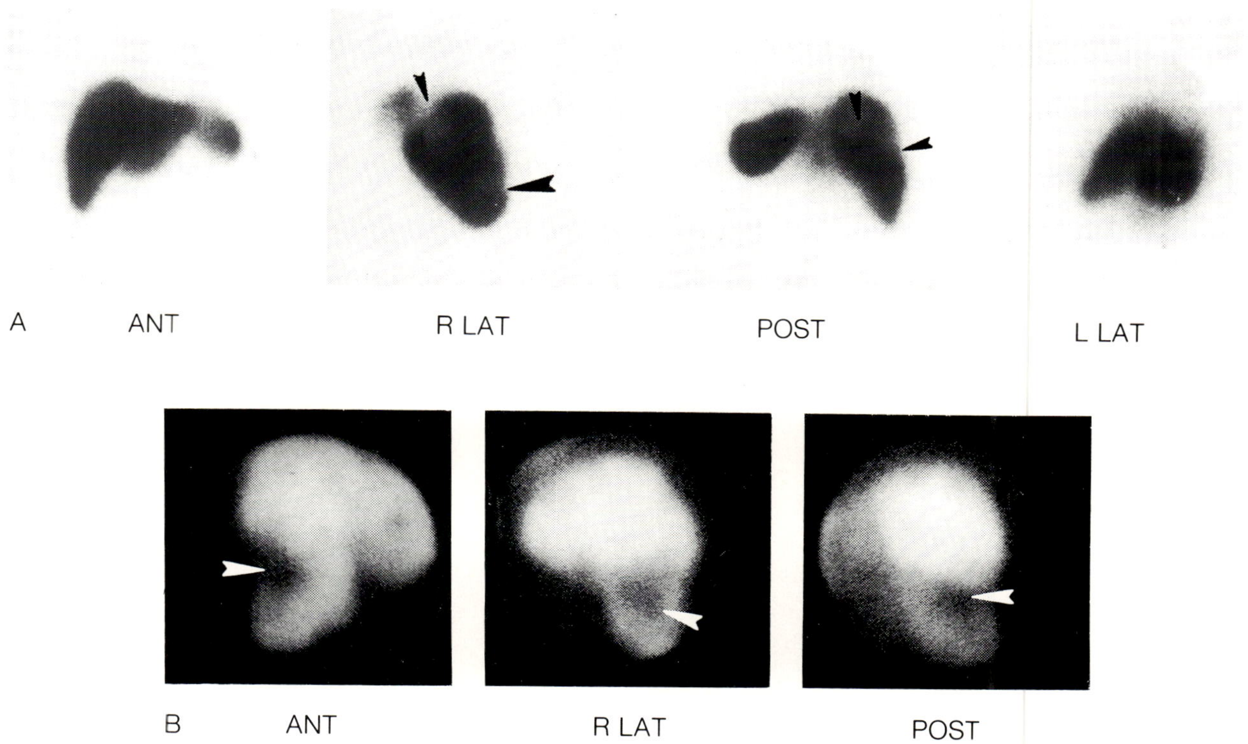


**FIG. 28. DETECTION OF METASTASES IMPROVED IN RIGHT LATERAL AND POSTERIOR POSITIONS.** Although in most cases hepatic metastases can be detected in the anterior position, improved identification can often be made in the right lateral and posterior positions. **A.** In this case, the area of reduced radioactivity in the superior portion of the right lobe as seen in the anterior position resembles a breast artifact. In the posterior position, the two metastatic lesions are sharply outlined (arrows). The far posterior location of the involved areas is demonstrated in the right lateral image (arrow). A Riedel's lobe is present, and the lobar separation ( larger arrow ) in the anterior and right lateral positions should not be confused with a space-occupying lesion (primary: carcinoma of breast). **B.** Several space-occupying lesions are seen in this patient with carcinoma of the breast. The large right lobe lesion (arrow) becomes more clearly outlined in the right lateral and posterior positions. Imaging in multiple positions helps to dispel any impression that a Riedel's lobe might be present.

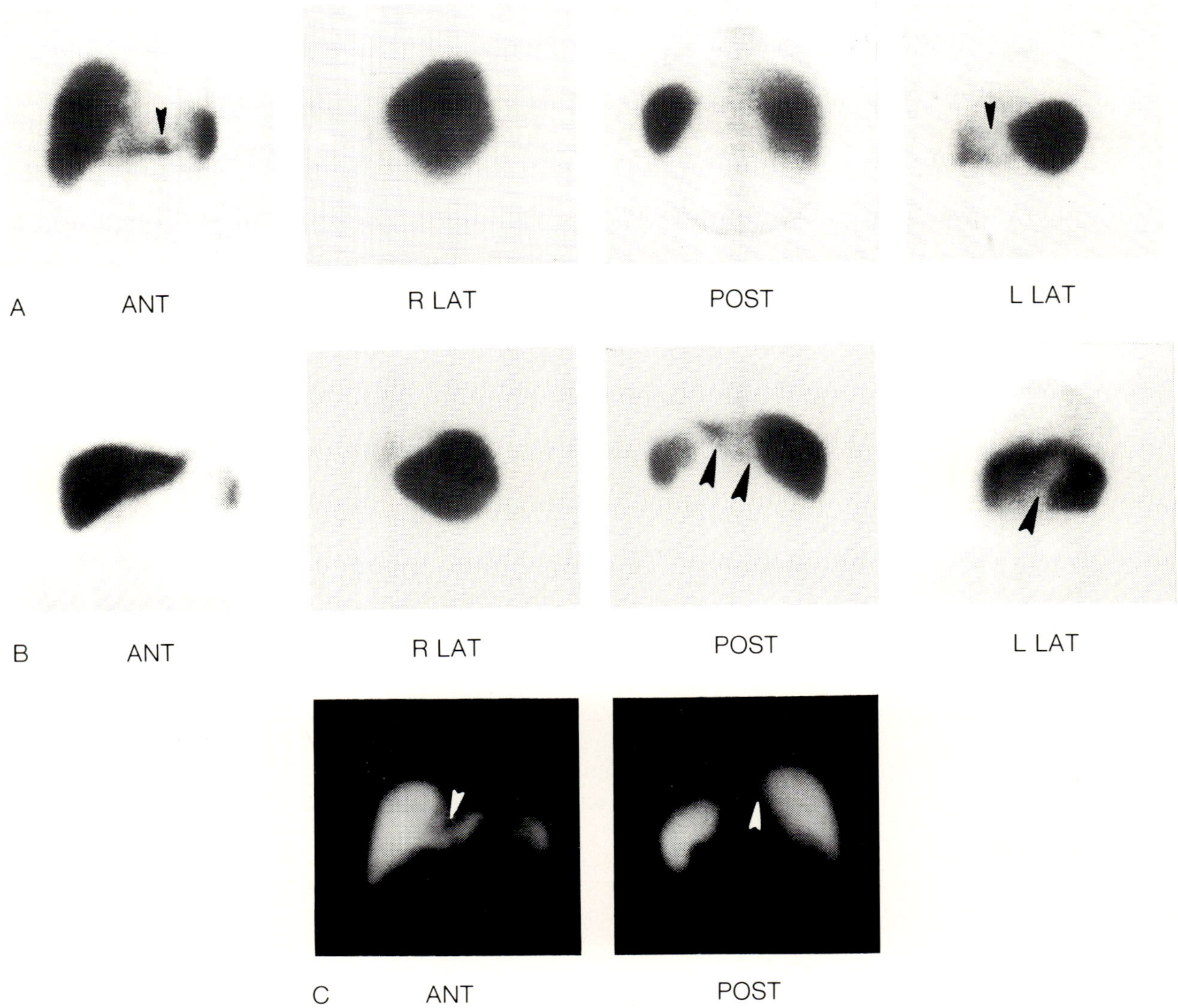


**FIG. 29. PRINCIPALLY LEFT LOBE INVOLVEMENT.** Left lobe lesions are sometimes difficult to identify because of the usual reduced radioactivity compared to that of the right lobe. Nonetheless, metastatic lesions in this region are usually sharply demarcated and can often be demonstrated in the left lateral as well as the anterior position. **A.** Extensive metastatic involvement of the left lobe is clearly seen in the anterior position (arrow). Reduced radioactivity in the left lateral position (arrow), anterior to the spleen, is a further indication of hepatic tissue replacement. The failure to visualize the left lobe in the posterior position is a common finding in the normal patient and does not necessarily signify tumor replacement (primary: carcinoma of the breast). **B.** The imaging of the site of metastatic replacement in the left lobe (arrow) is more subtle than in **A.** In this case, left lobe involvement is visible in the posterior position as well as in the left lateral view (primary: carcinoma of the lung). **C.** Involvement of superior portion of left lobe (arrow) due to metastases from carcinoma of breast. Although the site of reduced activity coinciding with the lesion is seen in the posterior position (arrow), the latter is certainly not diagnostic and could easily be overlooked.

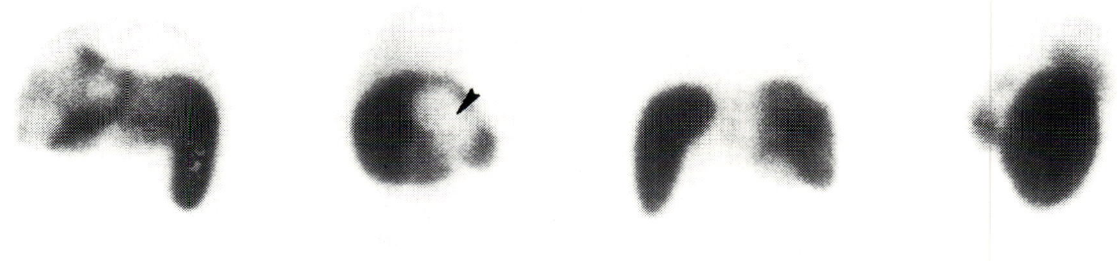

A ANT R LAT POST L LAT

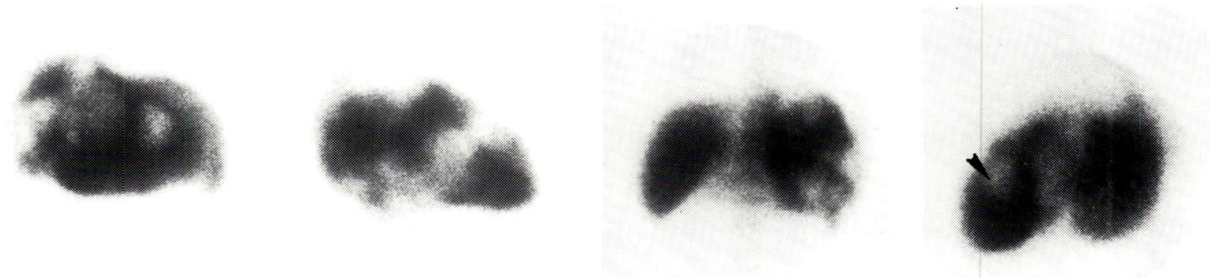

B ANT R LAT POST L LAT

**FIG. 30.** MULTIPLE METASTASES. **A.** There is extensive involvement of both the right and left lobes of the liver. That the involvement is predominantly anterior can be seen from imaging in the right lateral position. Note the absent radioactivity anteriorly (arrow) while relatively increased activity, signifying uninvolved liver, is seen posterior to the tumor area. Note how much better the lesions are identified in the anterior position compared to what is seen in the posterior position (primary: carcinoma of the colon). **B.** Moderate architectural distortion with extensive tumor involvement. There is compression of remaining functioning hepatic tissue as seen in the interspersed areas of increased activity. The far anterior identification of the left lobe metastases (arrow) can be seen in the left lateral position (arrow) (primary: bronchogenic carcinoma).

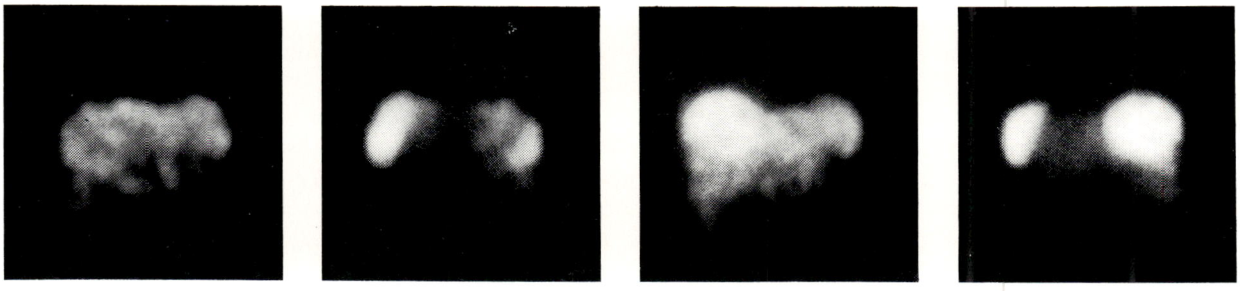

A ANT POST B ANT POST

**FIG. 31.** MULTIPLE, IRREGULAR METASTASES. The multiple areas of involvement are characterized by irregular, interspersed areas of tumor involvement in **A**, in a patient with oat cell carcinoma of the lung, and in **B**, a case of malignant melanoma.

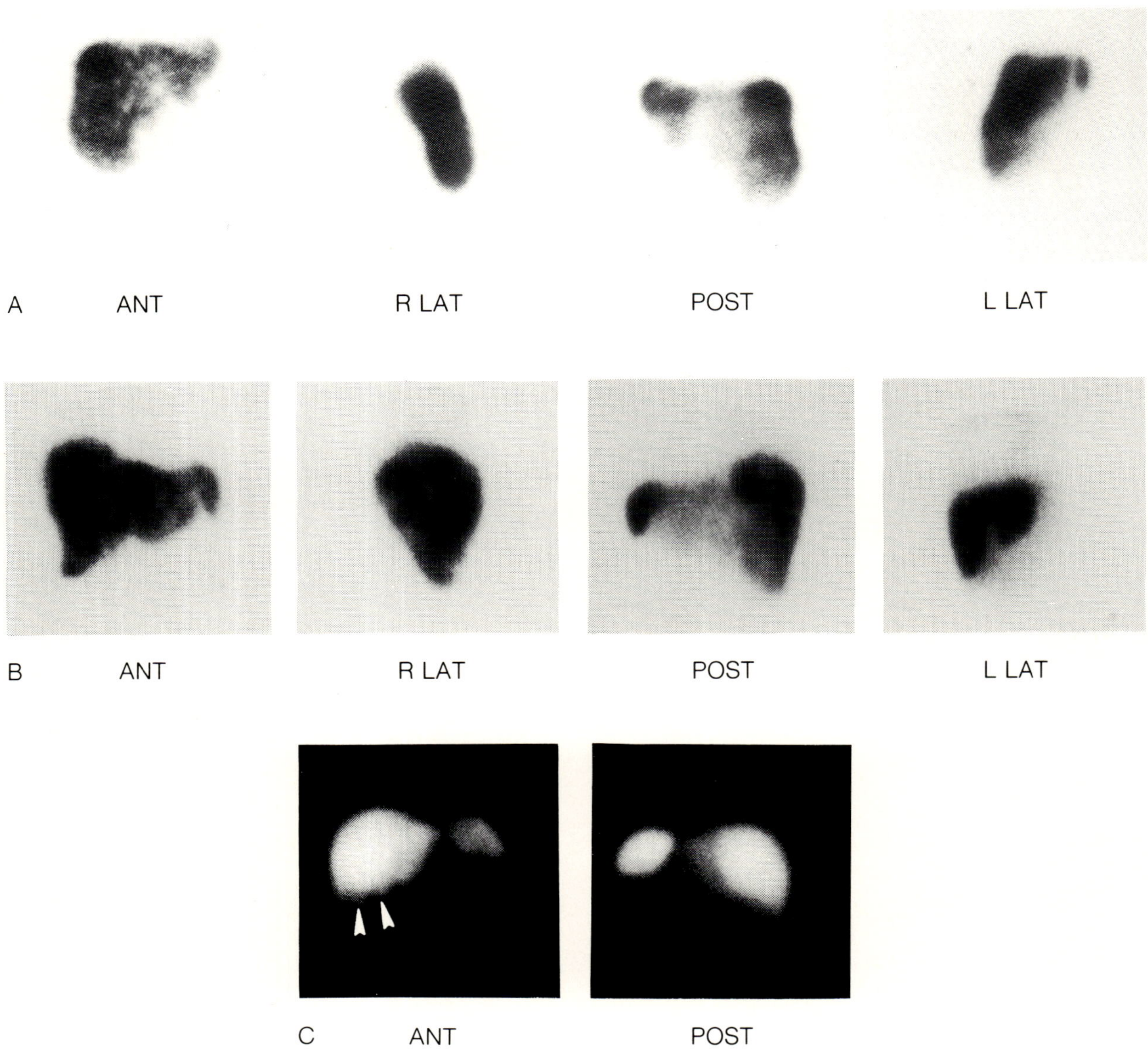


**FIG. 32. MULTIPLE METASTASES. Fine, Nodular Involvement.** The multiple, small metastatic foci are sometimes difficult to identify and may appear in a fine, reticulated pattern. The findings may be similar to those observed with extensive involvement of the liver in Hodgkin's disease. **A.** Multiple small metastases in a patient with carcinoma of the colon. **B.** Enlarged liver with somewhat irregular, fine areas of absent radioactivity due to metastases from bronchogenic carcinoma. **C.** Metastatic involvement along the inferior aspect of the liver only. Such involvement (arrows), as in this patient with breast carcinoma, is difficult to identify because of both the location and size of the lesions.

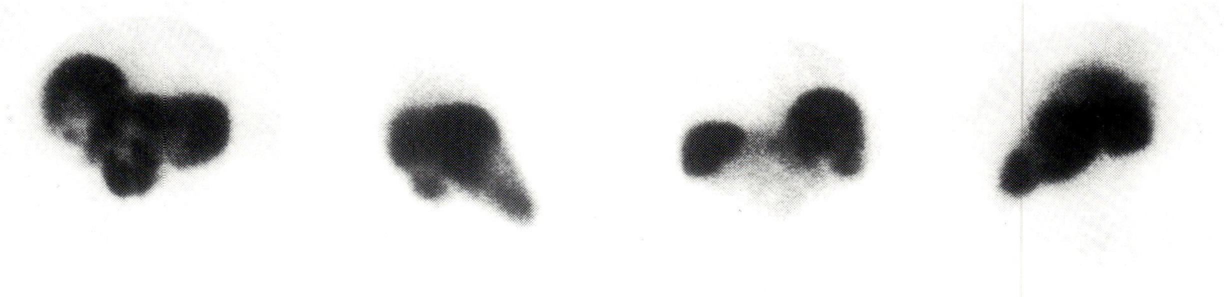


**FIG. 33. MASSIVE ARCHITECTURAL DISTORTION AND METASTATIC INVOLVEMENT.** The liver image may be barely recognizable in some cases of widespread replacement and displacement of hepatic tissue by tumor. Multiple metastases have resulted in absent visualization of a large portion of the right lobe. Imaging in the right lateral position makes orientation difficult.

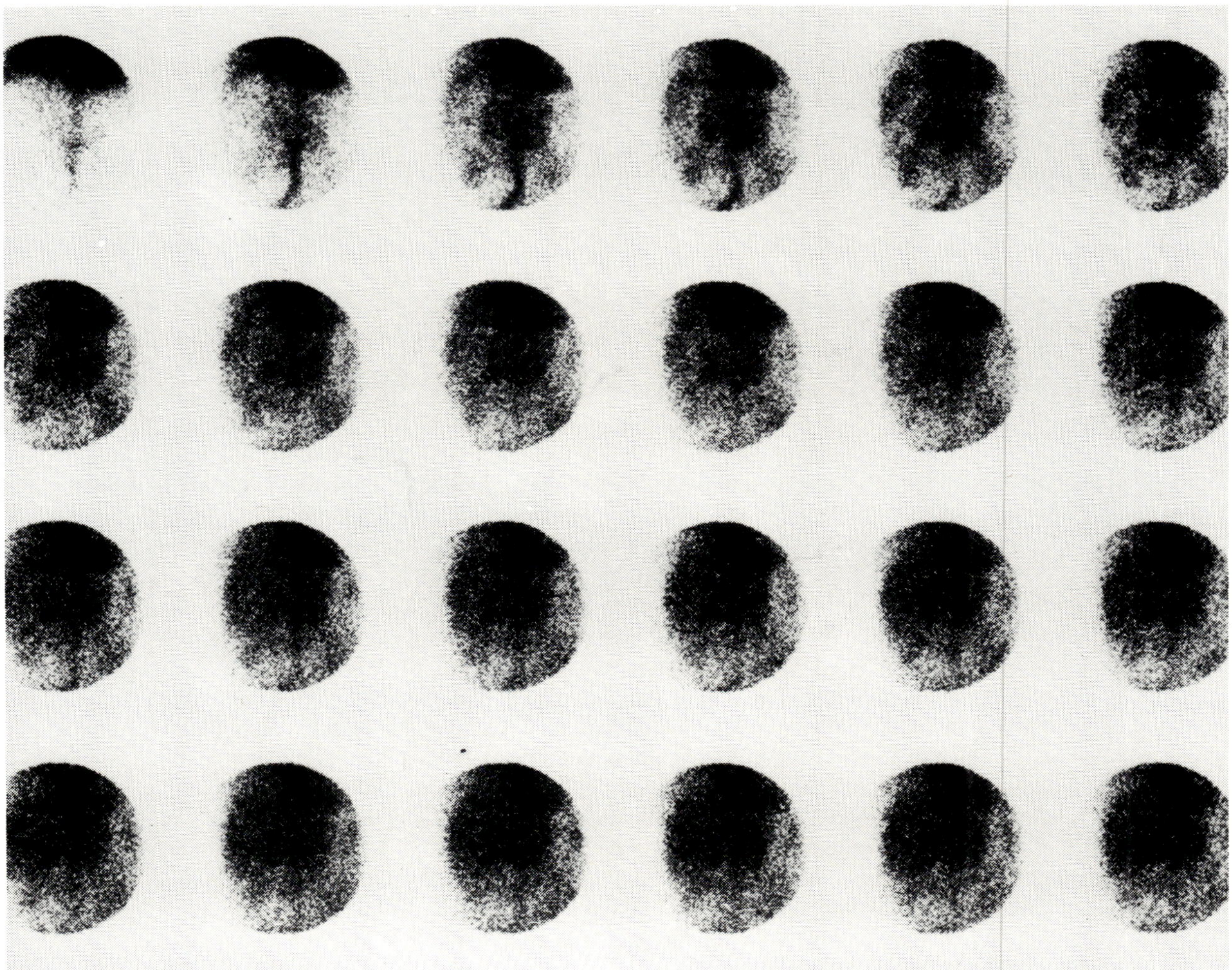

**FIG. 34. A.** Blood Flow Study (See legend next page)

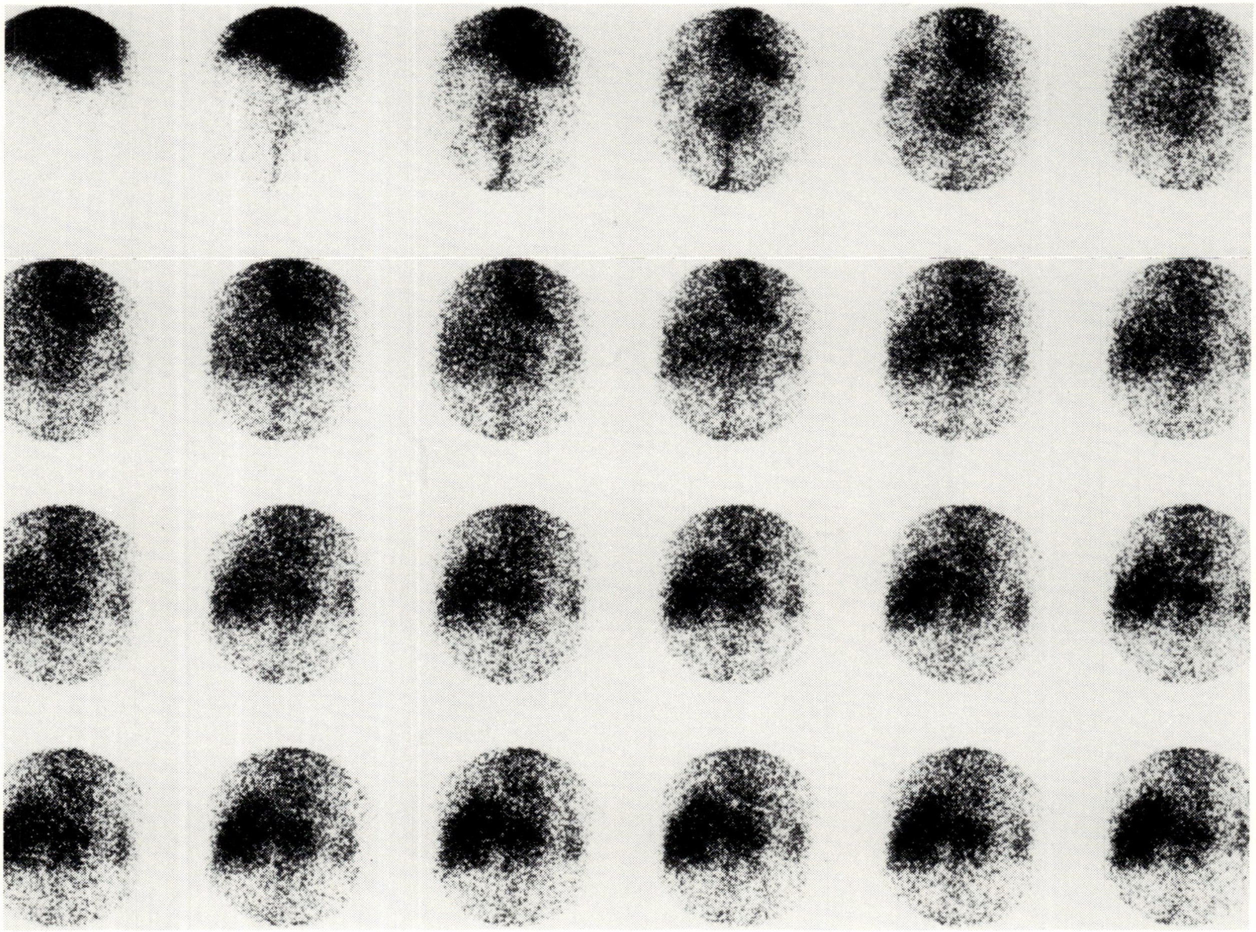

B Blood Flow Study

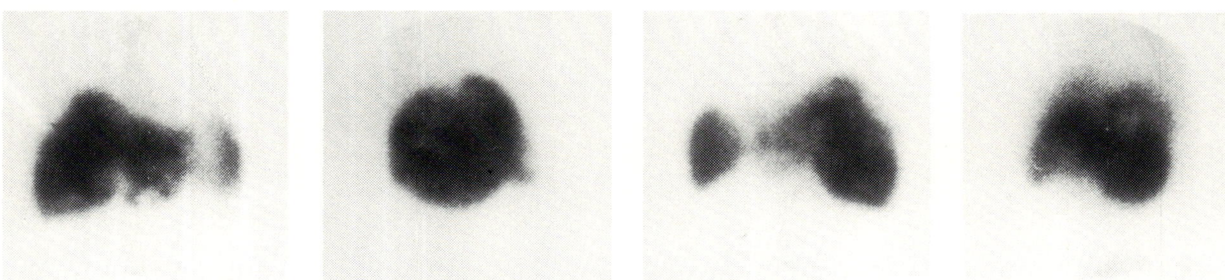

C ANT R LAT POST L LAT

**FIG. 34. HEPATIC ARTERY LIGATION AND LIVER VISUALIZATION.** The majority of Tc-99m SC that is phagocytized by the Kupffer cells is delivered to the liver by the portal venous system. Thus, interruption of the main hepatic artery has little effect on liver imaging in this patient with carcinoma of the gall bladder and extensive liver metastases. **A.** Blood flow study with Tc-99m sodium pertechnetate. There is hardly any hepatic imaging during the arterial phase (frames 1 to 3). During the venous phase the hepatic blood pool can be identified. **B.** Blood flow studies with Tc-99m SC show similar findings as in **A** during the arterial phase (frames 1 to 4). During the venous phase, there is phagocytosis of Tc-99m SC, and a hepatic image is discerned. **C.** Static imaging shows evidence of multiple metastases. Imaging is not degraded by the hepatic artery ligation.

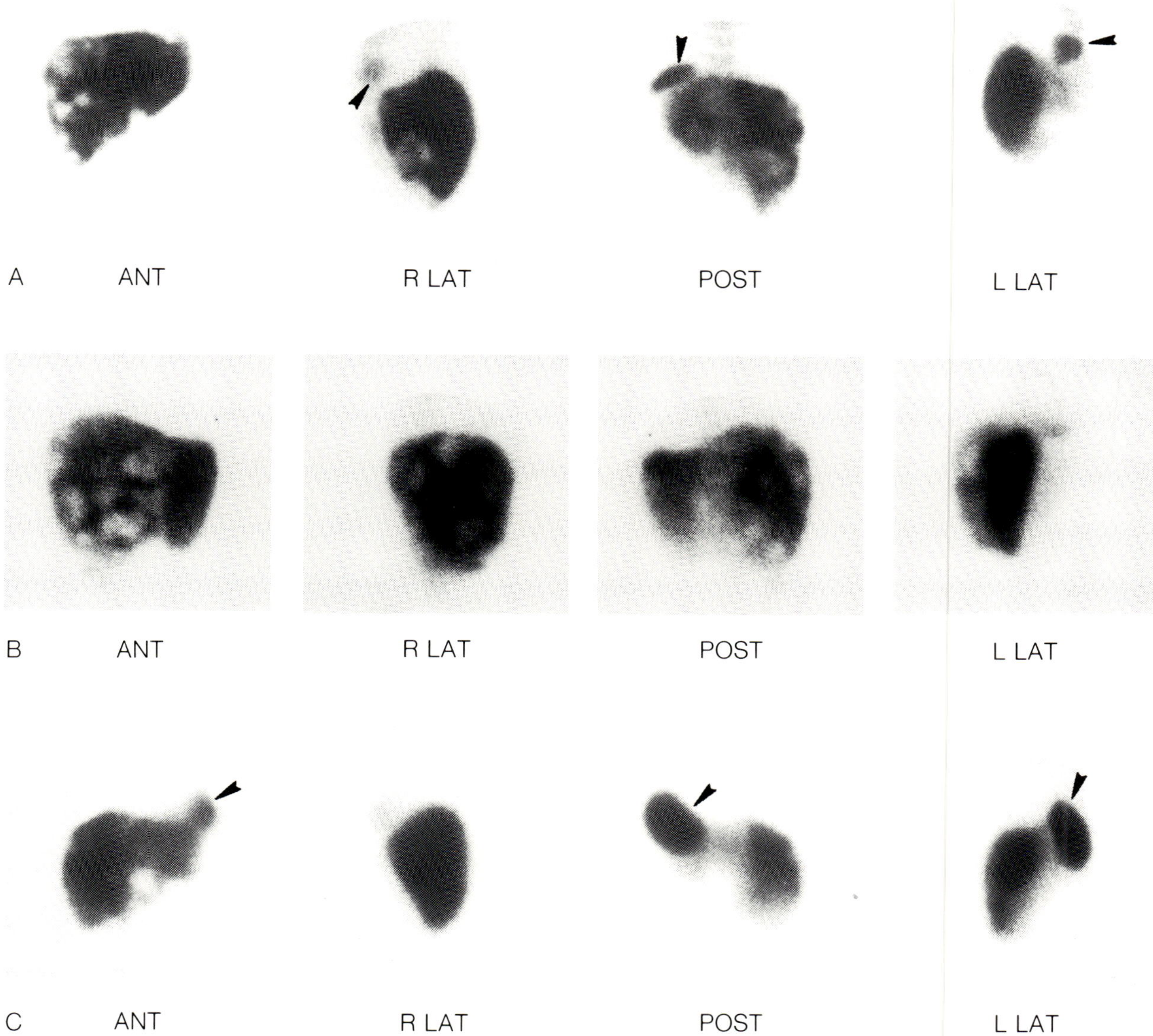


**FIG. 35. MULTIPLE METASTASES AND ORGAN DISPLACEMENT. A.** Extensive metastatic involvement of the liver is seen in both left and right lobes. The enlarged, tumor-laden liver causes the spleen (arrow) to be displaced superiorly. The flattening of the subdiaphragmatic portion of the right lobe, seen best in the anterior and posterior positions, is secondary to pulmonary involvement in this patient with bronchogenic carcinoma. **B.** Extensive metastatic involvement with anterior displacement of a markedly enlarged spleen. The massive involvement of the left lobe of the liver has progressively displaced the spleen forward (primary: carcinoma of the colon). **C.** Marked elevation of spleen associated with displacement of the left lobe farther toward the left upper quadrant. The extensive involvement of both hepatic lobes is difficult to appreciate from imaging alone. The involved, enlarged left lobe has resulted in mass displacement and elevation of the spleen (arrow) (primary: carcinoma of breast).

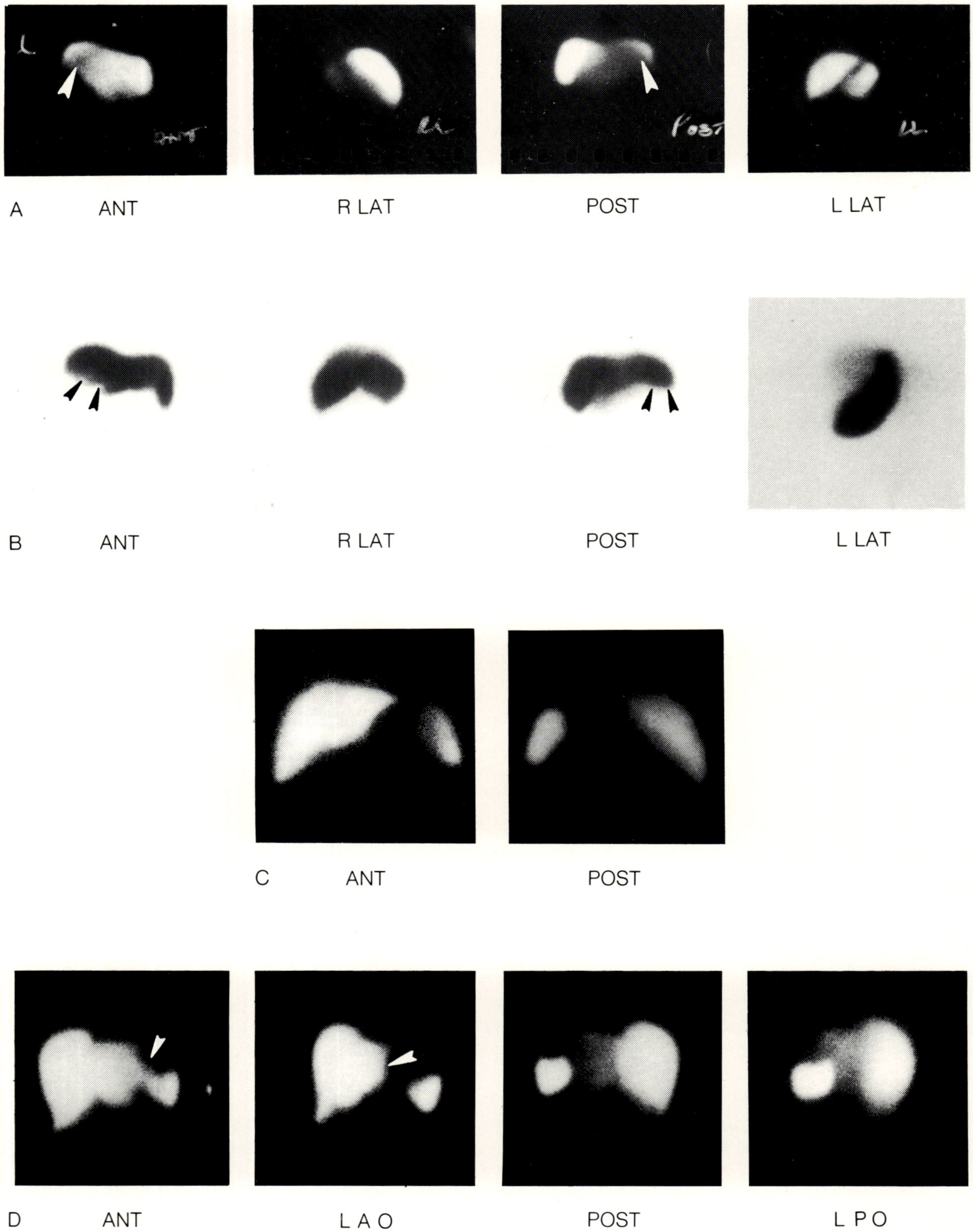


**FIG. 36. A–D.** (See legend next page)

**FIG. 36. LIVER DISPLACEMENT BY AN EXTRINSIC MASS.** This type of abnormality is sometimes produced by the growth of tumors in neighboring organs, such as in neoplasms of the kidney. However, it is sometimes difficult or impossible to distinguish imaging changes due to extrinsic masses from those due to involvement in the liver itself. **A.** Superior and anterior displacement and distortion of the right lobe by a Wilms' tumor of the right kidney. Increased activity due to compression is seen in the subdiaphragmatic portion of the right lobe. The area of the renal tumor is easily seen in the anterior and posterior positions (arrows). The anterior displacement is clearly visible in the right lateral position, with the tumor situated posteriorly. There was no metastatic involvement of the liver. **B.** Superior and anterior displacement in another patient with Wilms' tumor of the right kidney. Note the apparent irregularity inferiorly in the anterior position. The sharp outlines at the site of tumor compression (arrows) make the interpretation that there is an extrinsic mass rather than intrinsic involvement easier to arrive at. **C.** Concave reduction of radioactivity along the medial aspect of the left lobe from an extrinsic abdominal metastasis in a patient with carcinoma of the prostate. This is a subtle abnormality, close to normal in appearance. **D.** Duplication cyst of the esophagus displacing the spleen inferiorly and compressing the medial border of the left lobe, with an associated concave reduction in radioactivity, the latter emphasized in the LAO position (arrows).

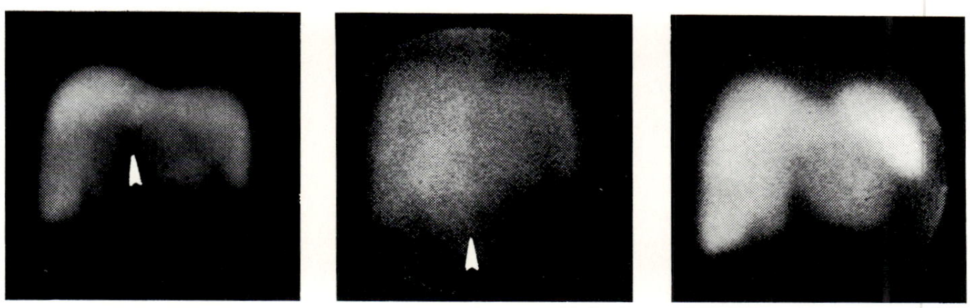

A ANT 99mTc- SC B ANT 67- Ga C ANT 99mTc- SC

**FIG. 37. ACCENTUATION OF THE LOBAR SEPARATION BY AN EXTRINSIC MASS. A.** Initial imaging shows marked accentuation of the lobar separation (arrow) . This was due to the impingement on the liver of an extrinsic mass, which was found to be an abdominal lymphoma. **B.** Identification of the lymphoma involvement (arrow) is made on Ga-67 imaging, performed 72 hours following radionuclide injection. **C.** Repeat liver imaging following successful chemotherapy, 7 months after the initial Tc-99m SC and Ga-67 imaging continues to show the enlarged liver but there is no longer any evidence of the effects of the lymphoma, now greatly reduced in size.

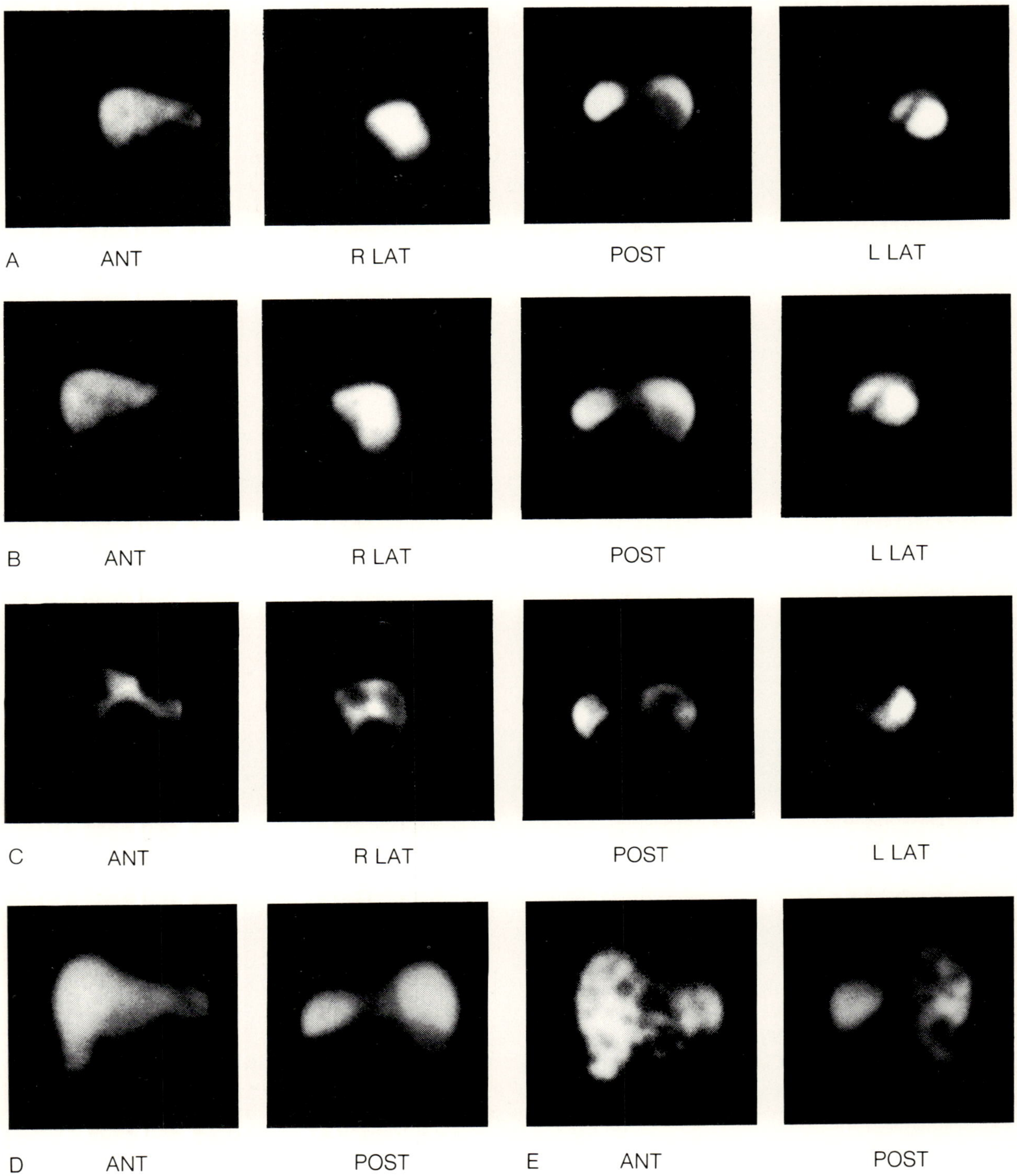


**FIG. 38. PROGRESSION OF METASTASES.** Hepatic images taken over a short period of time sometimes show remarkable changes demonstrating metastases that had barely been detectable. In many cases only by comparison of older images with more recent ones can the suspected areas of involvement be appreciated. **A.** Initial imaging shows several areas of reduced radioactivity in the anterior position that are of questionable sig-

nificance. No similar abnormalities are seen in the other positions. **B.** Imaging 6 months later shows several linear areas free of radioactivity due to biliary dilatation secondary to extrahepatic biliary obstruction by tumor. There is still no manifestation of intrinsic liver metastases at this time. **C.** Hepatic enlargement with widespread metastatic involvement 9 months after initial imaging. There is no hint on the earlier studies of the extensive hepatic involvement finally demonstrated (primary: carcinoma of pancreas). **D.** Initial imaging in another patient shows no well defined space-occupying lesion, although there is perceptible reduction in radioactivity in the left lobe. **E.** Imaging 10 months later shows well defined metastatic lesions in both lobes of the liver in the absence of any marked change in hepatic size (primary: carcinoma of the breast).

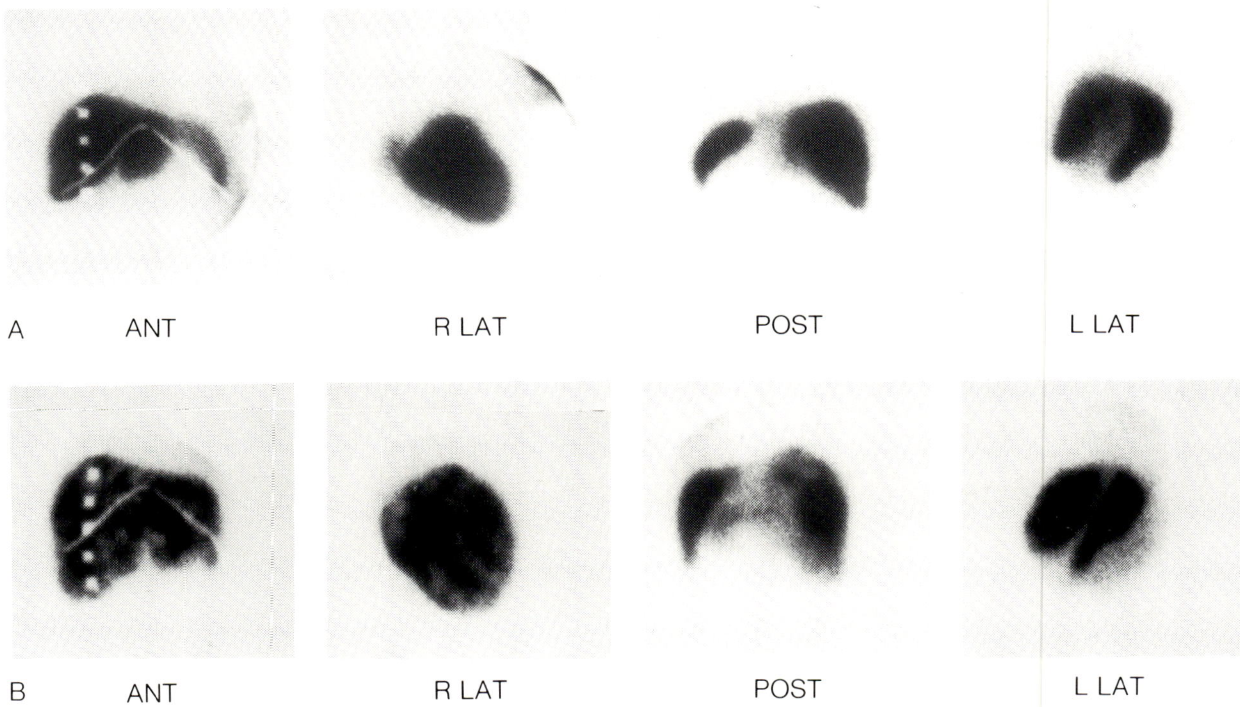


**FIG. 39. PROGRESSION OF METASTASES AND HEPATIC ENLARGEMENT.** Metastatic involvement is often associated with marked hepatomegaly, the hepatic size increasing over a relatively short period of time. Progressive increase in size of the liver with no obvious cause in a patient with a primary malignancy should be considered to be metastatic until proven otherwise. **A.** Initial imaging shows the liver to measure approximately 17 cm vertically. Note the position of the right costal margin marker. There is no evidence of metastatic disease at this time. There is straightening of the subdiaphragmatic portion of the right lobe secondary to a right-sided pleural effusion. **B.** Five months later, the liver has undergone rapid enlargement (22 cm vertically) with evidence of multiple metastases in both lobes. The spleen has also increased in size. Note the position of the right costal margin marker now compared with **A** (primary: carcinoma of breast).

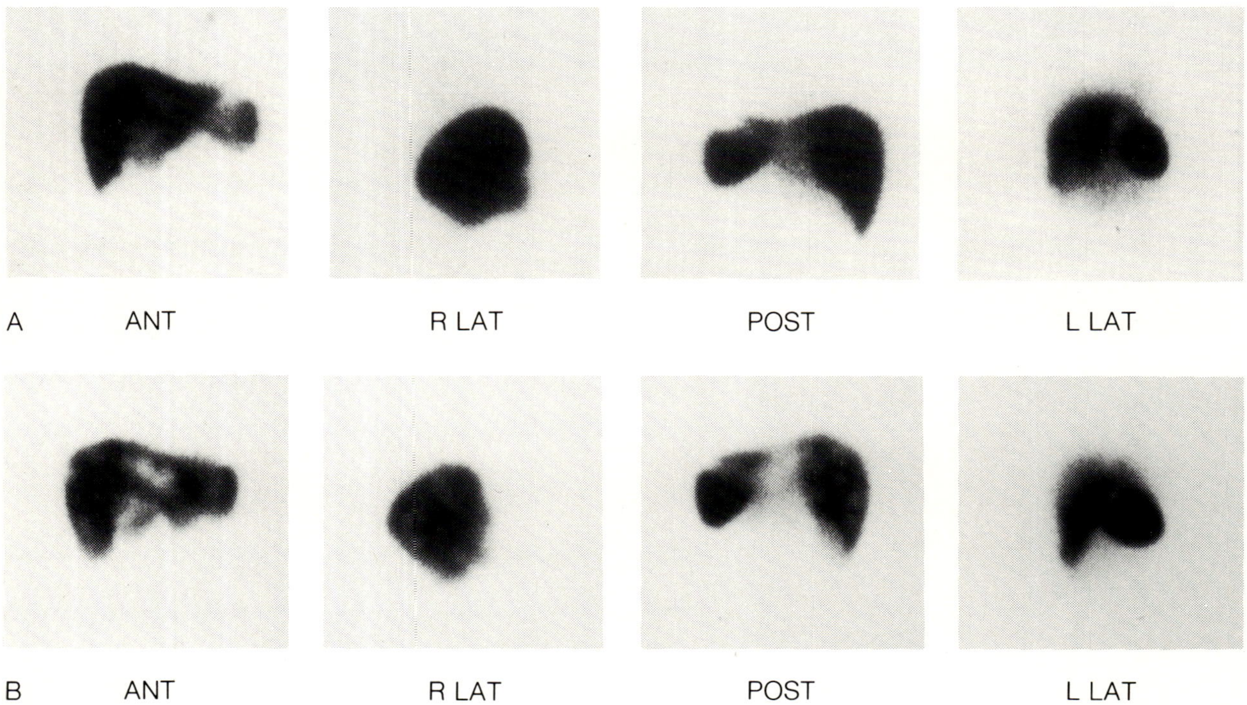


**FIG. 40. PROGRESSION OF METASTASES. Accentuation of Areas of Involvement with Serial Imaging. A.** Initial imaging shows multiple areas of absent radioactivity, indicating metastases in this young man with an embryonal cell carcinoma of the testis. **B.** Imaging 3 months later shows clarification of the initially identified areas with evidence of further extension. Although such manifestations may be due, in part, to reduced film intensity on the second study, the amount of liver involved has increased since the earlier imaging.

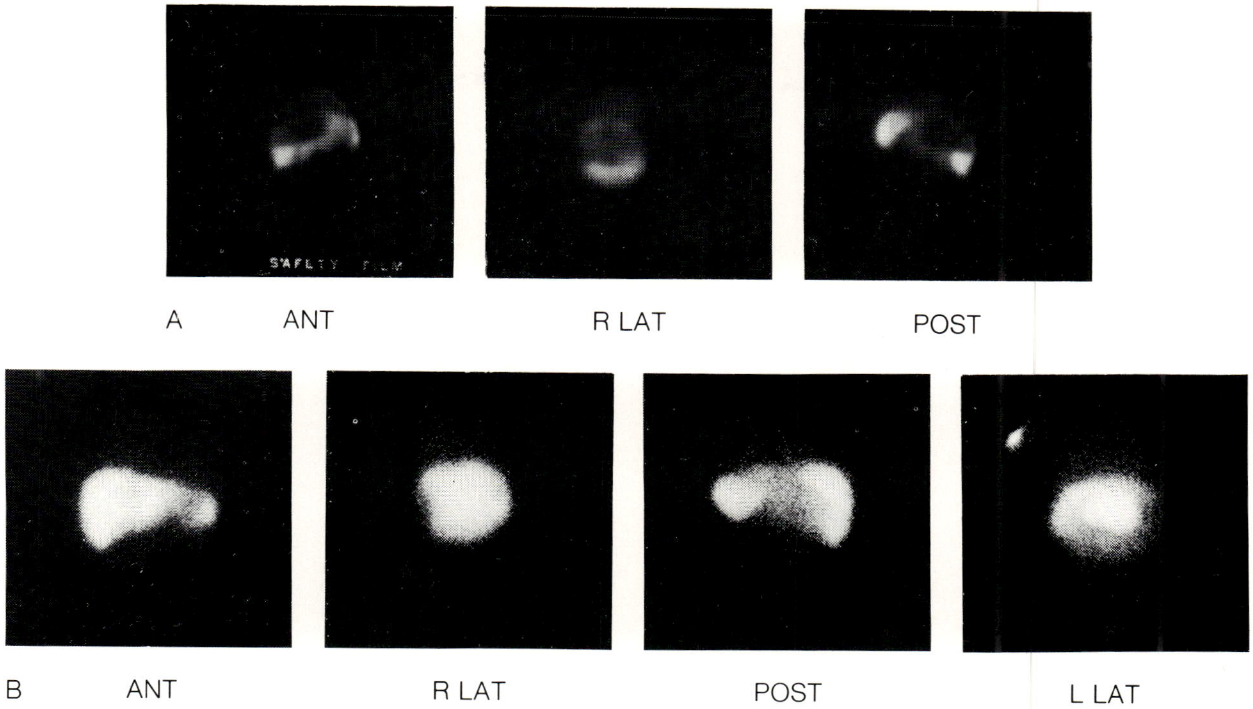


**FIG. 41. FAVORABLE RESPONSE TO CHEMOTHERAPY AND IMPROVEMENT ON LIVER IMAGING.** One of the objective methods of determining if chemotherapy has been beneficial is through the changing appearance of hepatic metastases on liver imaging. **A.** Extensive metastatic involvement in a child with Wilms' tumor. **B.** Four years later, the metastases are no longer detectable.

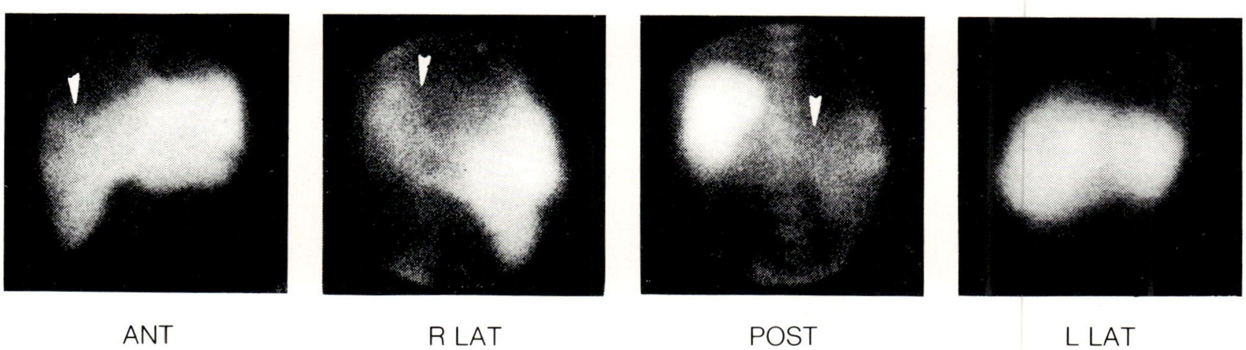


**FIG. 42. NEOPLASTIC INVOLVEMENT WITH DIRECT EXTENSION FROM LUNG.** Direct extension to the liver from bronchogenic carcinoma in the right lower lobe of the lung is clearly visible in the anterior and posterior positions. The direct extension of the tumor through the diaphragm is somewhat irregular. This is best seen in the right lateral position. The patient also has Laennec's cirrhosis.

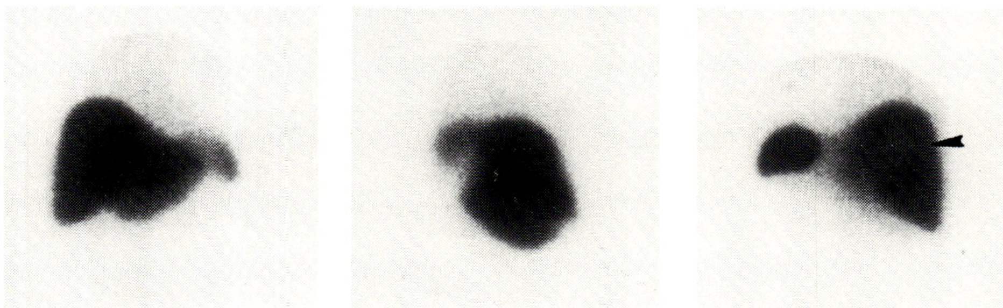

A ANT R LAT POST

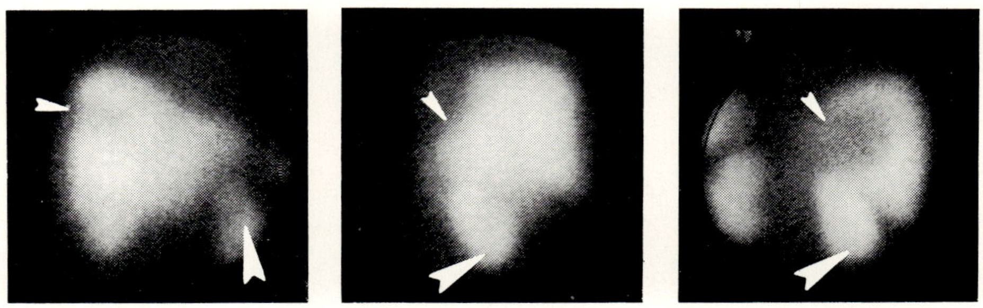

B ANT R LAT POST

**FIG. 43. COMBINED LIVER–KIDNEY IMAGING FOR IDENTIFICATION OF METASTASIS. A.** Initial liver imaging in the anterior, right lateral, and posterior positions shows evidence of a space-occupying lesion, posteriorly located, in the right lobe of the liver (arrows). In the posterior position, the abnormality might be confused with accentuation of the renal impression. **B.** Combined liver imaging (Tc-99m SC) and renal imaging (Tc-99m DTPA) clearly identify the kidney (larger arrow) as lying well below the involved area (arrow).

A ANT R LAT POST

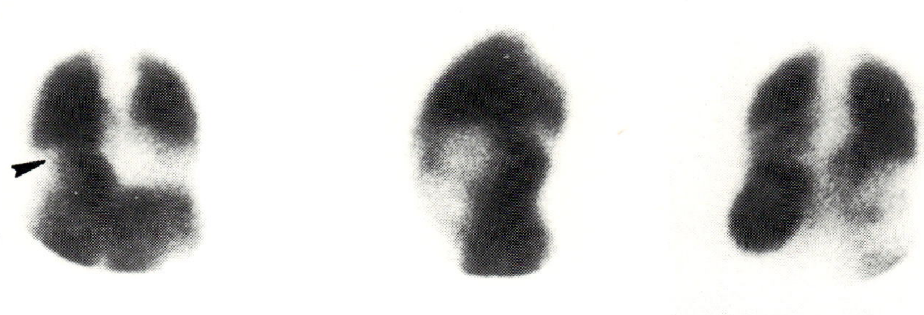

B ANT R LAT POST

**FIG. 44.** (See legend next page)

**FIG. 44. MULTIPLE METASTASES. COMBINED LUNG–LIVER IMAGING AND IMPROVED VISUALIZATION OF LESIONS. A.** Initial liver imaging in the anterior position shows reduced radioactivity along the lateral aspect of the right lobe (arrow), but the full extent of the lesion cannot be well appreciated. The posterior metastases are seen well in the right lateral and posterior positions. **B.** Combined lung–liver imaging helps accentuate the demonstration of the lesion in the anterior position (arrow). Combined imaging may help in the demonstration of metastases when imaging can be performed in the anterior position only.

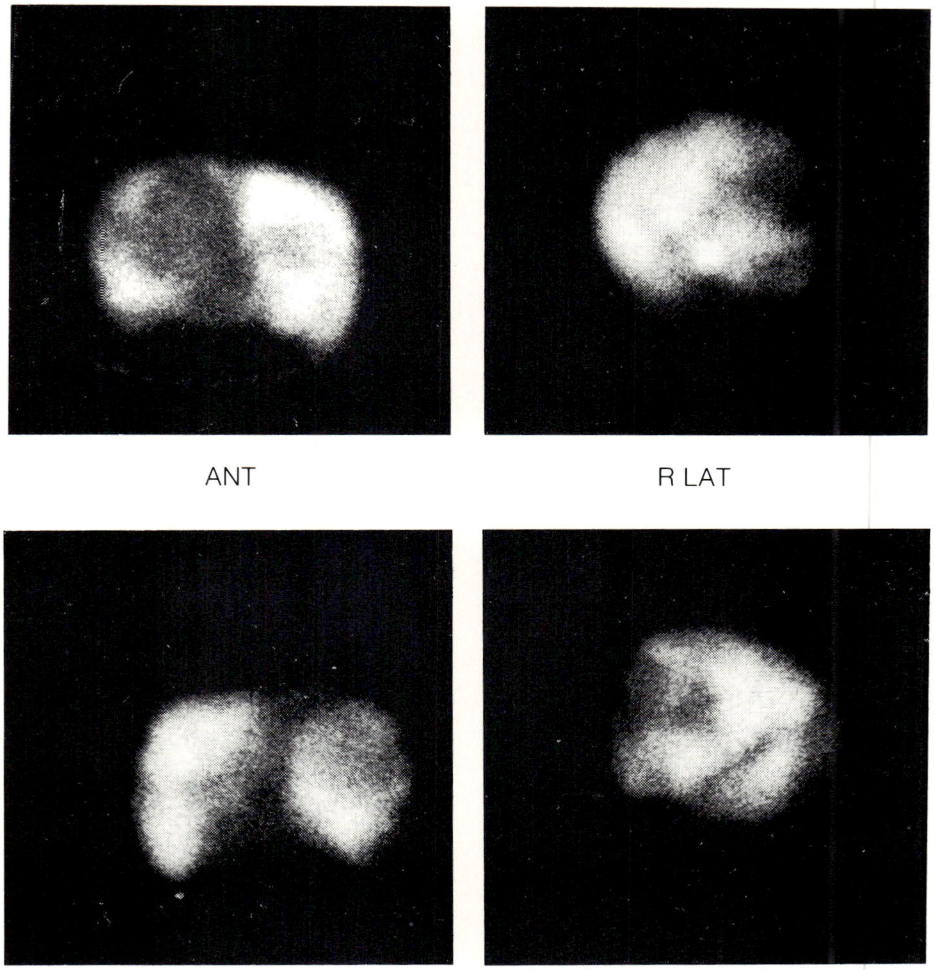


**FIG. 45. HEMANGIOENDOTHELIOMA.** Since this is a true neoplasm and is composed, for the most part, of masses of endothelial cells, resulting in hepatic tissue replacement, involvement in the liver is associated with absent radioactivity. In this 7-month-old patient, there is extensive hepatic tissue replacement by the tumor in both the right and left lobes.

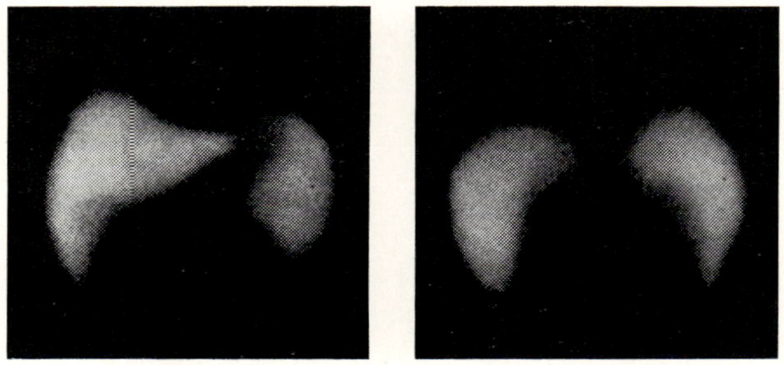

ANT POST

**FIG. 46. MULTIPLE MYELOMA.** There has been diffuse infiltration of myeloma cells into the hepatic sinusoids and throughout the spleen, resulting in both hepatic and splenic enlargement. Both the histologic and imaging findings are similar to those seen with chronic granulocytic leukemia when both liver and spleen are involved. In other cases of liver involvement in multiple myeloma, infiltration of the liver by plasma cells may be in the form of tumor-forming nodules.

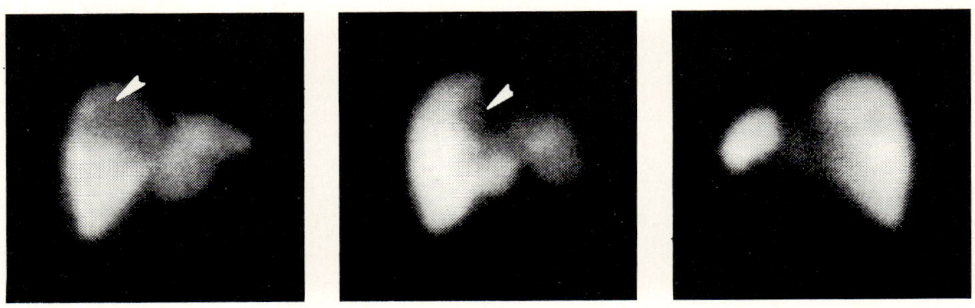

A ANT R A O POST

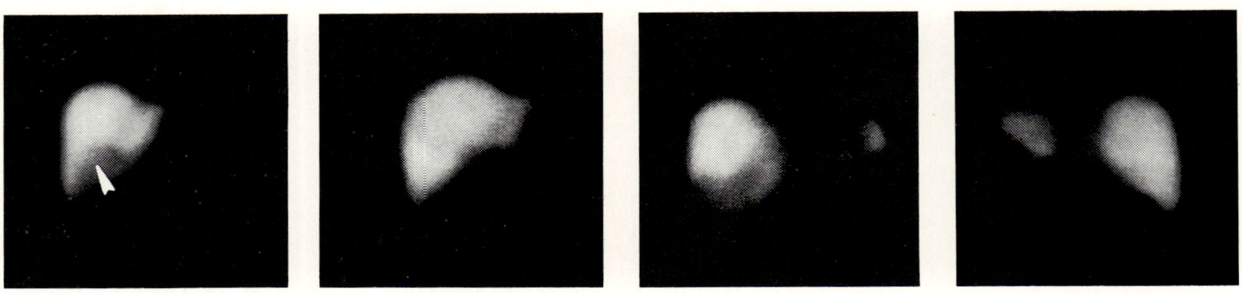

B ANT R A O L A O POST

**FIG. 47.** (See legend next page)

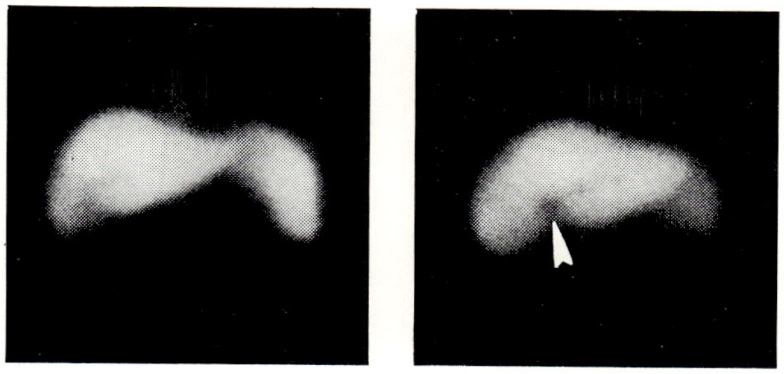

C ANT RAO

**FIG. 47.** IMPROVEMENT IN IMAGING IN OBLIQUE POSITIONS. Although liver–spleen imaging is commonly performed in the anterior, posterior, and both lateral positions, additional imaging in one or more oblique positions is sometimes essential and often helpful in the delineation of an abnormality, in the clarification of hepatic architecture in cases with unusual configurations of the liver, and in the separation of hepatic and splenic images. **A.** Improved demonstration of space-occupying lesion. Imaging in the anterior position shows the area of reduced activity in the right lobe, but in the right anterior oblique position the extent of the metastatic involvement is more clearly shown (primary: carcinoma of breast). **B.** Clarification of reduced radioactivity in right lobe. Because of the posterior position and reduced mass of the posterior portion of the right lobe, as it forms a fossa-like area, reduced radioactivity (arrow) is seen. As the entire right lobe is moved forward in the right anterior oblique position, the area of reduced activity is no longer detected. Note the prominence of the breast artifact in the RAO position. Also note the unusual orientation of the spleen in both the anterior and posterior positions (upside-down spleen). **C.** Identification of biliary dilatation secondary to extrahepatic biliary obstruction due to carcinoma of the pancreas improved in the RAO position. The relatively reduced radioactivity in the right lobe of the liver in the anterior position is a source of confusion in this image. However, the distraction of the right lobe is no longer a problem in the RAO position, and the dilated biliary tree is more clearly defined (arrow).

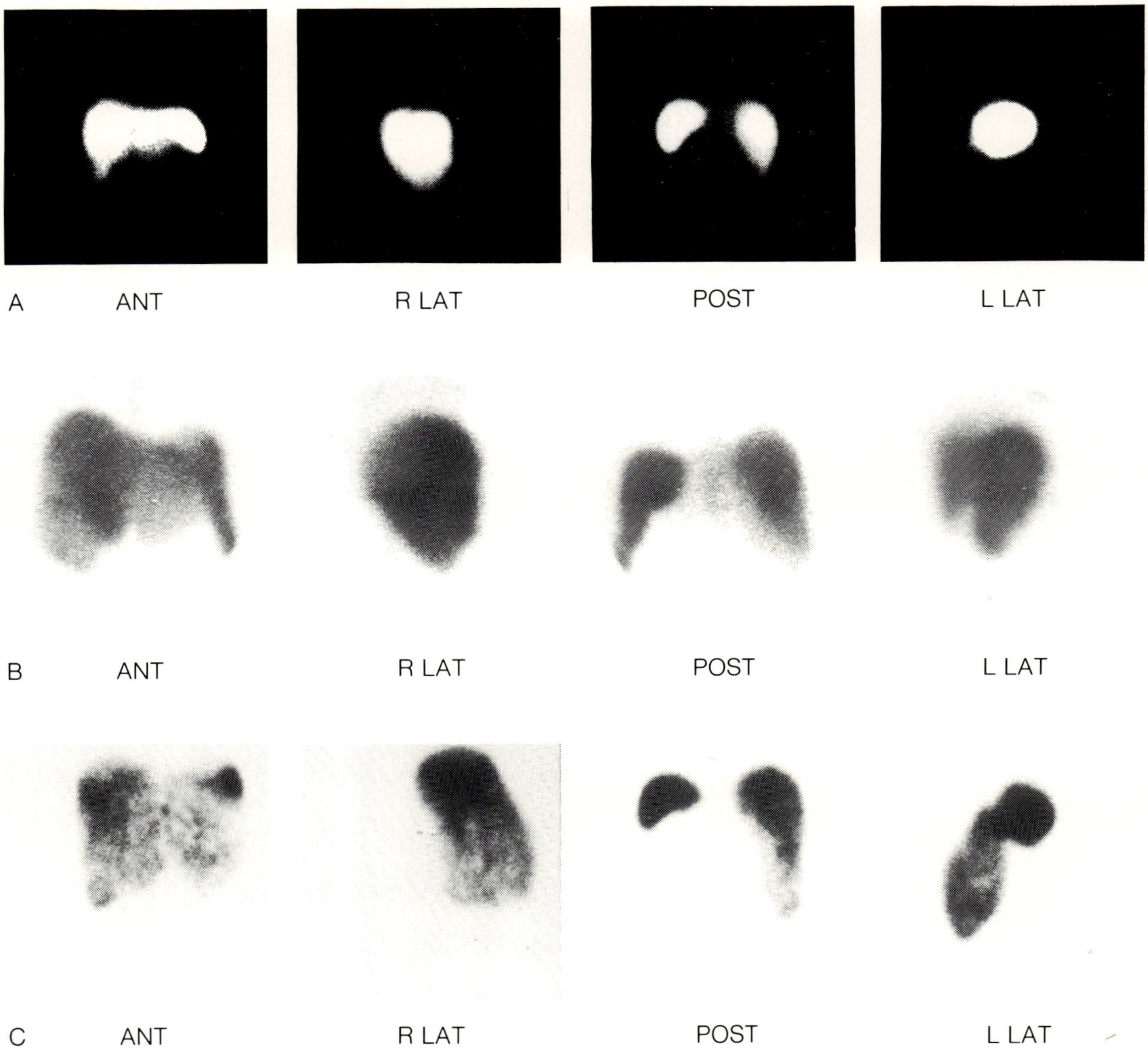


**FIG. 48.** **LYMPHOMA.** The liver is involved in approximately 70 percent of patients with Hodgkin's disease. Tumor tissue accumulates in the portal zones and spreads out from these sites. Though the entire organ is usually involved prior to hepatic infiltration, imaging may show increased radioactivity only in the spleen compared to the liver, as seen in **A** (see Fig. 88). The liver may become diffusely involved with lymphoma with the microscopic presence of tumor tissue at the portal areas. In such cases, no discrete space-occupying lesions can be detected on imaging despite the widespread involvement, as seen in **B.** Both the liver and spleen are enlarged but the characteristic manifestations of hepatic metastases are not visible. In this case, the individual areas of tumor involvement are too small to be detected. **C.** Multiple space-occupying lesions in a patient with Burkitt's lymphoma.

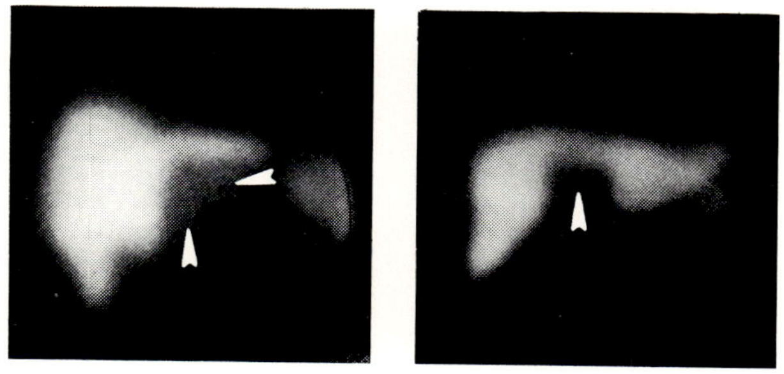

A ANT B ANT

**FIG. 49. CHANGES SECONDARY TO RADIATION THERAPY.** The Kupffer cells in that portion of the liver uninvolved with tumor are in the area of the portal at which the radiation therapy is directed. As a result of the radiation they undergo destructive and fibrotic changes. Thus they can no longer phagocytize Tc-99m SC in that region of the liver, and the area of treatment is clearly identified as a localized area of absent radioactivity. **A.** Rectangular area of absent radioactivity, corresponding to the therapy portal (arrows) in a patient with carcinoma of the bile ducts. **B.** Rectangular area of absent radioactivity due to radiation therapy for carcinoma of the head of the pancreas. Note the normal uptake in those portions of the liver unaffected by the radiation treatment.

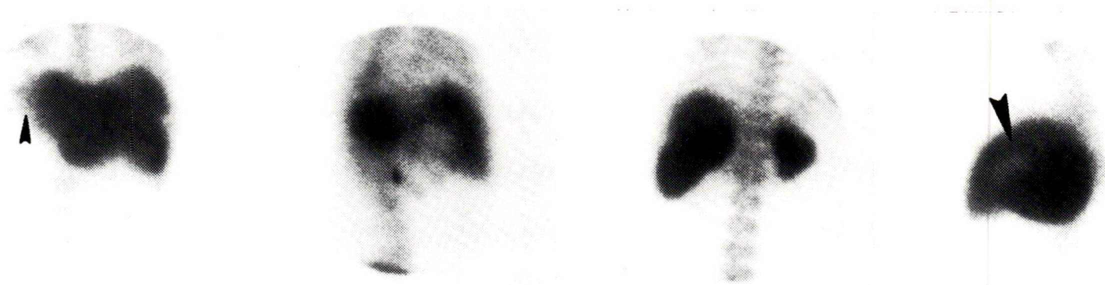

A ANT R LAT POST L LAT

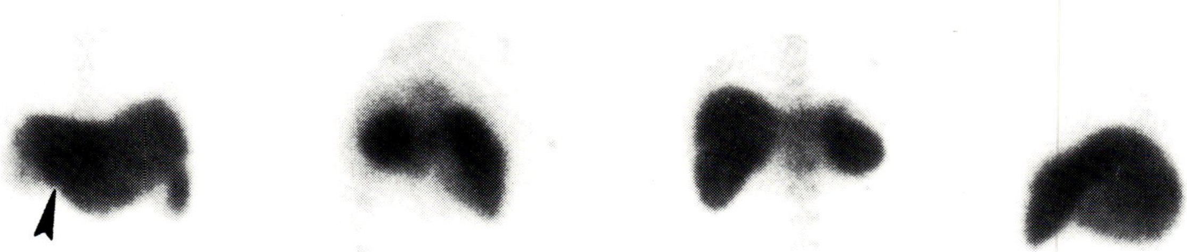

B ANT R LAT POST L LAT

**FIG. 50. A, B.** (See legend next page)

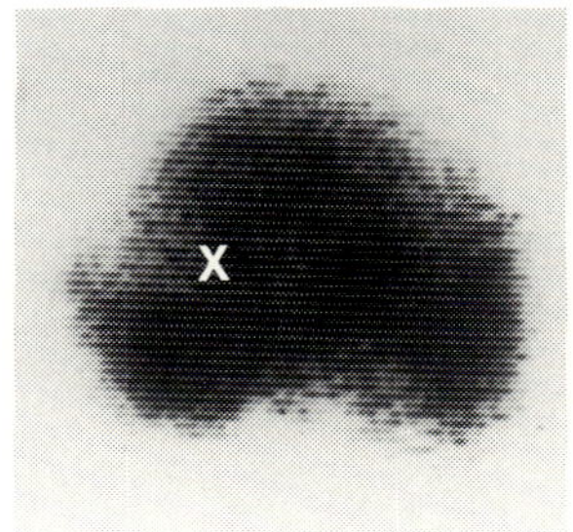


C ANT

**FIG. 50. PARTIAL HEPATECTOMY (Right Lobe Removed).** Following a right lobe hepatectomy, there is usually absent radioactivity in the right lobe area, some distortion of the hepatic image because of the right lobe removal, and some evidence of compensatory hypertrophy of the remaining left lobe. The latter sometimes may not be demonstrated on radionuclide imaging until 2 or 3 months have elapsed. **A.** Right hepatectomy following trauma. The right lobe area shows absent radioactivity (arrow) in the anterior position. Note the position of the left lobe (larger arrow) in the left lateral position, superior and anterior to the spleen. **B.** Same patient 6 weeks later showing some evidence of compensatory hypertrophy of left lobe (larger arrow). The patient also has Laennec's cirrhosis, as seen by the uptake of radioactive colloid by the RE cells of the bone marrow and the increased activity in the spleen. **C.** Anterior scan in a patient with a right hepatic lobectomy for a solitary right lobe metastasis 3 months earlier. There is now extensive enlargement of the remaining portion of the liver. Arrow indicates right body wall and the xiphoid is marked (X).

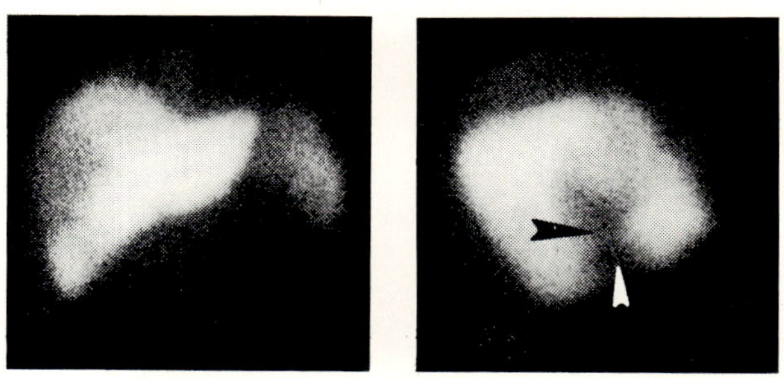

ANT R LAT

**FIG. 51. POSTOPERATIVE CHANGES.** Surgical intervention within the liver or hepatic bed usually results in unusual and augmented areas of absent radioactivity. Insertion of drains and packs contributes to the imaging abnormalities. Absent radioactivity associated with a cholecystectomy (small arrow) and a focal lesion (larger arrow) due to a metastatic lesion are visible in the right lateral position.

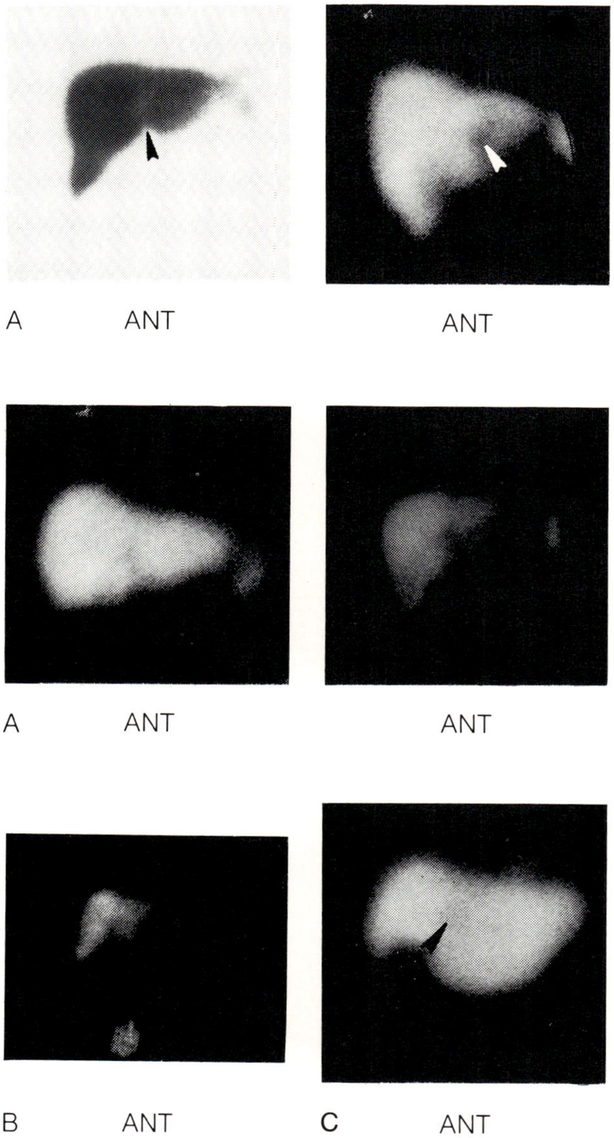


**FIG. 52.** BILIARY DILATATION. Although imaging abnormalities of the biliary tract are best seen with hepatobiliary agents such as Tc-99m iminodiacetic acid (IDA), (see page 64), evidence of extrahepatic biliary obstruction causing dilatation of the biliary tree also may be detected on Tc-99m SC liver imaging as a localized area of reduced or absent radioactivity. The reduction in radioactivity is often stellate in shape, but this is not a constant finding. The configuration of the abnormality is simply a reflection of the accompanying dilatation in the biliary tree, which appears on the radionuclide image as a localized area of reduced radioactivity akin to a space-occupying lesion. These findings are usually detected in the anterior position only. **A.** Clearly identified stellate-shaped area of absent radioactivity (arrow) is associated in each of four different patients with biliary obstruction due to carcinoma of the pancreas. **B.** Y-shaped area of absent radioactivity in the region of the porta hepatis. Extrahepatic biliary obstruction with subsequent biliary dilation was caused by carcinoma of common duct. **C.** Reduced radioactivity due to biliary dilatation is caused by carcinoma of the pancreas obstructing the extrahepatic biliary tract. In each of these patients, the reduction in radioactivity is not of the characteristic stellate-shaped variety. However, with the jaundiced patient, biliary dilatation should be considered in the event of such a localized reduction in radioactivity. **D.** Absent radioactivity due to biliary dilatation in a patient with carcinoma of the head of the pancreas. Note the unusual configuration of the irregularly dilated ducts of both the right and left lobes. **E.** Obstructing carcinoma at ampulla of Vater causing marked intrahepatic biliary dilatation (arrow). **F.** Irregular reduction in radioactivity (arrow) with biliary dilatation.

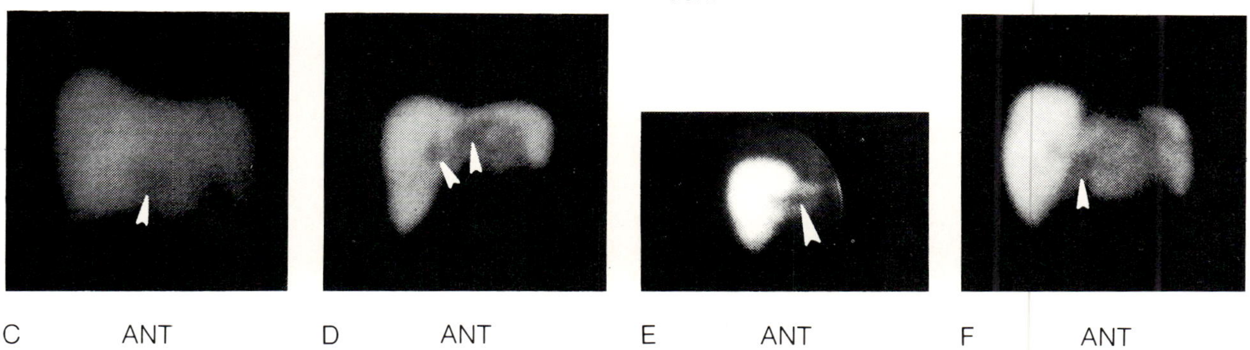

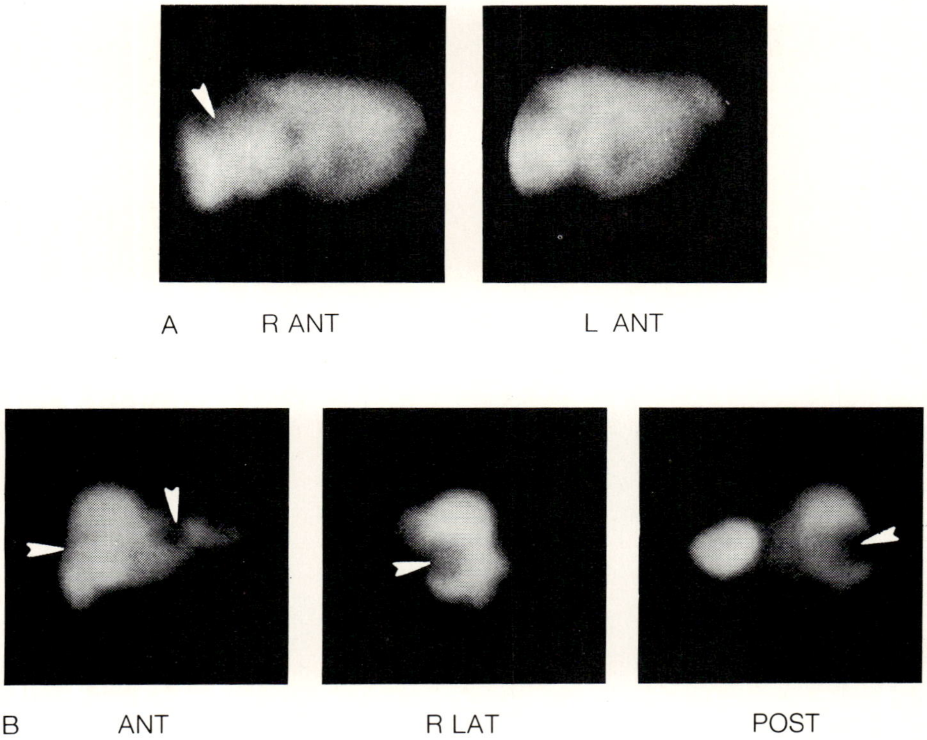


**FIG. 53. POLYCYSTIC DISEASE OF THE LIVER.** Multiple areas of absent radioactivity, both small and large, are seen throughout the liver. There are no characteristic features on static imaging to distinguish the polycystic involvement from the liver with multiple abscesses or metastases. **A.** Extensive involvement in subdiaphragmatic portion of right lobe (arrow). **B.** Large cystic lesions in the left lobe (arrow) and posterior portion of right lobe (arrow).

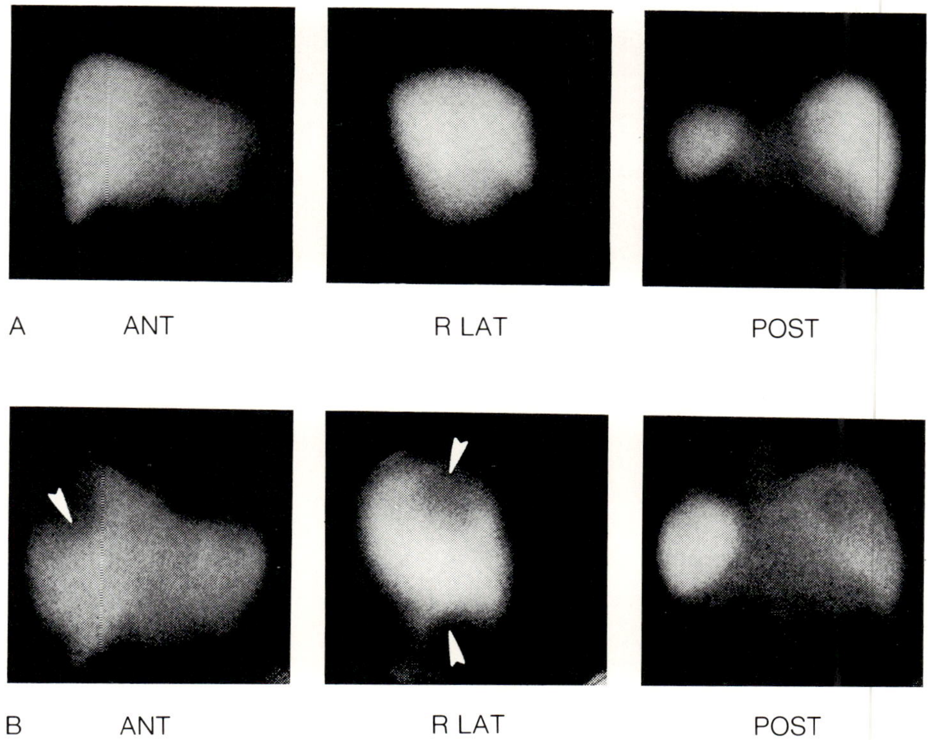


**FIG. 54. INTRAHEPATIC AND SUBHEPATIC ABSCESSES FOLLOWING ABDOMINAL SURGERY. A.** Preoperative imaging in this patient with Crohn's disease shows an enlarged liver with no evidence of space-occupying lesions. Following this, surgery was performed that included a partial small bowel resection and ileostomy. **B.** Postoperative imaging shows two discrete, somewhat rounded areas of absent radioactivity (arrows) due to abscess formation. The lesion in the subdiaphragmatic portion of the right lobe is intrahepatic and is seen to be girded in the anterior and right lateral positions by a least a rim of hepatic tissue. Only the superior border of the subhepatic lesion can be identified, and this failure to demonstrate hepatic radioactivity inferior to it helps establish the diagnosis of a subhepatic lesion. Note the relative anterior position of both lesions. The causative organ was not identified.

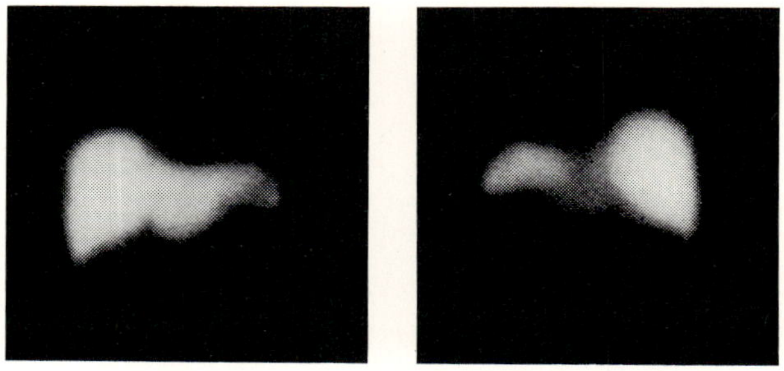

A ANT Liver POST Liver

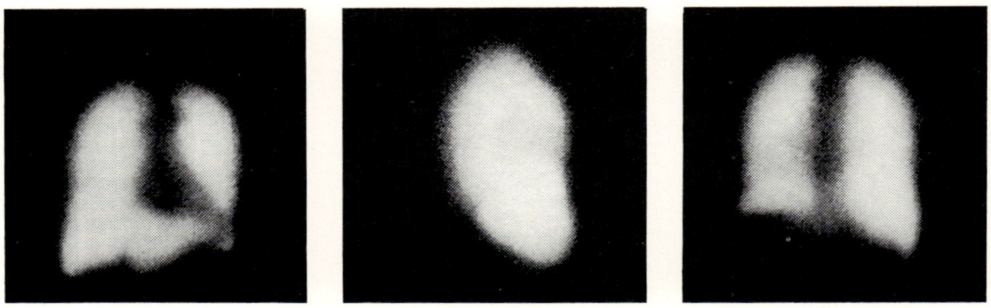

ANT Lung–Liver R LAT Lung–Liver POST Lung–Liver

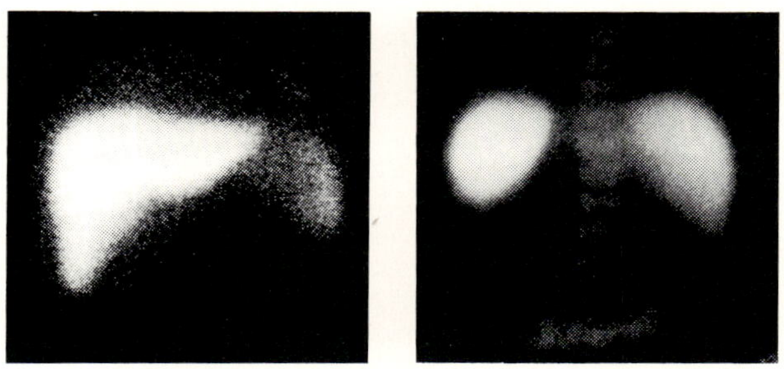

B ANT Liver POST Liver

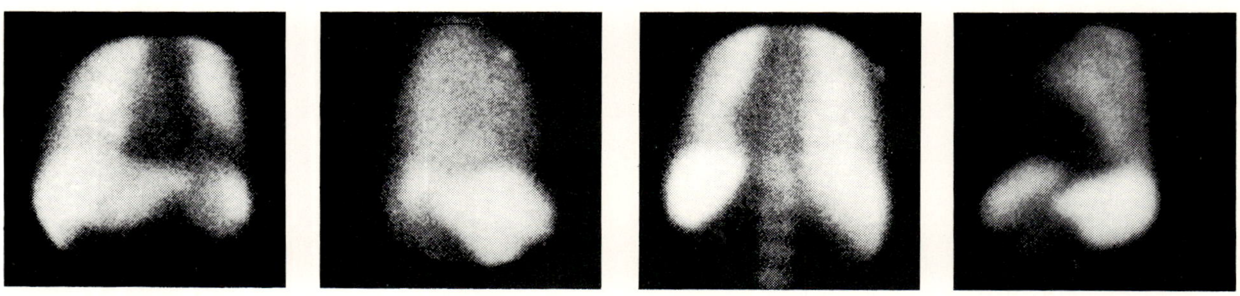

ANT Lung–Liver R LAT Lung–Liver POST Lung–Liver L LAT Lung–Liver

**FIG. 55. A, B.** (See legend on page 50)

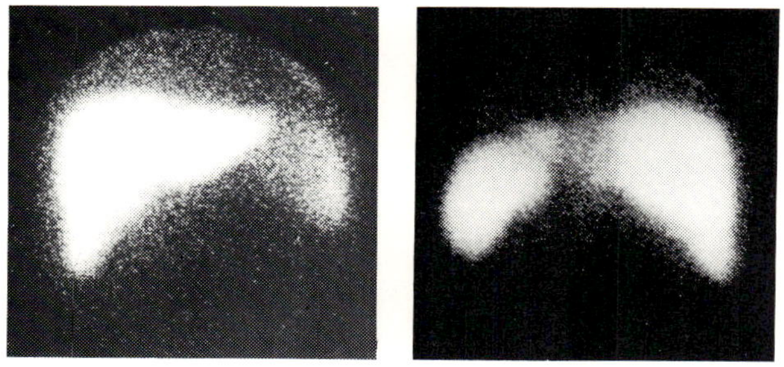

C ANT Liver POST Liver

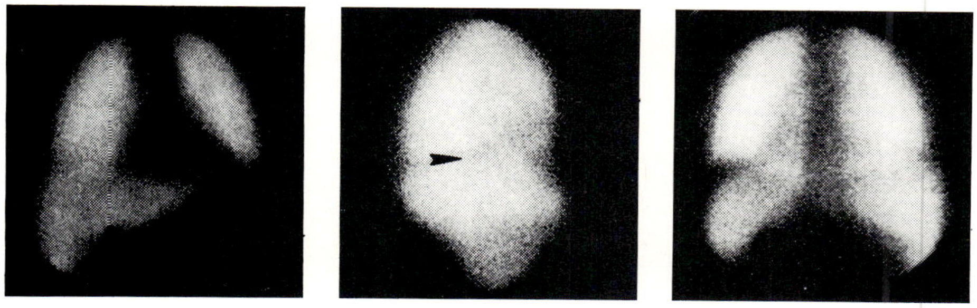

ANT Lung–Liver R LAT Lung–Liver POST Lung–Liver

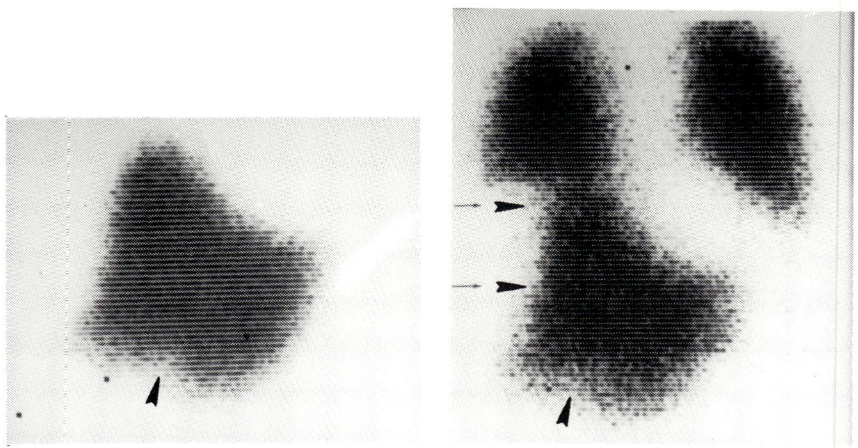

D ANT Liver ANT Lung–Liver

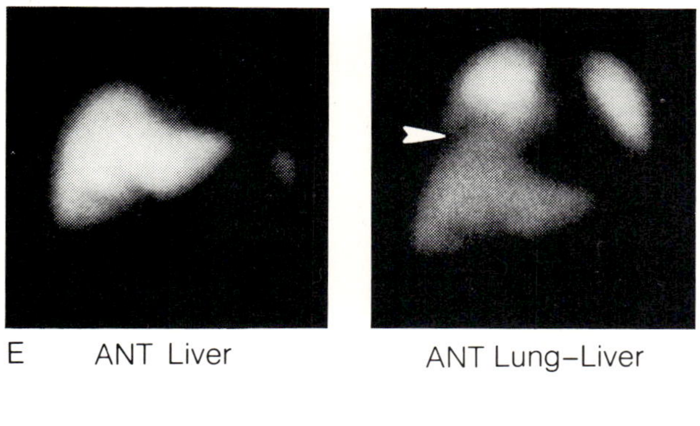

E ANT Liver ANT Lung–Liver

**FIG. 55. C–E.**
(See legend next page)

**FIG. 55.** **COMBINED LUNG–LIVER IMAGING.** Simultaneous imaging of both the liver and lungs may be useful in the detection of a subdiaphragmatic abscess. However, *any* pulmonary abnormality in the right lower lung field will probably be associated with reduced radioactivity, thus compromising the usefulness of combined imaging. Normally, as the subdiaphragmatic portion of the right lobe of the liver is enveloped and draped by the right lung, no area of absent radioactivity in this location is detected. **A.** Normal lung–liver imaging. Note the failure to visualize any reduction in radioactivity between the right lung and liver in any position. **B.** Normal lung–liver imaging. Reduced radioactivity between the left lobe and the spleen may be seen normally. Incidentally, the patient has cirrhosis. **C.** Right pleural effusion. This has resulted in a somewhat linear area of absent radioactivity (arrow), best seen in the right lateral position. **D.** Subdiaphragmatic abscess. Liver imaging in the anterior position suggests that a subdiaphragmatic abnormality lateral to the pointed dome is present. However, combined imaging helps define the extent of the subdiaphragmatic collection. A subhepatic abscess is also present. **E.** Subdiaphragmatic abscess. Initial hepatic imaging alone discloses no sharply defined evidence of a subdiaphragmatic abscess. However, combined imaging emphasizes a slight irregularity along the lateral portion of the right lobe, superiorly (arrow), which was found to be the site of an abscess.

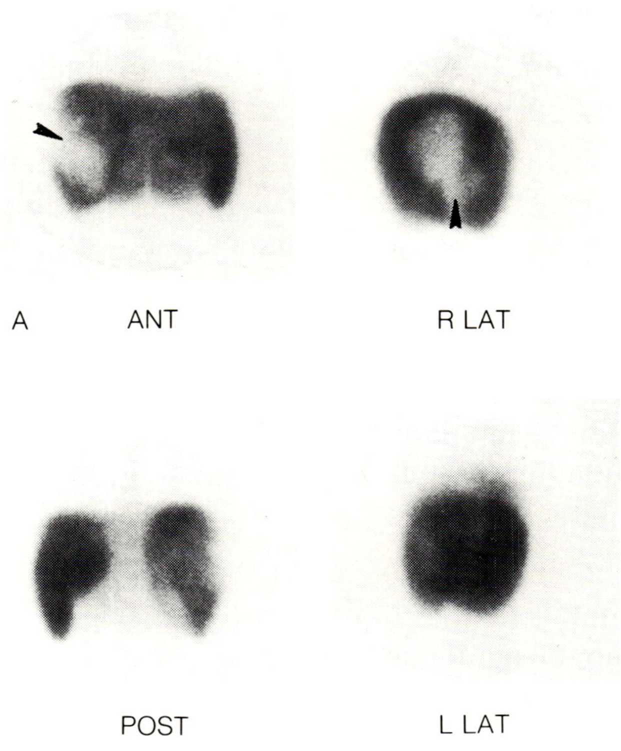


**FIG. 56. A.** (See legend next page)

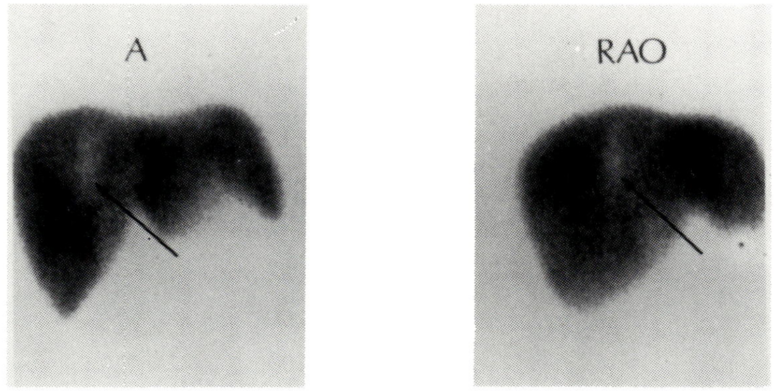


B ANT RAO

**FIG. 56. CHANGES SECONDARY TO TRAUMA. A.** A large hematoma (arrow) developed and at surgery was found to be present in association with a tiny hepatocellular carcinoma. Note the large size of the hematoma, most clearly visible in the anterior and right lateral positions. Its widest extent is best seen in the latter view (Tc-99m SC). **B.** Hepatic laceration. The area of absent radioactivity (arrow) is due to a laceration of the liver as a result of an automobile–bicycle collision (Tc-99m IDA). (Courtesy of Dr. John R. Sty, Milwaukee Children's Hospital)

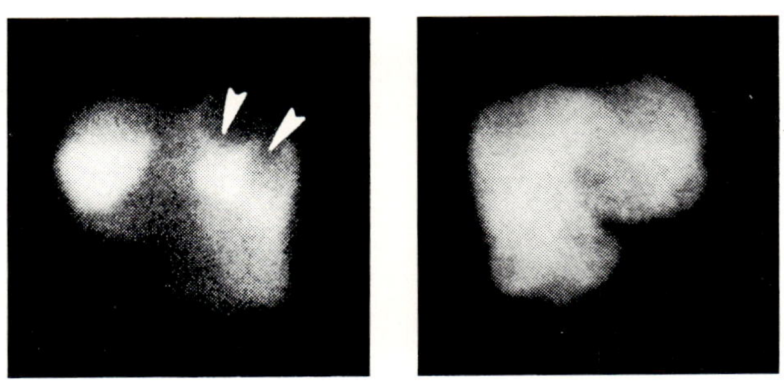

POST ANT

**FIG. 57. MULTIPLE HEPATIC ADENOMAS.** Multiple areas of absent radioactivity (arrows) in both the right and left lobes in a 16-year-old female are due to multiple hepatic adenomas. Although sometimes associated with the administration of oral contraceptive steroids, the lesions developed in this patient in the absence of such therapy. The rounded areas of absent radioactivity in the subdiaphragmatic portion of the right lobe ( large arrows) are due, in part, to surgical changes secondary to open biopsy of the tumors in that area. The adenomas are composed of polygonal cells and may show increased activity on I-131 rose bengal and Tc-99m IDA imaging.

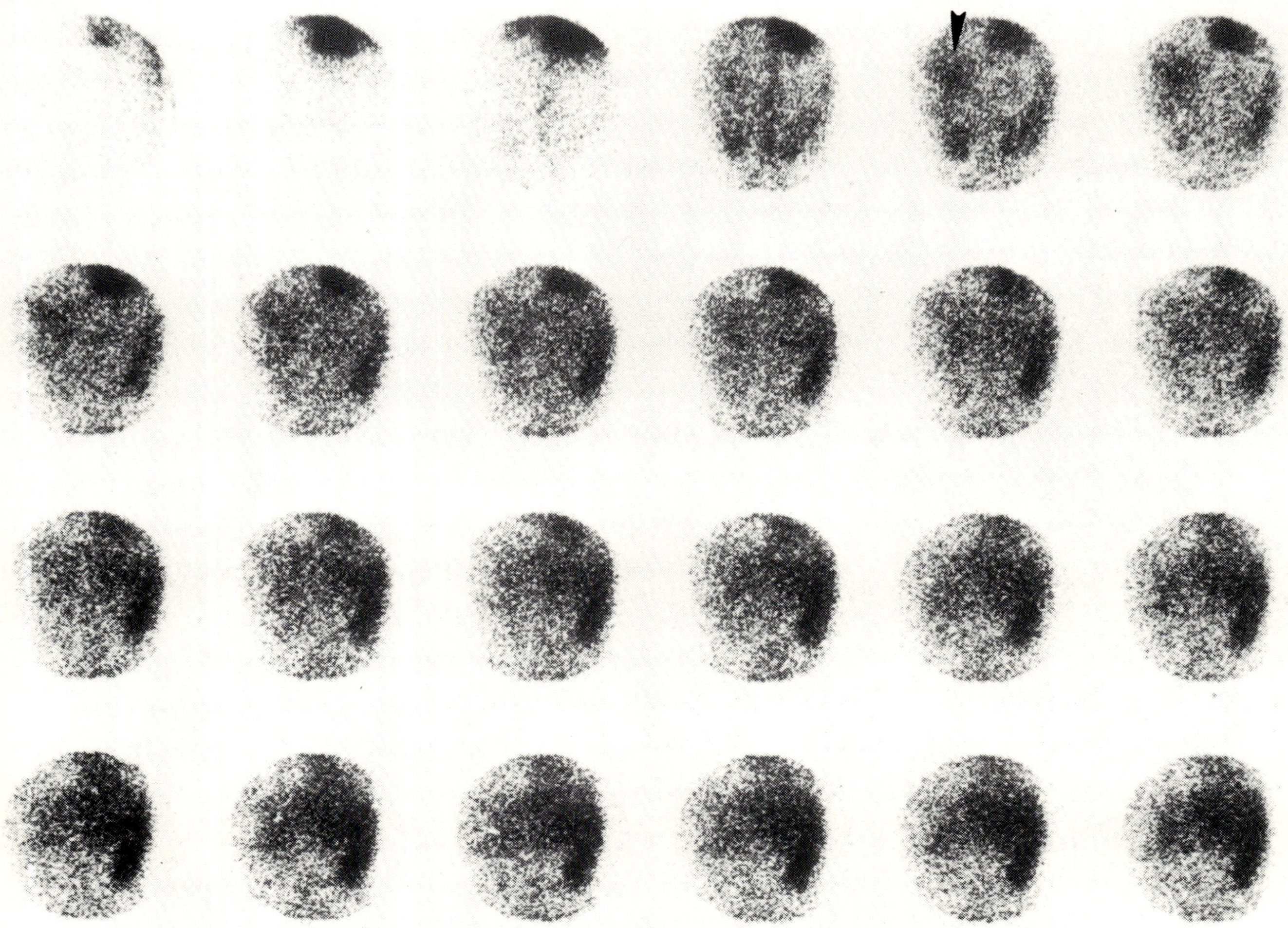

A Anterior Blood Flow

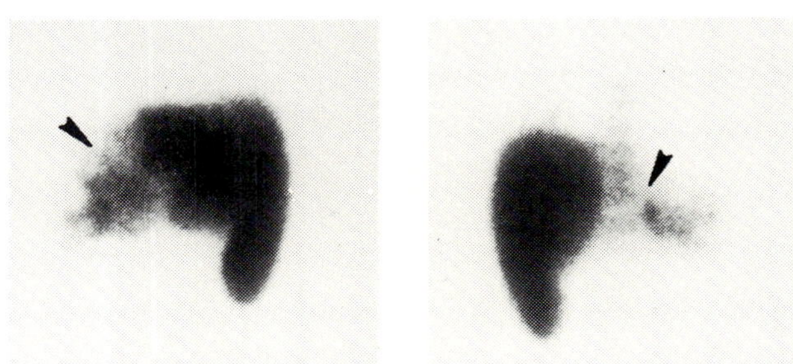

B ANT POST

**FIG. 58. INCREASED VASCULARITY IN HEPATOMA. A.** Blood flow study. Increased radioactivity (arrow) is visible during the arterial phase in the area of the malignant hepatoma. During the venous phase, at the time of phagocytosis of the radioactive colloid by the Kupffer cells, the same area of involvement shows absent activity (framing rate: 3 seconds/frame). **B.** Static imaging shows absent radioactivity (arrows) at the site of involvement.

## DIFFUSE HEPATIC DISEASE

The imaging findings in diffuse hepatic disease, such as cirrhosis, reflect both the pathological changes that have occurred in the liver and the resulting circulatory alterations.

In cirrhosis, following necrosis and disintegration of hepatic cells, extensive fibrotic tissue replacement occurs. There is also proliferation of hepatic cells adjacent to the fibrotic areas, resulting in the formation of regenerating nodules. Obstruction to portal venous flow occurs as a result of both the regenerating nodules and portal zone fibrosis, and the steps are set in motion for the development of increased portal venous pressure and subsequent shunting to systemic veins.

Shunting occurs at several levels. Venous sinusoids persist at the periphery of the regenerating nodules and shunting occurs from the portal zones to hepatic veins. Shunting also occurs through a number of large veins to the systemic venous circulation (e.g., left renal vein, left coronary vein, superior hemorrhoidal vein). Since the portal vein is formed by the union of the superior mesenteric and splenic veins, increased portal pressure will be reflected in elevated splenic vein pressure and congestive splenomegaly.

These changes have a profound effect on liver–spleen imaging. Areas of reduced radioactivity (due to replacement and destruction of Kupffer cells by fibrotic tissue) interspersed with areas of normal or increased activity (due to phagocytosis by Kupffer cells in regenerating nodules) characterize the radionuclide image. This is sometimes termed radioactive mottling. As a result of reduced portal flow to the liver, less Tc-99m SC is delivered to that organ, and the radioactivity present is even further reduced. The spleen usually shows increased radioactivity compared to the liver and varying degrees of splenic enlargement (due to increased portal pressure transmitted to the splenic vein and congestive splenomegaly).

It is common to visualize the bone marrow, as the shunting to the systemic circulation makes the radiocolloid available for phagocytosis elsewhere in the RES, such as in the RE cells of the bone marrow. In some cases, there is pulmonary visualization because of phagocytosis by alveolar lining cells.

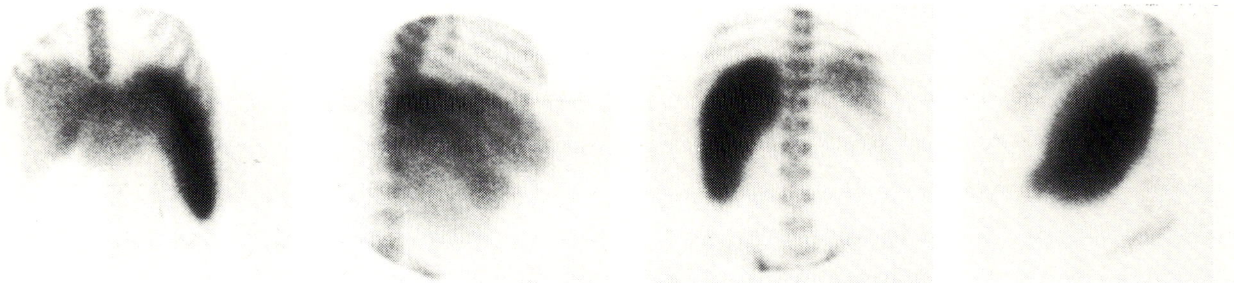

ANT R LAT POST L LAT

**FIG. 59. LAENNEC'S CIRRHOSIS AND SPLENOMEGALY.** This case illustrates many of the features that characterize Laennec's cirrhosis on radionuclide imaging: reduced radioactivity in an enlarged liver with relative sparing of the left lobe compared to the right; increase in splenic radioactivity and size (portal hypertension and congestive splenomegaly); presence of radioactive colloid in the bone marrow (associated with shunting from portal to systemic veins). Note the extensive bone marrow uptake and the remarkable structural identification of the sternum, ribs, vertebral column, and ilium. Some ascites is present, and this accounts for the separation of the lateral aspect of the right lobe, as seen in the anterior position, from the right lateral body wall. However, these changes are not so pronounced as those seen in Fig. 61A.

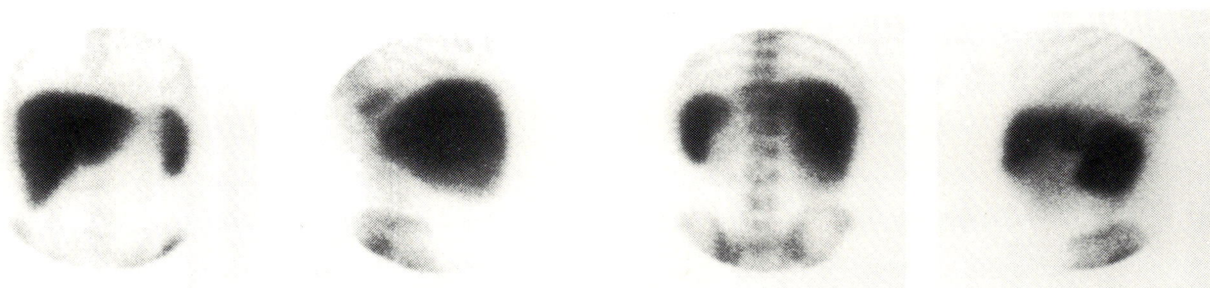

ANT R LAT POST L LAT

**FIG. 60. LAENNEC'S CIRRHOSIS WITHOUT OVERT HEPATIC CHANGES.** Although the liver is involved with cirrhosis, there are as yet no characteristic hepatic imaging changes, such as reduced liver radioactivity compared to the spleen, hepatomegaly, or relative sparing of the left lobe. Because of increased portal pressure, there is shunting from the portal to systemic veins, and this is responsible for the extensive uptake of radiocolloid in the bone marrow.

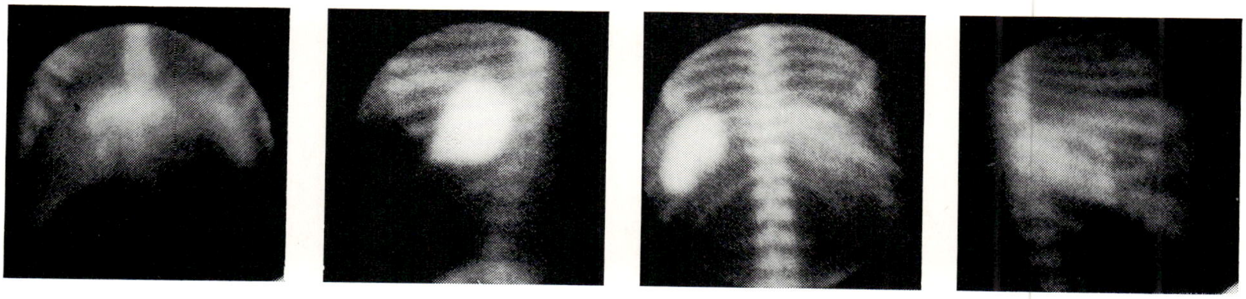

A ANT R LAT POST L LAT

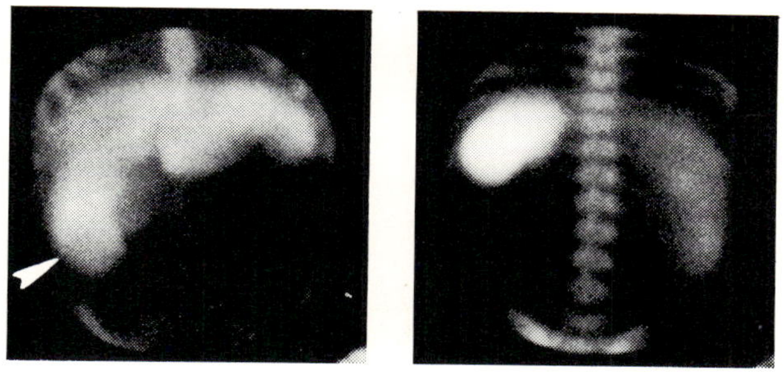

B ANT POST

**FIG. 61.** LAENNEC'S CIRRHOSIS AND EXTENSIVE BONE MARROW UPTAKE. **A.** There has been extensive fibrotic replacement of the right lobe and relative sparing of the left lobe. If there is a suspicion of tumor involvement of the right lobe, Ga-67 imaging should be performed. Note the exquisite costal marrow uptake of the Tc-99m SC. The separation of the ribs from the lateral border of the right lobe suggests ascites. **B.** Enlarged liver with a globular Riedel's lobe (arrow). Reduced radioactivity associated with right lobe involvement is visible.

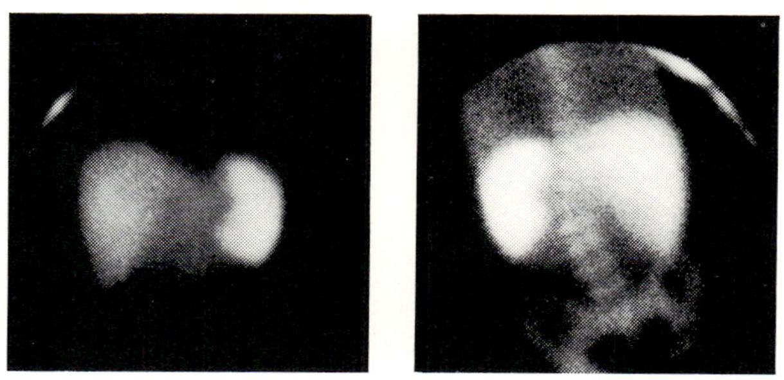

ANT POST

**FIG. 62.** CIRRHOSIS ASSOCIATED WITH MALNUTRITION. Cirrhosis developing on a nutritional basis has many of the features seen with Laennec's cirrhosis. The extensive portal fibrosis in this patient with Crohn's disease is associated with radioactive mottling. As a result of hepatic changes and increased portal pressure, the enlarged spleen shows increased radioactivity. Note the intense uptake of radiocolloid in the bone marrow.

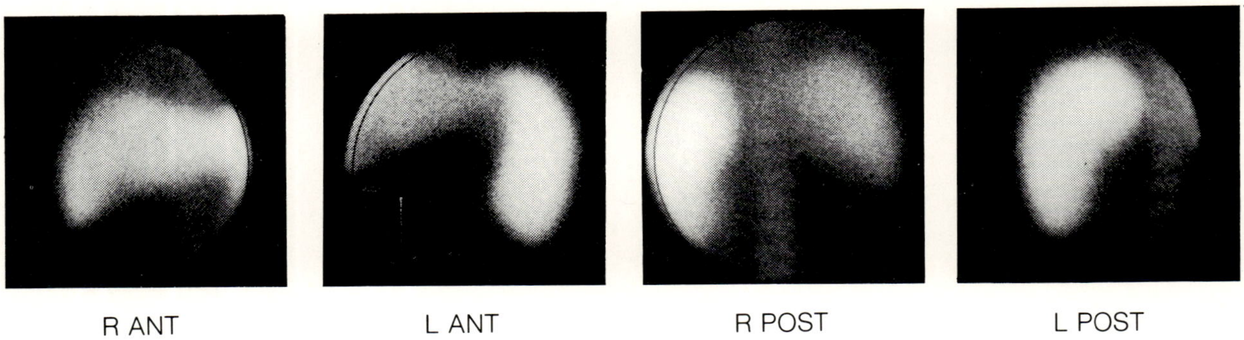


**FIG. 63. POSTNECROTIC CIRRHOSIS.** The imaging findings are usually similar to those seen in Laennec's cirrhosis. The shrunken liver with reduced radioactivity compared to that of the spleen is demonstrated. The enlarged spleen is a manifestation of portal hypertension and congestive splenomegaly.

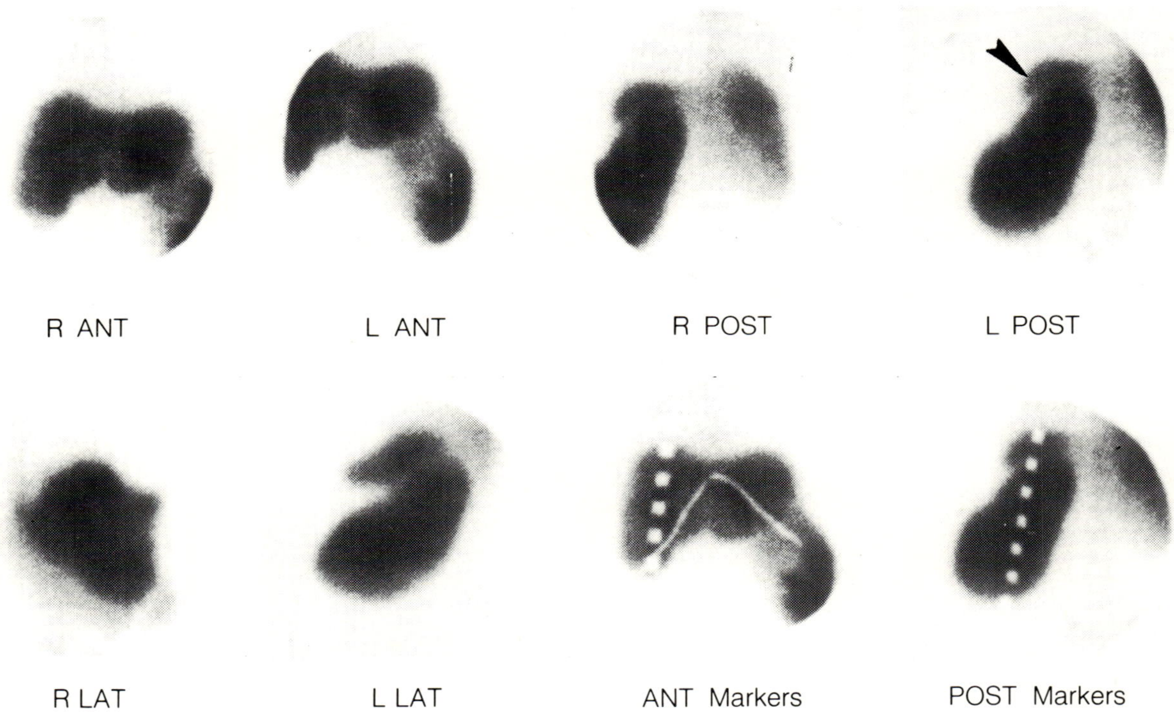


**FIG. 64. MACRONODULAR CIRRHOSIS AND ENORMOUS SPLEEN.** The areas of reduced radioactivity in the liver associated with macronodular cirrhosis are not nearly so impressive as the massive splenomegaly. The latter appears to be associated with increased portal pressure and marked congestive splenomegaly. Because of the posterior location of the upper pole of the spleen (compared to that of the left hepatic lobe) the splenic size cannot be appreciated in the anterior position. In the posterior position, a small area of left hepatic lobe ( large arrow) is identified. In the marker view, the spleen measures approximately 23 cm longitudinally.

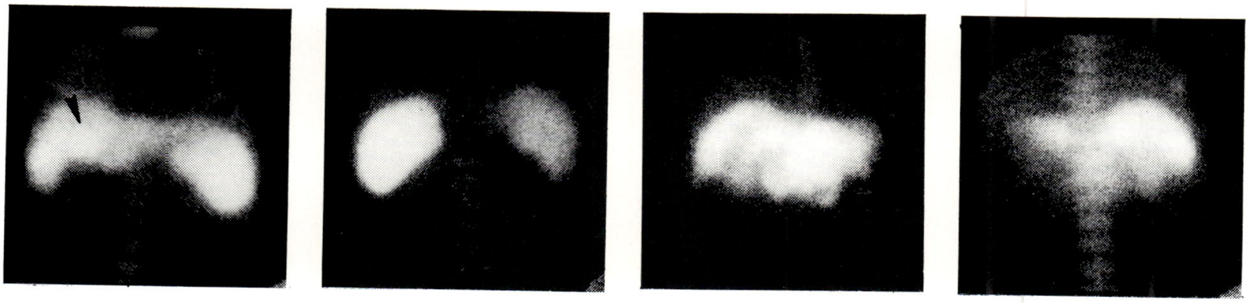

A ANT POST B ANT POST

**FIG. 65. LAENNEC'S CIRRHOSIS AND AREAS OF ABSENT RADIOACTIVITY RESEMBLING TUMOR.** Fibrotic changes may be extensive and have a somewhat nodular configuration. These fibrotic areas of hepatic tissue replacement may appear on imaging identical to multiple metastases. **A.** Somewhat rounded areas of radioactivity (arrow) are seen best in the anterior position in a patient with advanced cirrhosis. **B.** Irregular areas of absent radioactivity are due to cirrhotic changes. A portal–renal shunt had been performed on this patient along with a splenectomy.

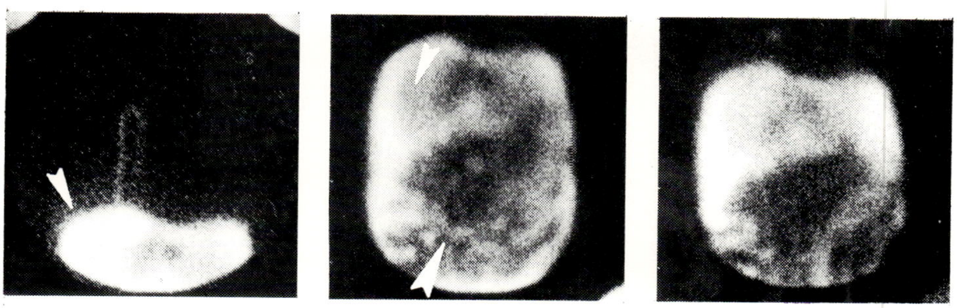

A ANT B ANT C ANT

**FIG. 66. DETERMINATION OF PATENCY OF LeVEEN SHUNT.** Following insertion of a shunt to drain ascitic fluid from the peritoneal cavity to the right jugular system, the shunt patency may be determined with Tc-99m SC. The radiocolloid is injected into the peritoneal cavity in the usual dose used for liver imaging. **A.** Five minutes later, imaging in the area of the right internal jugular vein shows increased activity as do other vascular structures in this region, indicating shunt patency and travel of the radioactive material from the peritoneal cavity to the systemic circulation. **B.** Imaging.at 15 minutes shows the hepatic image ( arrow ). Some radiocolloid has remained in the abdomen ( larger arrow ). **C.** Study at one hour shows satisfactory imaging of liver and spleen. The large area of absent radioactivity in the liver is due to fibrotic changes secondary to cirrhosis.

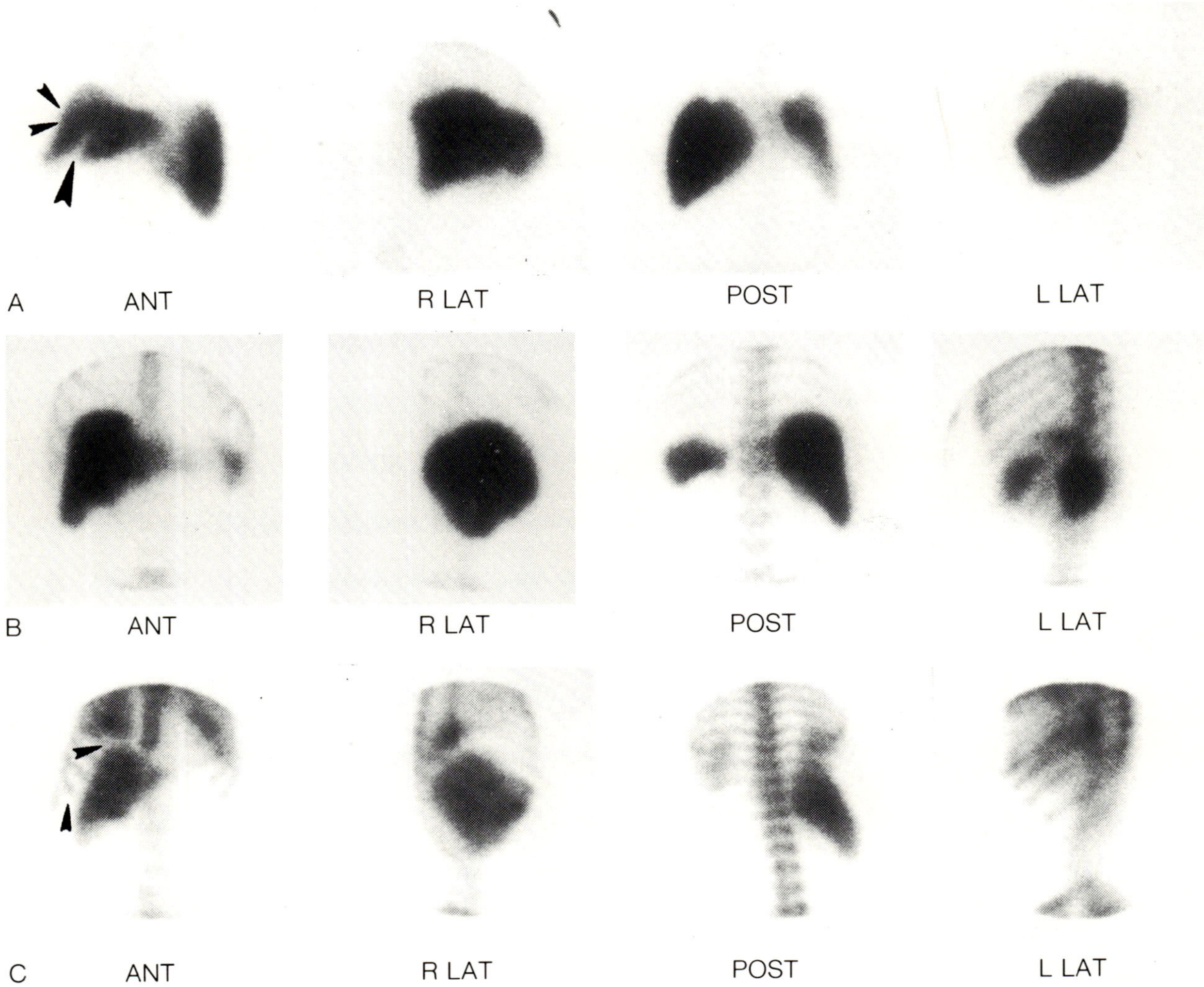


**FIG. 67.** CHANGES SECONDARY TO ASCITES. **A.** Ascites due to metastatic peritoneal implants from carcinoma of the vulva without liver metastases. The ascitic fluid is responsible for several positional changes on imaging. There is displacement of the lateral border of the right lobe of the liver from the right lateral body wall because of fluid interposition (arrows), and the lateral aspect of the right lobe of the liver appears to have a diagonal orientation. If a pulmonary image is present, there is a noticeable separation between the right lung and the superior portion of the right hepatic lobe. With the liver floating in a sea of ascitic fluid, marked accentuation of the lobar separation ( large arrow ) is visualized. There is a general foreshortening of the images because of fluid interposition, and estimation of organ size may be inaccurate. **B.** When there is a small amount of ascitic fluid, the changes are less prominent. The somewhat diagonal orientation of the lateral aspect of the right lobe and the separation from the right lateral body wall can be recognized. The reduced radioactivity in the left lobe in this patient with alcoholic cirrhosis is unusual. **C.** Ascites in a patient with cirrhosis who had a prior splenectomy. There is extensive extrahepatic uptake of Tc-99m SC in the bone marrow and alveolar lining cells of the lungs. Note the separation of the liver from the lateral body wall and lungs (arrows).

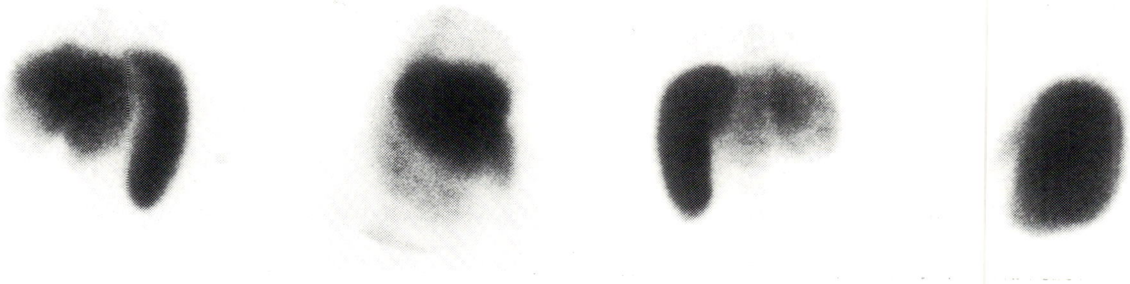

A ANT R LAT POST L LAT

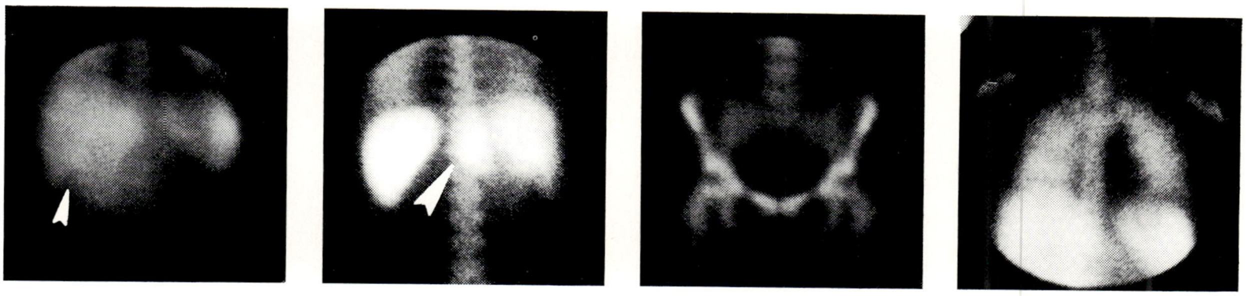

B ANT Abdomen POST Abdomen ANT Pelvis ANT Chest

**FIG. 68. HEPATIC VEIN THROMBOSIS (BUDD–CHIARI SYNDROME).** The imaging findings may be similar to those of cirrhosis. **A.** Although the liver is enlarged and tender, it appears smaller because of foreshortening by ascites. Other changes associated with ascites include the marked accentuation of the hepatic lobar separation and the displacement of the right lobe from the right abdominal wall. The reduced radioactivity in the right lobe is due in part to central necrosis of hepatic cells in this area. The marked congestive splenomegaly is usually seen with the more chronic form of the Budd–Chiari syndrome. **B.** The acute form is characterized clinically by hepatic failure with ascites. Accentuation of the lobar separation due to the ascitic fluid is easily identified (arrow). Areas of reduced activity in the liver are due to centrizonal necrosis. Since the venous drainage from the caudate lobe enters the inferior vena cava separately (rather than entering the hepatic veins involved with thrombosis), there is relatively increased activity in the caudate lobe ( large arrow ) when compared to the rest of the liver, where venous drainage is into the thrombosed hepatic veins. The caudate lobe is easily demonstrated in both the anterior and posterior positions. With the resulting increased portal pressure, there is massive shunting to the systemic veins with phagocytosis by RES cells in the bone marrow and even by the alveolar lining cells, which may become phagocytic. The latter phenomenon is responsible for the pulmonary visualization. Note the extent to which the vertebral and pelvic bone marrow are demonstrated.

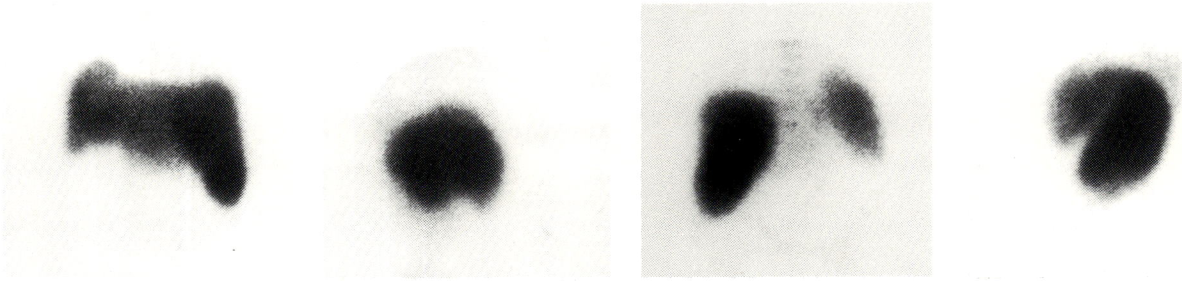

ANT R LAT POST L LAT

**FIG. 69. CHANGES SECONDARY TO CONGESTIVE HEART FAILURE WITH EARLY CARDIAC CIRRHOSIS.** This ultimately results in increased portal pressure and the ensuing imaging changes associated with hepatic fibrosis, shunting to the systemic veins, and congestive splenomegaly. The enlarged liver shows radioactive mottling. The uptake in the bone marrow is not so prominent as is customarily seen with Laennec's cirrhosis. The congested spleen is usually palpable and enlarged, as in this case.

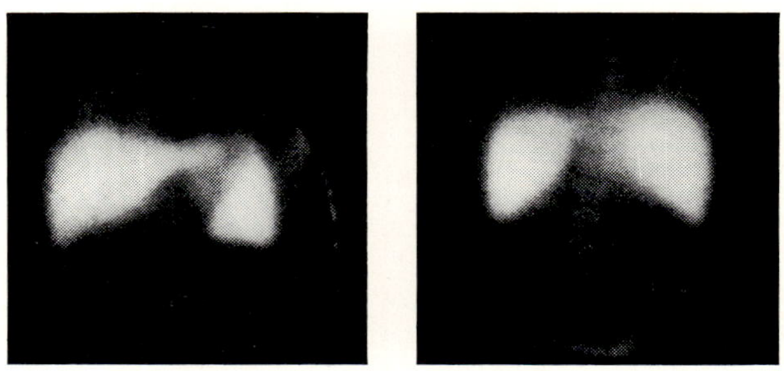

A ANT POST

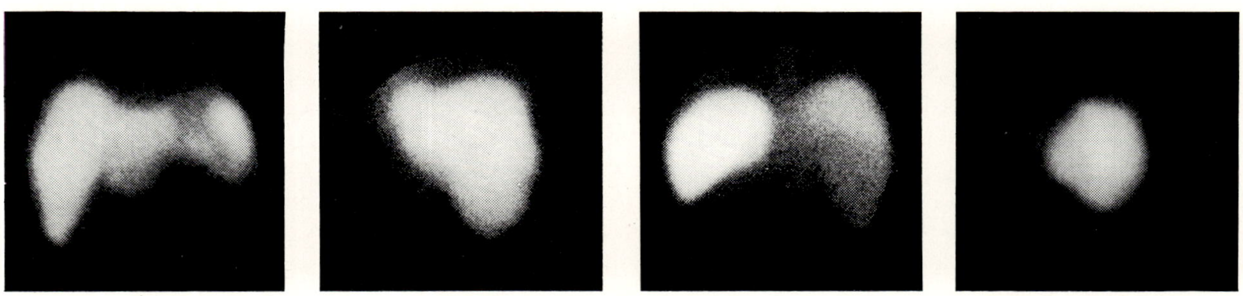

B ANT R LAT POST L LAT

**FIG. 70. VIRAL HEPATITIS.** Hepatic imaging may be normal in acute viral hepatitis; this is but a manifestation of the integrity of the Kupffer cells. With progression, fibrosis and replacement of Kupffer cells, and congestive splenomegaly, imaging may show evidence of splenic enlargement and uptake of Tc-99m SC elsewhere in the RES, as in **A** and **B**. However, it should be emphasized that it is unusual for viral hepatitis to show abnormalities on liver–spleen imaging.

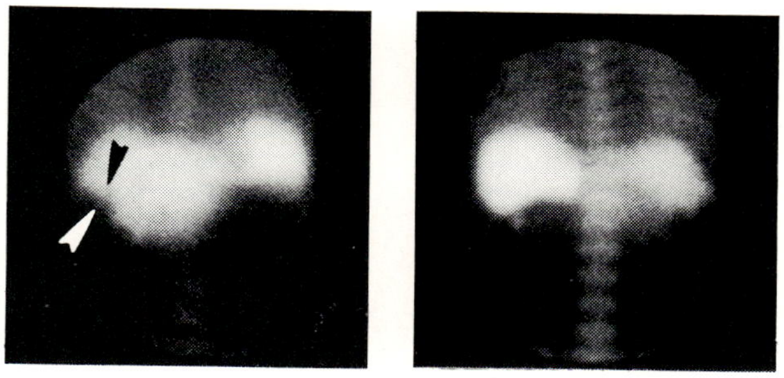


**FIG. 71.** BILIARY CIRRHOSIS. The imaging findings may be similar to those seen with Laennec's cirrhosis. There is destructive cholangitis in the liver, and among the characteristic pathological changes are focal accumulation of lymphocytes in the portal zones, associated with various degrees of bile duct damage and fibrotic replacement. In this patient with ascites, there is foreshortening of the hepatic image. Areas of absent radioactivity (arrows) due to granulomatous changes are seen, and the increased activity in the enlarged spleen is related to the increased portal pressure.

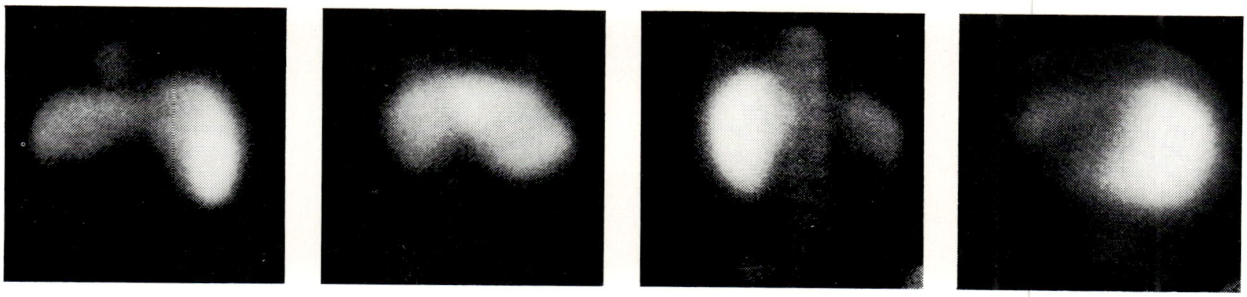


**FIG. 72.** HEMOCHROMATOSIS. As iron becomes deposited in the parenchymal cells of the liver, fibrotic changes occur. The pathological changes are similar to those of portal cirrhosis. Liver–spleen imaging reflects the fibrotic tissue replacement in the liver, the enlarged, congested spleen, and uptake of radiocolloid in the bone marrow. Note the similarity to Laennec's cirrhosis. When hemochromatosis is due to numerous blood transfusions, early deposition of iron occurs principally in the RES cells, and manifestations of liver involvement may not be striking; later, with iron deposition in hepatocytes and ensuing fibrotic changes, the imaging characteristics pictured above are similar for both idiopathic hemochromatosis and that due to multiple blood transfusions.

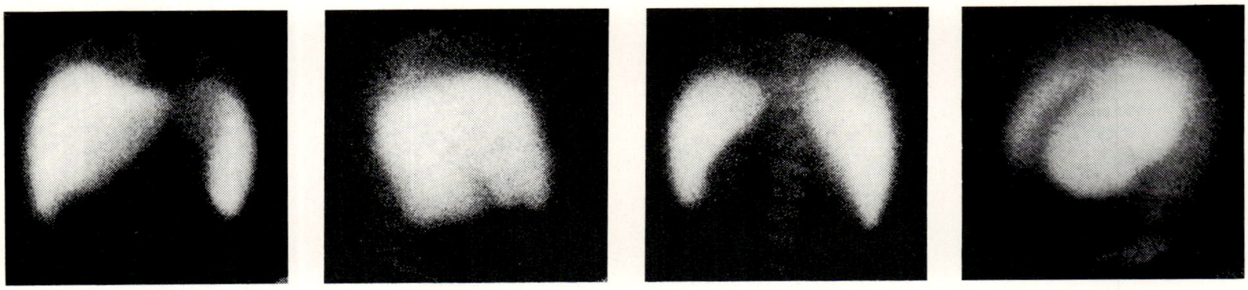

ANT R LAT POST L LAT

**FIG. 73.** **FATTY INFILTRATION IN HYPERLIPIDEMIA.** The imaging findings are similar to those seen with other diffuse liver disease. In this case there is extensive fatty infiltration in the liver associated with fibrotic changes. Visualization of the enlarged spleen and the bone marrow is related to the increased portal pressure.

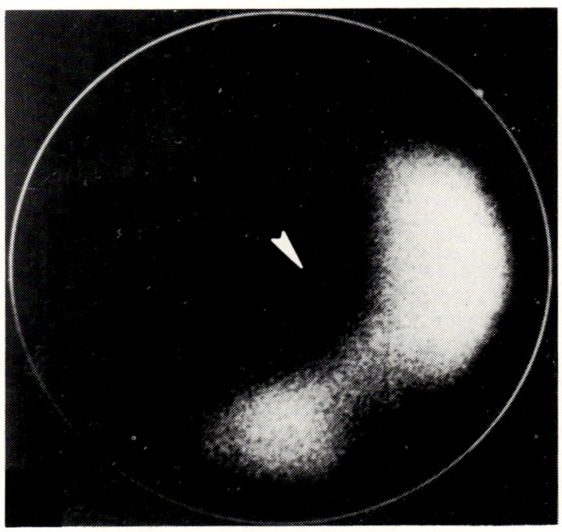

ANT

**FIG. 74.** **CONGENITAL CYST OF THE LIVER.** Such involvement can produce enormous cystic changes. However, unless there is sufficient clinical correlation, the etiology of the abnormality cannot be suggested by imaging alone (Tc-99m SC). (From Yeh SH: Clin Nucl Med 1:10, 1976)

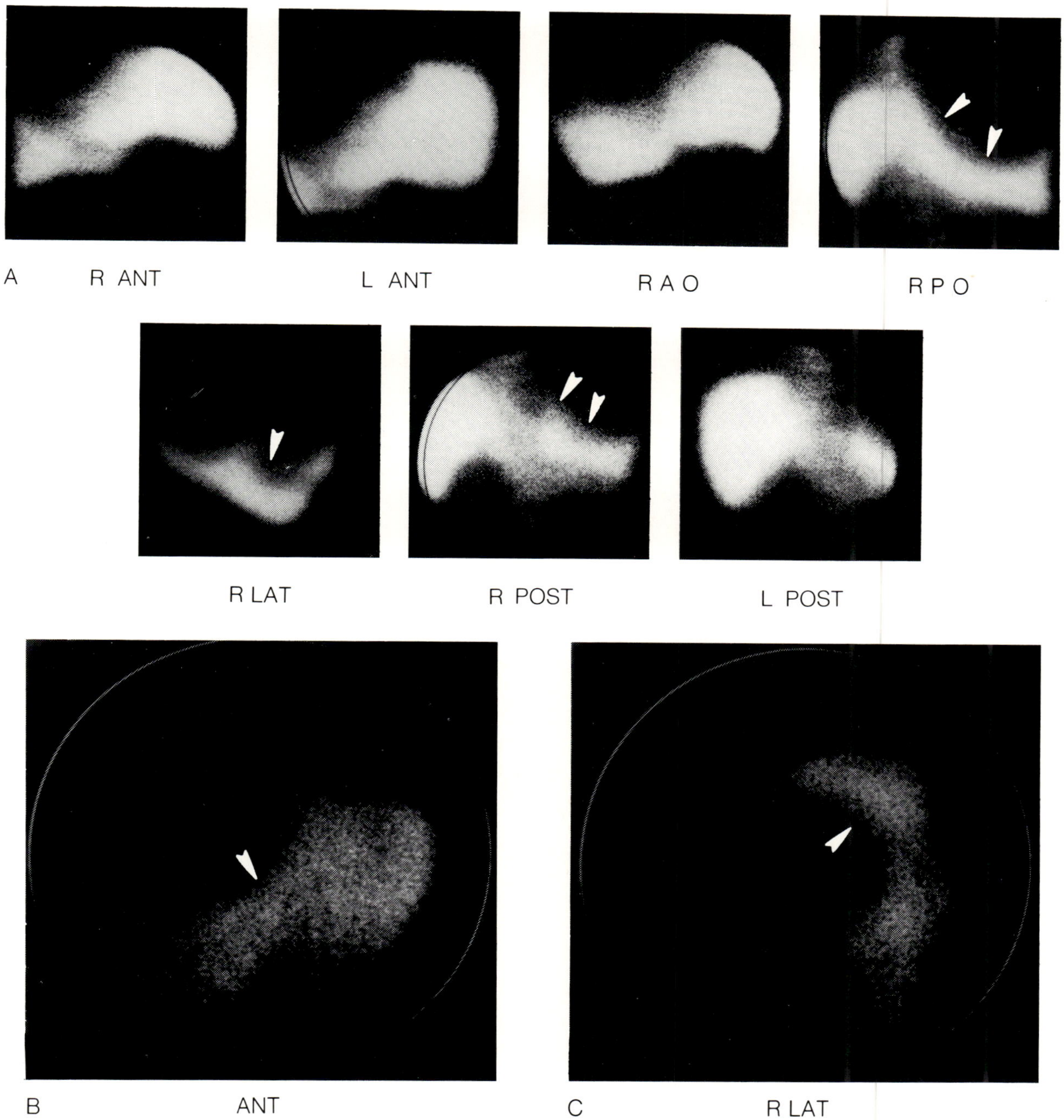


**FIG. 75. AMEBIC ABSCESS OF LIVER.** The imaging findings are identical to those seen with tumor. Although the surrounding hepatic tissue is often thin-walled, this feature is not in itself diagnostic. **A.** Amebic abscesses of the right lobe of the liver are associated with architectural distortion. The extensive involvement is seen in the anterior and right posterior oblique positions (arrows). The two large lesions (arrows) are delineated in the right lateral position. **B.** Large abscess (arrow) is visible in the anterior position. **C.** Right lateral image in another patient shows evidence of extensive hepatic tissue replacement (Tc-99m SC). (From Yeh SH: Clin Nucl Med 1:10, 1976)

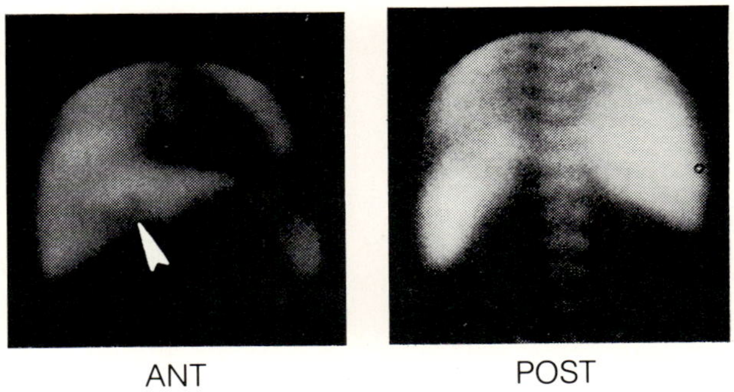


**FIG. 76.** HISTOPLASMOSIS. Involvement of the liver is readily identified at a site of infiltration (arrow). This disease characteristically involves the entire reticuloendothelial system. In addition to the delivery of radioactive colloid to the systemic circulation as a result of shunting in association with the increased portal pressure, there is also phagocytosis in the alveolar lining cells. This is seen with the presence of uniform radioactivity in the lungs.

## HEPATOBILIARY IMAGING

Tc-99m iminodiacetic acid (IDA) and related radionuclides are handled by the parenchymal cells of the liver in a manner similar to that of BSP. Following its intravenous administration, Tc-99m IDA is taken up and excreted by the hepatic parenchymal cells. Thus, the radionuclide may be employed for visualizing the major ducts in the biliary tree. The Tc-99m IDA becomes concentrated in the gallbladder, which is usually imaged about 2 hours following radionuclide injection. Evidence of obstruction in the biliary tree may be readily seen. In those situations in which function of the parenchymal cells of the liver is impaired, such as in hepatocellular disease, the clearing of the Tc-99m IDA is greatly reduced and the radionuclide is excreted through the kidneys. Renal images in such cases should not be confused with those of other structures in the hepatobiliary system. In those cases in which the total bilirubin is greater than 6 or 7 mg/dl, whatever the cause, there is insufficient uptake by the parenchymal cells to help determine whether or not the jaundice is associated with hepatocellular disease or mechanical obstruction somewhere in the biliary tree.

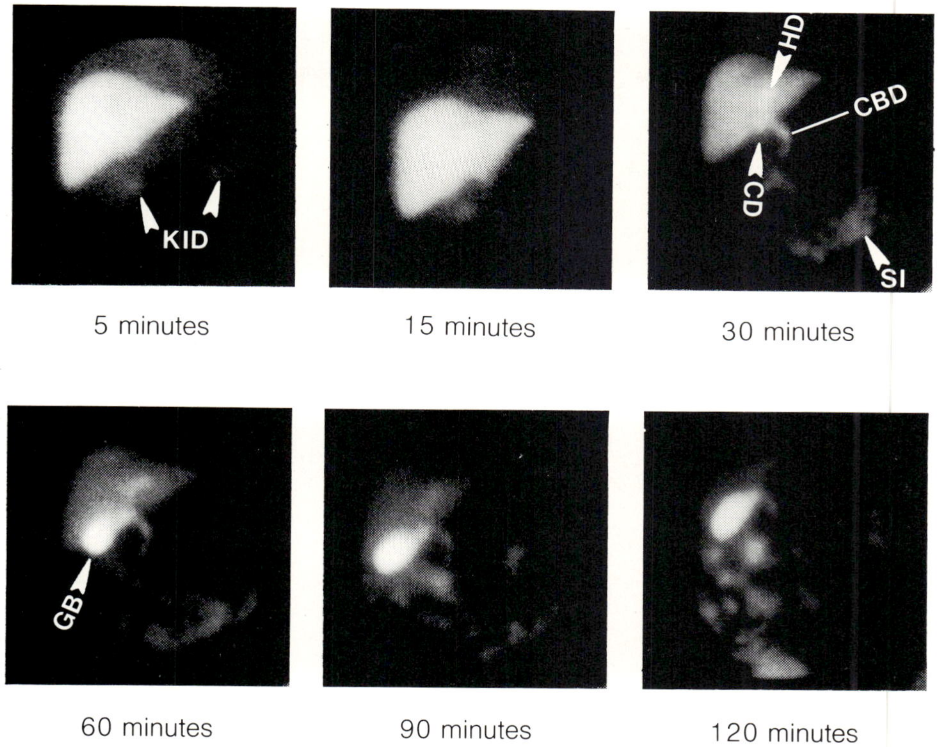


**FIG. 77. NORMAL HEPATOBILIARY AND GALLBLADDER IMAGING.** Imaging is started 5 minutes after the intravenous administration of 5 mCi of Tc-99m IDA, and the liver is clearly visualized. Note the renal (KID) visualization during early imaging. At 30 minutes, the common bile duct (CBD) is identified and radioactivity in the small intestine (SI) is detected. There may be visualization of the gallbladder at 30 minutes in some patients, but at 60 minutes, when most of the radioactive material has been excreted from the liver, the gallbladder (GB) itself is clearly visible. Note the cystic duct (CD) and hepatic duct (HD) and their union to form the common bile duct.

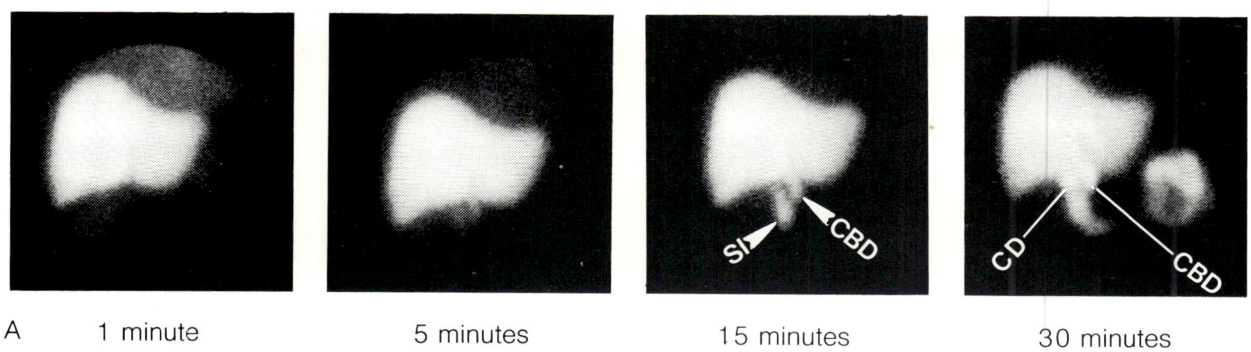


**FIG. 78 A. 1–4.** (See legend next on page 67)

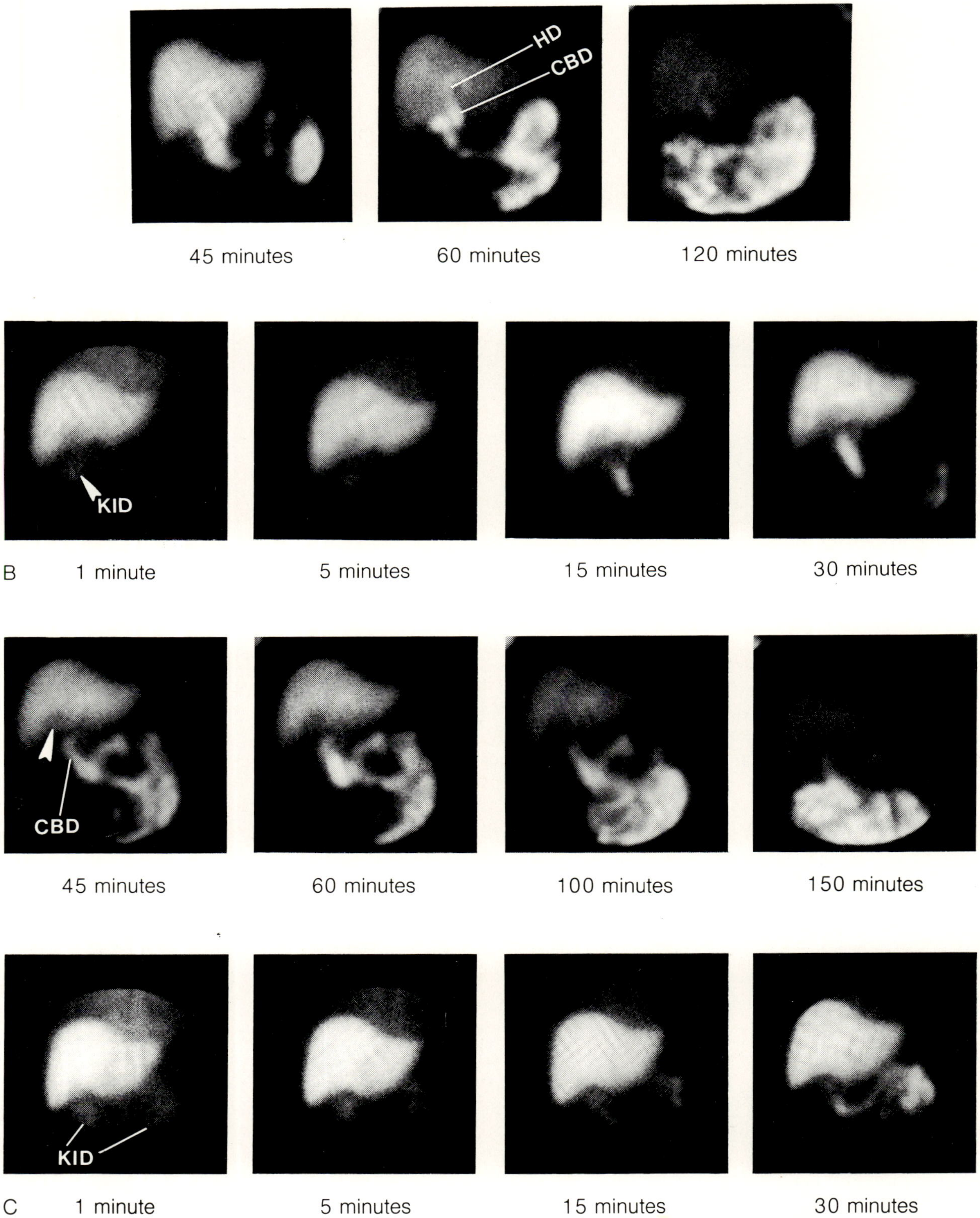


**FIG. 78. A.** 5–7, **B, C.**1–4 (See legend next page)

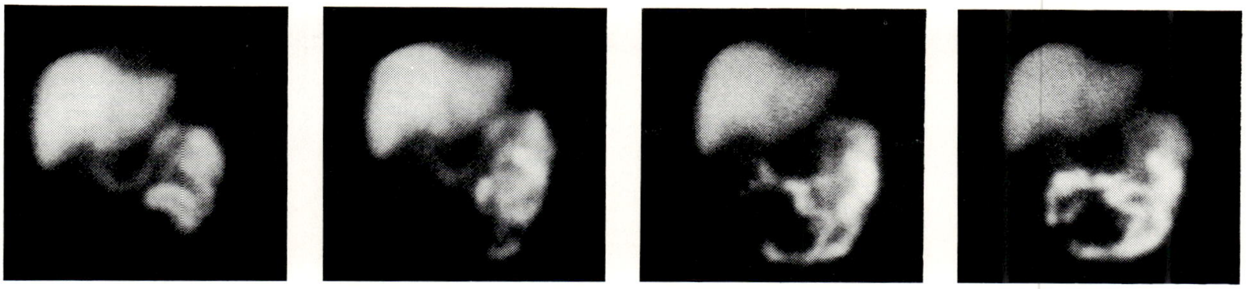

45 minutes | 60 minutes | 90 minutes | 120 minutes

**FIG. 78.** ACUTE CHOLECYSTITIS AND CHOLELITHIASIS. Serial imaging in each of three patients with cholecystitis and stones in the cystic duct results in failure to image the gallbladder because of obstructing cystic duct calculi. Although the inability to demonstrate the gallbladder is the common imaging finding in acute cholecystitis, the demonstration of other structures in the excretory apparatus of the liver (cystic duct, hepatic duct, and common bile duct) varies in these patients. **A.** Failure to visualize the gallbladder but sharp identification of other excretory ducts. Serial imaging shows early visualization of the distal portion of the hepatic duct (HD) and the common bile duct (CBD). At 30 minutes there is excellent visualization of the intrahepatic portion of the hepatic duct. At 30 minutes there is also identification of the distal cystic duct (CD); more proximal cystic duct visualization is prevented by a calculus at that site. The obstructing stone also prevents visualization of the gallbladder. Continued serial imaging shows gradual loss of radioactivity from the liver with progressive intestinal accumulation. **B.** Inability to visualize the gallbladder in another patient with cholecystitis. Early imaging shows renal (KID) activity. Thereafter, serial imaging up to 2.5 hours shows no evidence of gallbladder radioactivity. The gallbladder fossa (arrow) is seen as an area of reduced activity, inferiorly. **C.** Serial imaging shows failure of gallbladder visualization along with good excretion of Tc-99m IDA into the intestinal tract.

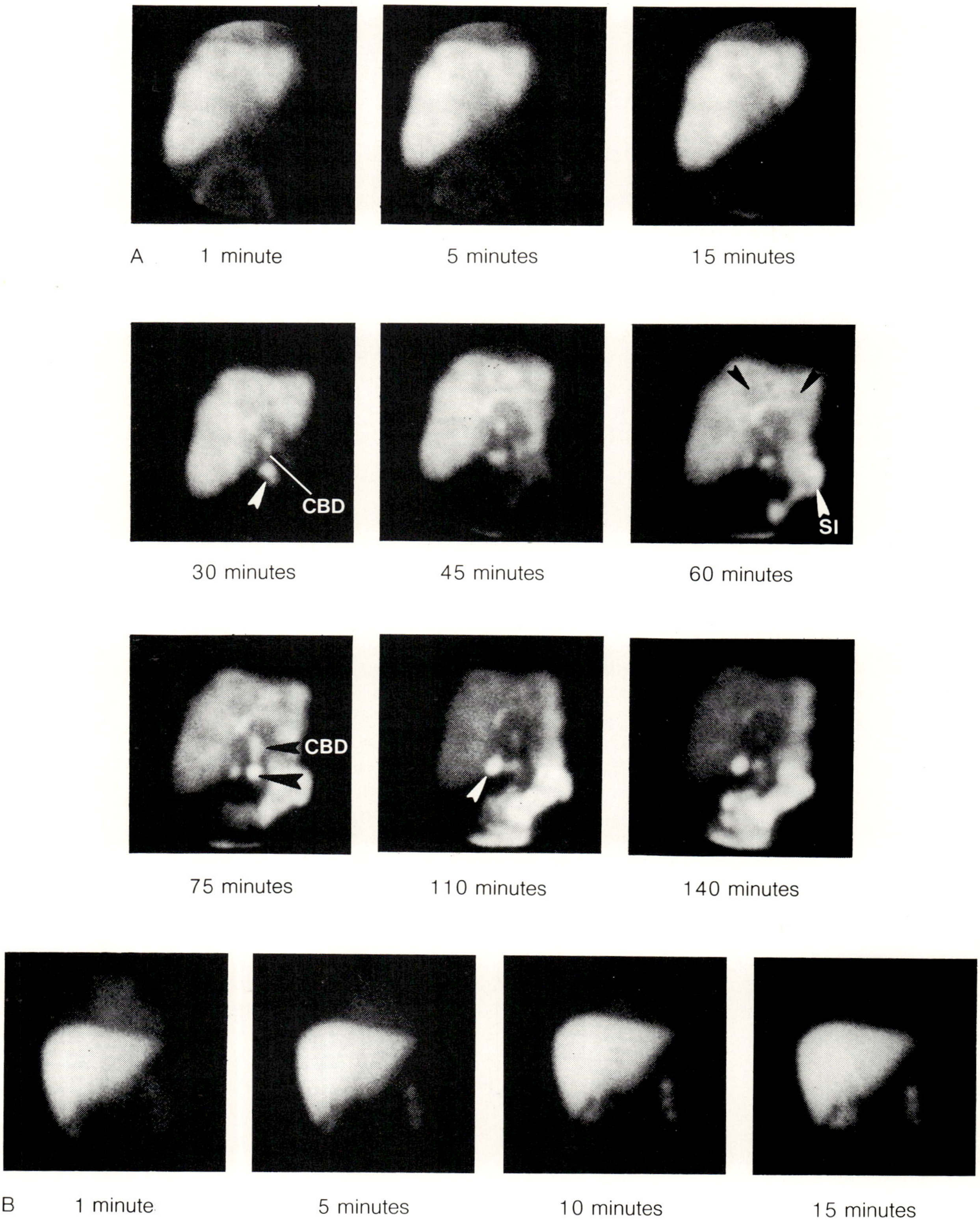


**FIG. 79. A, B. 1–4.** (See legend next page)

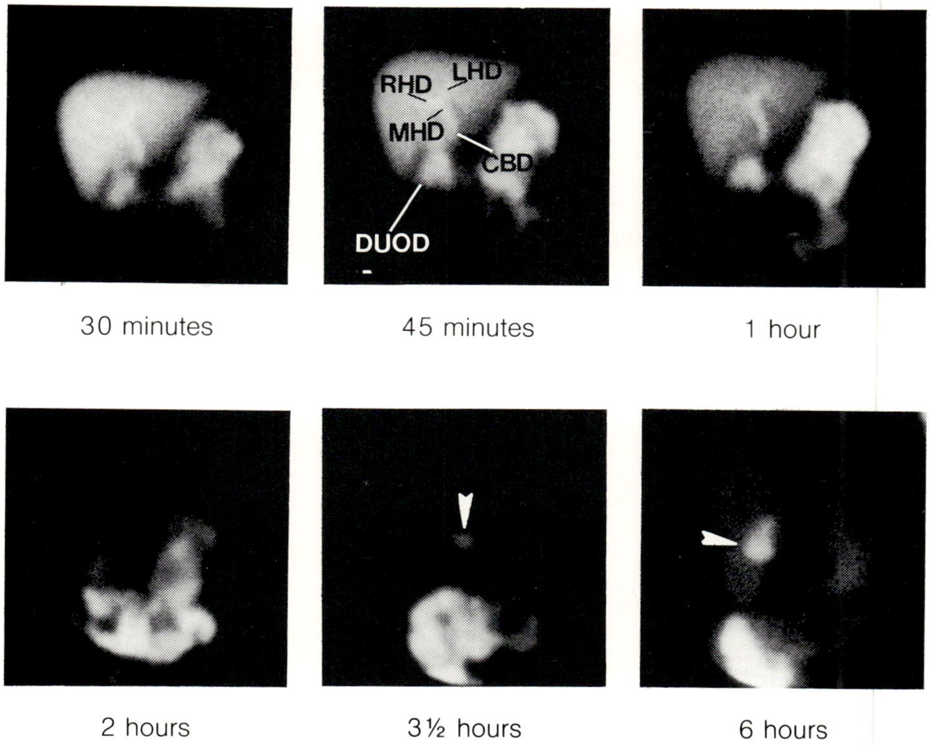


**FIG. 79.** GALLBLADDER AND BILIARY TRACT DISEASE. A. **Acute Cholecystitis and Partial Common Bile Duct Obstruction Due to Tumor.** In this patient with acute cholecystitis, who also has carcinoma of the colon and extensive hepatic metastases, there is failure to image the gallbladder on serial imaging. The latter is associated with cystic duct calculi. Multiple, rounded areas of absent radioactivity (arrows) in the liver indicate the metastases. The common bile duct (CBD) is identified at 30 minutes. At that time, incomplete obstruction of the distal common bile duct due to metastatic tumor to the region of the ampulla of Vater is seen. This is demonstrated by the accumulation of excreted radioactive material ( large arrow) at the site of the partially obstructing lesion. That the obstruction is incomplete is seen by the entry of the Tc-99m IDA into the small intestine (SI). **B. Chronic Cholecystitis.** This is characterized by very late visualization of the gallbladder. In this case, the gallbladder (arrow) may be seen at 3.5 hours but is not nearly so well defined as on the 6-hour image. Other structures demonstrated during the earlier portions of the study are the right hepatic duct (RHD), left hepatic duct (LHD), main hepatic duct (MHD), and common bile duct (CBD). The entry of radionuclide into the duodenum (DUOD) should not be confused with that of the gallbladder image.

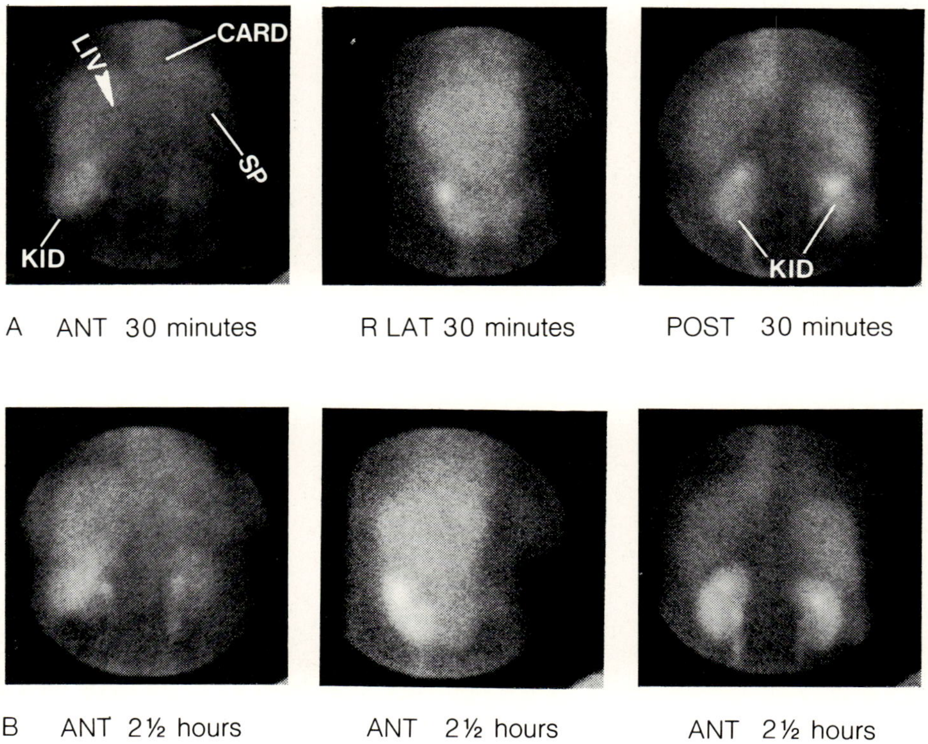


**FIG. 80.** Tc-99m IDA IMAGING IN HEPATOCELLULAR DISEASE. There is reduced clearing of the radioactive material from the blood resulting in high blood radioactivity in this patient with hepatitis. **A.** Imaging at 30 minutes discloses a poorly defined hepatic image (LIV). Renal images (KID) are identified in all three positions. The visualization of the spleen (SP) is purely a vascular phenomenon associated with elevated blood radioactivity; the cardiac blood pool (CARD) is also identified. **B.** Imaging at 2.5 hours discloses similar findings and on even more elegant renal image.

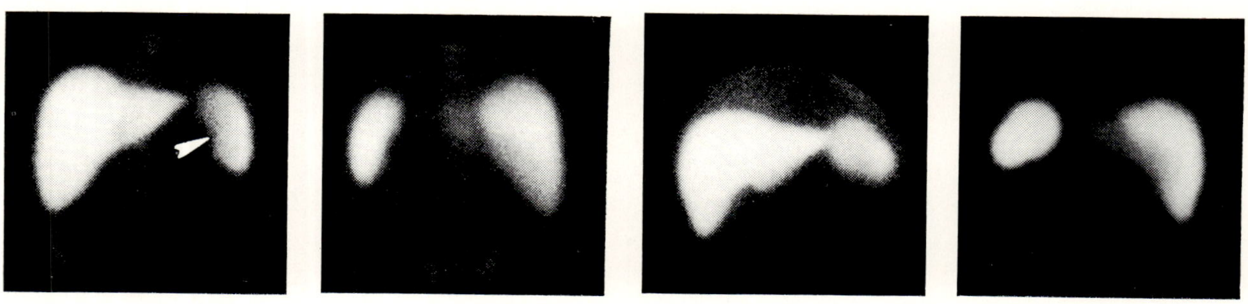

A ANT POST B ANT POST

**FIG. 81. A, B.** (See legend next page)

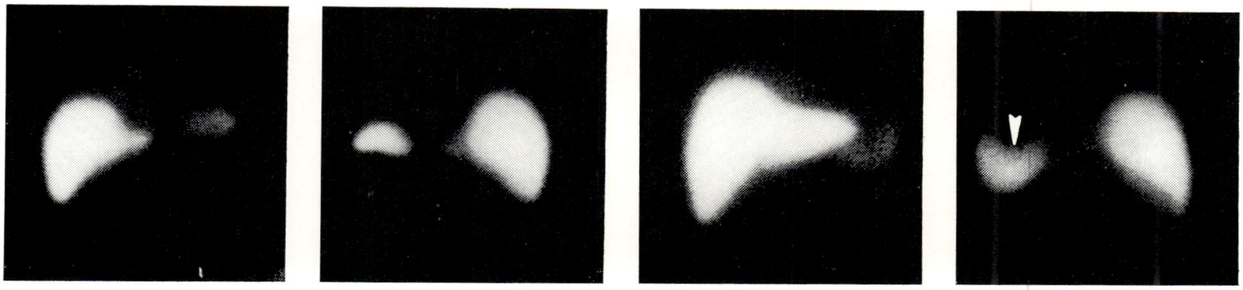

C ANT POST D ANT POST

## SPLENIC IMAGING

**FIG. 81.** SPLENIC ORIENTATION. The longitudinal axis of the spleen may be easily determined from inspection. **A, B.** The usual diagonal position of the longitudinal axis in two different patients is seen in the anterior and posterior positions. The medial location of the splenic hilus is identified by the arrow. **C.** Horizontal orientation of spleen. **D.** Upside-down spleen. The hilus (arrow) is situated on the superior surface of the spleen, and the hilar vessels have an anomalous position. This configuration should not be confused with changes secondary to trauma.

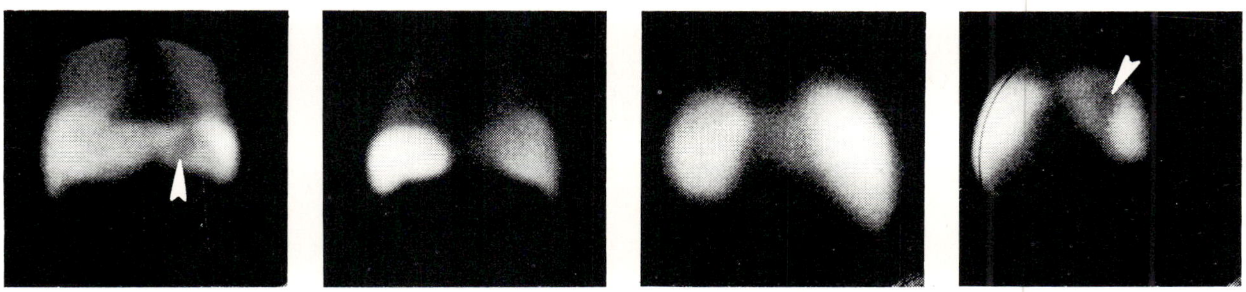

A ANT POST B L A O POST

**FIG. 82.** REDUCED ACTIVITY AT HILUS OF SPLEEN. Because of the fossal-like depression usually associated with the hilum, the imaging appearance may suggest a focal area of absent radioactivity. This is dependent, in part, on splenic position and the distance from the collimator. **A.** In the anterior position, the hilar area is seen as the region of reduced radioactivity (arrow). This spleen has a *somewhat* horizontal orientation and the lower pole has a relative anterior position; hence its relatively increased radioactivity. As the posterior portion of the spleen is visualized in the posterior position, the reduced radioactivity associated with the hilum is not seen. **B.** This spleen has the more common location with the longitudinal axis diagonal. The hilum is identified (arrow) in the POST position. Because of its relative anterior position, the lower pole shows increased activity.

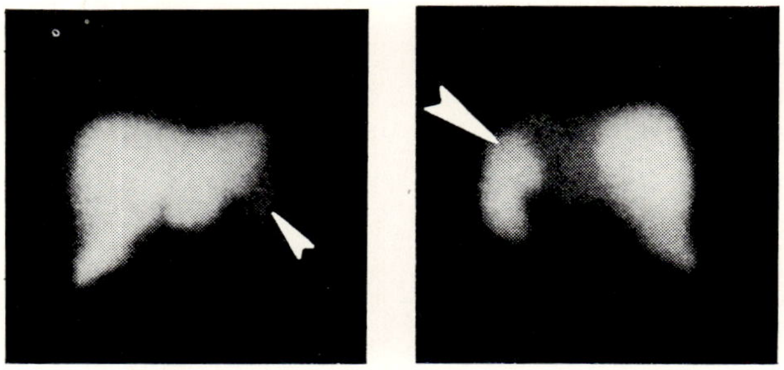

ANT POST

**FIG. 83. PROXIMITY OF LEFT LOBE OF LIVER AND SPLEEN.** A contiguous left hepatic lobe and spleen may be mistakenly interpreted as splenomegaly. Imaging in LAO and LPO positions may be necessary to image a zone of separation between liver and spleen. The relative posterior location of the spleen (arrow) is visible in the anterior position. With imaging in the posterior position, there may be difficulty in identifying the area of separation between the left lobe and spleen ( large arrow).

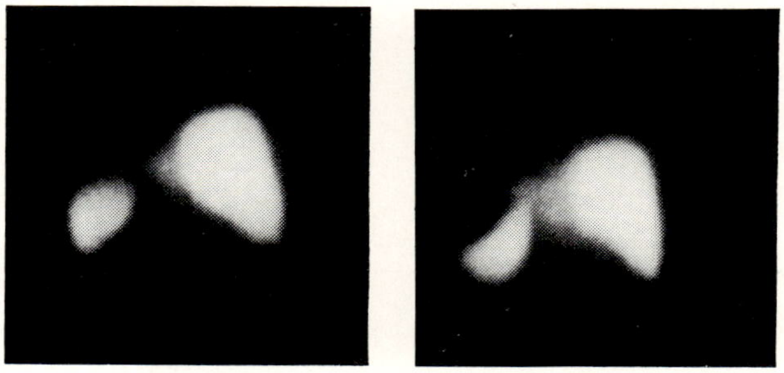

A POST Prone B POST Supine

**FIG. 84. CHANGES IN SPLENIC IMAGING RELATED TO PATIENT POSITION. A.** Study performed in the posterior position with the patient supine indicates no unusual imaging characteristics. **B.** Imaging with the patient prone results in relative medial and inferior displacement of the spleen associated with abdominal compression.

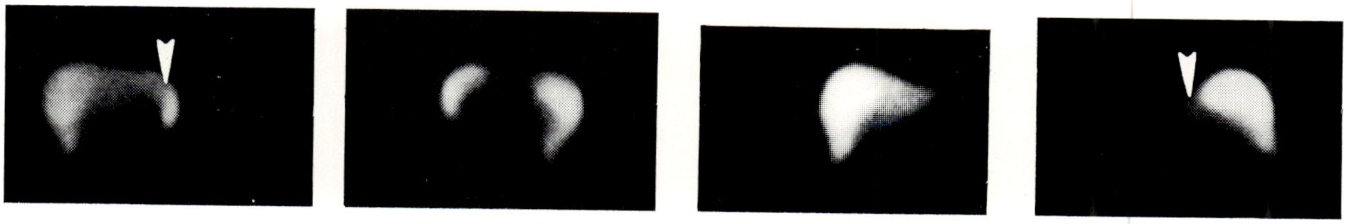

A Preoperative ANT — Preoperative POST — Postoperative ANT — Postoperative POST

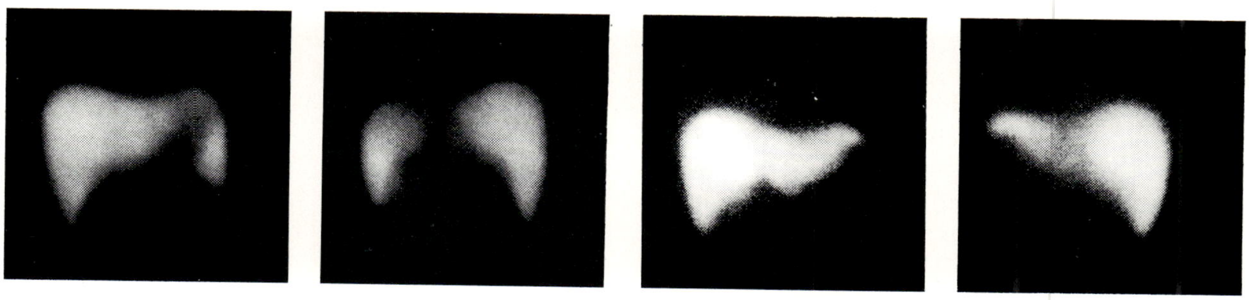

B Preoperative ANT — Preoperative POST — Postoperative ANT — Postoperative POST

**FIG. 85. CHANGES FOLLOWING SPLENECTOMY.** Following surgical removal of the spleen, alterations in hepatic configuration in the region of the left lobe are common. There is usually extension of the left lobe to the region formerly occupied by the spleen, and portions of the liver not previously seen with clarity on imaging may now be identified. **A.** Preoperative imaging in patient with Hodgkin's disease. The extension of the left lobe (arrow) is clearly visible in the anterior position, but its identification in the posterior position can be made only with difficulty. Postoperative imaging after splenectomy shows the extension to the left upper quadrant of the left lobe. Note the extension of the left lobe (arrow) that is now visible in the posterior position. Care must be exercised not to confuse this portion of the liver with what might be thought to be an accessory spleen. **B.** Following removal of the enlarged spleen in this patient with Hodgkin's disease, portions of the left lobe that were not clearly appreciated prior to surgery can be identified.

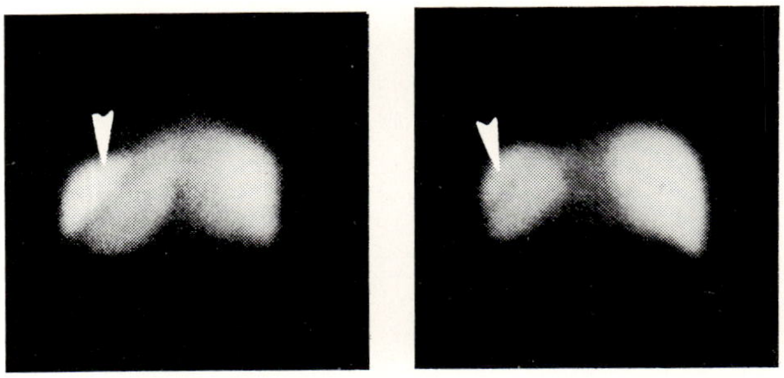

POST LPO

**FIG. 86. ACCESSORY SPLEEN.** It is usually difficult to identify an accessory spleen (or spleens) with Tc-99m SC. Oblique positions may be helpful in demonstrating such accessory organs and in distinguishing them from the left lobe of the liver and from the spleen itself. The accessory spleen extends posteriorly. The posterior image identifies the accessory spleen as the somewhat semilunar area of increased radioactivity (arrow) just lateral to the spleen. In the LPO position, the definition of the accessory spleen improves greatly (arrow), and its borders are well delineated.

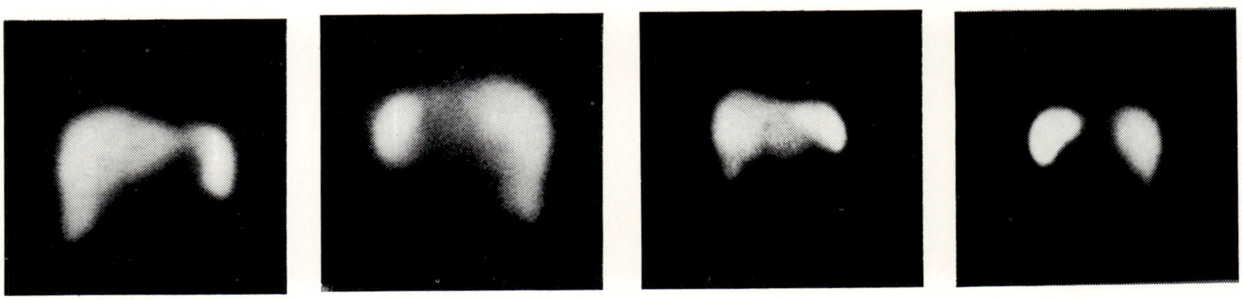

A ANT POST B ANT POST

**FIG. 87. INCREASED RADIOACTIVITY IN THE SPLEEN, AS COMPARED TO THAT IN THE LIVER.** This observation has been made in patients with lymphoma, malignant melanoma, and other neoplasms in the absence of known hepatic or splenic involvement or enlargement of either organ. It may be due to increased phagocytosis by the splenic macrophages. **A.** Increased radioactivity in the spleen compared to that in the liver in a patient with malignant melanoma. **B.** Increased splenic radioactivity in a patient with Hodgkin's disease.

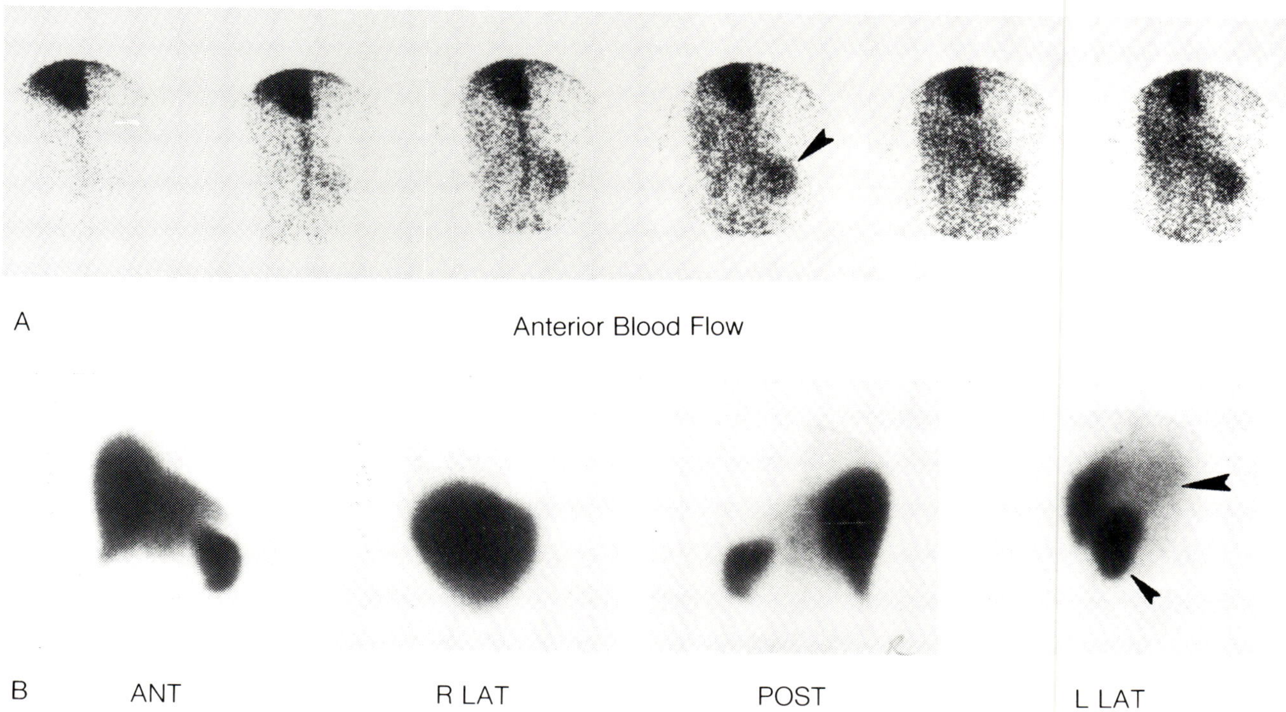


**FIG. 88. DISPLACEMENT OF SPLEEN.** There has been marked anterior and inferior displacement of the spleen by a retroperitoneal sarcoma. **A.** In the blood flow study, the spleen is identified (arrow) in an unusual inferior position. **B.** Note the relationship of the liver to the downward displaced spleen in the anterior position. Its forward displacement is indicated in the anterior position, as it appears to overlie the left hepatic lobe. In the left lateral position, the anterior location of the spleen (arrow) is visualized. Its usual position is identified by the large arrow.

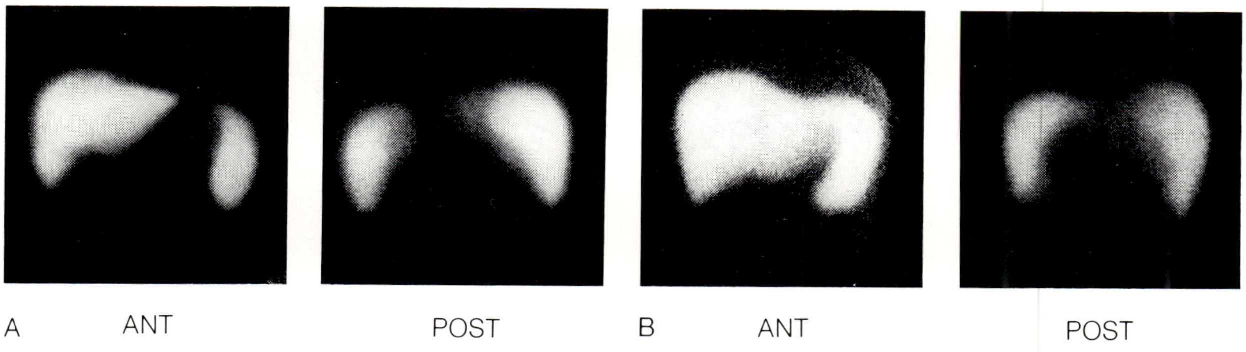


**FIG. 89. LYMPHOMA.** Various degrees of splenomegaly are common in lymphomas, sometimes in the absence of involvement of either the liver or spleen (see Fig. 68). There is often increased activity in the spleen compared to that in the liver, even when neither organ is enlarged. **A.** Enlarged spleen and a normal sized liver. **B.** Enlarged spleen shows relatively increased radioactivity because of its increased mass.

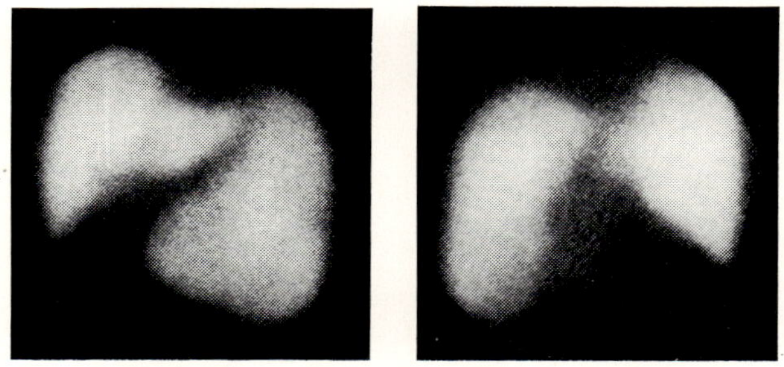

ANT POST

**FIG. 90. MALIGNANT LYMPHOMA.** Extensive involvement of the spleen caused by a poorly differentiated lymphocytic lymphoma has resulted in an enormous spleen. Its somewhat triangular shape in the anterior position is related, in part, to the position of the splenic hilus, which is situated in the center of the image. Markers indicated the unusual length in the posterior position to be 26 cm. The liver is of normal size, and there is no evidence of involvement in that organ.

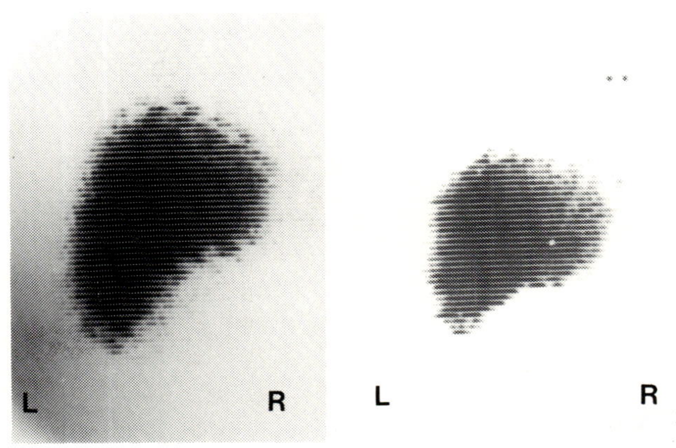


A ANT B POST

**FIG. 91. ACUTE MYELOGENOUS LEUKEMIA.** Massive splenomegaly seen on posterior scans before (**A**) and after (**B**) chemotherapy.

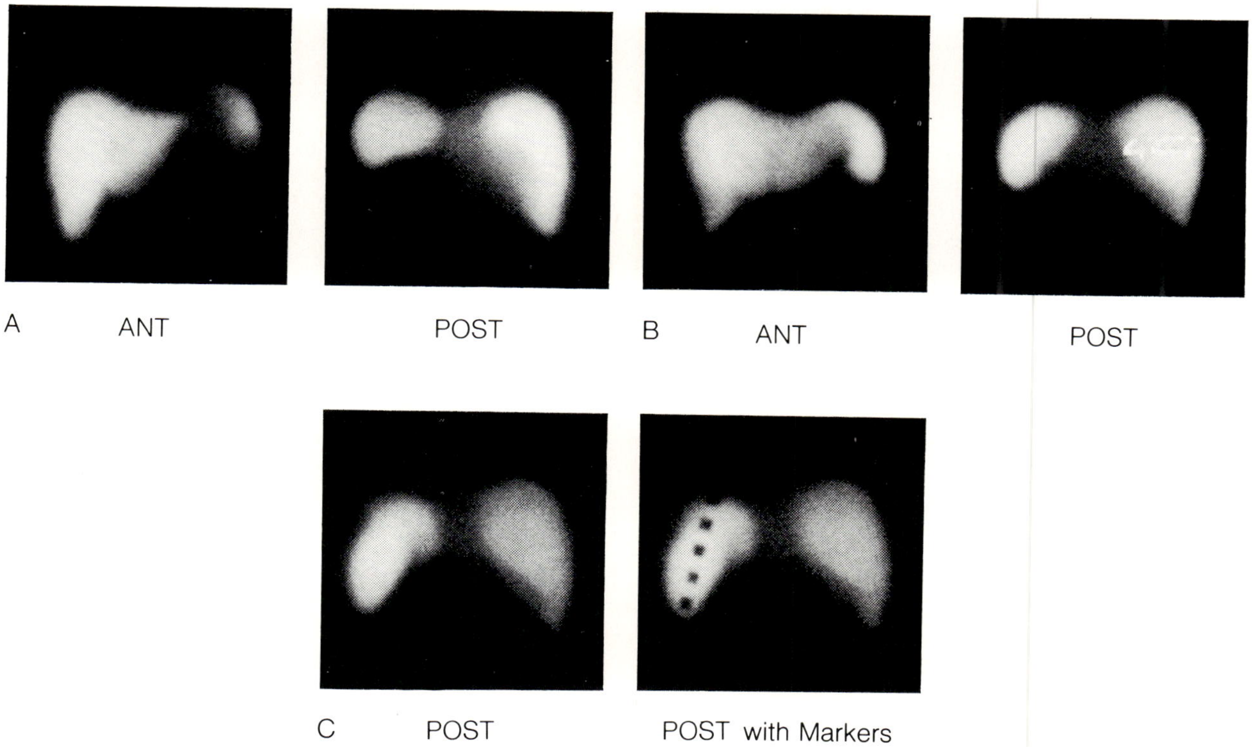


**FIG. 92.** CHRONIC MYELOGENOUS LEUKEMIA. Splenic enlargement usually occurs in association with infiltration of abnormal leukocytes and because of extramedullary hematopoiesis. **A.** Normal-sized spleen in patient under treatment for chronic myelogenous leukemia. **B.** Slightly enlarged spleen. **C.** Splenomegaly in patient with promyelocytic leukemia.

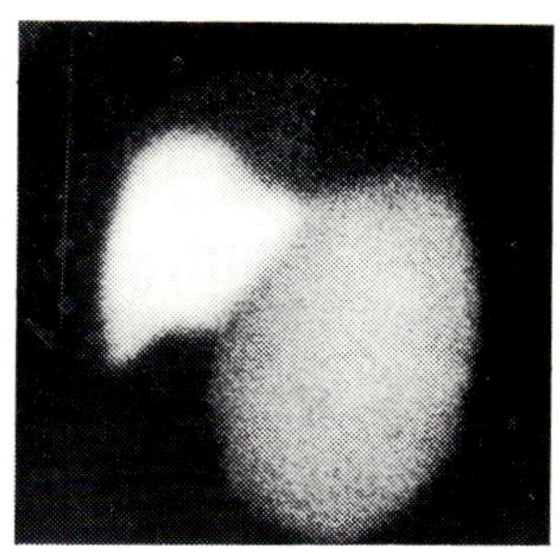


**FIG. 93.** LEUKEMIC RETICULOENDOTHELIOSIS (HAIRY CELL LEUKEMIA). There has been extensive infiltration in the spleen of atypical lymphocytes, and this has resulted in massive splenic enlargement. The splenic image is most clearly delineated in the anterior position. The uniform involvement of the spleen and its relative reduction in radioactivity throughout is characteristic of a diffuse infiltrative process; this is in contrast to increased splenic radioactivity and size seen with congestive splenomegaly.

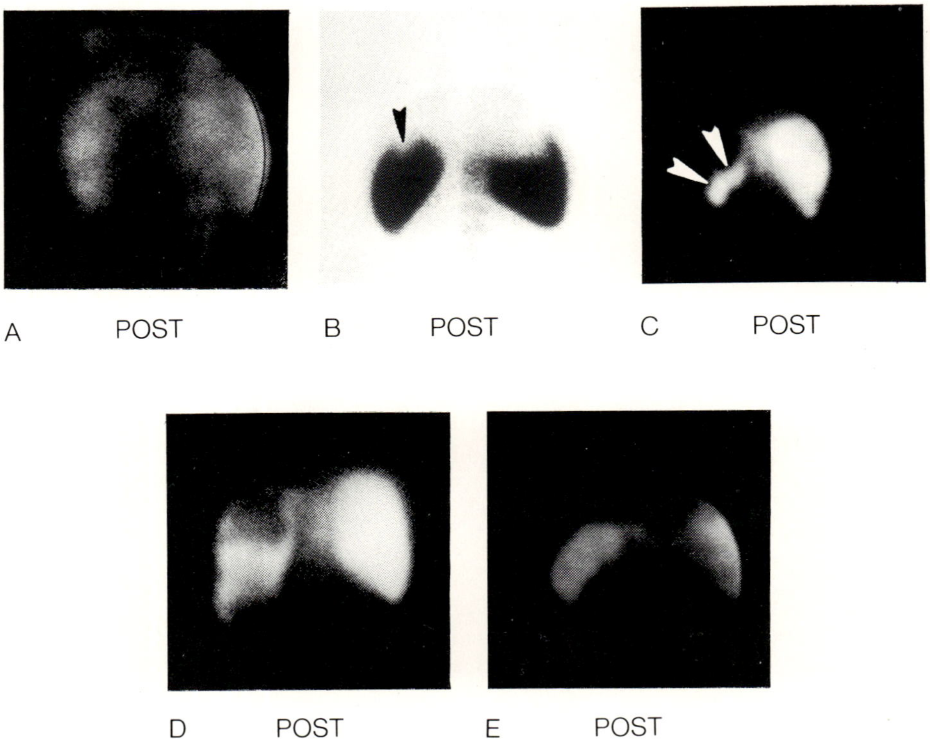


**FIG. 94. METASTASES TO SPLEEN.** Metastatic carcinoma involving the spleen is unusual. Aside from lymphomas, involvement of the spleen with tumor is rare. However, if a splenic metastasis is present, the diagnostic possibilities should include malignant melanoma as the primary site. **A.** Irregular and rounded areas of absent radioactivity are due to metastases from a malignant melanoma. The defects have no characteristic or regular appearance. **B.** Solitary area of absent radioactivity at upper pole of spleen is due to metastasis from a malignant melanoma. The site of involvement is most sharply delineated in the posterior position. **C.** In another patient with malignant melanoma, distinct, rounded areas of absent radioactivity in the spleen (arrows) are due to metastases. **D.** Extensive metastases in enlarged spleen from a malignant melanoma. **E.** Multiple, small focal areas of absent radioactivity due to metastatic foci from oat cell carcinoma of lung.

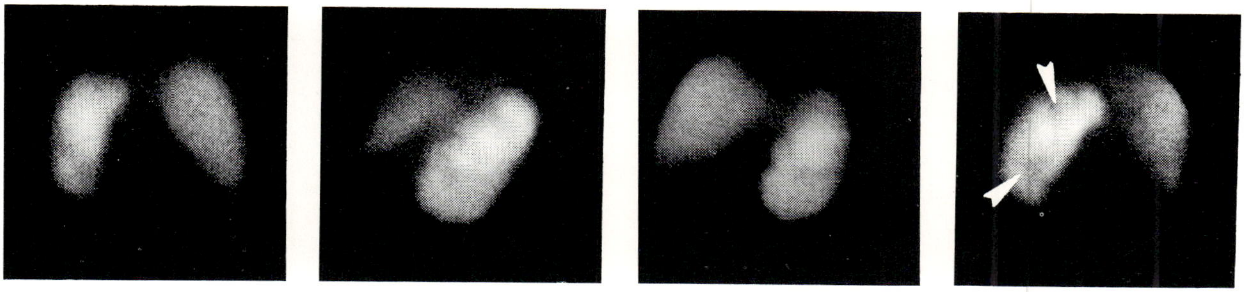

POST L LAT L A O L P O

**FIG. 95.** SPLENIC INFARCTION. One or more areas of absent radioactivity characterize vascular occlusion and resulting infarction of the spleen. In the patient with severe left upper quadrant pain and in whom splenic imaging shows one or more wedge-shaped areas of absent radioactivity, splenic infarction is a likely diagnosis.

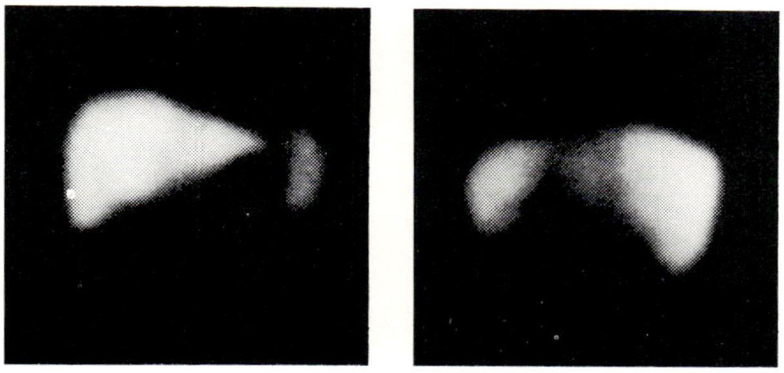

ANT POST

**FIG. 96.** POLYCYTHEMIA VERA. Although the spleen may show varying degrees of enlargement, splenic size is normal in this patient. The small, irregular areas of reduced radioactivity in the spleen are due to infarcts, thromboses, and sites of extramedullary hematopoiesis.

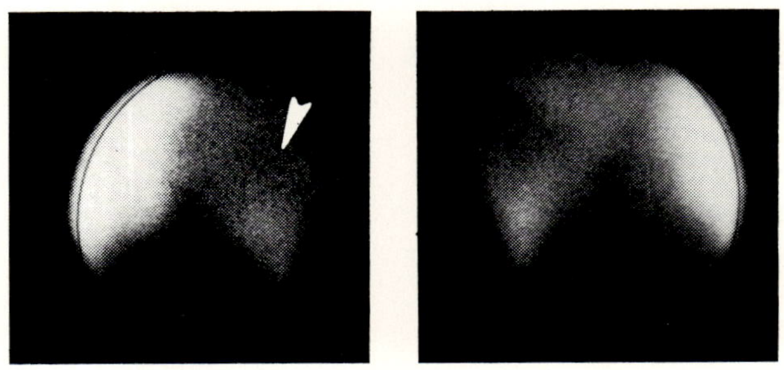

A ANT Liver POST Liver

Posttrauma

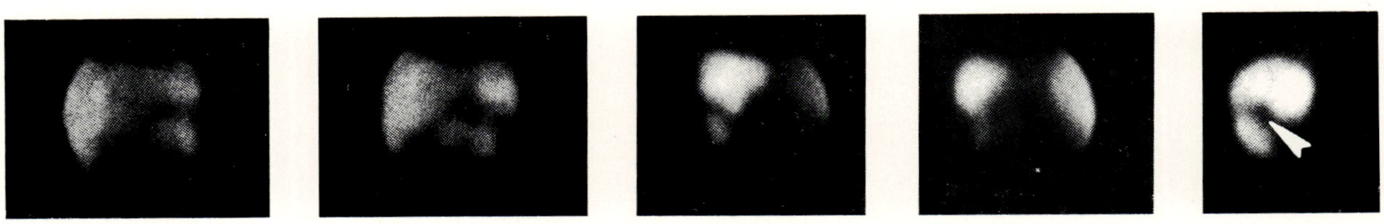

B ANT L A O L P O POST L LAT

Posttrauma

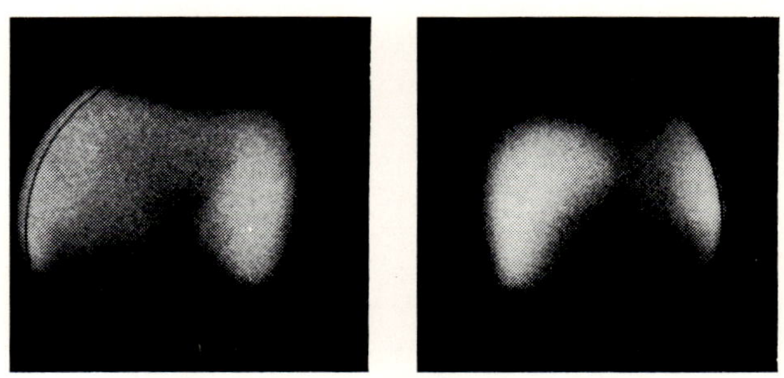

ANT POST

Pretrauma

**FIG. 97. A, B.** (See legend next page)

**FIG. 97. SPLENIC TRAUMA.** Following trauma or spontaneous rupture, a splenic hematoma can usually be identified as a focal area of absent radioactivity. Old, organized hematomas may result in imaging changes similar to the findings of more recent episodes. In the absence of an underlying disease that might involve the spleen, a site of absent radioactivity in the spleen in a patient exposed to abdominal trauma should be considered evidence of splenic hematoma or laceration until proven otherwise. **A.** Large area of absent radioactivity from a splenic laceration due to a crushing injury. The site of the hematoma (arrow) is more clearly visible in the anterior position. It is useful to image the patient in the left lateral, LPO, and LAO positions as well as in the anterior and posterior positions. In this case, the study had to be shortened because of the patient's condition. **B.** Splenic hematoma 2 weeks after automobile accident. There is a large hematoma involving the inferior half of the spleen. Its full extent is best appreciated in the posterior and LPO positions. Note the absent activity (arrow) in the left lateral position. Compare to the pretrauma images.

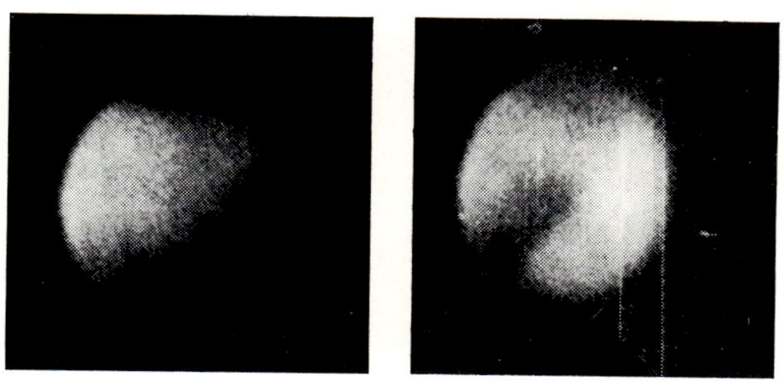

A ANT B ANT

**FIG. 98. FUNCTIONAL ASPLENIA.** During a sickle cell crisis, the increased blood viscosity results in markedly reduced perfusion to the spleen and failure to deliver the radioactive colloid to the organ. This in turn results in absent visualization of the organ at the time of crisis. Such a situation has been termed functional asplenia. It has been described for both hemoglobin SS and SC disease. With the resolution of the crisis, reduction in blood viscosity, and increased perfusion to the spleen, the organ may again be visualized. **A.** Absent radioactivity in the region of the spleen in a patient with splenomegaly and hemoglobin SC disease during a sickle cell crisis. This is functional asplenia. **B.** Visualization of enlarged spleen after resolution of sickle cell crisis, 3 days after initial study. (From Joshpe GP, Rothenberg SP, Baum S: Am J Med, 5:20, 1973)

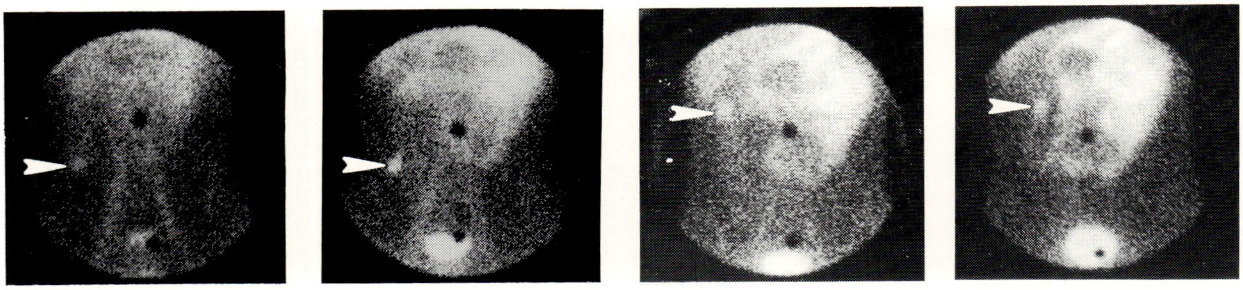

A ANT 5 minutes ANT 30 minutes ANT 60 minutes ANT 2 hours

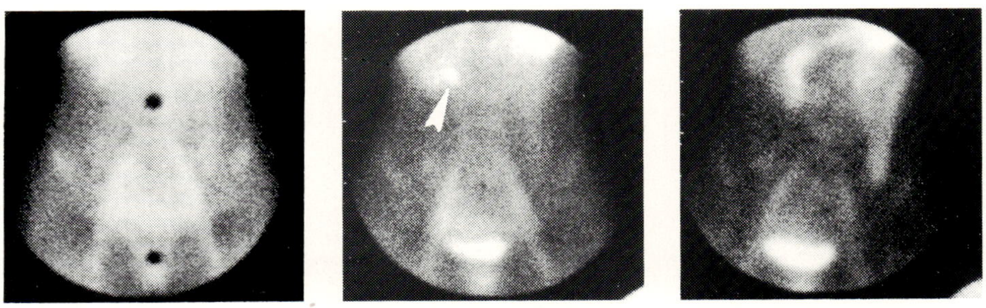

B ANT Immediate ANT 10 minutes ANT 40 minutes

## MECKEL'S IMAGING

**FIG. 99. IMAGING OF SECRETORY GASTRIC MUCOSA IN MECKEL'S DIVERTICULUM OF THE ILEUM.** The stomach may be imaged following the administration of Tc-99m sodium pertechnetate as the radionuclide is secreted in the gastric mucosa. Similarly, if ectopic gastric mucosa is present in a Meckel's diverticulum, imaging is possible because of the secretion of pertechnetate in the ectopic gastric mucosa. **A.** Identification of site of secretory gastric mucosa in a Meckel's diverticulum (arrow) sequentially over a period of 2 hours. Imaging appears best at 2 hours. The markers are on the umbilicus and pubis. Radionuclide identification was potentiated in this case by cimetidine, a potent $H_2$-receptor antagonist. Note the persistence of the abnormality. **B.** Normal study. Since the radionuclide is excreted in part by the kidneys, care must be exercised not to confuse increased activity in a renal pelvis, as in this case (arrow), with possible accumulation in ectopic gastric mucosa. The localization is transitory and is not seen after 10 minutes.

## Suggested Reading

Dyrbye M: Clinical evaluation of hepatic scintigraphy. Act Med Scand (Suppl) (624):88–92, 1979

Echevarria RA, Bonanno C: Value of routine abdominal nuclide angiography as part of liver scan. Clin Nucl Med 4:66–78, 1979

Fischer KC, Eraklis A, Rossello P, et al: Scintigraphy in follow-up of pediatric splenic trauma treated without surgery. J Nucl Med 19:3–9, 1978

Fonesca C, Rosenthall L, Greenberg D, et al: Differential diagnosis of jaundice by $^{99m}$Tc-IDA hepatobiliary imaging. Clin Nucl Med 4:135–142, 1979

Gold RP, Johnson PM: Efficacy of combined liver-lung scintillation imaging. Radiology 117:105–111, 1975

Henke CE, Wolff JM, Shafer RB: Vascular dynamics in liver scan "hot spot." Clin Nucl Med 3:267–270, 1978.

Huet PM, Chartrand R, Marleau D: Extrahepatic uptake of $^{99m}$Tc-phytate: its mechanism and significance in chronic liver disease. Gastroenterology 78:76–80, 1980

Petrokubi RJ, Baum S, Rohrer GV: Cimetidine administration resulting in improved pertechnetate imaging of Meckel's diverticulum. Clin Nucl Med 3:385–388, 1978

Rosenthall L, Shaffer EA, Lisbona R, et al: Diagnosis of hepatobiliary disease by $^{99m}$Tc-HIDA cholescintigraphy. Radiology 126:467–474, 1978

Sham R, Sain A, Silver L: Hypertrophic Riedel's lobe of the liver. Clin Nucl Med 3:79–81, 1978

Sober AJ, Mintzis MM, Lew RA, et al: The significance of augmented radiocolloid uptake by the spleen in patients with malignant melanoma. J Nucl Med 20:1232–1236, 1979

Sty JR, Babbitt DP, Boedecker RA: $^{99m}$Tc-PIPIDA biliary imaging in children. Clin Nucl Med 4:315–324, 1979

Weissmann HS, Frank MS, Bernstein LH, et al: Rapid and accurate diagnosis of acute cholecystitis with $^{99m}$Tc-HIDA cholescintigraphy. Am J Roentgenol 132:523–528, 1979

# 2/ Perfusion and Ventilation Lung Imaging

Perfusion lung imaging shows the regional distribution of pulmonary arterial blood flow throughout the lungs. Tc-99m-labeled particles, usually macroaggregated albumin (TcMAA) or human albumin microspheres (TcHAM) are injected intravenously and pass into the pulmonary vascular bed. Almost all of the particles are 10-40$\mu$ in size, lodge initially in precapillary arterioles, and are retained in the lungs for a half-time of about six hours. The pattern of pulmonary blood flow immediately following injection is in effect frozen in time, allowing gamma images to be obtained in multiple views.

Abnormal perfusion images are seen in diseases that directly affect the pulmonary vasculature, as well as in conditions that cause regional impairment of ventilation and reflex shunting of blood away to less hypoxic lung areas. Regions that are underperfused from any cause receive fewer radioactive particles, resulting in a defect in the lung image. Clearance of particles from the lungs probably results from enzymatic, chemical, and macrophage activity or breakdown into smaller fragments. Subcapillary-sized particles that pass through the lungs into the systemic circulation are eventually removed by phagocytosis, mainly in the liver and spleen.

When the study is interpreted, a three-dimensional image should be reconstructed in the viewer's mind, as with radiographs. Consideration should be given to size, shape, location, and orientation of the lesion and its relationship to normal anatomical structures. If serial studies are obtained, this additional temporal dimension may help to characterize the lesion. Most diseases are dynamic processes, evolving, spreading, or being modified by treatment and healing. Perfusion defects due to embolism, pneumonia, pulmonary edema, and bronchial asthma usually change over relatively short time intervals. Some diseases are typically unchanged over short or even long time intervals such as chronic obstructive pulmonary disease, parenchymal scarring, and regional fibrocalcific disease.

A current chest x-ray must always be reviewed in an attempt to explain perfusion defects and is especially helpful in cases of lung parenchymal disease. However, abnormal perfusion also results from diseases of the airways and extrapulmonary disorders that may not be apparent from simple x-ray examination. These conditions, sometimes unsuspected clinically, can be diagnosed using radioactive gases such as the xenon isotopes, Xenon 133(Xe-133) or Xenon 127(Xe-127).

Ventilation lung imaging provides a visible display representing the movement of air into and out of the various lung areas. This is a dynamic study providing regional information that can be compared with perfusion images. Suspicion of pulmonary embolism is the most common clinical indication for lung imaging. In this regard the probability of embolism is high in lungs having two or more segmental defects that are normally ventilated, and low with ventilation/perfusion defects that are well matched. The need for combined studies increases in the middle and later years of a patient's life, when disorders of ventilation are more prevalent, as well as in younger patients with a history of lung disease or smoking.

Inhalation lung imaging using radioaerosols is of value in the diagnosis of airway disease, but this study is not in general use and will not be discussed here.

## NORMAL LUNG PERFUSION AND VENTILATION

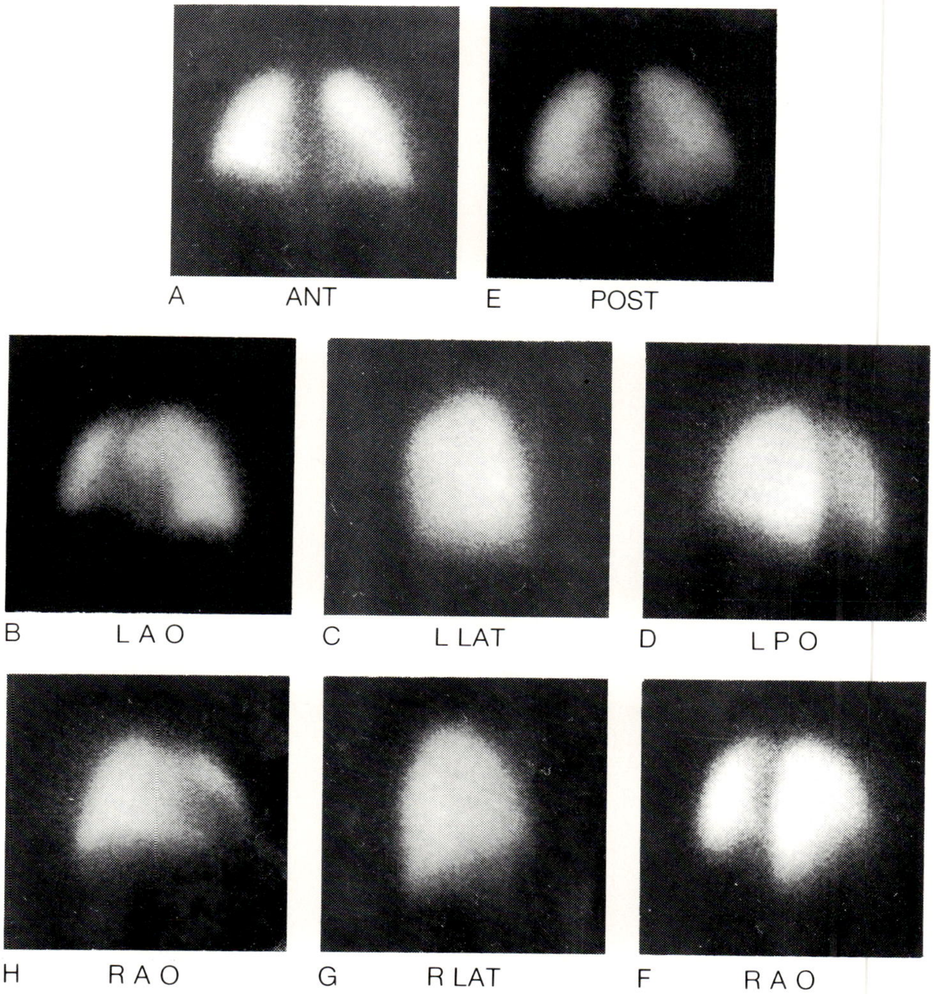


**FIG. 1.** NORMAL LUNG PERFUSION. An optimal routine examination includes 8 views (**A** through **H**). The posterior obliques (**D** and **F**) are the most valuable views, and the anterior obliques (**B** and **H**) are usually the least useful. When the patient is injected in the supine position, the radioactive particles are evenly distributed throughout the lungs, with a gently increasing gradient of activity from the upper anterior to the lower posterior lung fields. The cardiac and mediastinal spaces between the lungs have a configuration in the combined anterior and posterior views (**A** and **E**) that is similar to the respective area in the PA chest x-ray. Cardiomegaly and mediastinal masses will cause distortions that are common to both examinations. An enlarged cardiac space may be caused by cardiomegaly, and by effusions or other conditions of the pericardial sac and adjacent pleural cavity. When a diverging hole collimator is used, the oblique views show the nearer lung larger than the opposite lung. In the lateral views (**C** and **G**) the smaller image of the distant lung is superimposed on the closer lung

and normally is not identifiable if the patient is in the true lateral position. If rotated, the lung images may override and cause a false defect, which will disappear when the patient is repositioned accurately. However, a true lesion is unlikely if seen in only one view of a complete study. Faulty preparation of Tc-99m-MAA has free Tc-99m pertechnetate, which is concentrated in the thyroid gland and stomach (**I** through **K**). A patient with a cardiac pacemaker implanted in the right upper chest wall (**L** through **O**) has a rounded defect seen *enface* in the right anterior oblique view (**M**) but not in the other views because the diverging collimator (used here) sees the peripheral lung fields tangentially. In another patient (**P** through **S**) the pacemaker is on the left side. A small defect that changes from the left to right upper lung (**T** and **V**) is due to a metallic medallion worn on a necklace. In the anterior view (**U**) a small photon-deficient area could be seen in the background activity between the apices in the original reproduction.

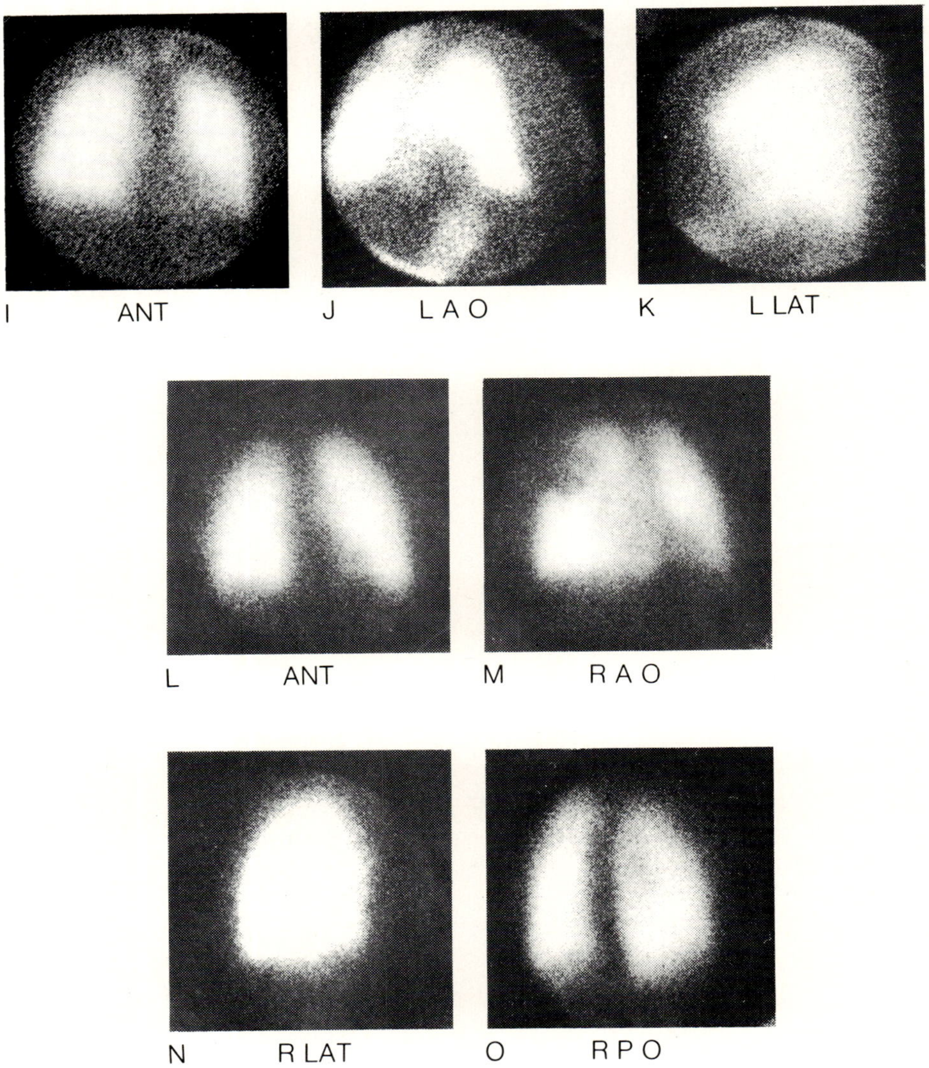


**FIG. 1. I–O.** (See legend page 87)

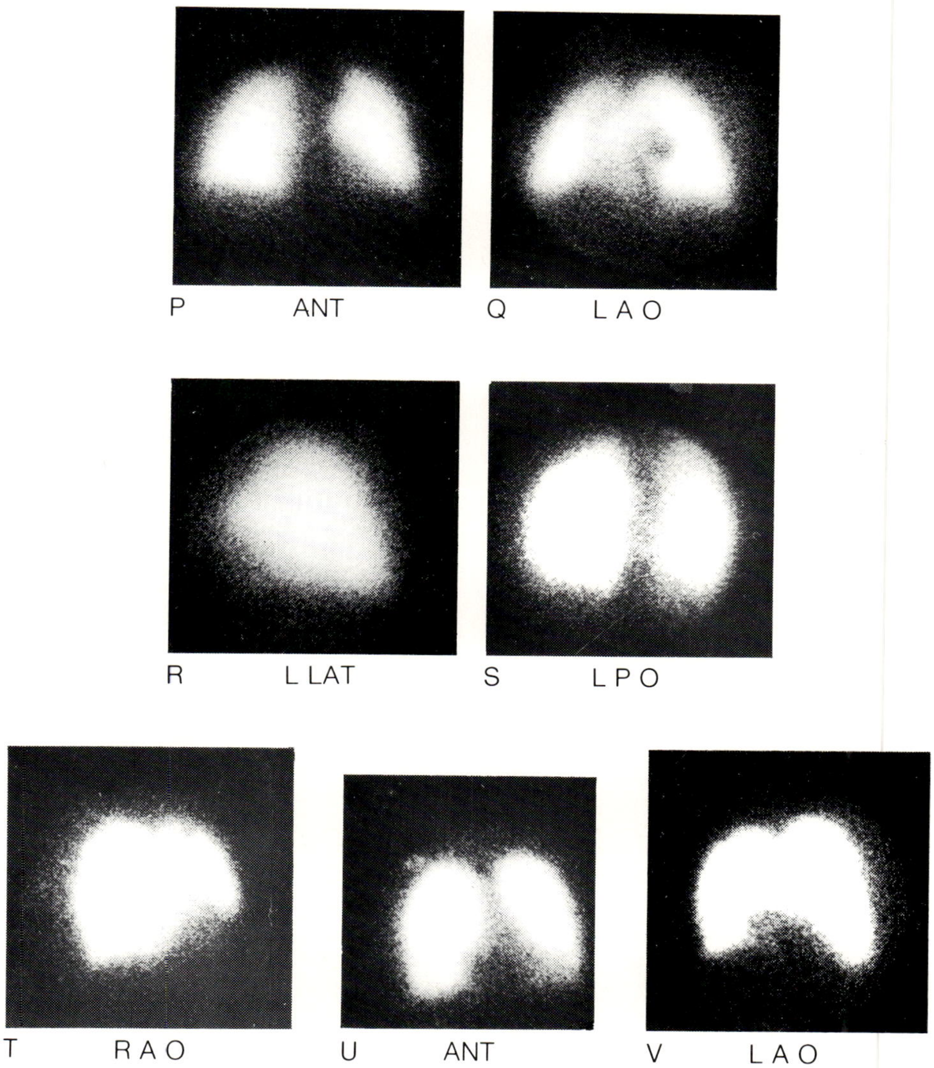


**FIG. 1. P–V.** (See legend pages 87–88)

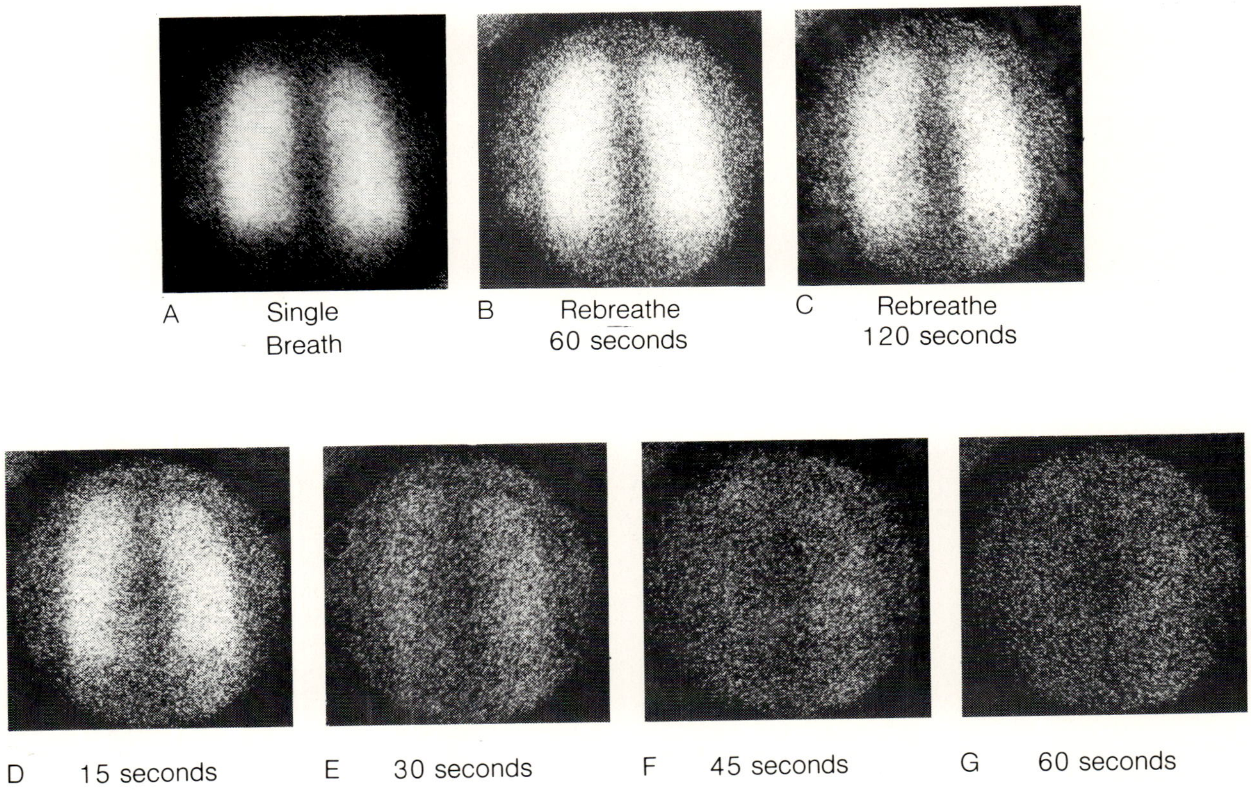


**FIG. 2. NORMAL LUNG VENTILATION.** With the patient's single full breath, inhaled radioxenon is evenly distributed to all lung areas, reaching the terminal airways and alveoli in the normal patient (**A**, posterior view). There is a less noticeable gradient of activity from the upper to lower lung fields than is seen in perfusion lung images. Fifteen-second images obtained during closed-system rebreathing of xenon-oxygen mixture show uniform distribution at 60 seconds (**B**) and 120 seconds (**C**). Serial 15-second frames after the patient's switching to room air breathing (**D** through **G**) show a homogeneous pattern of washout from all lung areas. Note that a small amount of alveolar xenon normally crosses the alveolar membrane to reach the blood and be distributed throughout the body. Because it is highly soluble in lipids, xenon accumulates in adipose tissue including the liver, which is faintly seen with prolonged rebreathing. Liver activity should not be mistaken for delayed washout of xenon from the base of the lung. Occasionally, splenic blood-pool radioactivity or swallowed xenon in the stomach may also be seen.

## PULMONARY VASCULAR DISORDERS

Lung perfusion defects caused by disorders affecting pulmonary arteries alone are usually accompanied by normal ventilation studies. Pulmonary artery lesions may be in the lumen (most commonly thromboembolism), the wall (branch coarctation or hypoplasia, vasculitis, etc.), or may be extrinsic and pressing on the artery (tumor, enlarged lymph nodes, fibrosis, hematoma, aneurysm).

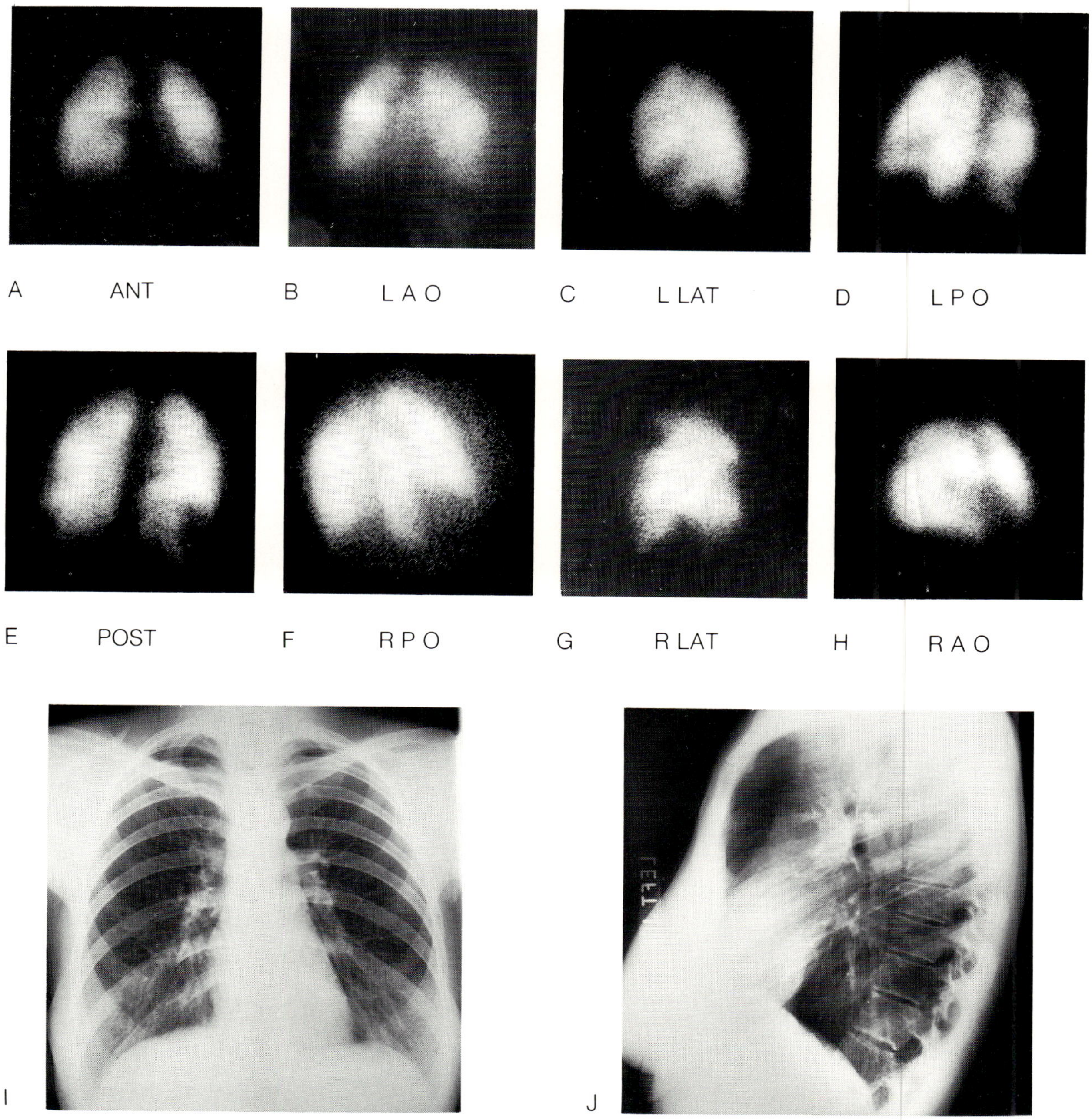


**FIG. 3.** PULMONARY THROMBOEMBOLISM. Many well defined segmental perfusion defects involving both lungs (**A** through **F**) with normal chest x-ray (**I** and **J**) and normal lung ventilation study. This is a classic pattern of pulmonary embolism.

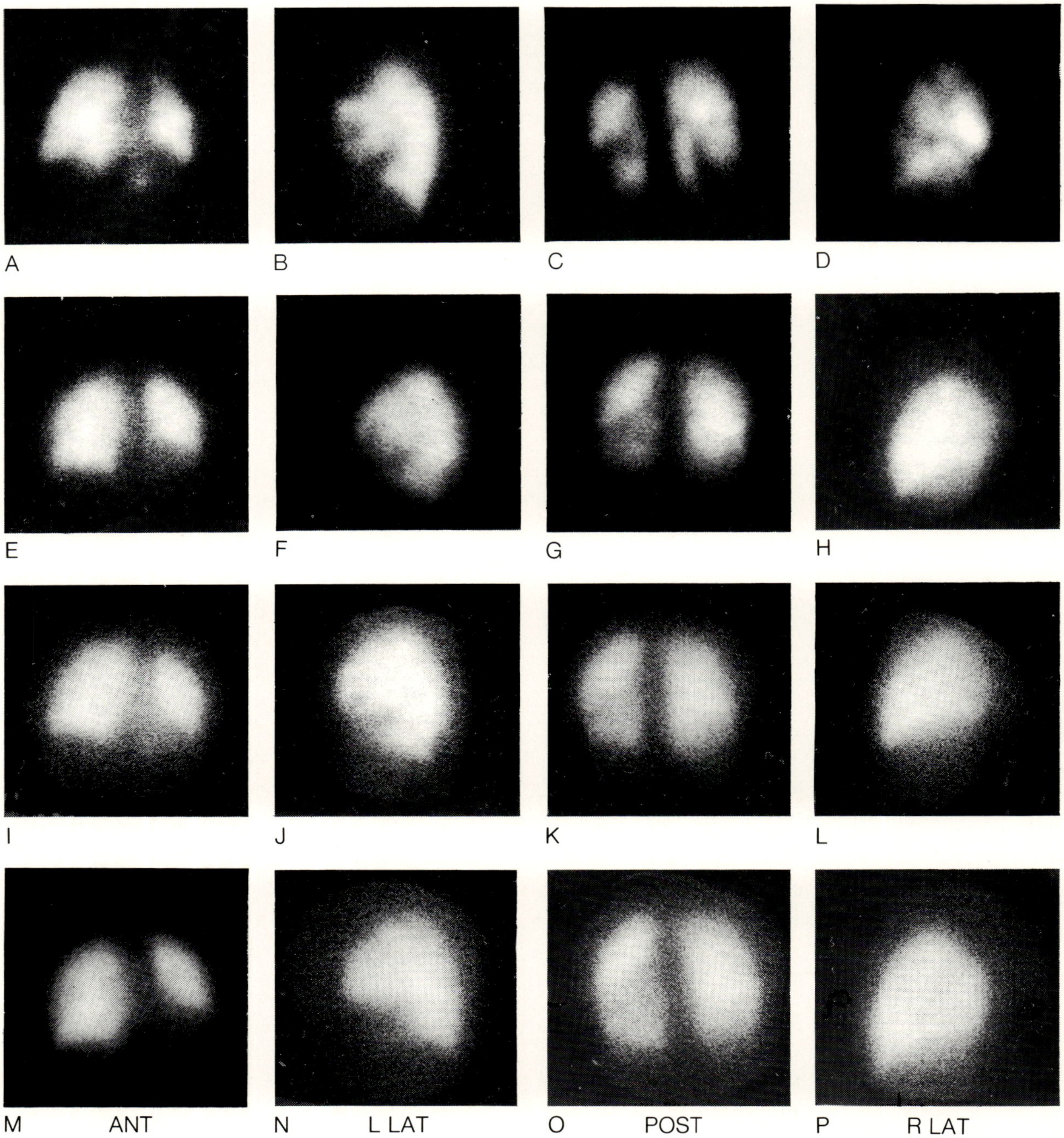


**FIG. 4. RESOLUTION OF PULMONARY EMBOLISM.** Selected frames from a series of studies of a patient with pulmonary embolism initially show multiple segmental perfusion defects (**A** through **D**). After 2 weeks (**E** through **H**) most of the regions are reperfused. Residual small defects show slight further improvement at 3 weeks (**I** through **L**) and 6 weeks (**M** through **P**). Pulmonary embolism may resolve slowly or incompletely in older patients with preexisting cardiopulmonary disease. In young, otherwise healthy patients, resolution is more rapid and defects may disappear within a few days with adequate therapy.

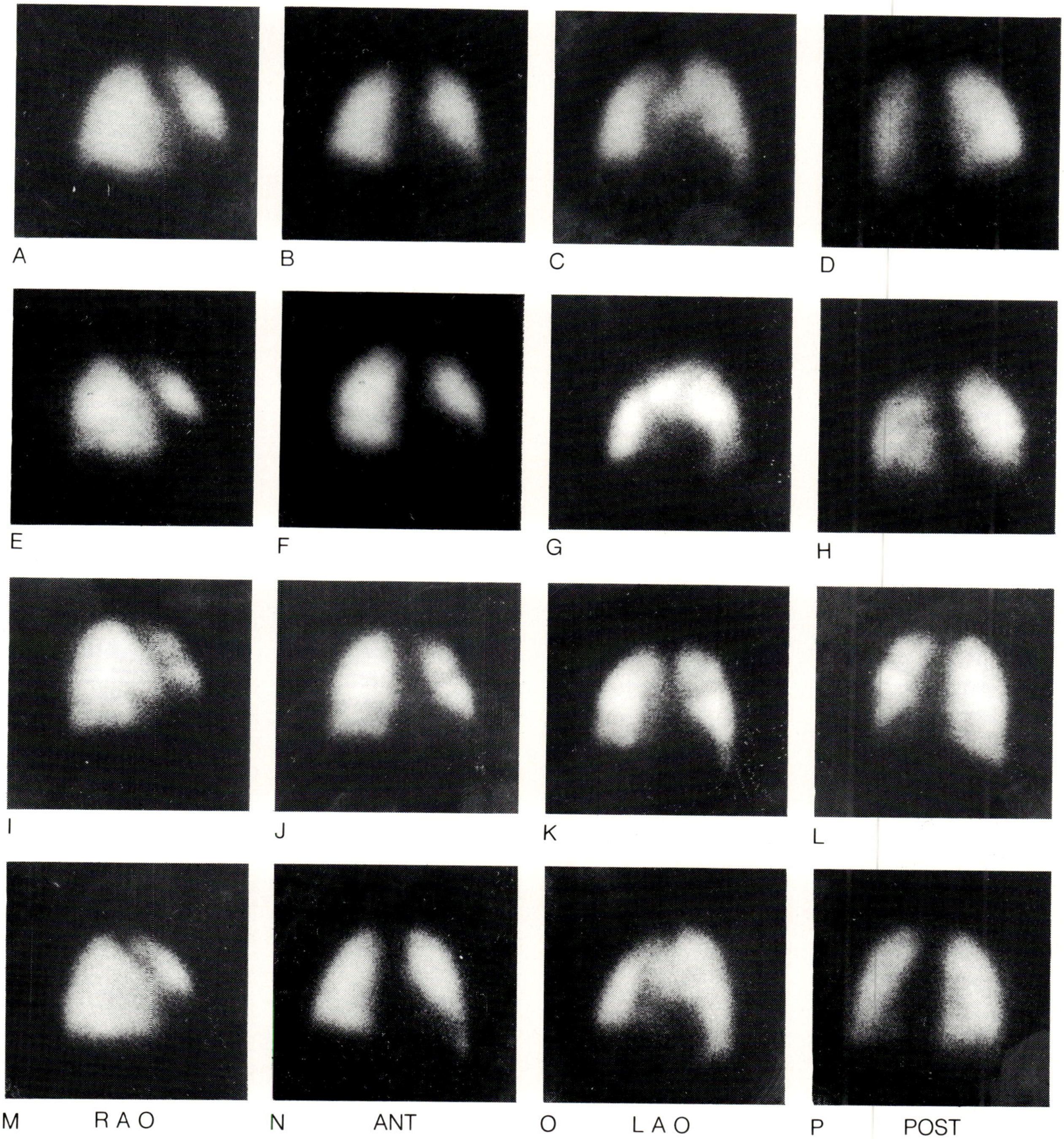


**FIG. 5. PROGRESSION AND RESOLUTION OF PULMONARY EMBOLISM.** Views of the baseline study (**A** through **D**) and 2 weeks later (**E** through **H**) show the appearance of several perfusion defects. At 3 weeks (**I** through **L**) some lesions have improved but new defects are present. These have resolved at 4 weeks (**M** through **P**). Note that sometimes a defect in one area of the lungs may appear to worsen when blood is redistributed to other lung areas where emboli resolve more rapidly. A partially occluded vessel, which decreases in size when blood flow to it decreases, may become totally occluded. The result is a change from decreased to absent perfusion of the supplied lung segment.

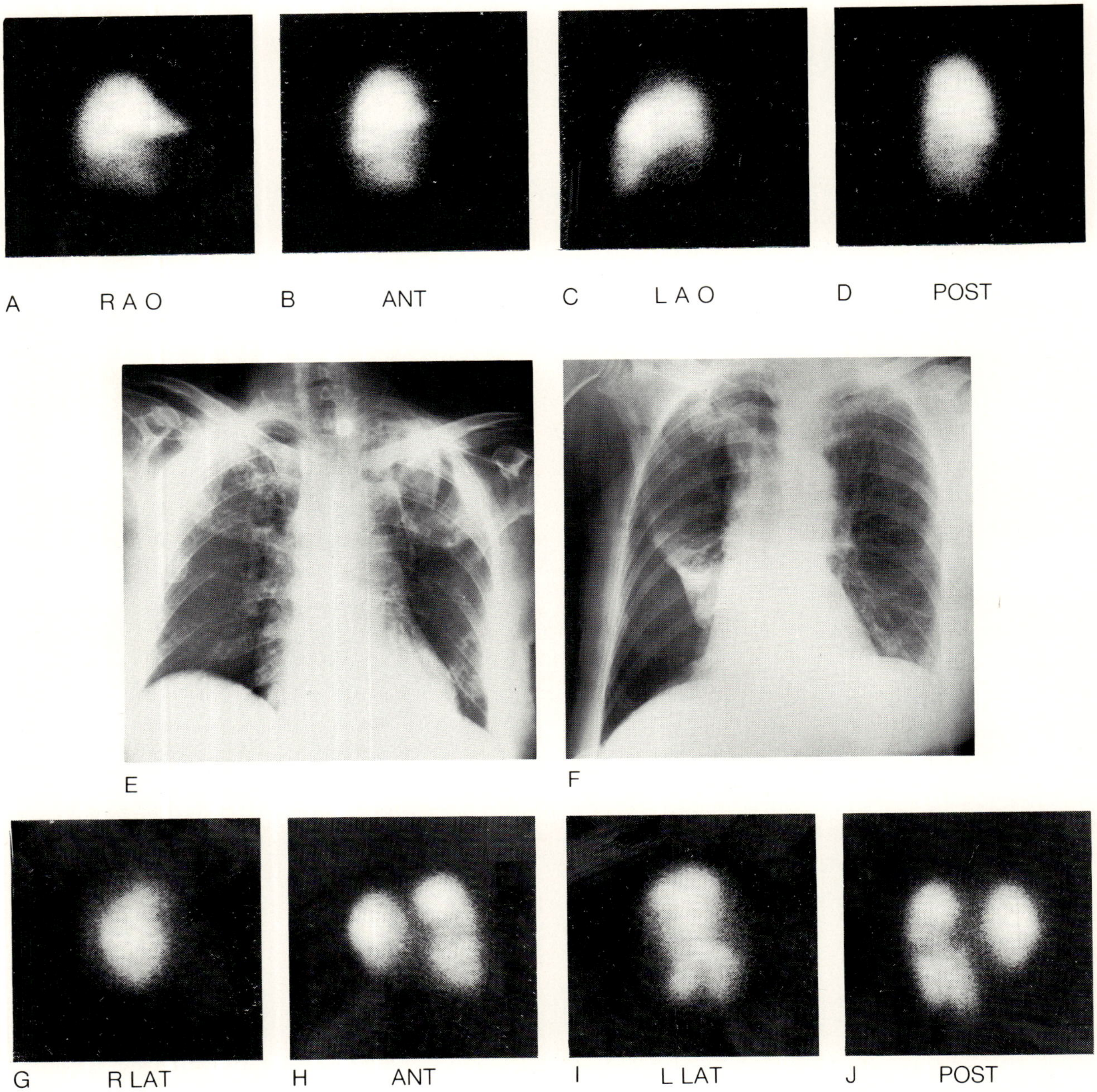


**FIG. 6. PULMONARY INFARCTION.** With pulmonary embolism alone, the ventilation study is normal and the chest x-ray may also be normal or show nonspecific findings. When pulmonary infarction occurs, a radiographic density is usually seen, often matched by a ventilation defect but without trapping, since xenon cannot enter collapsed or blood-filled alveoli. Pulmonary infarcts cannot be distinguished from pneumonia. However, patients with infarcts usually also have embolism to other lung areas and these will show unmatched perfusion defects. Non-perfusion of left lung due to massive embolism (**A** through **D**) is accompanied by x-ray density compatible with infarction (**E**). Perfusion defects in right lung without x-ray and ventilation abnormalities indicate embolism. Findings in left lung of another patient (**G** through **J**) are due to embolism. A right-sided pneumothorax (**F**) resulted from a blown-out infarct, which occurs rarely.

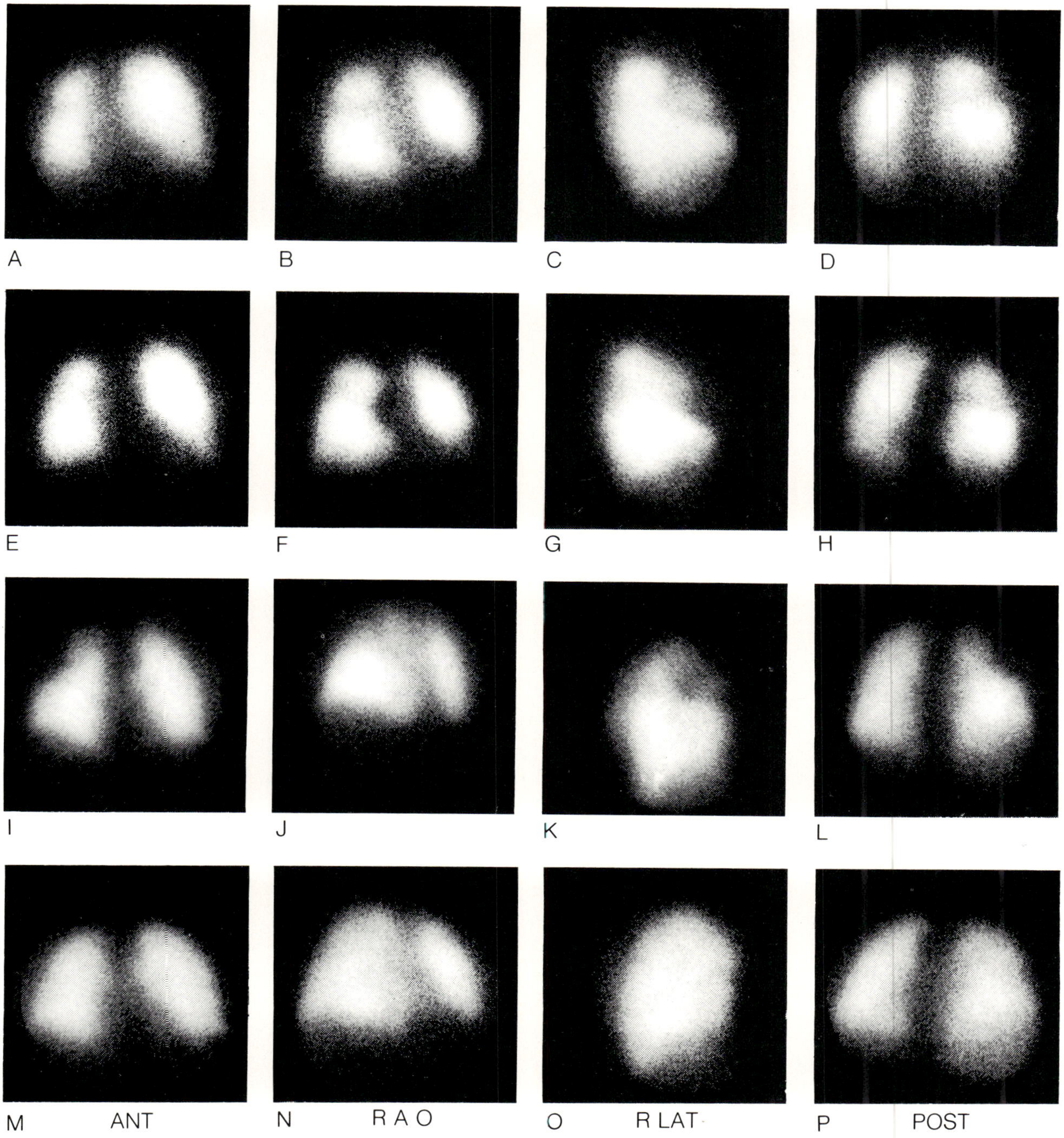


**FIG. 7.** SINGLE PERFUSION DEFECT. In a patient with normal radiographic and ventilation studies, a perfusion defect in only one area is much less likely to be due to thromboembolism than are two or more segmental defects in separate areas. Alternate considerations include narrowing or extrinsic pressure on a pulmonary artery, in which case the defect (**A** through **D**) may be unchanged with time (**E** through **H**, 6 weeks later). The relatively rare solitary embolus (**I** through **L**) should resolve within a few days (**M** through **P**, 6 days later), or other lesions should quickly appear.

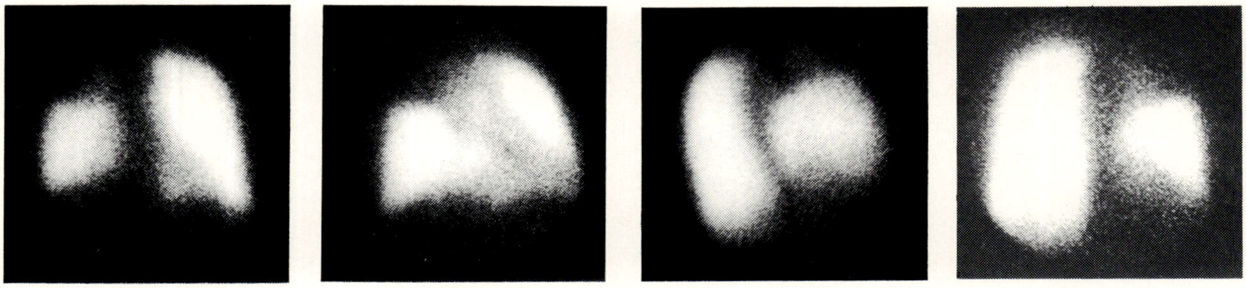

A ANT | B RAO | C RPO | D POST

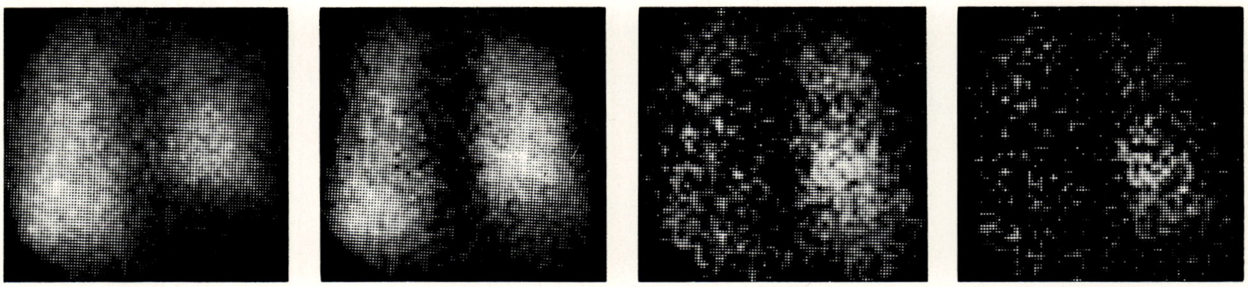

E Single Breath | F Rebreathe 120 seconds | G Washout 30-60 seconds | H Washout 60-90 seconds

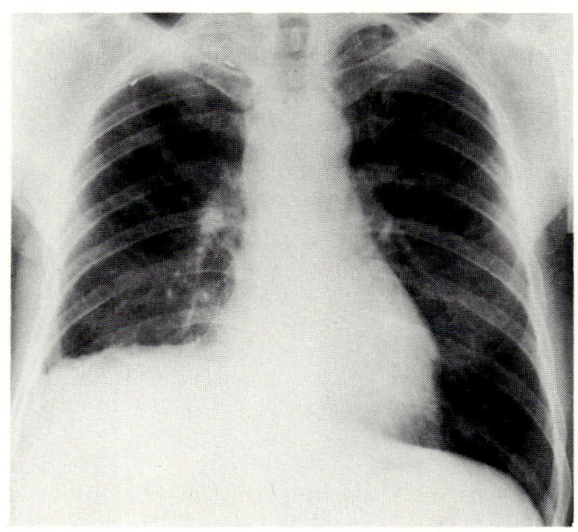

I

**FIG. 8. RADIATION DAMAGE.** A patient with squamous cell carcinomas in a cavitating lesion in the apex of the right lung and in the base of the tongue was treated with right upper lobectomy and 4 MeV radiation therapy. Eighteen months later, lung images show absent perfusion (**A** through **D**), normal ventilation (**E** through **H,** posterior views), and no significant x-ray findings (**I**) in an area of the right upper lung that was included in a portal used to deliver a tissue dose of 4750 rads in 65 days. The perfusion defect has a sharply defined transverse margin unrelated to normal segmental anatomy (guillotine sign). Note that the right hemidiaphragm and liver are high in position and that blood-borne radioxenon accumulates and is retained in the liver, not in the right lung base. Following radiation therapy, early and late clinical phases may appear; their severity will depend on the radiation dose and its rate of delivery, and on the volume of lung exposed. Radiation pneumonitis may be seen at 6 to 12 weeks, followed by clinical remission but gradual appearance of radiation fibrosis after 6 to 9 months. Damage and loss of capillaries, dense fibrosis, and distortion of normal architecture are present in this phase of disease. In this and probably most other cases of radiation fibrosis, regional oligemia is the most striking abnormality.

## DISORDERS OF SMALL AIRWAYS

Abnormal function of distal small airways prevents normal movement of gases into and out of alveoli. This and other factors cause regional alveolar hypoxia, which results in redistribution of pulmonary blood flow away from poorly ventilated areas. Matching defects are seen in both the ventilation and perfusion studies, whereas radiographic changes are usually less evident or absent. This group of disorders includes pulmonary emphysema and chronic bronchitis (chronic obstructive pulmonary disease), asthma, bronchiectasis, and inhalation burns. The last condition is unusual because the rare combination of abnormal ventilation and normal perfusion may be seen.

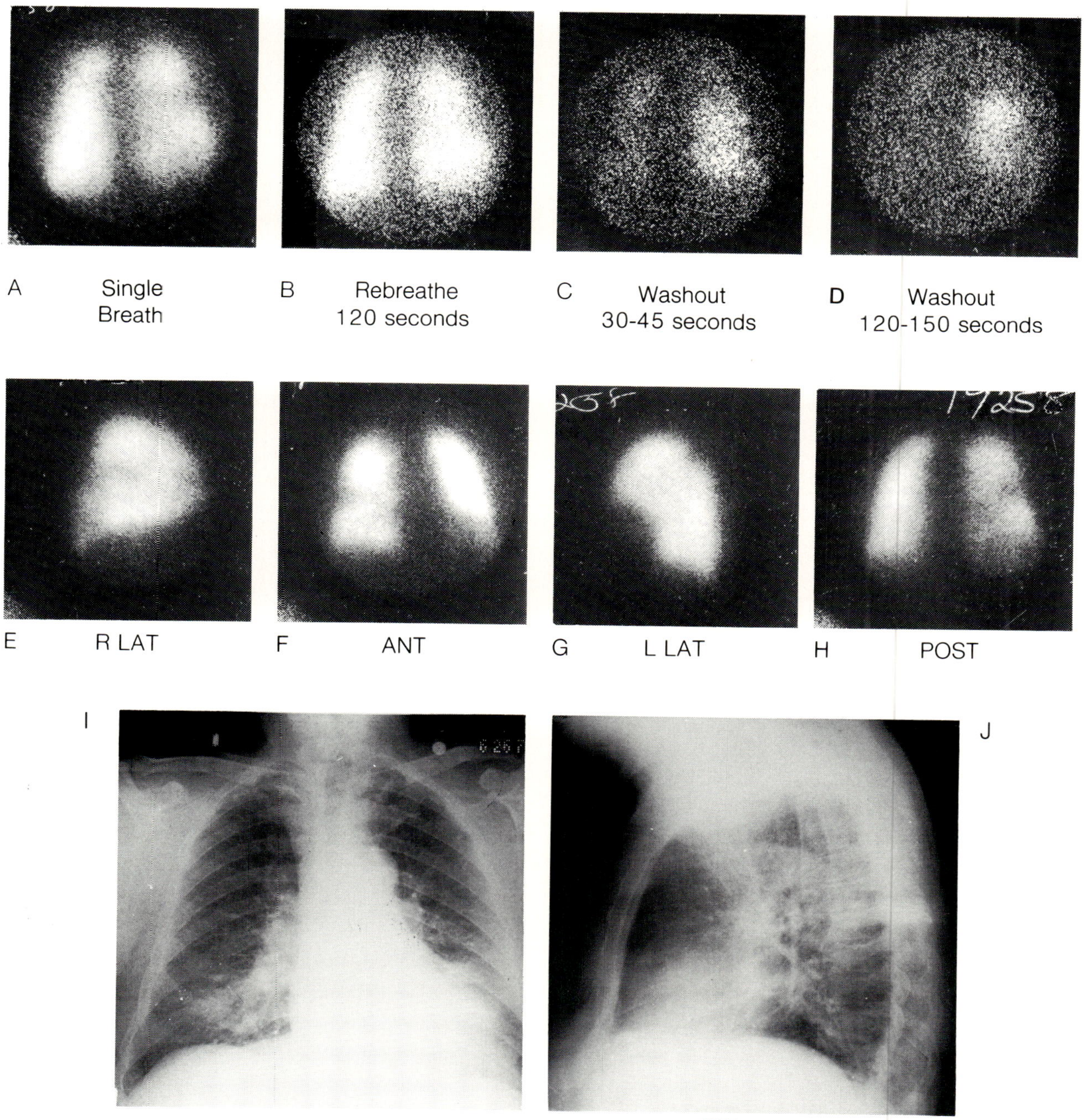


**FIG. 9.** A – J (See legend next page)

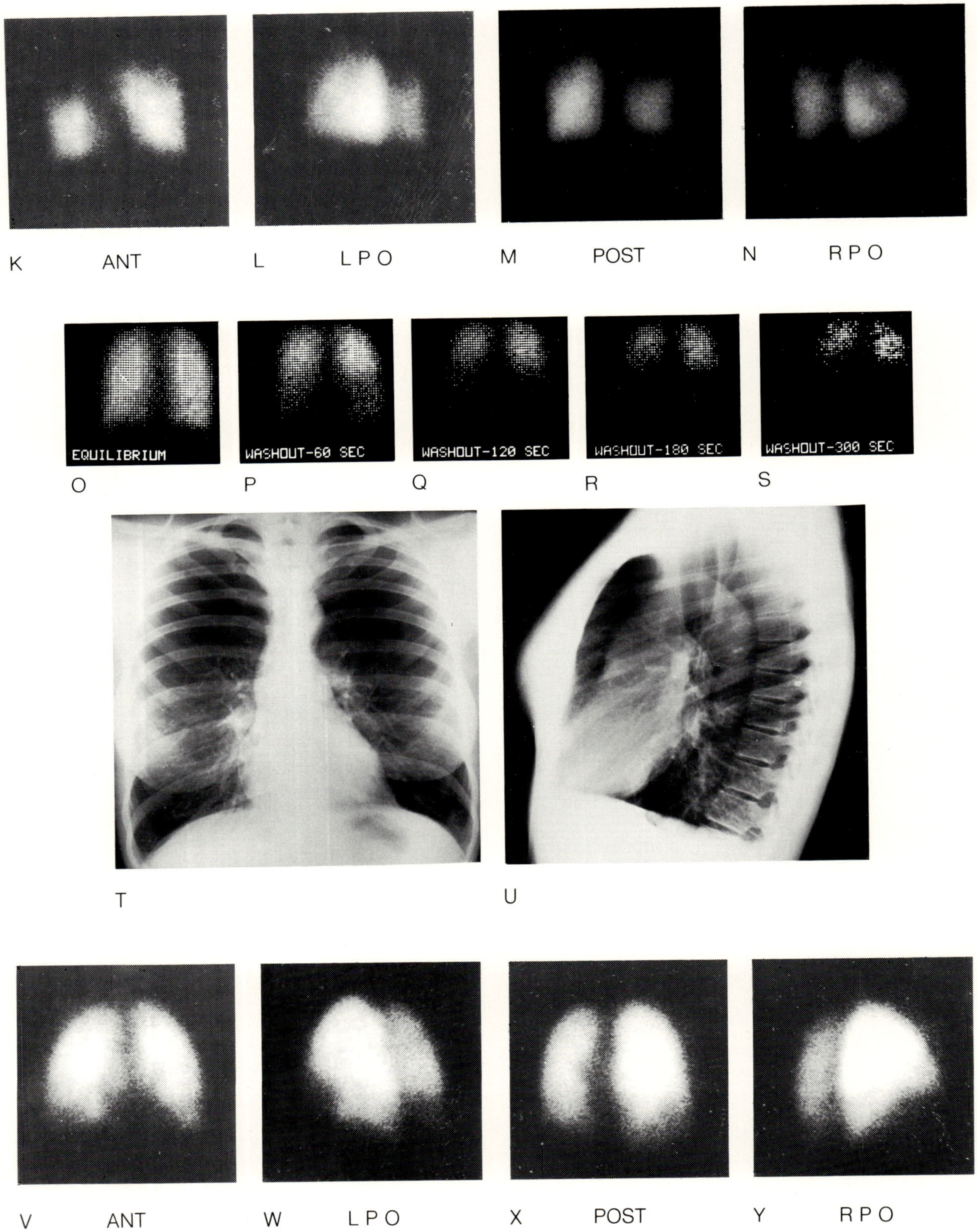


**FIG. 9. K–Y.** (See legend next page)

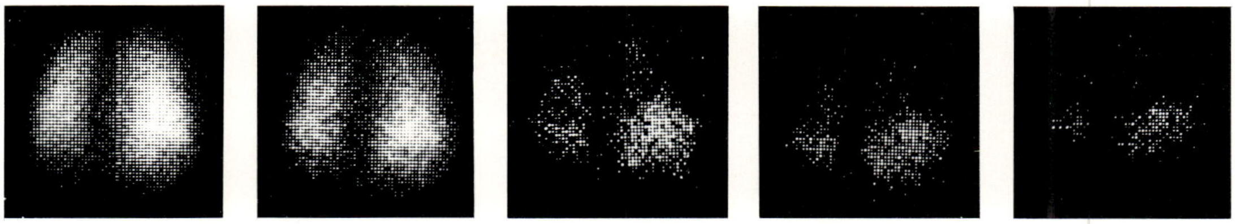

Z Equil. AA 30 seconds BB 90 seconds CC 150 seconds DD 300 seconds

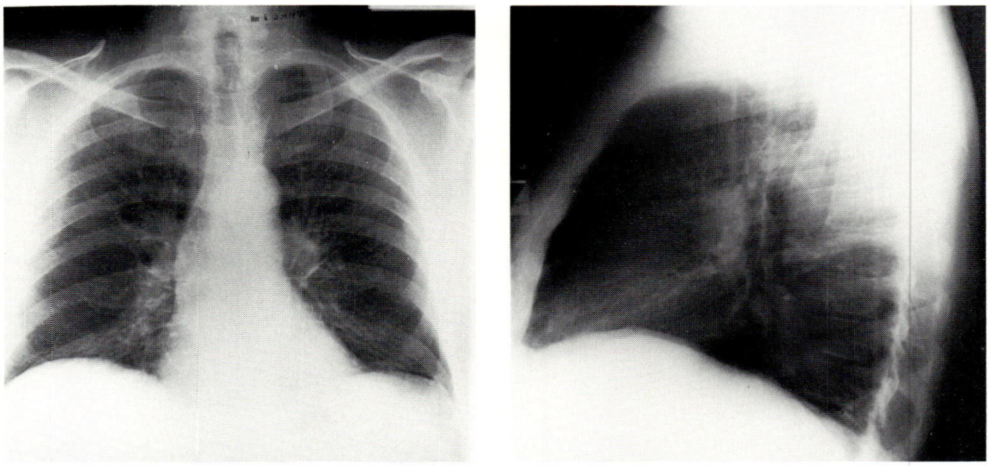

EE FF

**FIG. 9.** CHRONIC OBSTRUCTIVE PULMONARY DISEASE. Narrowing of multiple small airways due to increased tone, edema, fibrosis, or excessive secretions, and decreased elastic recoil of lung parenchyma with overinflation and breakdown of the walls of alveoli are some of the factors in chronic bronchitis and pulmonary emphysema that result in poor ventilation. Single breath lung image (**A,** posterior view) shows defects where gas entry is poor, but with rebreathing (**B,** posterior view) the defects fill in and the distribution becomes more uniform as obstructed airways are bypassed by collateral ventilation. The washout phase (**C** and **D,** posterior views) is most sensitive for the detection of air-trapping. These views show the distribution of regions from which the clearance of xenon is delayed. Decreased pulmonary blood flow to poorly ventilated areas results in perfusion defects with a similar distribution (**E** through **H**). Chest x-ray (**I** and **J**) shows little evidence of the extent and regional distribution of the disease. The clinical picture in this patient is chronic bronchitis. Centriacinar emphysema usually affects the upper parts of the lobes (**K** through **U**), whereas involvement of the lower lobes (**V** through **FF**) may be due to any constituent of COPD, especially basal panacinar emphysema in alpha$_1$ antitrypsin deficiency. However, the common pattern of COPD ranges from nonsegmental single area to widespread patchy involvement of both lungs. Note that the rate of washout of xenon depends on the rate and depth of breathing. In a patient without lung disease, xenon should be cleared evenly from all lung areas by 2 minutes, assuming a normal minute volume. A longer time may not be abnormal if a patient's breathing is slow and shallow during the study. Hence, all patients should be instructed and observed to be breathing in a manner that is natural for them.

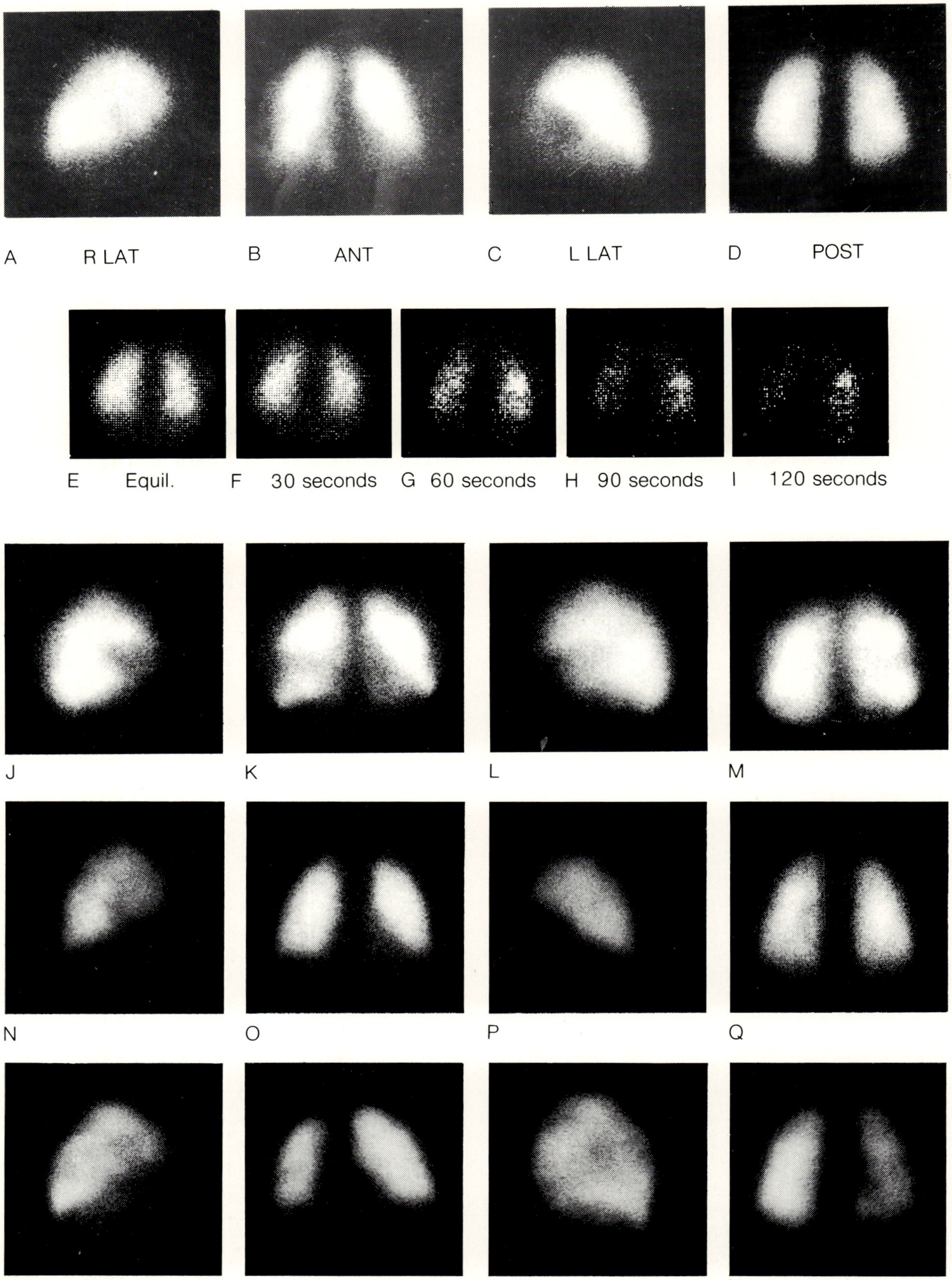


**FIG. 10. A–U.** (See legend next page)

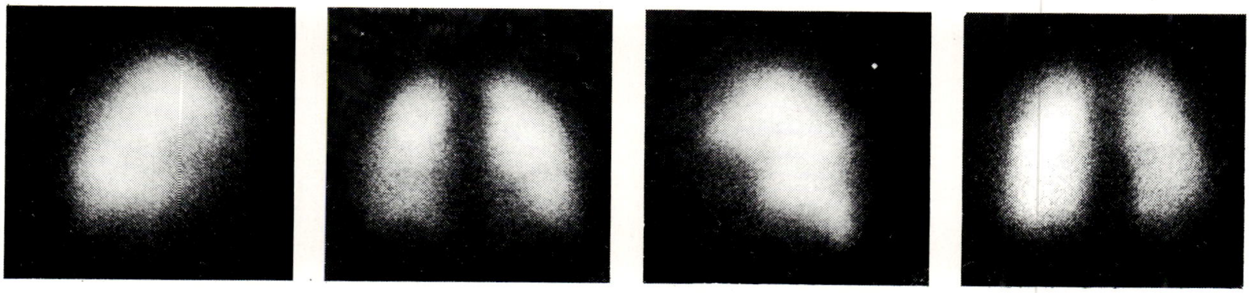

V R LAT W ANT X L LAT Y POST

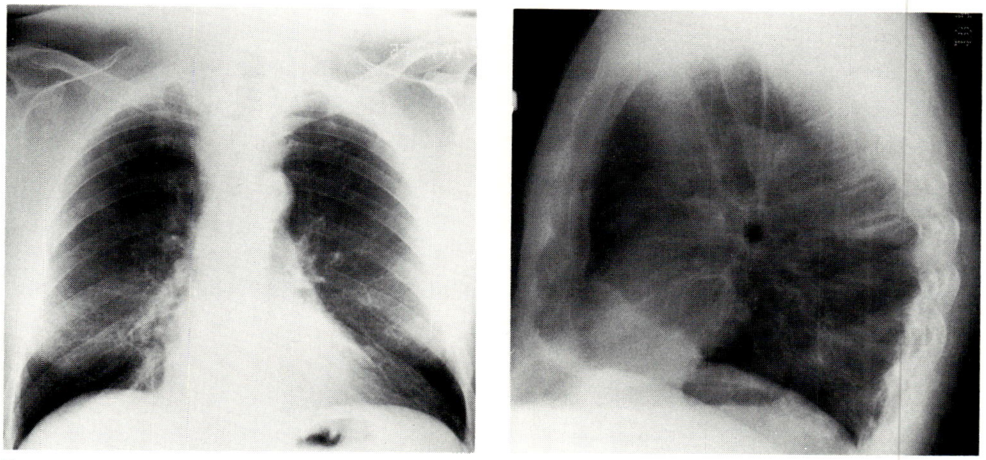

Z AA

**FIG. 10.** ASTHMA. In pulmonary emphysema, chronic bronchitis, asthma, and bronchiectasis, lung images show matched ventilation/perfusion defects with limited or sometimes absent changes in plain chest x-rays. In asthma, the defects may or may not relate to segmental anatomy and tend to vary in severity and distribution over the course of the disease. Even when the patient is relatively asymptomatic, defects may still be present, albeit less pronounced. In the other diseases listed above, the lesions are more stable and seldom reversible. A patient with asthma has areas of decreased pulmonary blood flow (**A** through **D**) and poor ventilation due to air-trapping (**E** through **I**). Note that after the patient's rebreathing xenon for 2 minutes the distribution of lung volume is uniform (**E**). This image provides regional information but does not evaluate *total* lung volume, which in asthma could be normal, or increased if air-trapping causes overinflation of the lungs. Compare perfusion images (**A** through **D**) with other studies in the same patient taken 12 months before (**J** through **M**), 8 months before (**N** through **Q**), 3 weeks after (**R** through **U**) and 3 months after (**V** through **Y**). Chest x-ray (**Z** and **AA**) was taken when patient was symptom-free and lung perfusion was normal (**N** through **Q**). Other images show a changing pattern of abnormal pulmonary blood flow. Matching ventilation/perfusion defects were present in each case, but for brevity selected perfusion images only are shown because lesions are better appreciated in the multiple views, which can be routinely obtained.

## DISORDERS OF LARGE AIRWAYS

Lesions that partially obstruct major airways may be intraluminal (foreign body, mucus plug, blood clot, malpositioned endotracheal tube, adenoma, or carcinoma), involve the bronchial wall (bronchospasm, fibrosis, infiltrating cancer), or cause extrinsic pressure on the bronchus (enlarged lymph nodes, tumor, aneurysm, abscess or hematoma, etc.). Some of these lesions may not be detected on plain chest x-rays if hidden in the hilar or mediastinal shadows. When airflow through a large airway is impeded, ventilation and matched perfusion defects confined to a single region are usually seen. Such a region may involve a segment, lobe, or entire lung depending on the level of obstruction. In contrast, small airway disorders tend to be multicentric and nonsegmental.

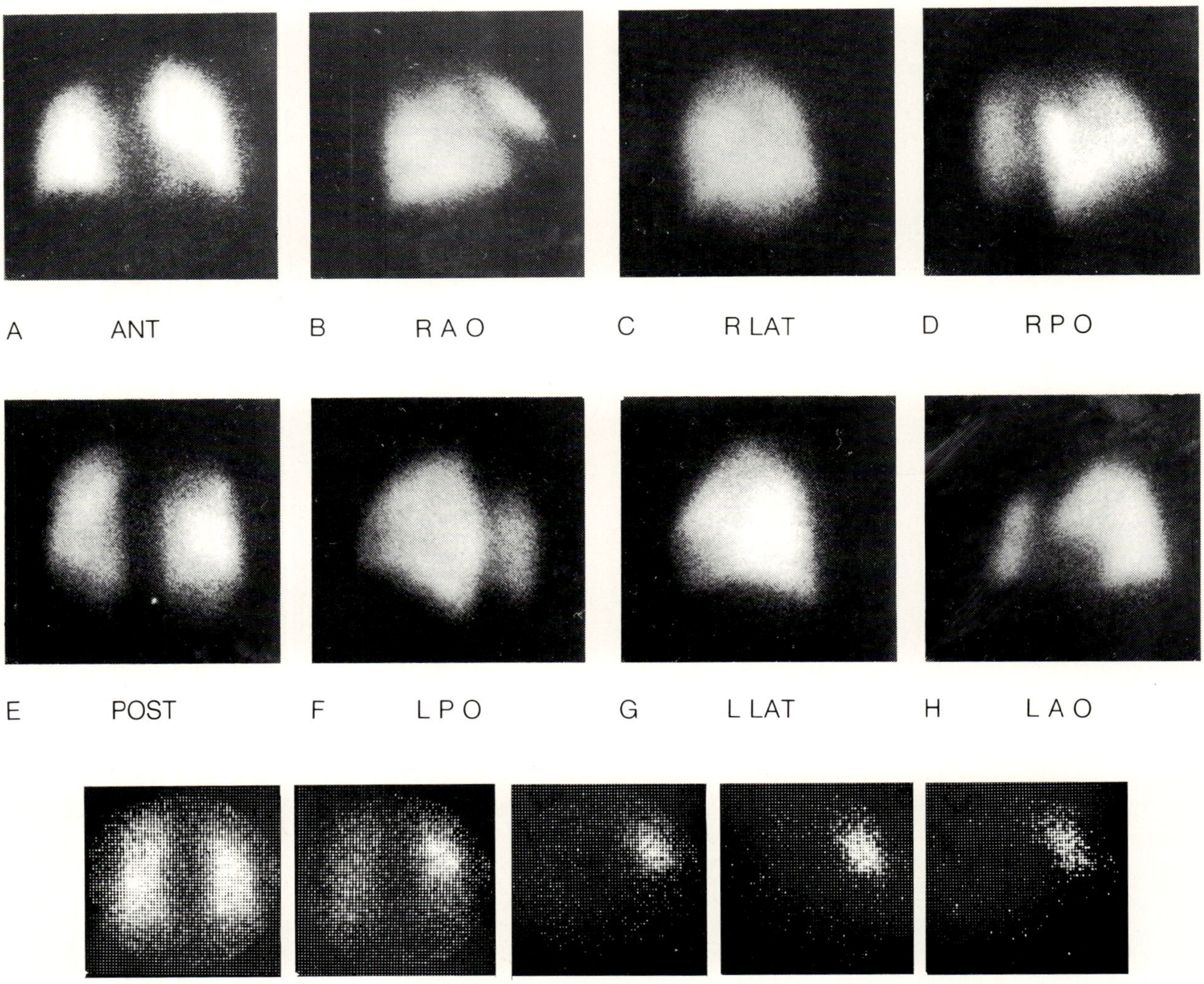

A ANT B RAO C R LAT D RPO

E POST F LPO G L LAT H LAO

I Equil. J 30 seconds K 90 seconds L 180 seconds M 330 seconds

All Views are Posterior

**FIG. 11. A–M.** (See legend next page)

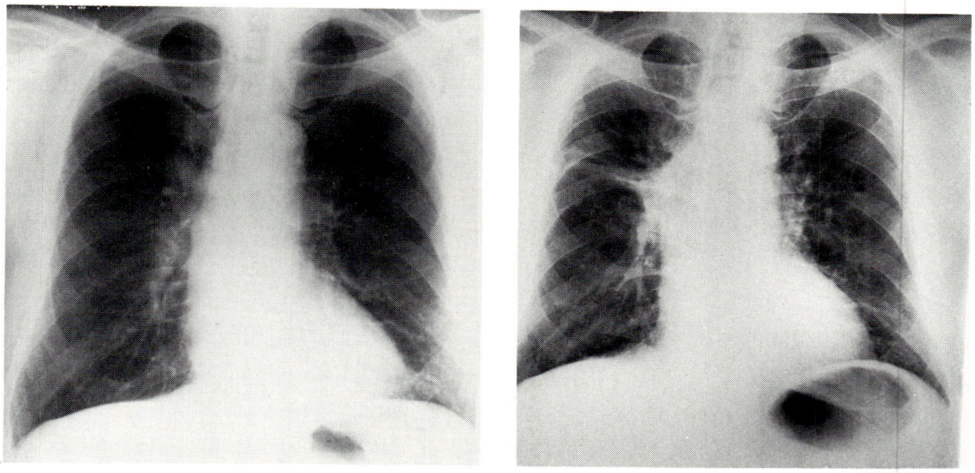

N O

**FIG. 11.** **CARCINOMA OF THE BRONCHUS.** A malignant tumor may obstruct or distort the lumen of a bronchus, or infiltrate the bronchial wall and prevent normal contraction and dilatation, thereby producing relatively diminished air flow. Outside the bronchus, a tumor may compress or invade pulmonary veins or, more rarely, pulmonary arteries. However, a perfusion defect will be present with airway obstruction alone, a condition resulting in redistribution of blood flow away from the area of alveolar hypoxia. A single right upper lobar perfusion defect (**A** through **H**) shows equilibration of xenon into the area after 2 minutes (**I**) but marked retention during the washout phase (**J** through **M**). Chest x-ray (**N**) has a suspicious area above the right hilus, but tomography, pulmonary angiography, and bronchoscopy failed to detect the presence of a tumor. The patient returned 9 months later with an unresectable carcinoma of the right upper lobe bronchus (**O**). At the time of the initial workup the lesion was probably confined to the wall of the bronchus, a position that caused relative airway obstruction by preventing normal bronchial dilatation but did not produce a visible mass. In other cases, a tumor or its metastases may primarily involve pulmonary blood vessels without significantly affecting lung ventilation. Lung imaging is useful before surgery or radiation therapy in helping to evaluate the extent of disease and appropriateness of treatment. Lung imaging may also prove to be useful in the early detection of carcinoma of the bronchus.

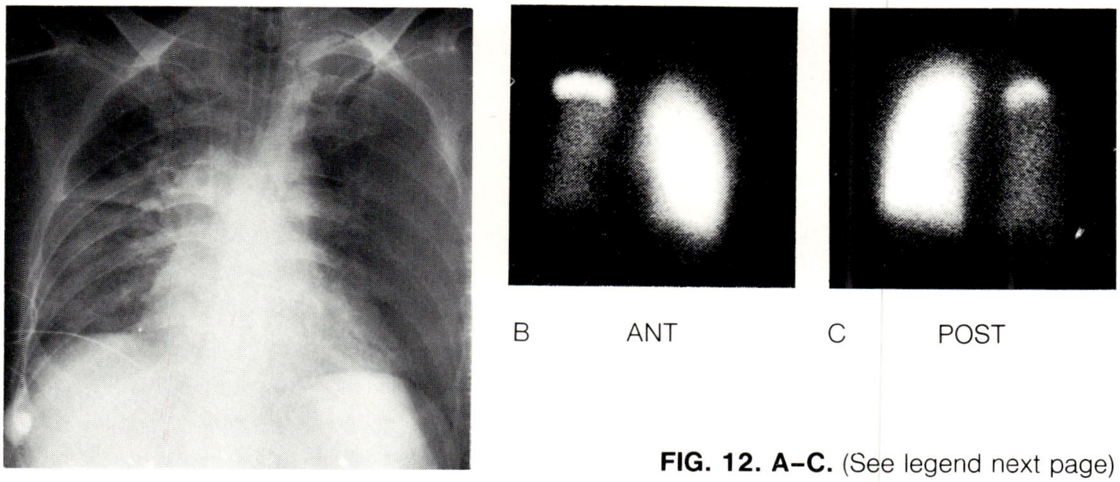

A B ANT C POST

**FIG. 12. A–C.** (See legend next page)

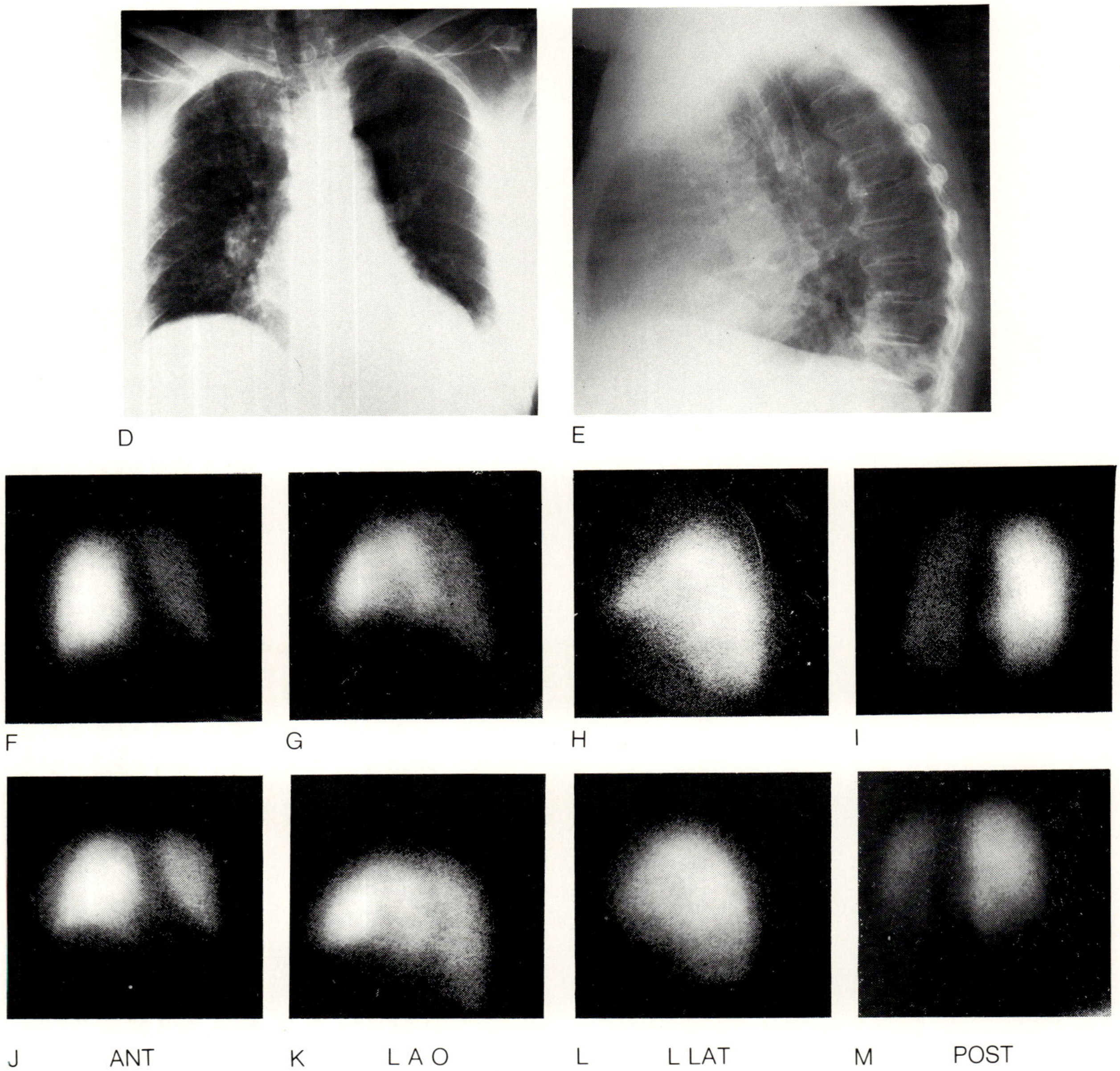


**FIG. 12.** **MUCUS PLUG.** Excessive secretions plugging a bronchus may result in abnormal ventilation and a perfusion defect similar to that caused by an obstructing tumor. With sudden occlusion of a mainstem bronchus, alveolar air is absorbed by the perfusing blood and the lung volume slowly decreases. The lung takes several hours to become airless because of the low solubility of nitrogen. (If pure oxygen is breathed, atelectasis is more rapid and may occur in a few minutes.) A patient with polymyositis and poor bronchial toilet has a pneumonic infiltrate in the right lung (**A**). Exudate and secretions collecting in the right mainstem bronchus interfere with ventilation, and as a result, perfusion images (**B** and **C**) show decreased volume and markedly reduced blood flow to the right lung. (Linear radioactivity at the top of the right lung is hung up in a CVP catheter used for injection of the radiopharmaceutical.) Underperfusion of an entire lung, lobe, or segment may similarly result from a blood clot, foreign body, or malpositioned endotracheal tube covering the ostium of a bronchus. An

elderly woman with unresolving pneumonia in the left lower lobe (**D** and **E**) and ghost image of the left lung (**F** through **I**) came to bronchoscopy, which discovered a piece of almond surrounded by intense inflammation of the adjacent left mainstem bronchus. She recalled eating chocolate-coated almonds without difficulty one month before. Two days after removal of the foreign body, the left lung perfusion has improved (**J** through **M**) but is not yet normal, probably because of residual inflammation and edema of the bronchial wall. Young children and peanuts have similar incompatibility.

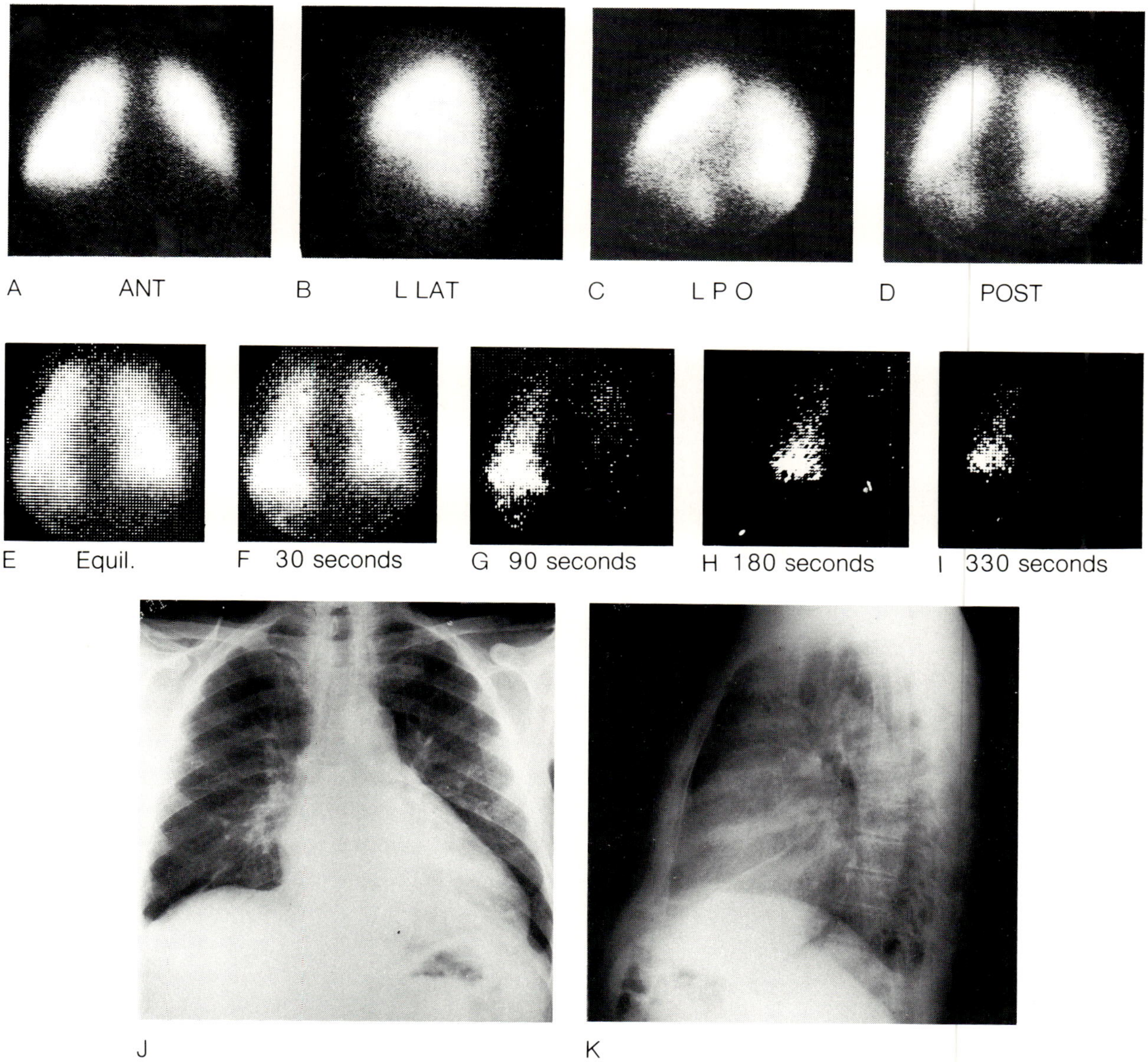


**FIG. 13. EXTRINSIC BRONCHIAL OBSTRUCTION.** A matched ventilation/perfusion defect is confined to the left lower lobe (**A** through **I**) in a patient with prolapse and insufficiency of the mitral valve. After a workup to exclude an endobronchial lesion, airway obstruction was attributed to extrinsic pressure on the left lower lobe bronchus by an enlarged left heart (**J** and **K**).

## ALVEOLAR AND INTERSTITIAL DISORDERS

In alveolar diseases such as various pneumonias, pulmonary edema, alveolar cell carcinoma, etc., the alveoli and alveolar ducts may be filled with fluid, exudate, or tumor cells. With interstitial diseases including some pneumonias and granulomatous diseases, diffuse interstitial fibrosis, and lymphangitic spread of malignant tumors, there may be edema, cellular infiltration, or fibrosis, which may distort, collapse, or obliterate alveoli and capillaries. Common to most alveolar and interstitial disorders is reduction or loss of peripheral airspace volume and absence of air-trapping. Because lung parenchyma is involved, chest x-rays are almost always abnormal, showing alveolar, interstitial, or other patterns that typify certain groups of diseases. Lung imaging defects, when present, show the involved regions to have decreased perfusion, decreased entry of xenon with the first breath and after equilibration, but no trapping during washout. These findings reflect diminished regional lung volume with unimpaired expiratory gas flow. In general, the x-ray findings are more obvious than the corresponding lung image defects, which may be subtle or on occasion virtually absent.

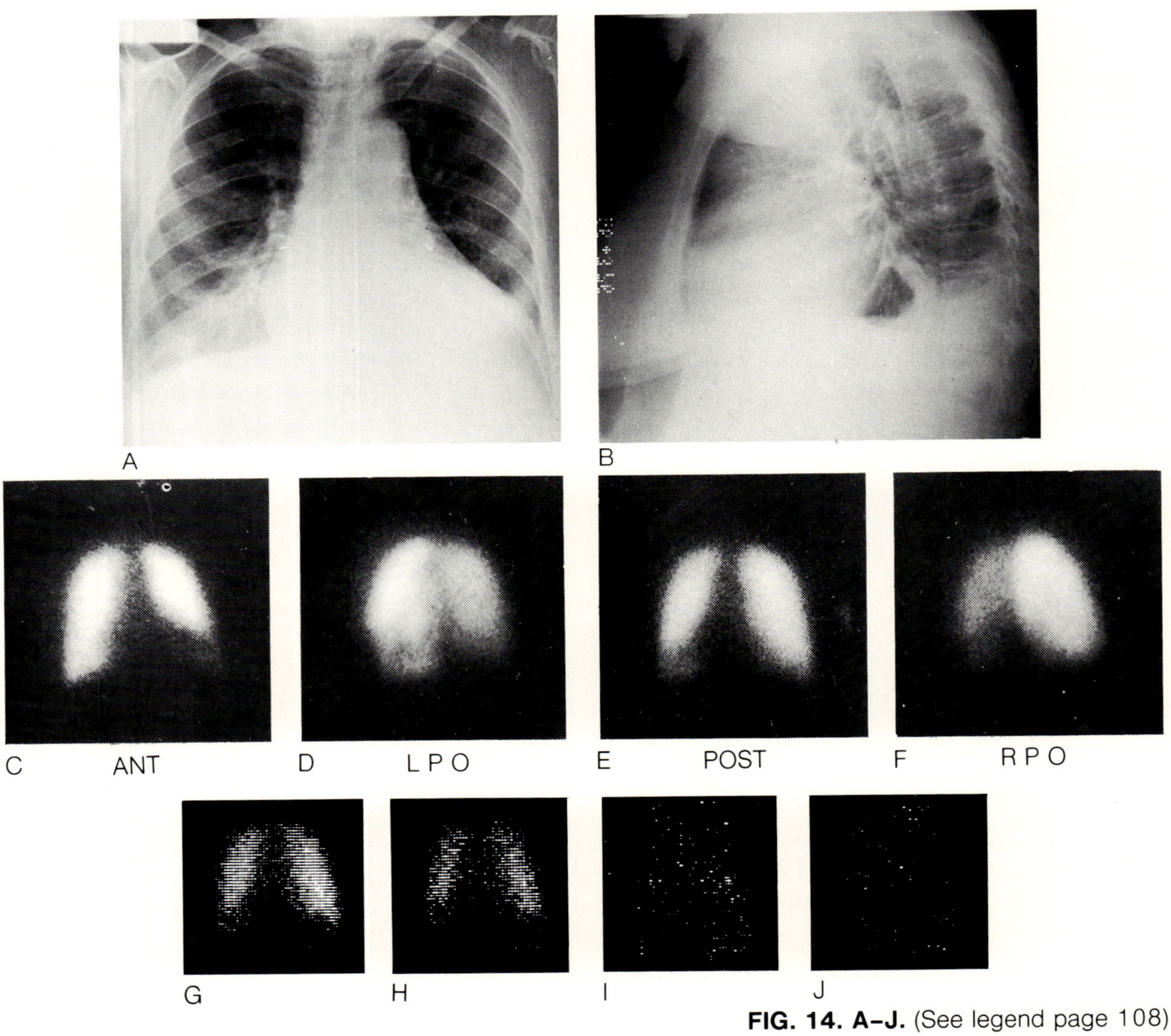


**FIG. 14. A–J.** (See legend page 108)

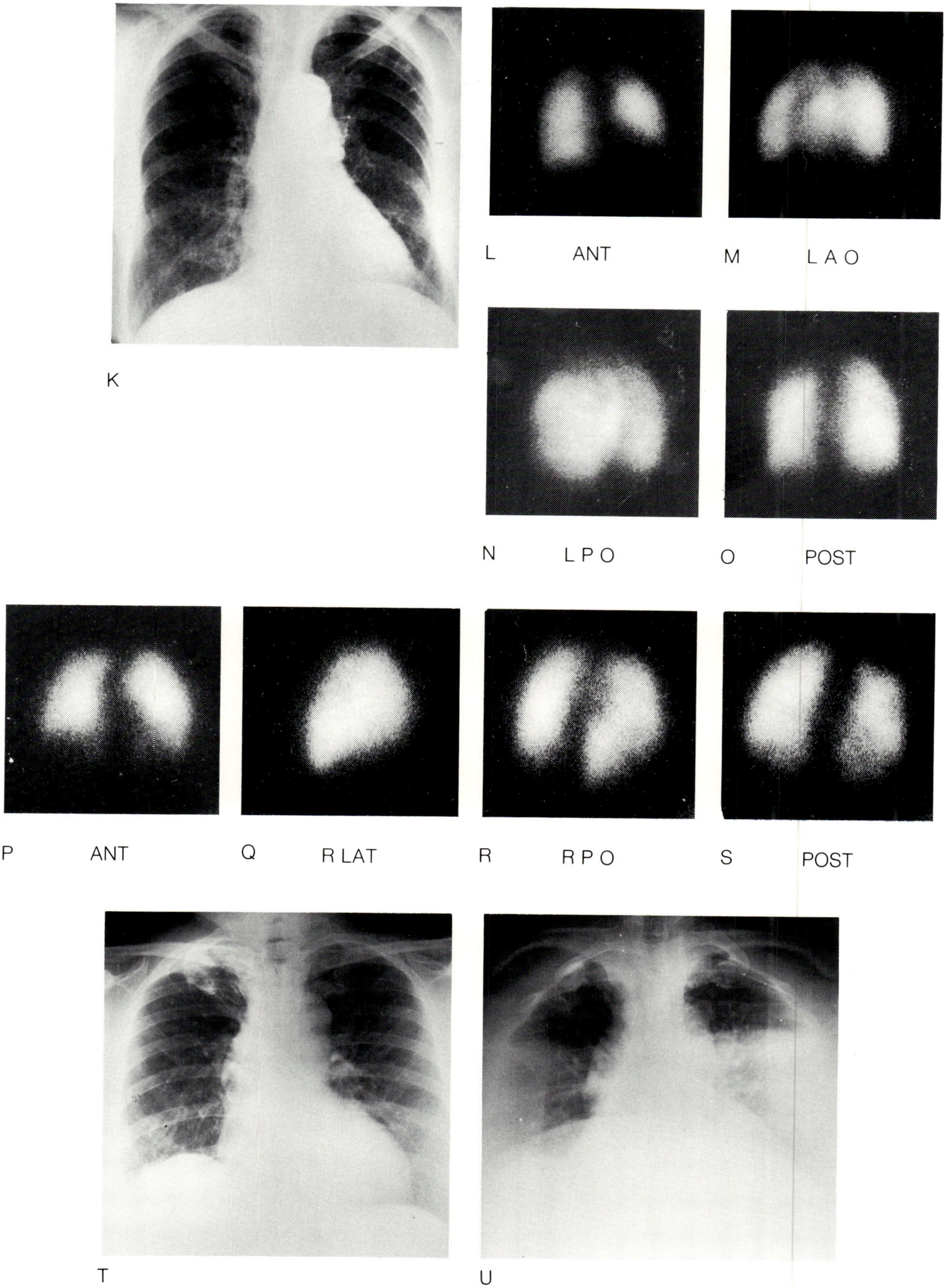


**FIG. 14. K–U.** (See legend next page)

**FIG. 14.** PNEUMONIA. Infiltrates in both lower lobes (**A** and **B**) are associated with diminished pulmonary perfusion in the same areas (**C** through **F**), and with decreased entry of xenon after rebreathing for two minutes (**G**, posterior view). Xenon cannot enter collapsed or liquid-filled alveoli. However, if some alveoli or alveolar ducts within an area of pneumonia are not filled with exudate, xenon may enter the remaining airspace but will be washed out without retention (**H** at 30 seconds, **I** at 60 seconds, **J** at 90 seconds). In cases where exudate spills into the more proximal airways or when bronchospasm occurs, impeded airflow may result in delayed washout of xenon, but this is not common in most pneumonias. In pneumonias and pulmonary edema, both of which normally resolve without leaving significant structural change, the abnormalities seen in chest x-rays and lung images correct themselves. Some infections and other diseases cause permanent damage to the lung, such as fibrocalcific changes and obliteration of capillaries (**K** through **O**, left upper lobe). Small parenchymal lesions may be seen as perfusion defects but escape detection on lower-resolution, single-view ventilation images. The patient's chest x-rays should be scrutinized for evidence of parenchymal disease to match the perfusion defects, lest these be misdiagnosed as a vascular disorder alone, for example as a (subsegmental) thromboembolism. X-rays should always be reviewed and special views taken if indicated. A perfusion defect in the right upper lobe (**P** through **S**) due to inactive tuberculosis (**T**) is better seen in lordotic view (**U**). In some cases, tomography may be necessary to define a lesion. Note that a pulmonary infarct cannot be differentiated from pneumonia on the basis of x-rays and lung images, though it is rare to have a single infarct without evidence of embolism to other lung areas.

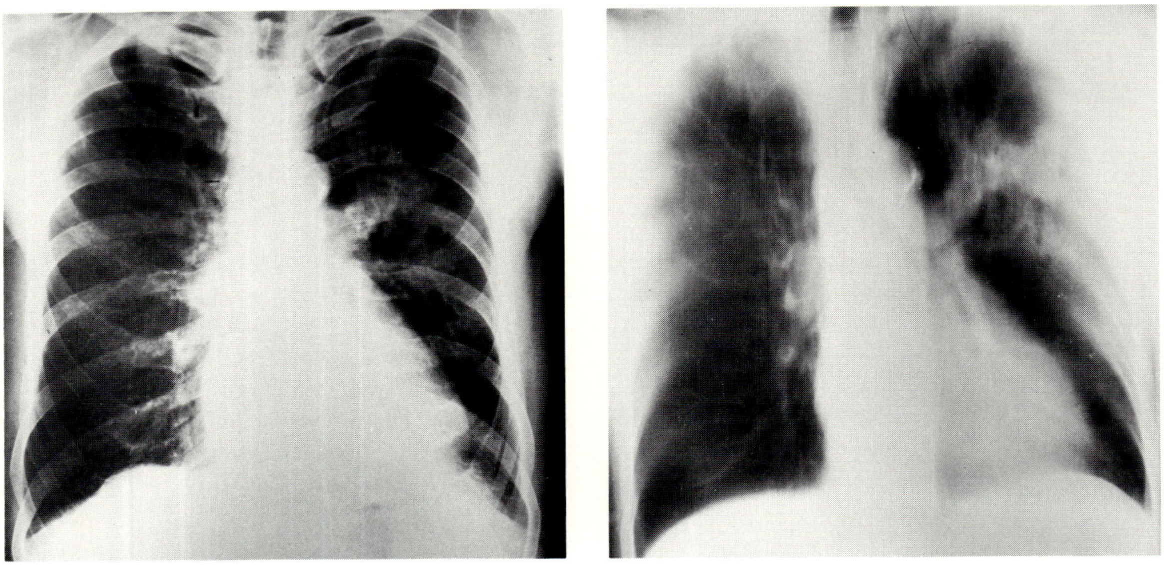

A

B

**FIG. 15. A, B.** (See legend next page)

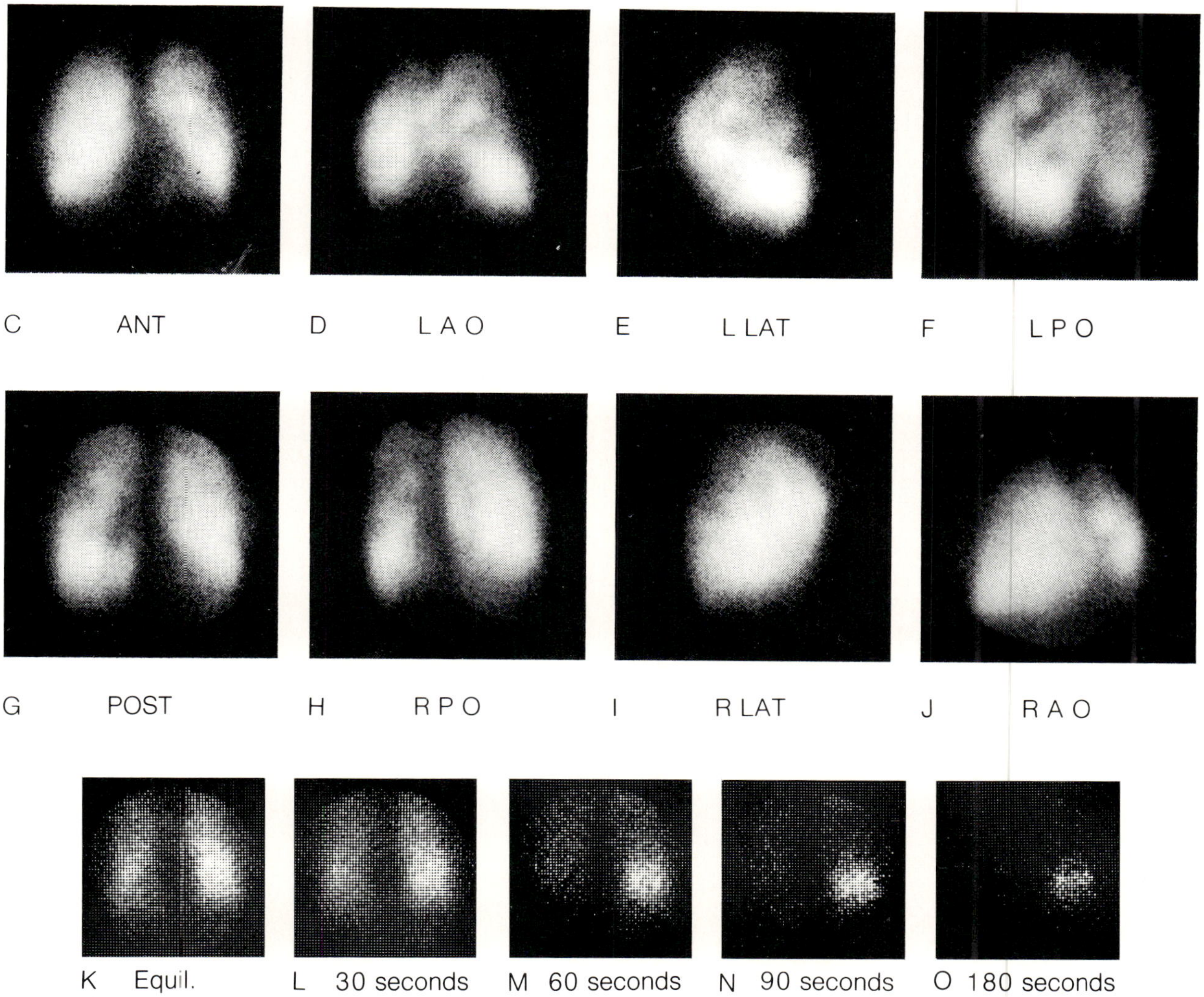


Ventilation Lung Images are Posterior Views

**FIG. 15.** ALVEOLAR CELL CARCINOMA. When acini are filled with tumor cells, the chest x-ray (**A**, and tomogram **B** showing density in the left mid-lung field and patent bronchus) and lung images (**C** through **O**) are similar to those seen with pneumonia. In contrast to carcinoma of the bronchus, major airway obstruction is not a feature of alveolar cell carcinoma unless caused by metastases to hilar lymph nodes, or by plugging of the bronchus with secretions and desquamated tumor cells. Note that this patient has evidence of other abnormalities, including obstructive airway disease in the right lower lung field, which may be of importance to the surgeon contemplating left pneumonectomy.

## CARDIOVASCULAR DISORDERS

Lung imaging is not usually performed in adults for evaluation of cardiac disorders, but since these patients may at some time be suspected of having pulmonary embolism, the abnormal pattern due to each condition should be recognized, if present. Lung shape, contour, or size may be mechanically altered by cardiomegaly, aortic aneurysm, pleural effusion, etc. When hemodynamic disturbances occur, either with increased pulmonary blood flow (left-to-right shunts), decreased flow (e.g., pulmonary stenosis), or increased pulmonary resistance (pre- or postcapillary, such as idiopathic pulmonary hypertension, left ventricular failure, or mitral valve disease), alterations in the pulmonary vasculature are often detected on chest x-rays. However, perfusion lung images will only show abnormalities of *regional* blood flow, or an imbalance of blood supply to the right and left lungs, and cannot detect an overall increase or decrease of pulmonary circulation. Ventilation images are of value only in differentiating other diseases involving the lungs.

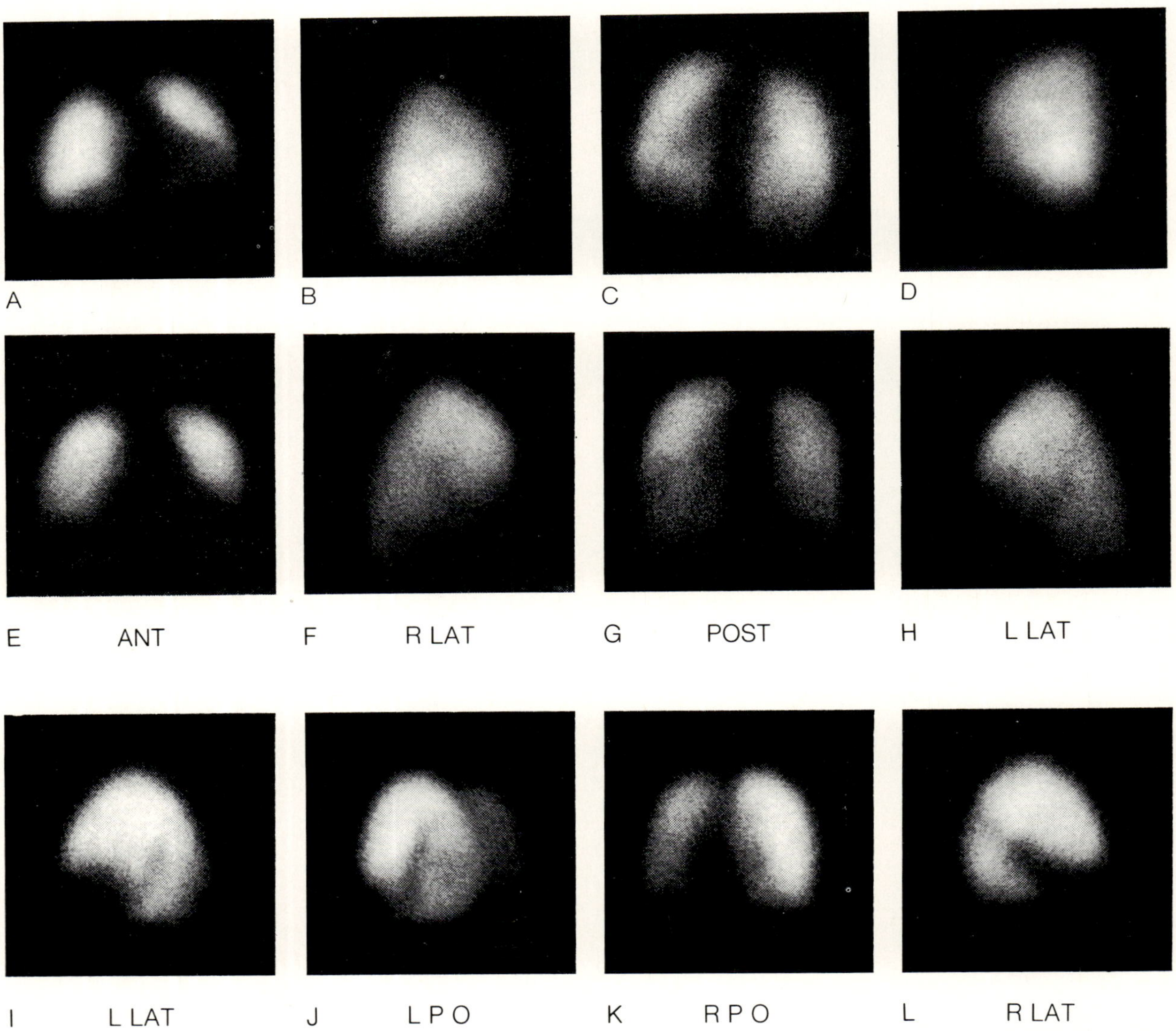


**FIG. 16. A–L.** (See legend next page)

**FIG. 16. CONGESTIVE CARDIAC FAILURE.** When cardiomegaly is present without cardiac failure, perfusion lung images (**A** through **D**) show enlargement of the cardiac space and preservation of the normally increasing gradient of activity from the upper to lower lung fields. With failure of the left ventricle, the pulmonary veins become distended, pulmonary venous pressure rises, and blood flow is usually redistributed from the lower to the upper lung fields (from posterior base to anterior apex, locally mediated by uncertain mechanisms), this last resulting in images showing reversal of the normal gradient of radioactivity (**E** through **H**, same patient 8 months later). Pulmonary edema, like pneumonia, causes patchy areas which are underperfused and poorly ventilated. Pleural effusions produce mechanical effects on the lungs, and depending on the mobility of pleural fluid surrounding the lung or entering the fissures, the defects may change with the position of the patient or be fixed relevant to pooling of the effusion at the time of injection. Rounding of the lung contours and fissure signs (**I** through **L**), as well as diminished volume, ventilation, and perfusion of a lobe or an entire lung, may occur depending on the quantity of effusion. Lung image defects are often explained by chest x-ray findings. Of course, positional differences of the patient in each examination must be borne in mind.

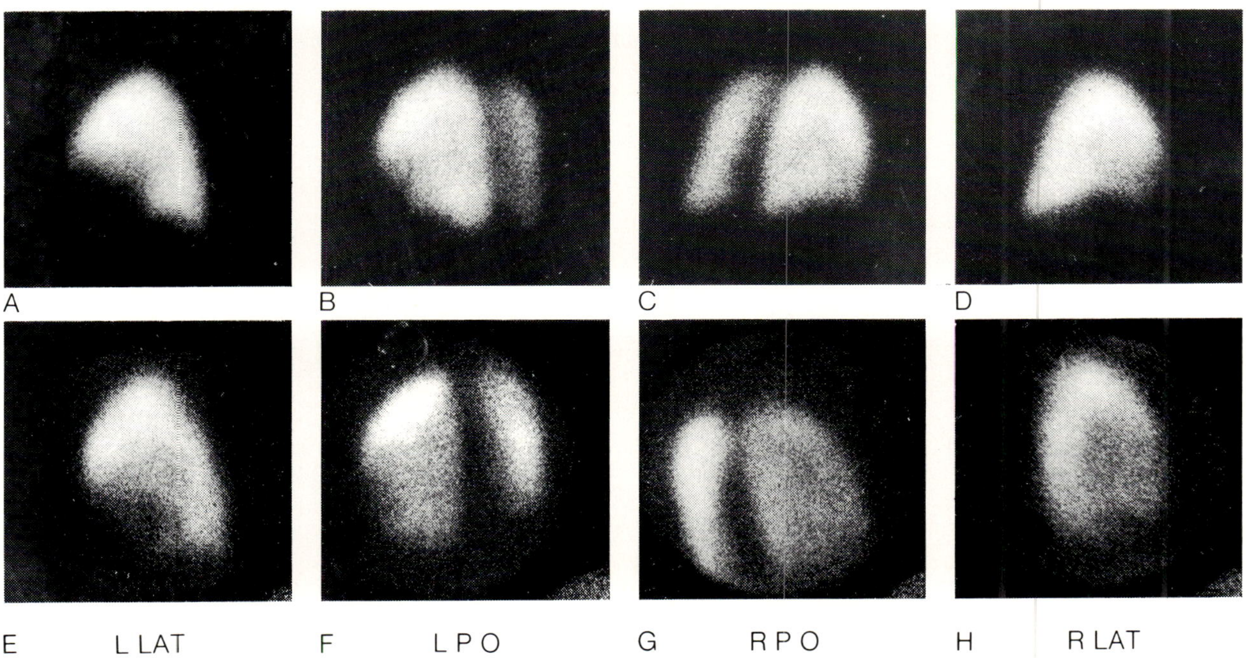


**FIG. 17. MITRAL VALVE DISEASE.** In patients with mitral valve disease, there is good correlation of left atrial pressure with the ratio of pulmonary blood flow to the upper and lower lung fields. Reversal of the gradient of activity is seen in a patient with mitral stenosis who was injected supine, before (**A** through **D**) and during an episode of cardiac failure (**E** through **H**), when the findings are more pronounced. Gradient reversal is nonspecific and also seen with other causes of pulmonary venous hypertension. In mitral valve disease, additional focal perfusion defects have also been described, especially in the right middle lobe, as well as ventilation abnormalities that are not of diagnostic value. When pulmonary embolism is suspected in these patients, angiography may be necessary to avoid confusion.

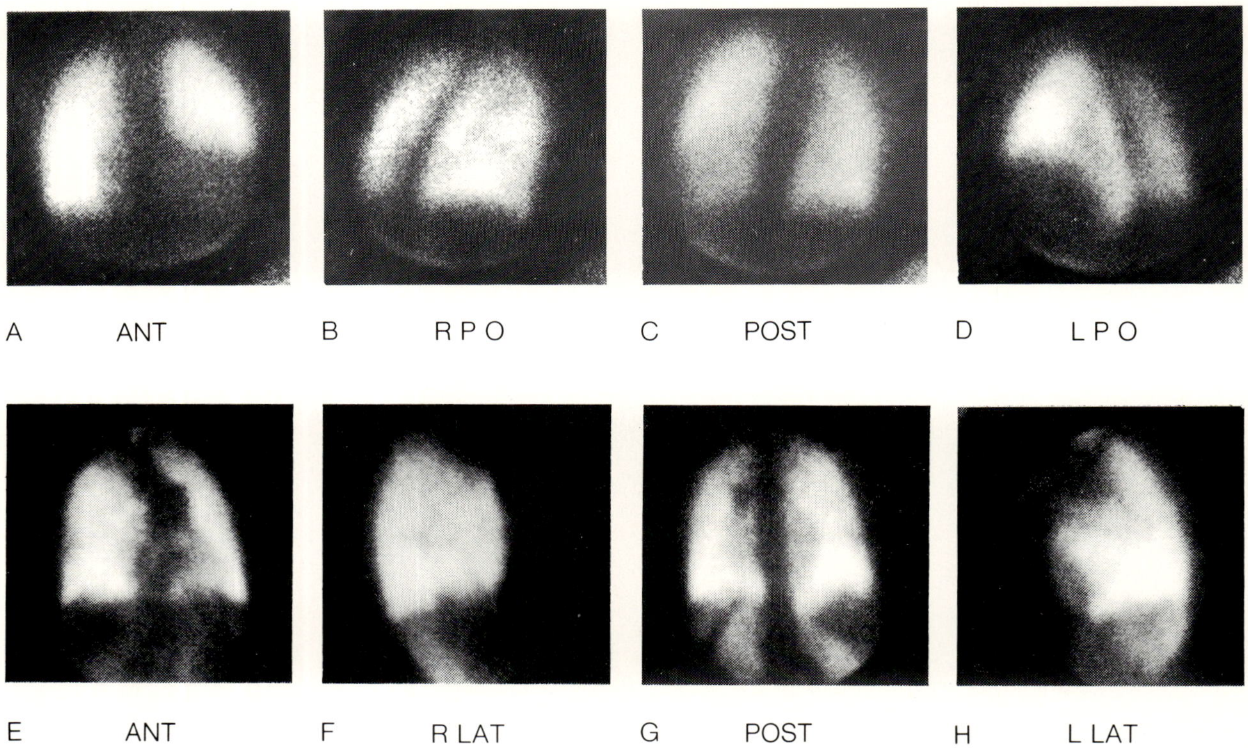


**FIG. 18. CONGENITAL HEART DISEASE.** Uneven distribution of macroaggregates in the right and left lungs may be seen when there are abnormal vascular pathways, either congenital or surgically created, or when branch stenoses cause diminished regional blood flow. Valvular stenoses and dilated cardiac chambers, which produce an angular relationship of the heart to the pulmonary arteries, may cause selective jetting of blood into either artery. Shunts, which allow a chronic pressure or volume overload of the pulmonary vasculature, may lead to structural changes in the lungs and uneven distribution of blood flow. Abnormal perfusion images are seen in a 23-year-old male with untreated truncus arteriosus (**A** through **D**). The right upper lung field is oligemic but normally ventilated (not shown). The reason for abnormal perfusion in any patient with congenital heart disease may be recognized with further workup but sometimes remains unclear. The individual congenital disorders will not be reviewed here. In patients with right-to-left shunts, particles that enter the systemic circulation become trapped in the small vessels of structures supplied by the aorta, in amounts proportional to their share of the cardiac output. If the kidneys are clearly visible on perfusion lung images, a right-to-left shunt should be suspected (**E** through **H**, a 52-year-old woman with "reopened" atrial septal defect). Because of the dual blood supply to the liver, particles may reach the liver via the hepatic artery but not via the portal vein (which normally provides 75 to 80 percent of the blood supply to the liver). They are filtered out by the splanchnic arteriolar-capillary bed and spleen. If the liver and spleen are visible but not the kidneys, then the preparation of macroaggregates contains excessive numbers of small particles that have passed through the pulmonary capillary bed to be phagocytosed by the reticuloendothelial system. The same results would be reproduced in other patients receiving the same preparation.

## DISORDERS OF THE CHEST WALL AND PLEURA

Poor exchange of respiratory gases may result from extrapulmonary disorders, which restrict the ability of the thoracic cage to act as a bellows. Kyphoscoliosis, ankylosing spondylitis, intercostal muscle spasm with rib fractures, pleural fibrosis, empyema or effusion, mesothelioma, and neuromuscular disorders are some of the conditions that may impair lung ventilation. When involvement is asymmetric, lung images show diminished ventilation and perfusion of the affected lung compared to the more normal contralateral lung. In most cases, the reason is evident from the chest x-ray.

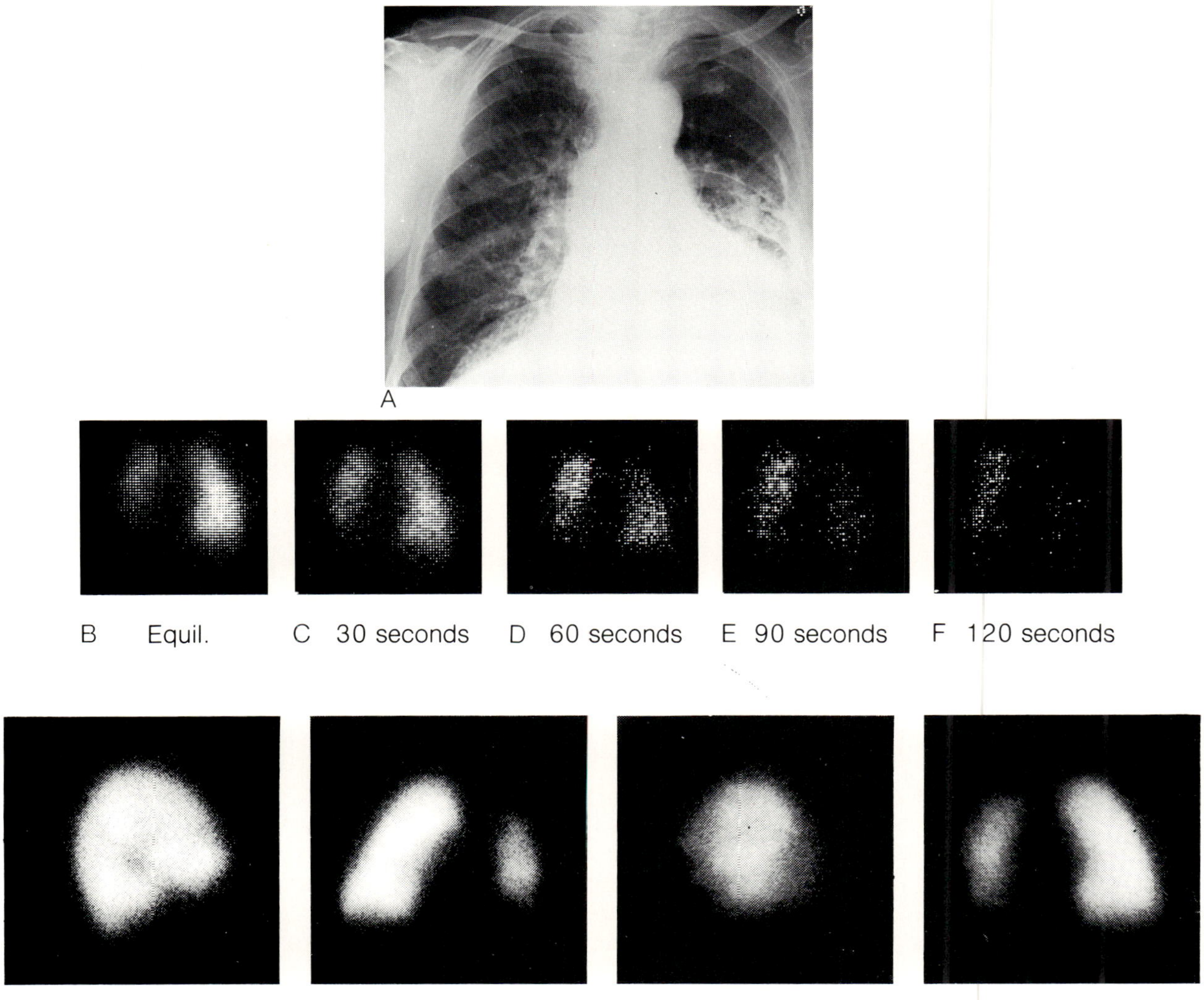


**FIG. 19. PLEURAL FIBROSIS.** Calcification of the pleura with small left hemithorax (**A**) results in decreased left lung volume and poor gas entry after rebreathing xenon for two minutes (**B,** posterior view). Delayed washout relative to the opposite lung (**C** through **F,** posterior views) is due to rigidity of the pleura, not to airway obstruction. Imbalanced perfusion results (**G** through **J**).

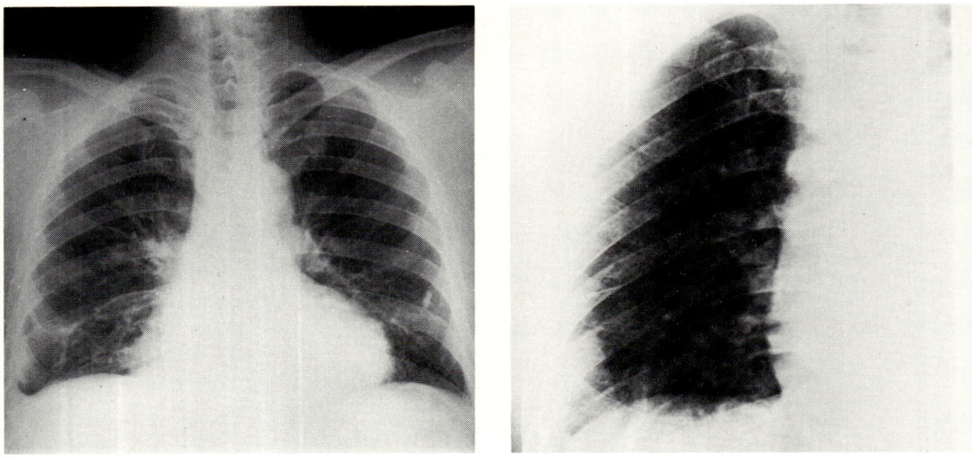

A B

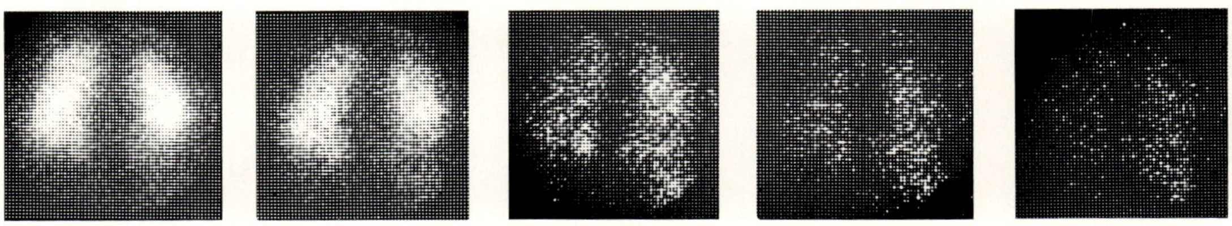

C Equil. D 30 seconds E 60 seconds F 90 seconds G 120 seconds

All Views are Posterior

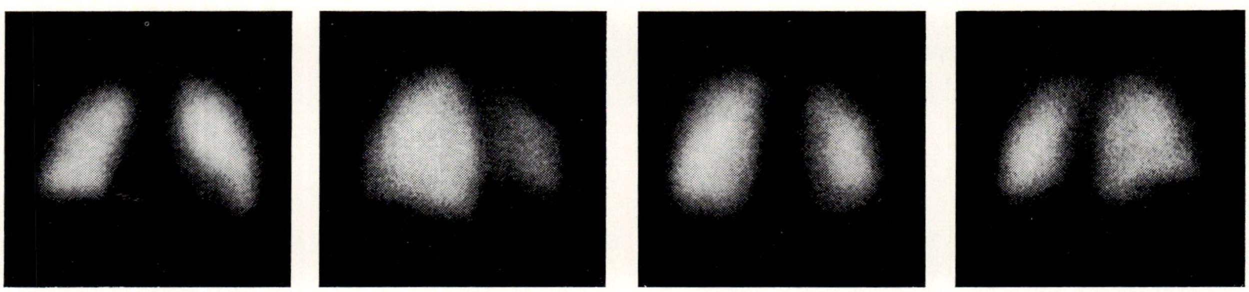

H ANT I LPO J POST K RPO

**FIG. 20.** **PLEURITIS.** A patient with right-sided pleuritic chest pain has radiographic findings of blunted right costophrenic angle and thickened pleura along adjacent chest wall (**A** and **B**), and slightly delayed washout of xenon (**C** through **G**) with subtle underperfusion (**H** through **K**) of the right lung compared to left. The findings may be transient and return to normal after acute pleural infections and trauma, which cause splinting of the chest wall and, thus, impairment of lung ventilation.

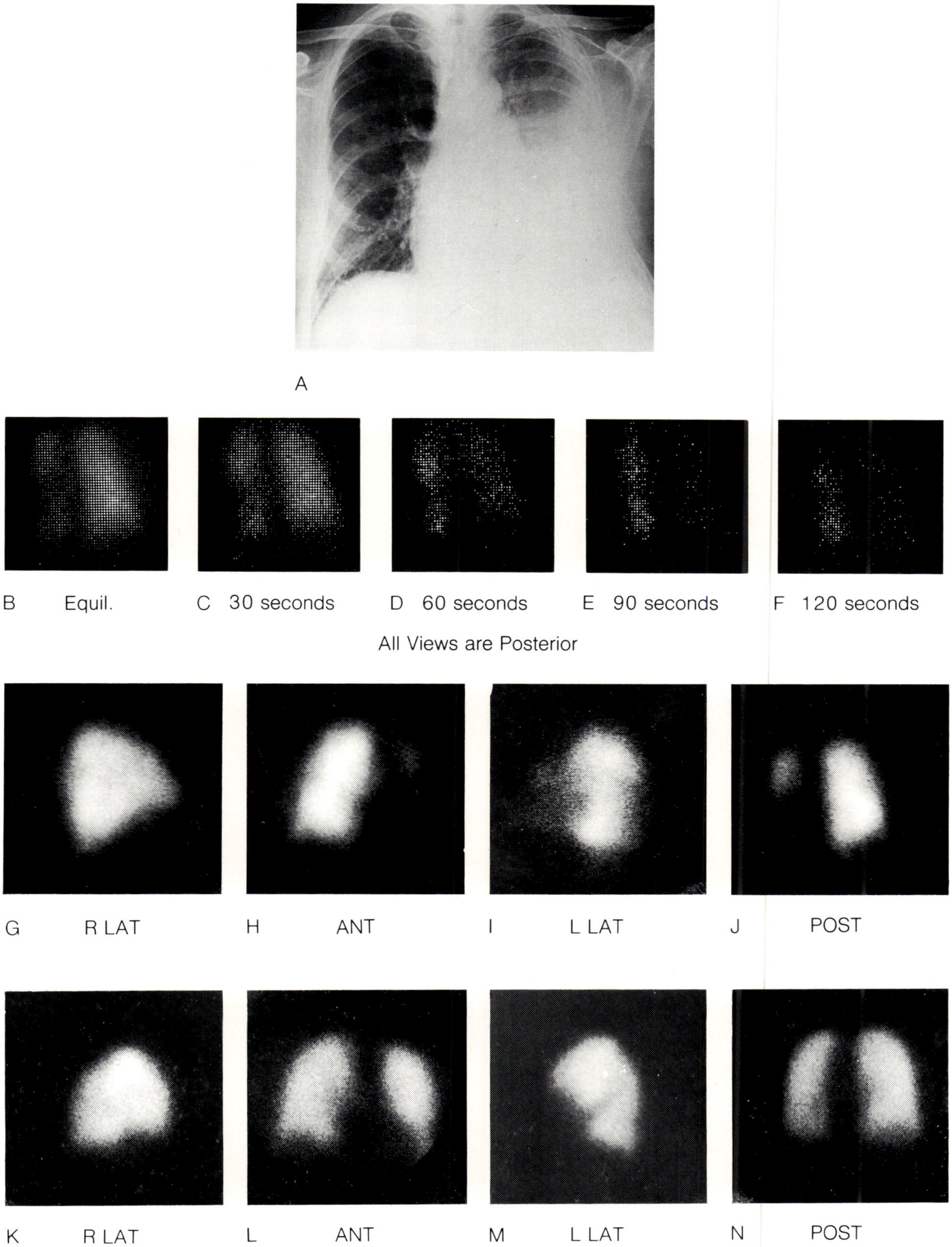


**FIG. 21. A–N.** (See legend next page)

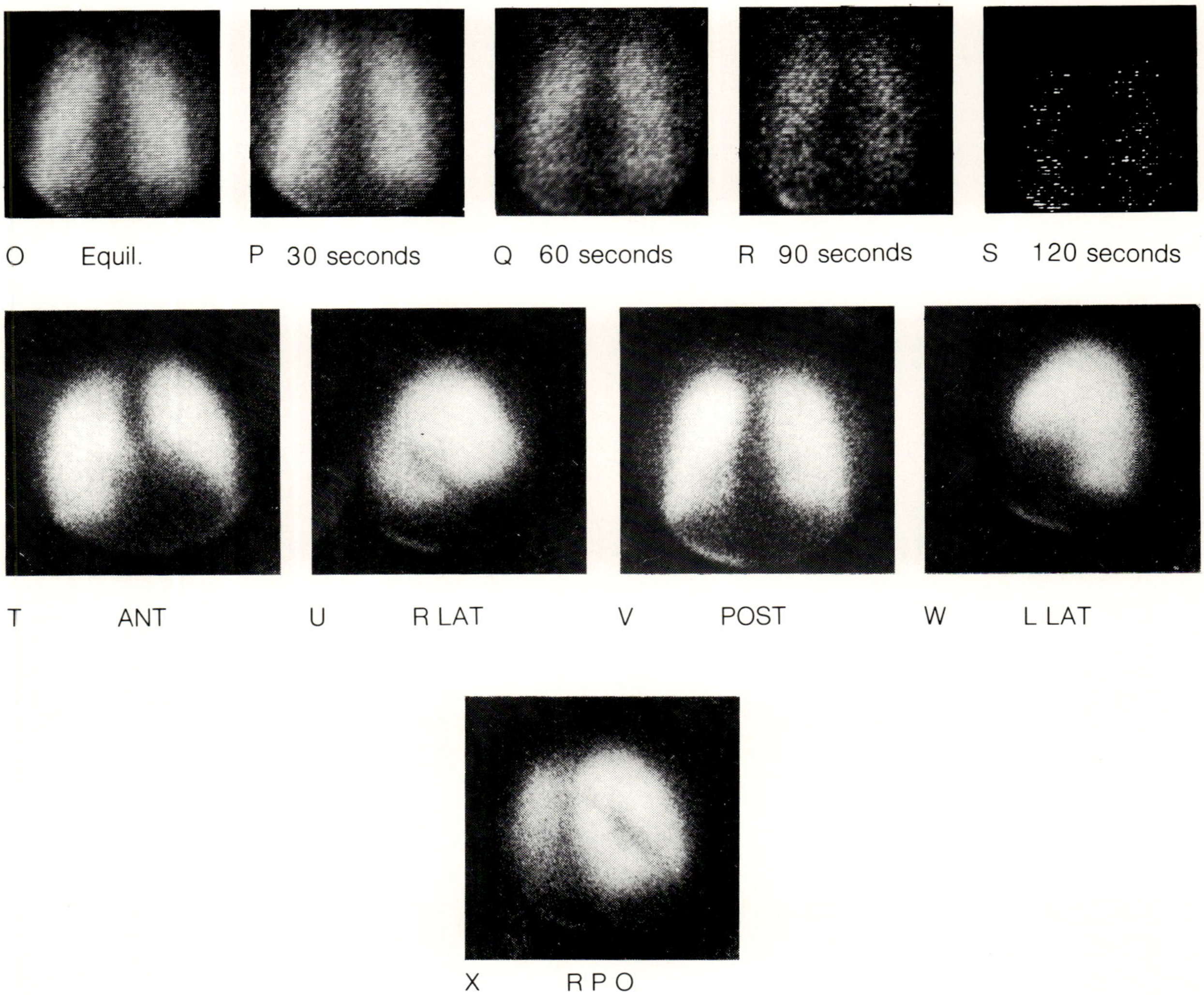


**FIG. 21. PLEURAL EFFUSION.** Excess fluid in the pleural space may result from cardiac failure (see Fig. 16) where the effects of both failure and effusion are seen in the lung images and x-rays. A massive effusion (**A**) will severely restrict the ability of a lung to expand, and thus cause decreased lung volume, poor alveolar gas exchange, and a shift of ventilation (**B** through **F**) and of perfusion (**G** through **J**) to the opposite lung. Small, mobile effusions of any etiology may gravitate to different regions of the pleural space relevant to the position of the patient at the time of examination. The result is varying or mismatched lesions in perfusion lung images and x-rays. No matching defect may be seen in the ventilation images because in the usual posterior view, the sheetlike effusion offers little photon attenuation. The physician must be careful not to interpret these unmatched perfusion defects as a pulmonary vascular disorder (including embolism). A small effusion in the left oblique fissure is seen only in the recumbent left lateral view (**M**) of perfusion images (**K** through **N**, from an eight-view study), but was not detectable in ventilation images or chest x-rays taken with the patient erect, until decubitus films were subsequently obtained. In another patient with normal ventilation images (**O** through **S**, posterior views) a defect seen in the left lateral view (**W**) of the perfusion study (**T** through **X**, from an eight-view study) could be misinterpreted as

occlusion of the pulmonary artery supplying the anterior basal segment if other views were not obtained, which would show the lesion to occupy the full length of the oblique fissure (**X**). With appropriate positioning of the patient, chest x-rays would show this fissure sign to be due to a pleural effusion.

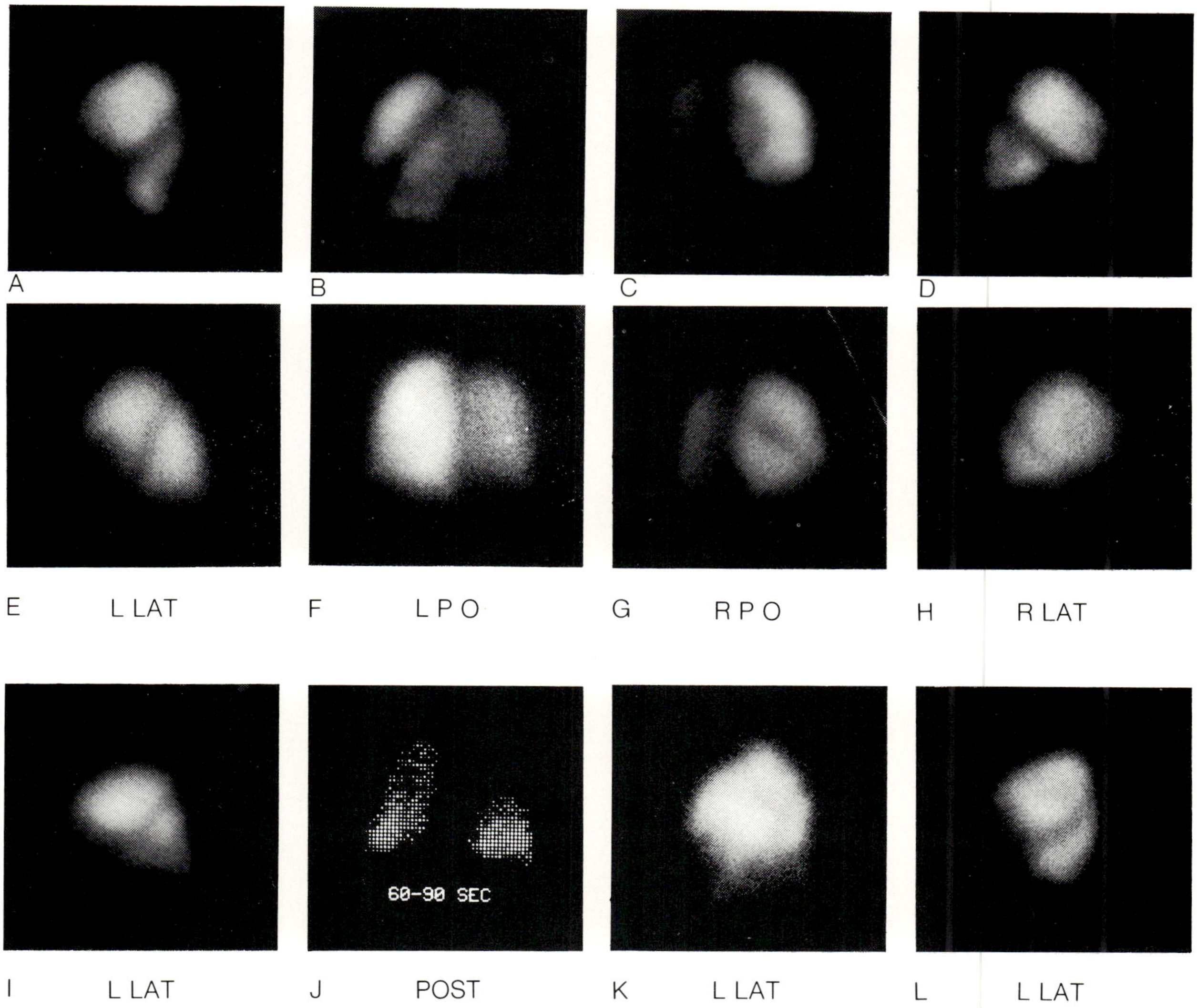


**FIG. 22.** FISSURE SIGN. A linear defect corresponding to a partial or full- length lung fissure may be due to fluid or fibrosis separating the lobes, or to these and other diseases that cause poor ventilation and/or perfusion of lung bordering the fissure. Thickening of the interlobar fissure, excess pleural fluid with cardiac failure (**A** through **D**) or without (**E** through **H**, another patient, but note in both cases changing defects due to shifting effusion when patient is repositioned), chronic obstructive pulmonary disease (**I**, and radioxenon washout **J**), major emboli with breakup into smaller fragments (**K**, with **L** taken 10 days later), and the rare cases of microemboli alone may all produce this nonspecific defect. Its main importance is that it should not be misdiagnosed as a segmental perfusion defect in the lung.

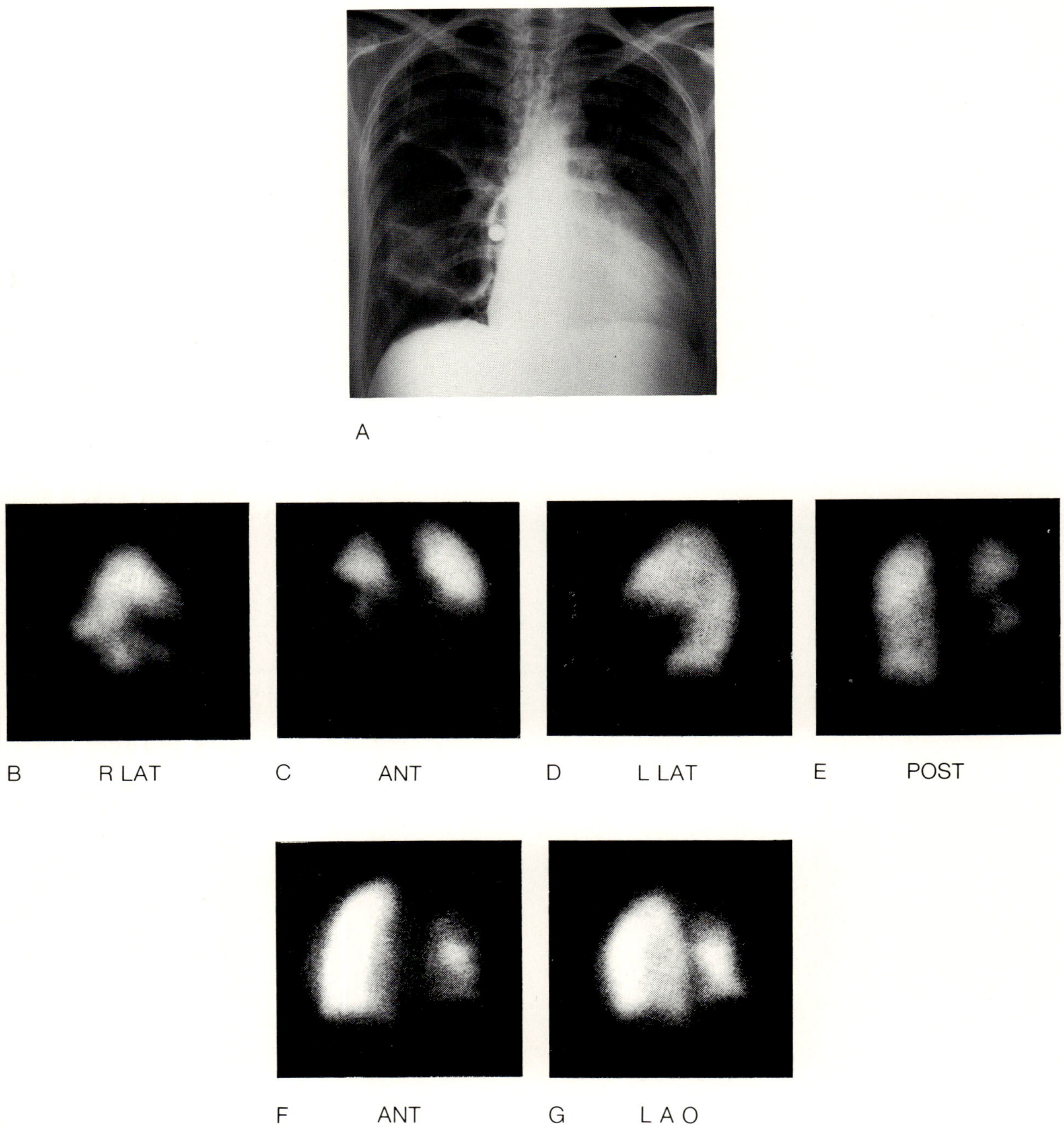


**FIG. 23. PNEUMOTHORAX.** Air in the pleural cavity allows the lung to collapse away from the chest wall and may prevent full expansion of the lung, resulting in impaired ventilation and perfusion. Pneumothorax in the presence of pleural adhesions may cause bizarre distortions of the normal lung appearance (**A** through **E**), whereas stiffness of the lung due to pulmonary edema or extensive pneumonic infiltrate tends to preserve the shape of the lung (albeit smaller, **F** and **G**) when complete collapse does not occur. In any case, the key to diagnosing concurrent pulmonary embolism is the finding of unmatched segmental perfusion defects in the opposite lung (see Fig. 6).

## DISORDERS OF THE DIAPHRAGM

Neurologic and various other diseases affecting the skeletal musculature of the chest wall, abdomen, or diaphragm may cause mild to severe impairment of lung ventilation. Poliomyelitis, muscular dystrophy, myasthenia gravis, high cervical trauma, and other diseases affecting ventilation of both lungs as a unit will not be considered here since lung imaging is better suited to analysis of regional abnormality.

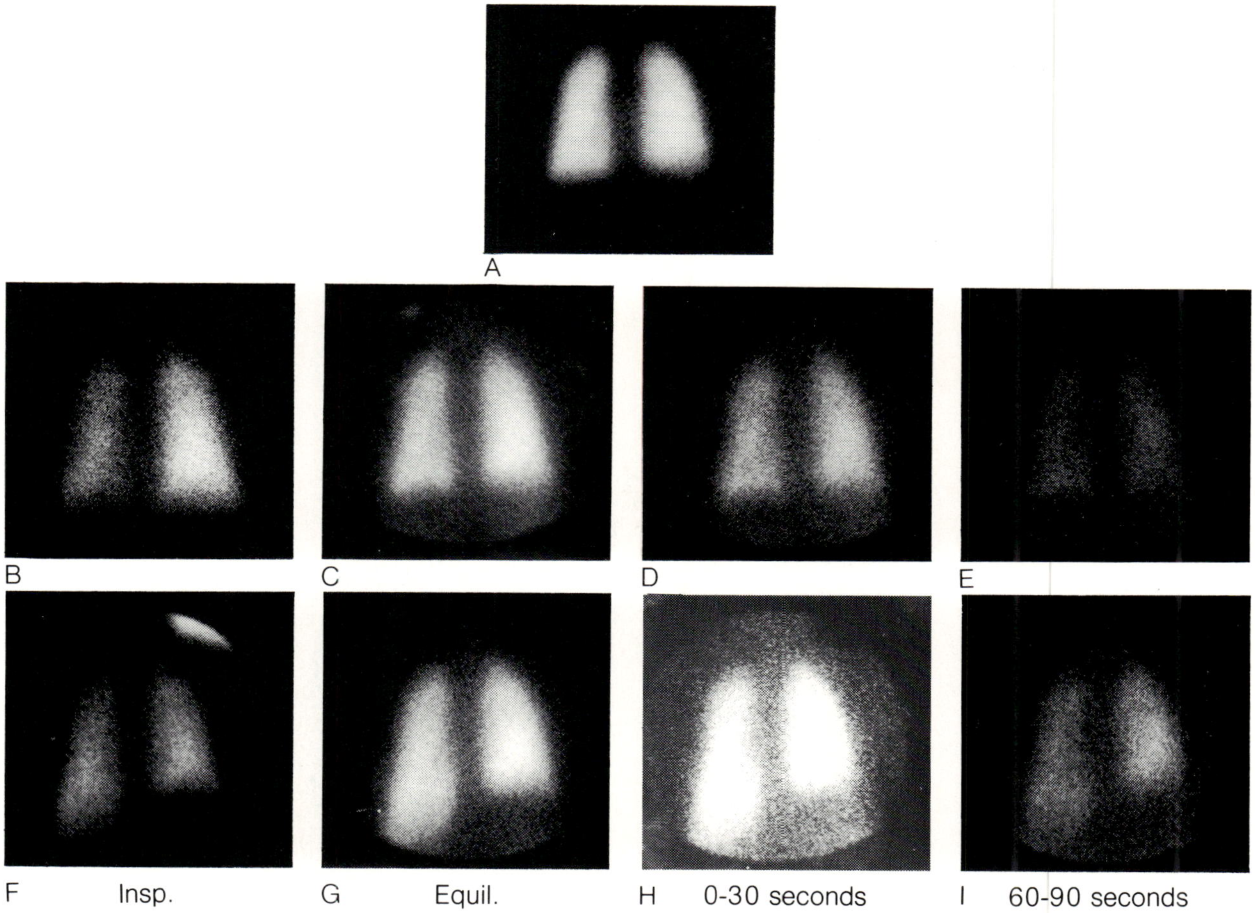


All Views are Posterior

**FIG. 24. PHRENIC NERVE PACING.** A 16-year-old patient with central hypoventilation syndrome probably resulting from encephalitis five years prior, offers an opportunity for the observation of the effects of phrenic nerve stimulation. Resting perfusion image is normal (**A**). Following overnight stimulation of the left phrenic nerve at the rate of 12 per minute but with the pacer off at the time of study, single breath ventilation image (**B**) shows poor entry of xenon into the left lung due to fatigue of the left hemidiaphragm compared to unstimulated right hemidiaphragm. Images after the patient's unassisted rebreathing of xenon (**C**) and during washout (**D** and **E**) show approximately equal lung volumes and symmetric ventilation. Repeat study with left phrenic nerve stimulation (**F** through **I**) shows that contraction of left hemidiaphragm causes an increased left lung volume at the expense of the right, and slightly better ventilation of the left lung compared to the right. (Images courtesy of Dr. William W. L. Glenn, Dr. Alexander Gottschalk, and Dr. Robert C. Lange.)

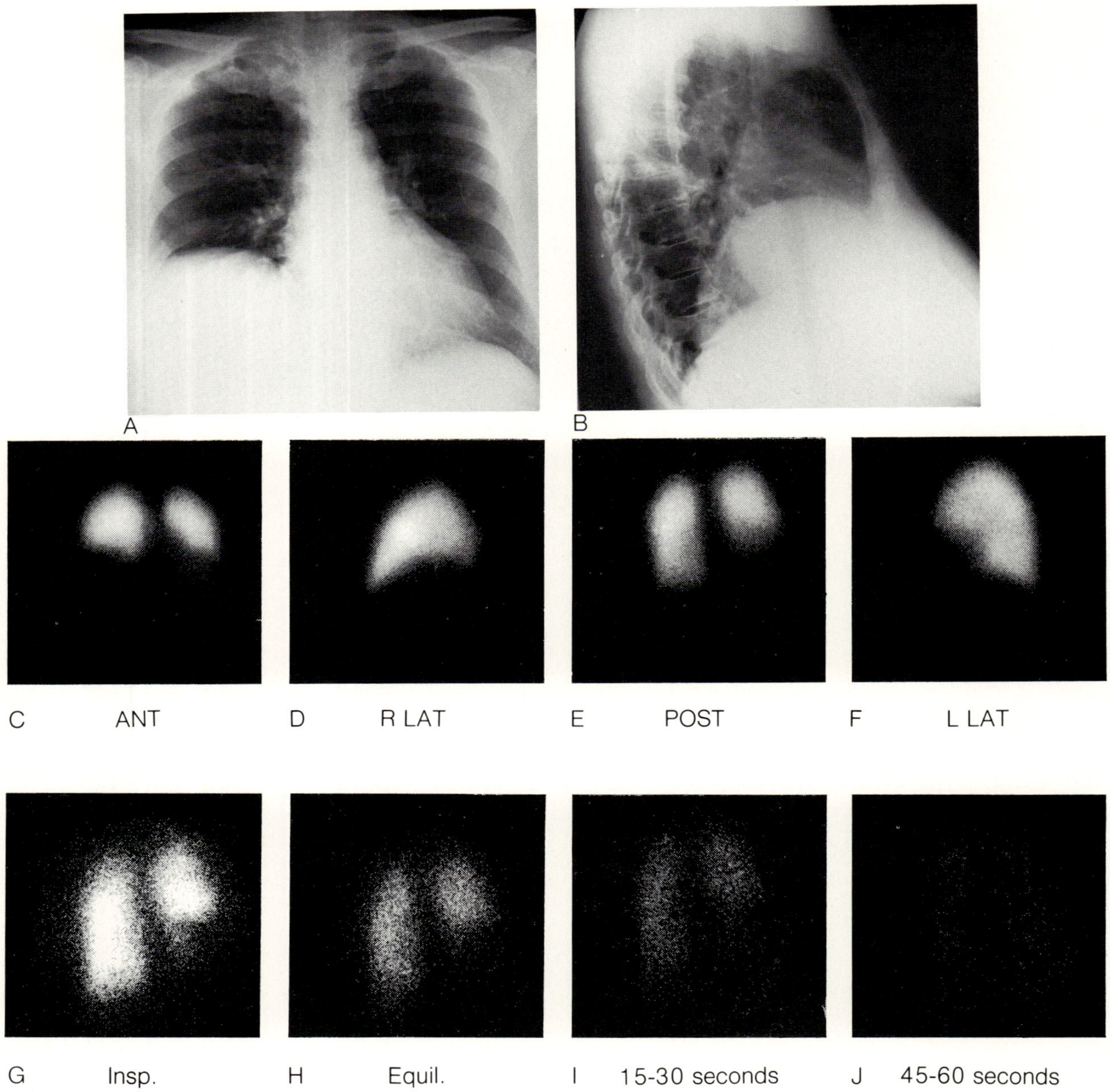


**FIG. 25. EVENTRATION OF THE DIAPHRAGM.** Eventration or paralysis of a hemidiaphragm results in a high position of the liver and/or other abdominal contents, and decreased lung volume (**A** and **B**), which is matched in perfusion (**C** through **F**) and ventilation images (**G** through **J**, posterior views). Note that the normally concave contour of the lung base is preserved but with a more acute posterior costophrenic angle. In contrast, a subpulmonary effusion will often change its location in the various positions of the patient and cause rounding and hypoperfusion of the lung base. Localized eventration and herniations of the diaphragm permit upward protrusion of portions of abdominal viscera such as liver, stomach, or intestine, a condition usually causing focal concave defects in the images of the adjacent lung. If Tc-99m sulphur colloid or pertechnetate are administered, normal liver or stomach can be shown to occupy the area of the lung defect, unless the lung defect is due to a mass lesion in the lung itself.

## Suggested Reading


Bateman NT, Coakley AJ, Croft DN, et al: Ventilation-perfusion lung scans for pulmonary emboli. Accuracy of Reporting. Eur J Nucl Med 2:201–203, 1977

Bianco JA, Shafer RB: Implications of liver activity associated with $^{133}$Xe ventilation lung scans. Clin Nucl Med 3:176–178, 1978

Biello DR, Mattar AG, McKnight RC, et al: Ventilation-perfusion studies in suspected pulmonary embolism. AJR 133:1033–1037, 1979

Biello DR, Mattar AG, Csei-Wusu A,et al: Interpretation of indeterminate lung scintigrams. Radiology 133:189–194, 1979

Chervu LR, Vallabhajosula SR, Blaufox MD: Quality control of technetium-labelled lung imaging agents. Int J Nucl Med Biol 4:201–203, 1977

Ciofetta G, Pratt TA, Hughes JM: Regional pulmonary perfusion assessed with continuous intravenous infusion of Kr-81m; a comparison with Tc-99m macroaggregates. J Nucl Med 19:1126–1130, 1978

Coates G, Nahmias C: Xenon-127. Prog Nucl Med 5:47–68, 1978

Diagnostic Decision-Process in Suspected Pulmonary Embolism. Report of the Herlev Hospital Study Group. Lancet 1. 8130:1336–1338, 1979

Dziuk B, Reuter TD: Diagnostic usefulness of difference between the results of functional ventilation scanning and perfusion scanning of the lungs. Radiol Diagn (Berl) 18:533–542, 1977

Fazio F, Lavender JP, Steiner RE: $^{81m}$Kr Ventilation and $^{99m}$Tc perfusion scans in chest disease: comparison with standard radiographs. AJR 130:421–428, 1978

Fazio F, Lavender JP, Steiner RE: Radioisotopes, chest radiology and lung physiology. J Belge Radiol 61:219–228, 1978

Fairshter RD, Riley CA: Acute respiratory failure: a rare complication of perfusion photoscintigraphy in a patient with bullous emphysema. Am J Med Sci 275:193–197, 1978

Fischer KC, McNeil BJ: The indeterminate lung scan: its characteristics and its association with pulmonary embolism. Eur J Nucl Med 4:49–53, 1979

Godfrey S, McKenzie S: The place of radioisotopic lung function studies in paediatrics. Arch Dis Child 52:859–864, 1977

Li DK, Treves S. Heyman S, et al: Krypton-81m: a better radiopharmaceutical for assessment of regional lung function in children. Radiology 130:741–747, 1979

McGoldrick PJ, Rudd TG, Figley MM, et al: What becomes of pulmonary infarcts. AJR 133:1039–1045, 1979

McLaughlin GL, Burt RW, Depalma B, et al: Effect of ventilation images on observer interpretation of lung perfusion examinations. AJR 128:1037–1038, 1977

Makhija MC, Bronfman HJ, Lange RC, et al: Ventilation patterns mimicking COPD in patients with diaphragmatic pacing for Ondine's Curse. Radiology 129:111–116, 1978

Mizuno M, Miyakawa K, Mizutani A, et al: The use of pulmonary scintigraphy for endobronchial foreign bodies. Auris Nasus Larynx 5:49–53, 1978

Nielsen PE, Kirchner PT, Cerber FH: Oblique views in lung perfusion scanning: clinical utility and limitations. J Nucl Med 18:967–972, 1977

Rabinovitch M, Rosenthal A, Sade RH, et al: Regional lung function studies and radionuclide angiography in d-transposition of the great arteries. Pediatr Res 11:1117–1121, 1977

Ramos M, Baumann HR, Muhlberger F: Perfusion and ventilation imaging in pulmonary tuberculosis. Clin Nucl Med 3:233–242, 1978

Reba RC, Secker-Walker RH, Poulose KP: Nuclear medicine procedures in diagnosis of pulmonary diseases. Primary Care 5:465–485, 1978

Reichel J: Pulmonary embolism. Med Clin North Am 61:1309–1318, 1977

Savoca CJ, Gamsu G, Brito AC: The effect of acute pulmonary edema on pulmonary vascular resistance: significance for the interpretation of dilated upper lobe vessels on chest radiographs. Invest Radiol 12:488–495, 1977

Schall GL, McDonald HD, Carr LB, et al: Xenon ventilation-perfusion lung scans. The early diagnosis of inhalation injury. JAMA 240:2441–2445, 1978

Seaton D, Ogilvie CM: Regional lung function in asymptomatic cigarette smokers. Am Rev Respir Dis 118:265–270, 1978

Secker-Walker RH: Pulmonary physiology, pathology, and ventilation-perfusion studies. J Nucl Med 19:961–968, 1978

Susskind H, Atkins HL, Klopper JF, et al: Xenon-127 ventilation studies. Prog Nucl Med 5:144–170, 1978

Susskind H, Ellis KJ, Atkins HL, et al: Studies of whole-body retention and clearance of inhaled noble gases. Prog Nucl Med 5:13–34, 1978

Taplin GV: The history of lung imaging with radionuclides. Semin Nucl Med 9:178–185, 1979

Taplin GV, Chopra SK: Inhalation lung imaging with radioactive aerosols and gases, Prog Nucl Med 5:119–143, 1978

Taplin GV, Chopra SK: Lung perfusion-inhalation scintigraphy in obstructive airway disease and pulmonary embolism. Radiol Clin North Am 16:491–513, 1978

Tsou B: Pulmonary embolism: dilemmas in diagnosis and therapy. Primary Care 5:397–409, 1978

Viamonte M, Jr., Koolpe H, Janowitz W, et al: Pulmonary thromboembolism—update. JAMA 243:2229–2234, 1980

# 3/Thyroid Imaging

Currently, most thyroid imaging is performed with iodine-123 sodium iodide or Tc-99m sodium pertechnetate. Thyroid imaging performed following the oral administration of radioactive sodium iodide is, in large part, a representation of thyroid function. The greater the radioactive iodine uptake, the greater will be the quantity of tracer delivered to the gland. Hence, the definition and size of the thyroid image will vary with the ability of the thyroid to take up the radioactive material. Following the trapping of the radioiodide and its subsequent organification, the radioiodine becomes incorporated into thyroid hormone as it is stored in the gland, and it is in this form that the radionuclide image of the thyroid is obtained. Several isotopes of iodine have been employed for clinical imaging: I-123, I-125 and I-131.

In the past, since I-131 was commonly used in the determination of the thyroidal radioactive iodine uptake, most thyroid imaging had been performed with this tracer. Since a dose in excess of 25 μCi of I-131 sodium iodide is usually given for imaging, the radiation exposure from this tracer should be borne in mind. In patients with a radioactive iodine uptake in the normal range, the radiation dose to the thyroid from I-131 is about 2 rads/μCi.

With the increasing availability of cyclotron-produced isotopes in recent years, I-123 has been steadily replacing I-131 for thyroid studies. There are a number of favorable characteristics associated with I-123: a relatively short half-life of 13 hours, no emission of beta radiation, and a low radiation dose to the thyroid. Following the oral administration of I-123 sodium iodide, the radiation dose to the thyroid in the normal individual is about 0.02 rads/μCi while for I-131 the radiation dose is almost 100 times greater. Moreover, the principal gamma energy of I-123 at 159 KeV makes it an attractive radioisotope for imaging with both the gamma camera and rectilinear scanner. The usual adult dose of I-123 sodium iodide is about 100 to 400 μCi.

The employment of I-125 for thyroid imaging has been limited. Although it is not a beta emitter, its very low gamma energy and relatively long half-life have not been considered favorable characteristics for purposes of imaging.

During the past several years, Tc-99m sodium pertechnetate has been frequently used for thyroid imaging. Unlike iodide, the pertechnetate ion ($TcO_4^-$) becomes trapped in the thyroid but does not become organified. The usual adult dose is about 5 mCi administered intravenously approximately 15 to 30 minutes prior to imaging.

There is some controversy concerning pertechnetate thyroid imaging in regard to the imaging of thyroid nodules. Disparate results have been reported in a number of instances in which a nodule was found to be ''cold'' or nonfunctioning on radioiodine imaging while on the Tc-99m study the same area showed normal or even increased radioactivity. Since one of the cardinal uses of thyroid imaging is to determine whether or not a nodule is ''cold,'' or nonfunctioning, and therefore whether or not the possibility of thyroid neoplasm should be considered, the reliability of pertechnetate imaging in the patient with a thyroid nodule has been open to question. I-123 sodium iodide appears to be a more dependable agent.

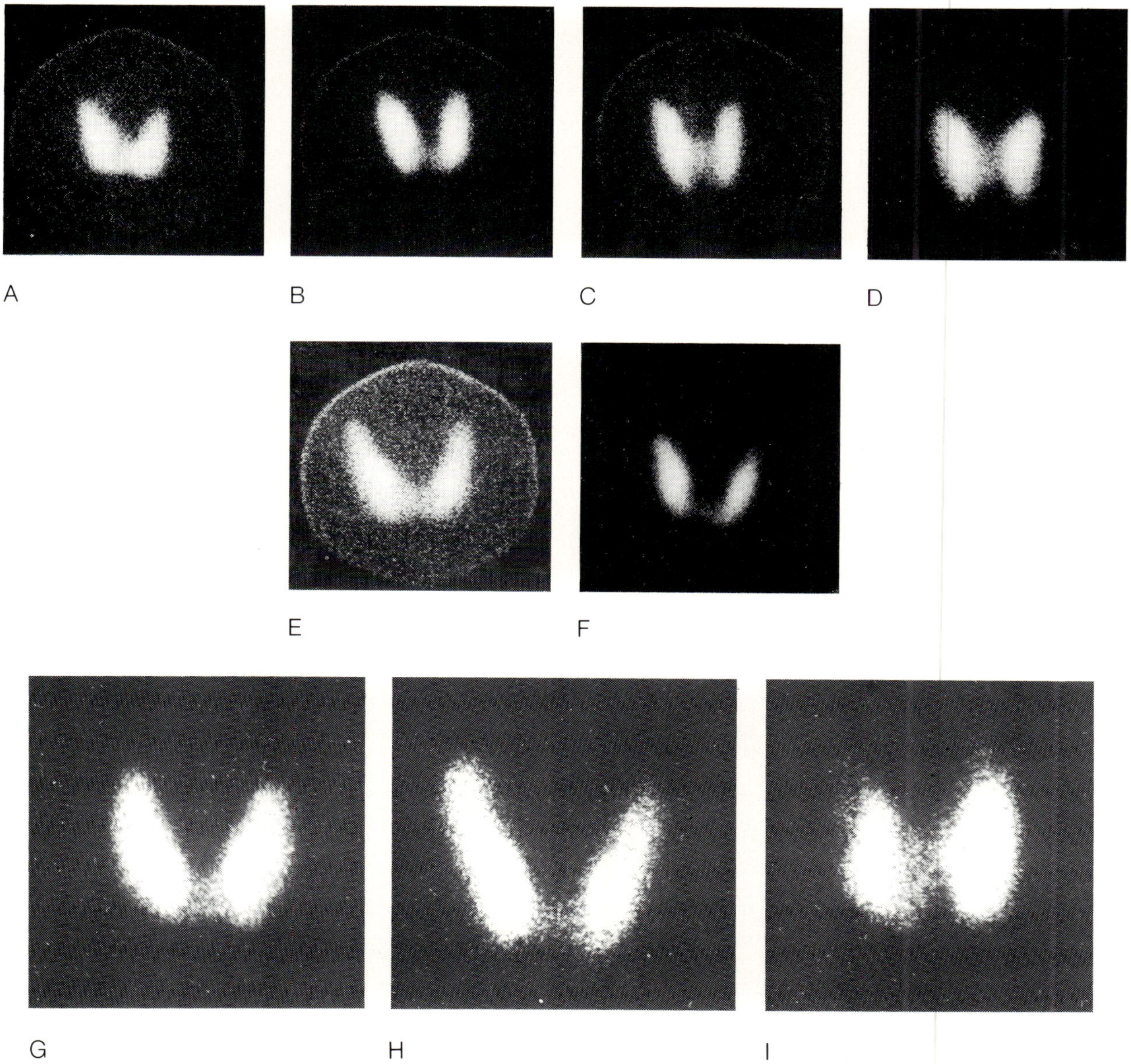


**FIG. 1. NORMAL THYROID IMAGING.** There is great variability among patients in both thyroid size and configuration. In the patient with relatively symmetrical lobes, each lobe measures approximately 3 to 5.5 cm longitudinally; this is, in part, related to body build. Where the mass of each lobe is greatest centrally, there will be relatively increased radioactivity. With reduced mass at the extremes of both lower and upper poles, reduced radioactivity is visible. There is sometimes clear-cut demonstration of the isthmus (I-123 sodium iodide).

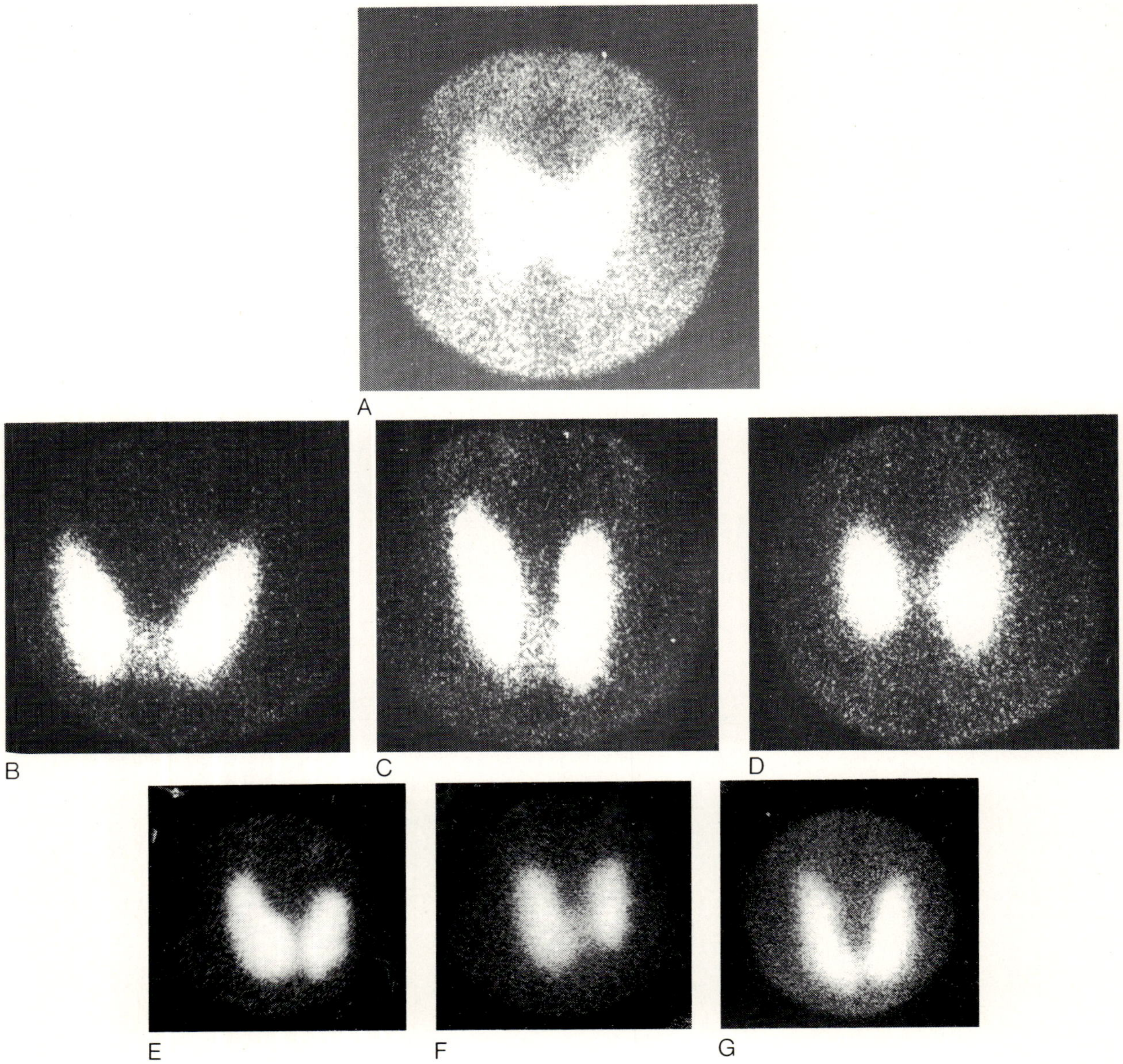


**FIG. 2. NORMAL THYROID IMAGING WITH Tc-99m SODIUM PERTECHNETATE.** Unlike thyroid imaging with radioiodine, areas of increased radioactivity outside the thyroid gland may be seen in the field of view with pertechnetate imaging. These include the salivary glands, the entry and presence of salivary secretions in a number of structures (buccal and oral cavities, esophagus), and the blood background radioactivity. The last is especially noted in cases of low thyroid uptake of pertechnetate. **A.** Normal thyroid imaging. Note the blood background radioactivity. **B.** Symmetrical gland in which the isthmus is well defined. **C.** Both lobes are elongated, with slight elevation of the right as compared to the left. **D.** Suggestion of small pyramidal lobe at left upper pole. **E** through **G.** Less background radioactivity.

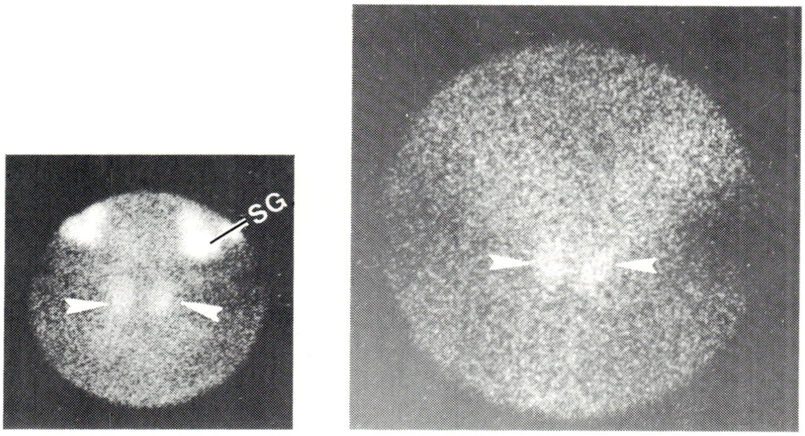


A B

**FIG. 3. IDENTIFYING THE PRESENCE OF A THYROID GLAND IN INFANTS WITH Tc-99m SODIUM PERTECHNETATE.** Since the radiation dose is so low, pertechnetate imaging is useful in showing that functioning thyroid tissue is indeed present in an infant and in demonstrating its location. Although the imaging is not elegant, the presence and location of the thyroid gland (arrow) is, nevertheless, identified (SG—submandibular gland).

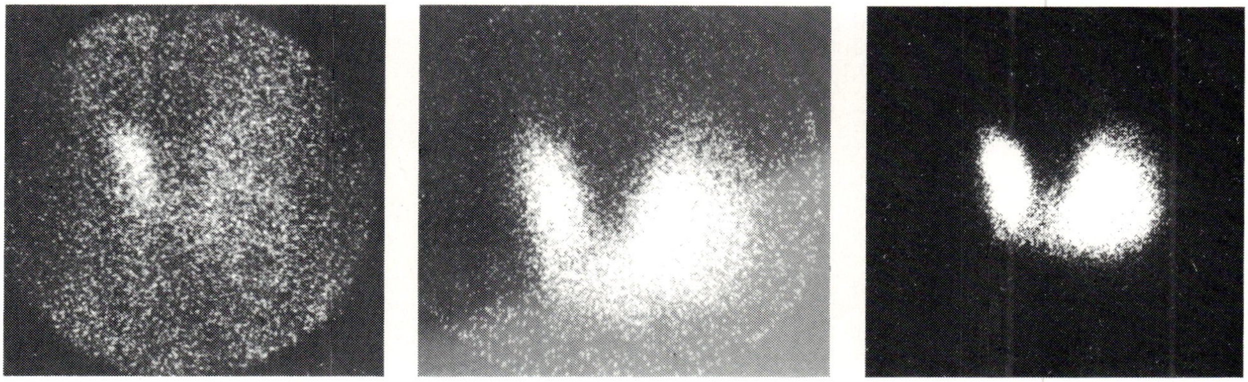

A B C

**FIG. 4. DISPARATE IMAGING BETWEEN PERTECHNETATE AND RADIOIODINE.** Imaging was performed because of a palpable nodule in the region of the left lobe. **A.** Imaging with Tc-99m sodium pertechnetate shows radioactivity relatively reduced and absent in the left lobe and in the area coinciding with the palpable nodule. **B.** Study performed with I-131 sodium iodide shows evidence of functioning thyroid tissue related to the palpable nodule, with no suggestion of a nonfunctioning or cold nodule. **C.** Imaging done with I-123 sodium iodide shows findings somewhat similar to those seen with I-131, but the imaging characteristics are improved with I-123.

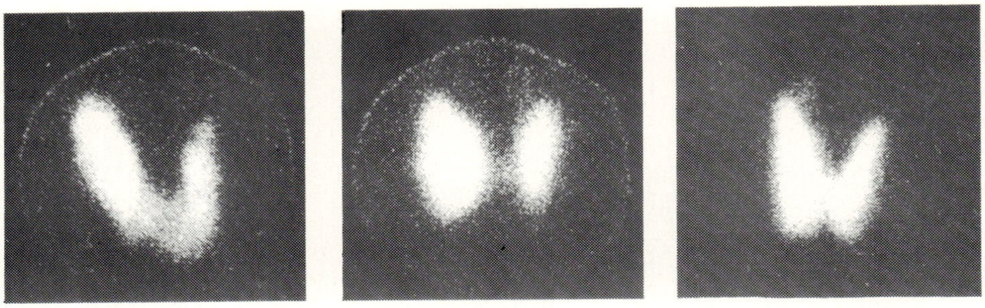

A

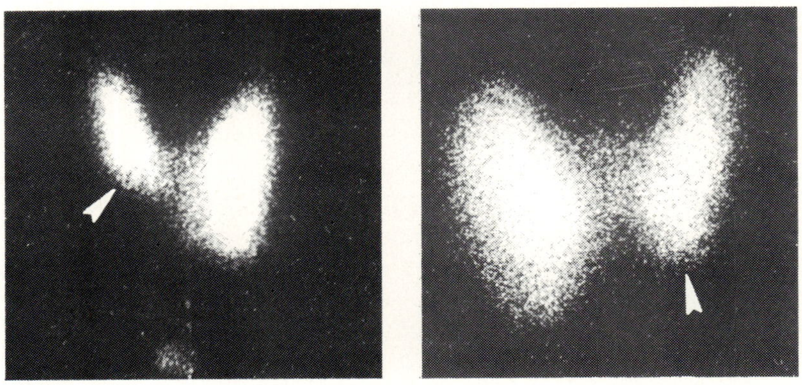

B

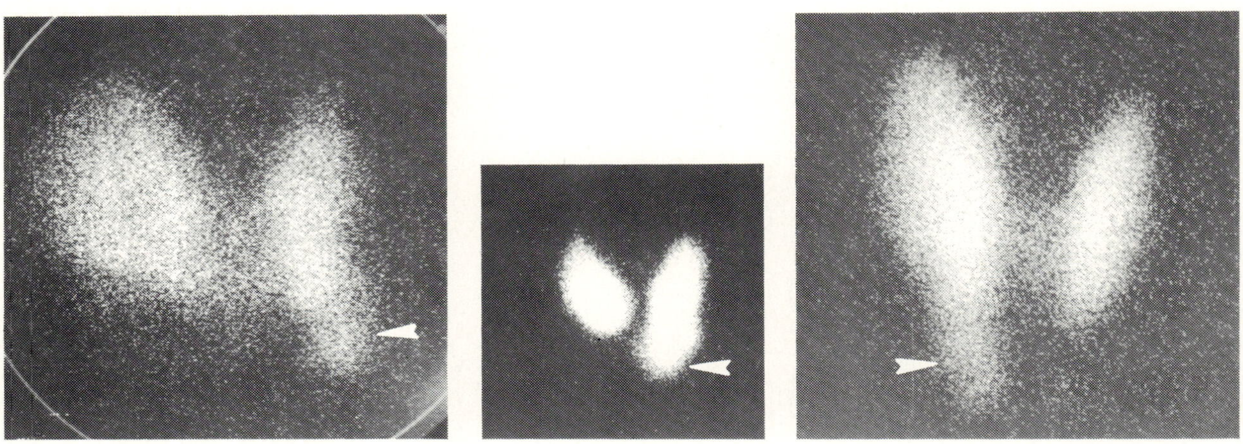

C

**FIG. 5. ASYMMETRY IN A NORMAL THYROID GLAND.** It is not uncommon to visualize a marked disparity in size between the two lobes. The absence of radioactivity inferior to the smaller lobe may be mistakenly associated with a nonfunctioning or "cold" nodule. Asymmetry is also seen with marked elevation or downward extension of one of the lobes. **A.** Right lobe larger than the left (I-123). **B.** Asymmetry which may lead to false impression that the absence of radioactivity (arrow) inferior to the smaller lobe may be due to a nonfunctioning nodule (I-123). **C.** Asymmetry associated with accessory lobes (arrow) related to a lower pole (I-123).

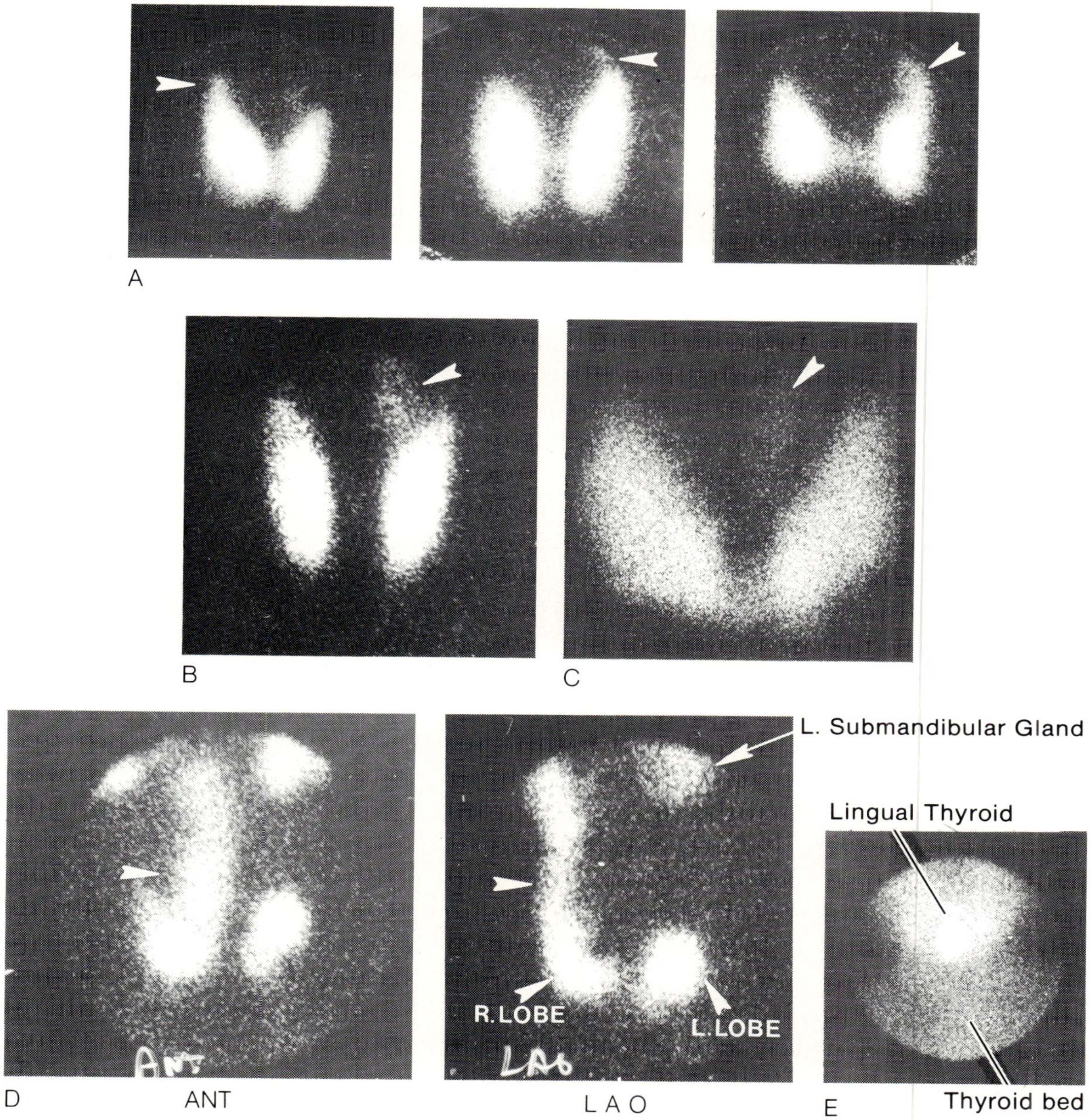


## ACCESSORY LOBES

**FIG. 6.** PYRAMIDAL LOBES. Additional thyroid lobes usually develop in remnants of thyroid tissue remaining in the course of the obliterated thyroglossal duct. A pyramidal lobe may extend from the isthmus or an upper pole to the region of the hyoid bone. Most commonly, only small portions of the pyramidal lobe become developed. The uptake in pyramidal lobes may be very low, and this accounts for their frequent visualization in the hyperthyroid patient or those patients who have received a large dose of radioactive material. **A.** Pyramidal lobes (arrows) related to an upper pole (I-123). **B.** Pyramidal lobe (arrow) related to the left upper pole (Tc-99m). **C.** Pyramidal lobe (arrow) realized extending toward the isthmus (I-123). **D.**

Pyramidal lobe (arrow) extending from hyoid area to right upper pole seen in both the anterior and left anterior oblique positions. In the latter view, the relation of the pyramidal lobe to the right upper pole is clearly visible (Tc-99m). **E.** Lingual thyroid (Tc-99m).

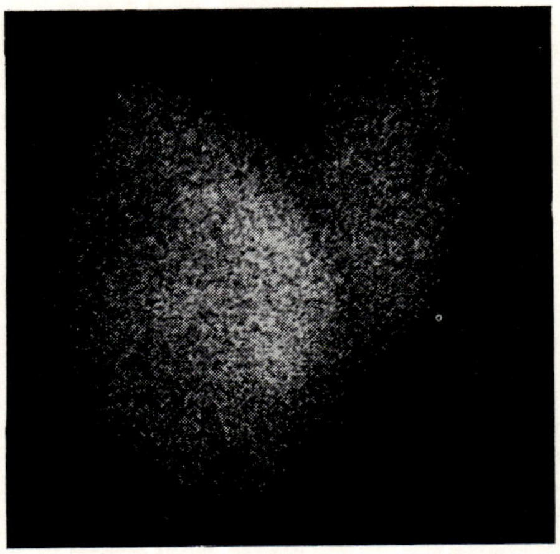

A.1. Static

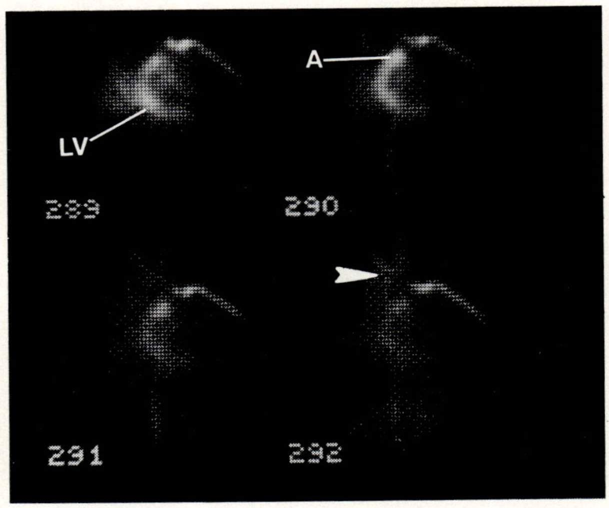


A.2. Blood Flow

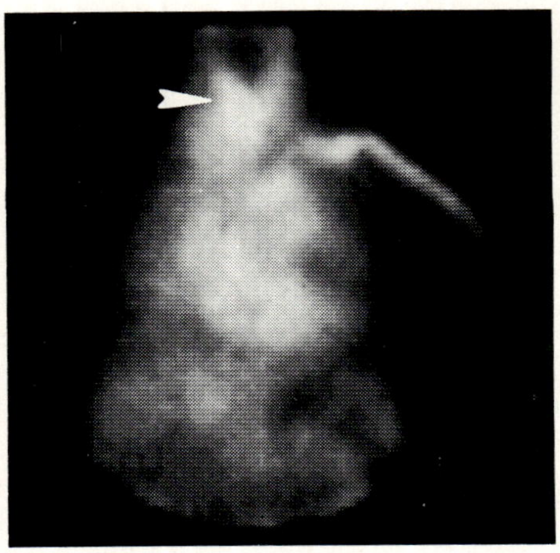

A.3. Composite Blood Flow

**FIG. 7.** (See legend next page)

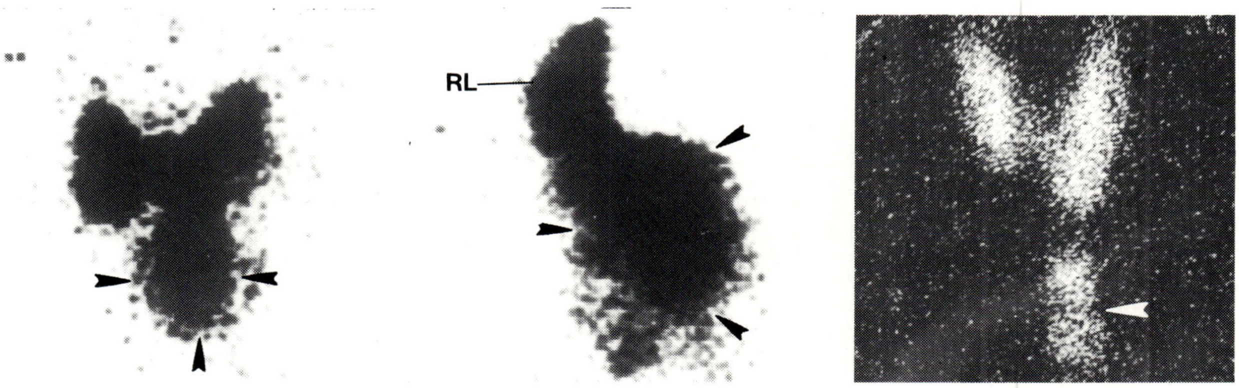


B C D

**FIG. 7. SUBSTERNAL EXTENSION.** Substernal or retrosternal extension of the thyroid gland is usually manifested on the chest x-ray with the appearance of an anterior mediastinal mass. To assist in the detection of these extensions, the suprasternal notch should be marked on the scan. Substernal extensions may involve one or both lobes or may be associated with an accessory lobe. They vary in size and may be small and asymptomatic or very large and responsible for severe symptoms, such as those due to tracheal compression. **A.** Substernal extension of one lobe. **1.** Static imaging performed in the anterior position identifies the inferior extension (arrow) of the right lobe. The suprasternal notch (X) is marked and the downward elongation of the right lobe is readily appreciated (I-123). **2.** Selected sequential frames in the same patient from the computerized readout of the blood flow study using Tc-99m sodium pertechnetate, in which images were obtained at intervals of 2 seconds, starting with the entry of Tc-99m into the left ventricle (LV). The ascending aorta (A) is clearly seen in the next frame, and in the final frame the substernal thyroid is identified (arrow). **3.** The composite, computerized radionuclide blood flow study demonstrates the mediastinal mass even more clearly as a substernal thyroid (arrow). **B.** Distinct accessory lobe clearly identified (arrows) as it extends into the chest (I-131). **C.** Enormous accessory lobe (arrows), which resulted in marked tracheal compression when patient was recumbent. Because of respiratory problems, the left lobe had been surgically removed previously, and the remaining right lobe (RL) is closely related to the accessory, retrosternal portion (I-131). **D.** Accessory lobe with noticeable separation from the left lower pole (I-123).

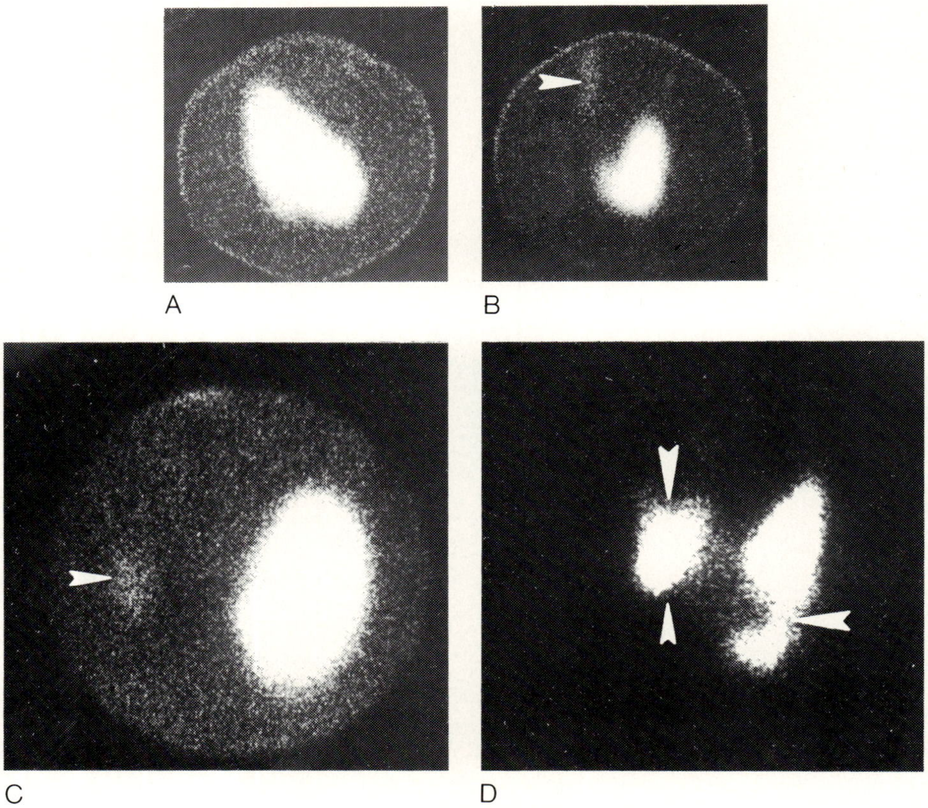


**FIG. 8. POSTOPERATIVE CHANGES.** Following surgical intervention there is often gross architectural distortion of the thyroid, with the removal of entire lobes or portions of lobes. In some patients further architectural distortions are associated with hypertrophy and hyperplasia of the remaining tissue, especially if surgery had been performed for hyperthyroidism. From the scan appearance itself, it is usually impossible to tell whether the defects present have been caused by previous operations or if there has been localized displacement or replacement of thyroid tissue by underlying disease. **A.** Surgical absence of the left lobe. Only the right lobe is visualized, and there is no hint of activity in the region of the extirpated lobe. These imaging findings are identical to those seen in congenital absence of a lobe (I-123). **B.** Surgical removal of the right lobe with isthmus remaining. Also remaining is the faintly visualized pyramidal lobe (arrow), which had been related to the right upper pole (I-123). **C.** Partial thyroidectomy of right lobe with some residual thyroid tissue (arrow) remaining in the area of the removed lobe. It is sometimes impossible to remove *all* of the lobe to be excised, and the presence of residual thyroid tissue can be seen on imaging (Tc-99m). **D.** Architectural distortion associated with partial thyroidectomy in a patient with a multinodular goiter. The areas of absent radioactivity are associated with both removed thyroid (small arrow) and remaining multiple benign nodules ( larger arrows) (I-123).

## AUTONOMOUSLY FUNCTIONING NODULES

The autonomously functioning thyroid nodule secretes thyroid hormone on its own, without stimulation from a tropic hormone, and the resulting level of thyroid hormone in the blood leads to the shutting off of the secretion of endogenous TSH by the pituitary gland. As a consequence, there is little or no secretion of thyroid hormone in the gland outside the autonomously functioning thyroid nodule, and these areas are said to be suppressed by the functioning portion of the thyroid gland. Thyroid imaging is usually performed in these patients following the detection of a nodule on physical examination, or because of symptoms of hyperthyroidism.

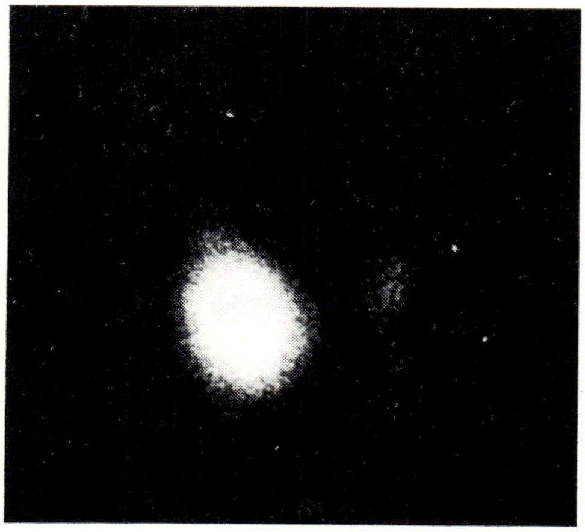

A

**FIG. 9.** NONTOXIC, AUTONOMOUSLY FUNCTIONING NODULES. **A.** Solitary, autonomously functioning nodule. Only a small, somewhat rounded area of radioactivity is seen in the region of the right lower pole; this corresponds to the site of a palpable nodule. The remainder of the right lobe and the entire left lobe are being suppressed by the autonomously functioning nodule. The latter secretes thyroid hormone independently and is not under the control of the pituitary gland. The level of thyroid hormone in the blood is sufficient to result in little or no secretion of TSH by the pituitary gland and, as a result, little or no radioiodine is taken up in the suppressed portions of the gland. Imaging methods to help confirm the diagnosis of autonomously functioning nodules through TSH stimulation or triiodothyronine (T3) suppression are shown in Figs. 10 and 11 (I-123). **B.** Solitary autonomously functioning nodule with ovoid configuration. Although these nodules are characteristically rounded, they sometimes have the shape of an entire thyroid lobe (I-123). **C.** Solitary, autonomously functioning nodule with a somewhat irregular contour (I-123). **D.** Multiple autonomously functioning thyroid nodules. Both nodules are situated in the right lobe; there is barely any visualization of the remaining right lobe and the left lobe (I-123). **E.** Multiple autonomously functioning nodules, both lobes. A portion of thyroid tissue superior to the left-sided nodule continued to be visualized (I-123). **F.** Multiple autonomously functioning nodules (arrows) related to the isthmus are seen. Both the right and left lobes ( larger arrows) are faintly imaged (I-123).

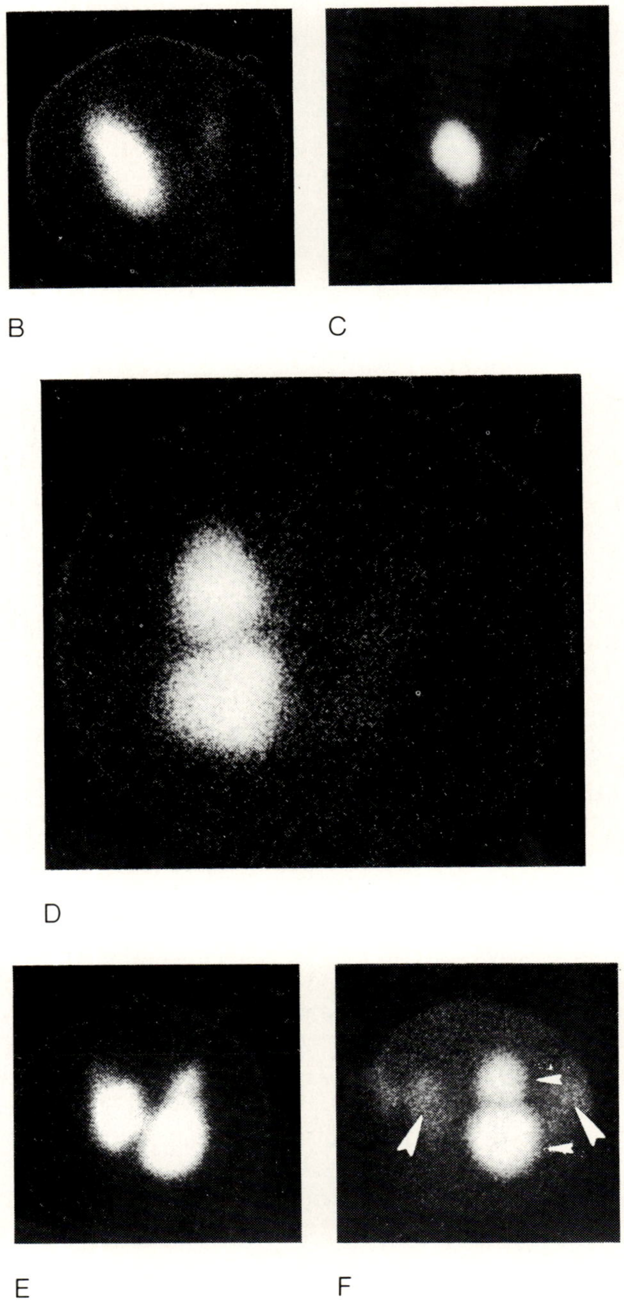


**FIG. 9. B–F.** (See legend on previous page)

A

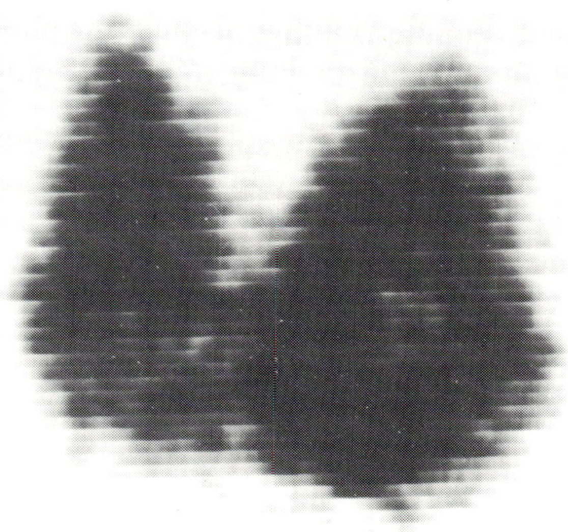

B

**FIG. 10. AUTONOMOUSLY FUNCTIONING NODULE AND TSH STIMULATION.** In the initial study **A,** the only visualized portion of the gland is in the region of the left lower pole. This underlies the palpable left-sided nodule. **B.** TSH stimulation imaging. The patient was given 10 units of TSH intramuscularly daily for 3 days and on the third day the patient also received an oral dose of I-131 sodium iodide. Imaging was performed 24 hours later. With the exogenous TSH leading to depletion of the thyroid hormone by those portions of the gland under pituitary control, uptake of radioactive iodine is now visible in the right lobe and remainder of the left lobe not previously visualized and helps establish that these portions of the thyroid gland have indeed been suppressed. Since the patient with an autonomously functioning nodule may become hyperthyroid, extreme caution should be exercised in performing the TSH stimulation studies because of the possibility of inducing a hyperthyroid crisis. To help establish a diagnosis of autonomous function, the method of thyroid suppression shown in Fig. 11 is usually preferred.

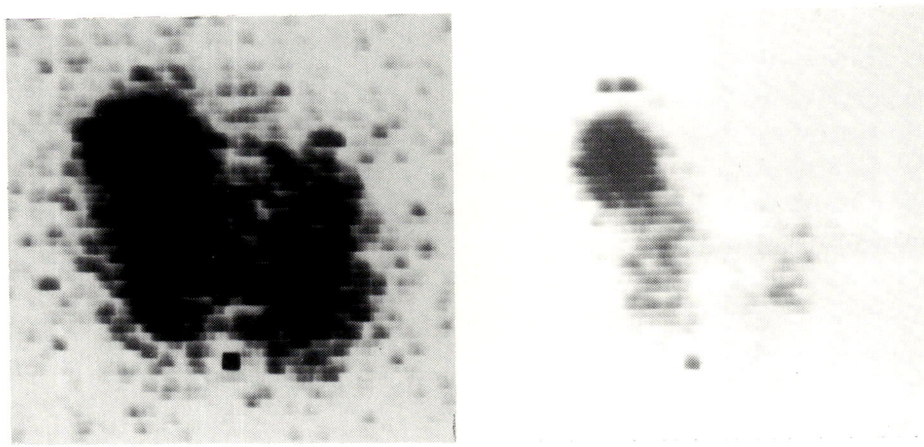

A B

**FIG. 11.** AUTONOMOUSLY FUNCTIONING NODULE AND T3 SUPPRESSION. **A.** Thyroid scan shows evidence of relative hyperfunction in the region of the right upper pole. **B.** Imaging following T3 suppression. The patient was given 25 $\mu$g of triiodothyronine (T3) p.o. t.i.d. for 8 days and on the eighth day also received an oral dose of I-131. Imaging performed 24 hours later clearly outlines the autonomously functioning nodule at the right upper pole. By the reducing or shutting off of the secretion of endogenous TSH through the administration of T3, the uptake of radioiodine is unaffected in the autonomously functioning nodule but is markedly suppressed in the remainder of the gland.

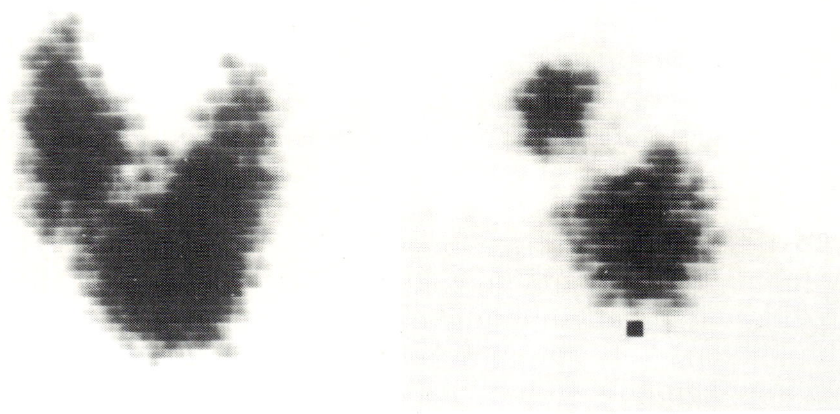

A B

**FIG. 12.** MULTIPLE AUTONOMOUSLY FUNCTIONING NODULES AND TSH STIMULATION. **A.** Before TSH stimulation, autonomously functioning nodules are identified at the right upper and left lower poles. **B.** After TSH stimulation, the remaining portions of the gland are visualized. Multiple autonomously functioning nodules are encountered less frequently than the single variety.

**FIG. 13. TOXIC AUTONOMOUSLY FUNCTIONING NODULE.** The imaging appearance of the autonomously functioning nodule in a patient with hyperthyroidism may be identical to that of nontoxic nodules. Such patients should not receive TSH to help establish the diagnosis, lest a hyperthyroid crisis ensue. There appears to be almost complete suppression of the entire left lobe and the uninvolved portion of the right lobe.

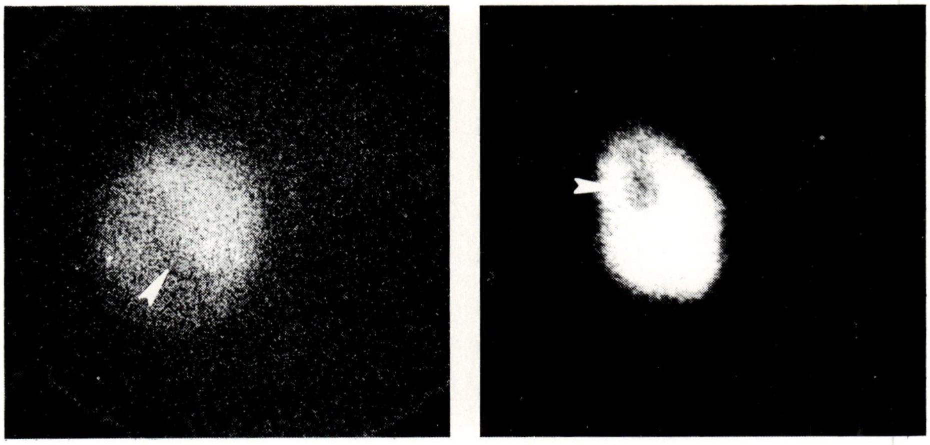

**FIG. 14. DEGENERATIVE CHANGES IN AN AUTONOMOUSLY FUNCTIONING NODULE.** Areas of absent activity in these nodules may be due to cystic, hemorrhagic, ischemic, or even neoplastic degeneration. The development of hyperthyroidism in the patient with an autonomously functioning nodule often abates following such degenerative changes (arrows) (I-123).

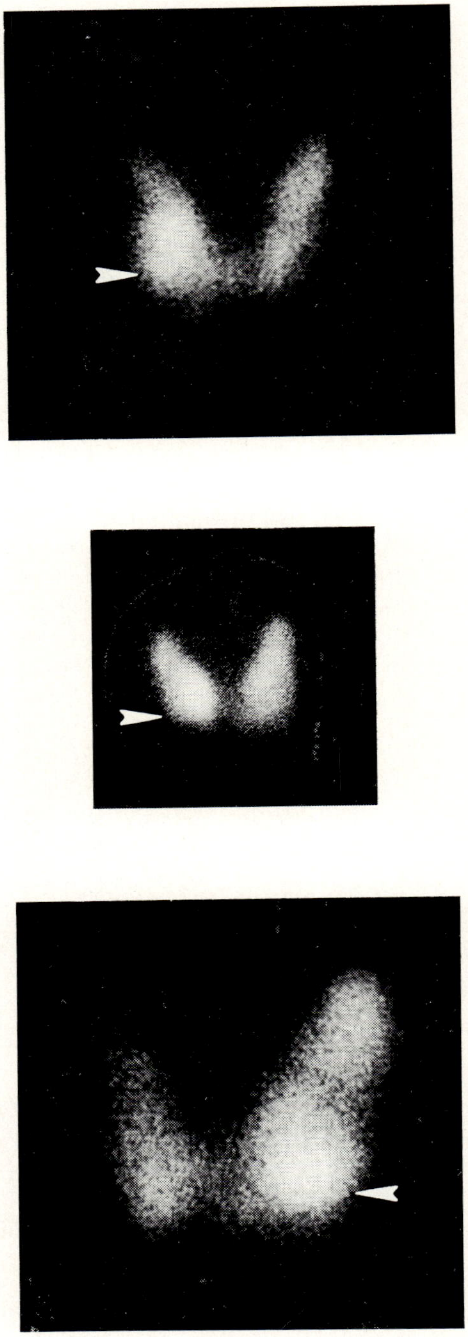

**FIG. 15. AREAS OF RELATIVE HYPERFUNCTION NOT CAUSING COMPLETE SUPPRESSION.** Solitary, palpable nodules may be associated with areas that show relative hyperfunction when compared with the remainder of the gland. The involved regions are discrete (arrows) and may or may not be associated with hyperthyroidism (I-123).

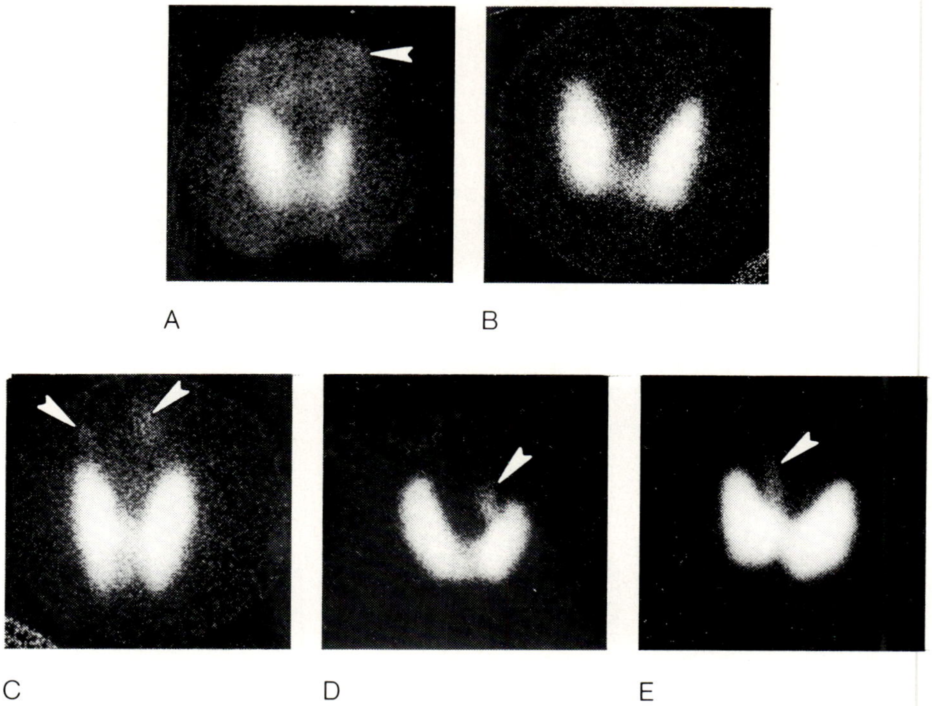

**FIG. 16. GRAVES' DISEASE.** Among the manifestations of Graves' disease that may be reflected on radionuclide imaging are the diffusely enlarged gland, due to diffuse hyperplasia of the thyroid, and the elevated radionuclide uptake associated with the hyperthyroid state. The excellent definition of images obtained with either pertechnetate or radioiodine is related to this increased uptake. The latter is associated with the frequent visualization of pyramidal lobes that would otherwise escape detection in the patient without an elevated uptake. The uniform involvement in each of these cases of Graves' disease is a further manifestation of the smooth, diffusely enlarged gland with absence of nodularity. **A.** Right lobe larger than the left but both diffusely involved. Note the submandibular glands (arrows) (Tc-99m). **B.** Anatomy is clearly defined, including the isthmus (I-123). **C.** Visualization of pyramidal lobes related to midline and right upper pole (arrows) (I-123). **D.** Elongated right lobe. A pyramidal lobe (arrow) related to the left upper pole is seen (I-123). **E.** Symmetrical gland with pyramidal lobe (arrow) seen somewhat related to the midline (I-123).

## NONFUNCTIONING OR "COLD" NODULES

For the most part, areas of nonfunction or absent radioactivity on thyroid images are associated with replacement, destruction, or invasion of thyroid tissue at these sites. Such abnormalities may be single or multiple, benign or malignant. The solitary palpable thyroid nodule, which is manifested on imaging as an area of nonfunctioning thyroid tissue, is a cause for concern because of the possibility of neoplasm. The incidence of malignancy in solitary nonfunctioning thyroid nodules is in the neighborhood of 4 percent. It must also be borne in mind that countless other entities may cause localized destruction or replacement of thyroid tissue (e.g., cyst, infarction, necrosis, hemorrhage, benign adenoma, thyroiditis, nodular goiter). Occasionally, the scan appearance of a solitary region of nonfunction, corresponding to the site of the palpable nodule, is not clearly defined. This abnormal appearance may sometimes be further clarified with the use either of thyroid-stimulating hormone (TSH), which helps increase radioactive iodine uptake to the thyroid and thereby improves imaging, or of a larger dose of radioactive material.

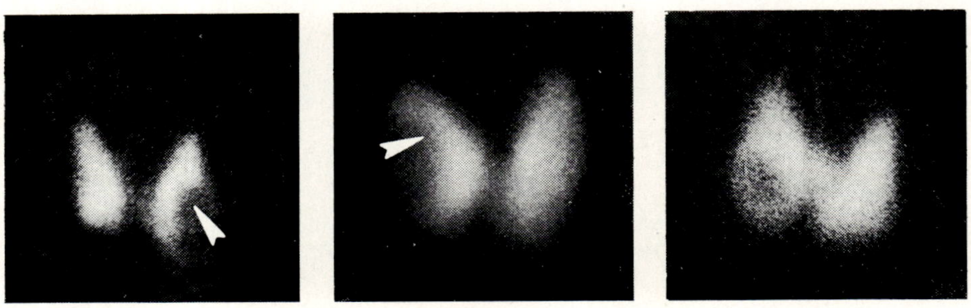

A B C

**FIG. 17. FOLLICULAR ADENOMAS.** Most benign tumors of the thyroid gland are adenomas and arise from the epithelium lining the thyroid follicle. These follicular adenomas are often designated in terms of the type of follicle from which the tumor is formed. Thus, the microfollicular adenoma (fetal adenoma) is composed of small, poorly formed follicles, while the macrofollicular adenoma (colloid adenoma) is characterized by enlarged follicles greatly distended with colloid. These tumors are usually solitary and are well encapsulated. The discrete, localized area of absent radioactivity in each of these patients coincided with a solitary palpable nodule, found upon surgery to be a follicular adenoma. **A.** Large, well-defined area of absent radioactivity (arrow) in left lobe. This 34-year-old female had received radiation therapy to the thymus gland as an infant (I-123). **B.** Large area of involvement (arrow) in the right lobe (Tc-99m). **C.** Sharply defined area of absent radioactivity within the right lobe toward the lower pole (I-123).

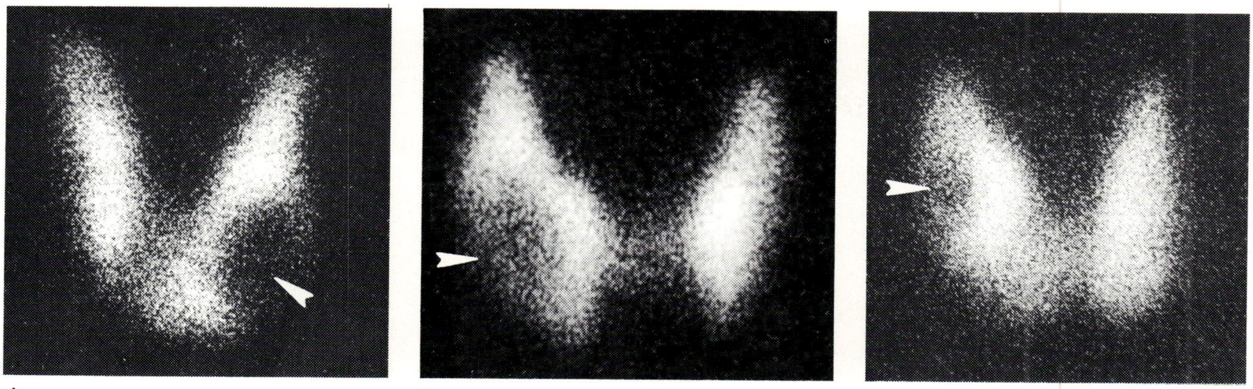

A B C

**FIG. 18. FOLLICULAR ADENOMAS, CLEARLY DEFINED.** The sharply outlined areas of absent radioactivity are not particularly characteristic of adenomas; these findings could be seen with countless other solitary thyroid lesions, such as malignancy, cyst, or thyroiditis. **A.** Solitary, ovoid area of absent radioactivity (arrow) at left lower pole. It is difficult to appreciate the extent of such a lesion from physical examination alone, and its appearance prior to imaging may suggest involvement of the entire lobe (I-123). **B.** Somewhat irregular area of absent radioactivity (arrow) in a patient in whom the entire right lobe was palpable (I-123). **C.** Identification of a small, discrete, rounded area of absent radioactivity (arrow) in the right lobe (I-123).

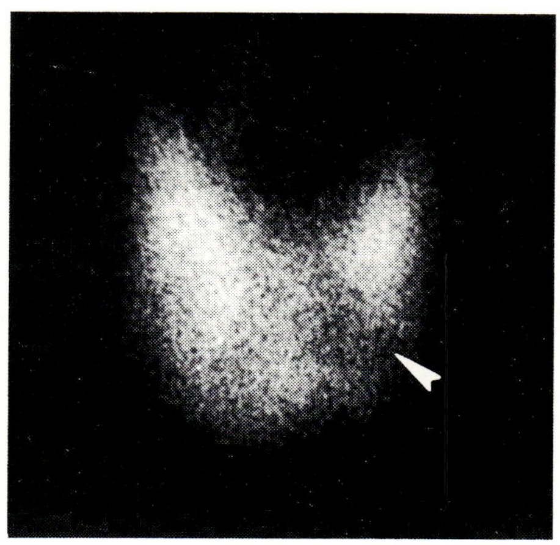

**FIG. 19. FOLLICULAR ADENOMA LESS CLEARLY DEFINED.** Not all adenomas can be seen on radionuclide imaging nor are all that are demonstrated sharply outlined. The clarity with which the site of absent radioactivity (arrow) is visible in this patient does not approach that of the images shown in Figs. 17 and 18.

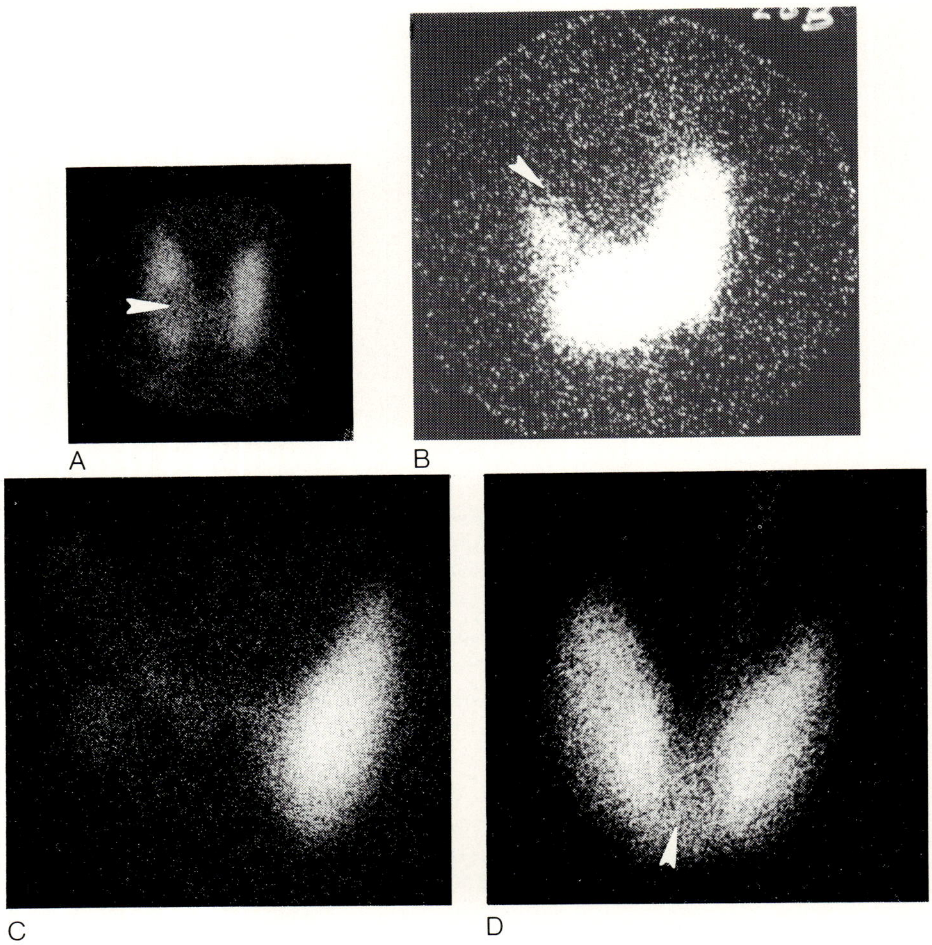

**FIG. 20. PAPILLARY ADENOCARCINOMA.** The papillary adenocarcinoma is the most commonly encountered malignant neoplasm of the thyroid, comprising about 50 percent of thyroid cancer, and has the lowest grade of malignancy of these tumors. The tumor is extremely slow growing and is well differentiated. Papillary adenocarcinoma spreads by lymphatic invasion to other sites within the thyroid gland and to regional lymph nodes. Distant metastases are rare. Most commonly, these tumors are mixed and are composed of both papillary and follicular elements, the tumor type depending on which form predominates. There are no distinctive imaging characteristics. **A.** Papillary adenocarcinoma sharply defined. The somewhat ovoid area absent of radioactivity in the right lobe (arrow) corresponds to a solitary, palpable nodule at that site (Tc-99m). **B.** Involvement of right lobe. The area absent of activity (arrow), which coincides with a right-sided nodule, is related to a large portion of the right lobe. Although the imaging abnormality does not suggest a circumscribed, localized lesion, this is what was found at surgery (I-123). **C.** Extensive involvement and replacement of the right lobe. Only a few small areas of functioning tissue remain in the right lobe. The large areas of absent radioactivity indicate the extensive tumor involvement (I-123). **D.** Evidence of tumor barely perceptible. A rounded nodule is palpable over the isthmus. The reduction in radioactivity (arrow) commonly seen in that region is, in this case, due to a papillary adenocarcinoma (I-123).

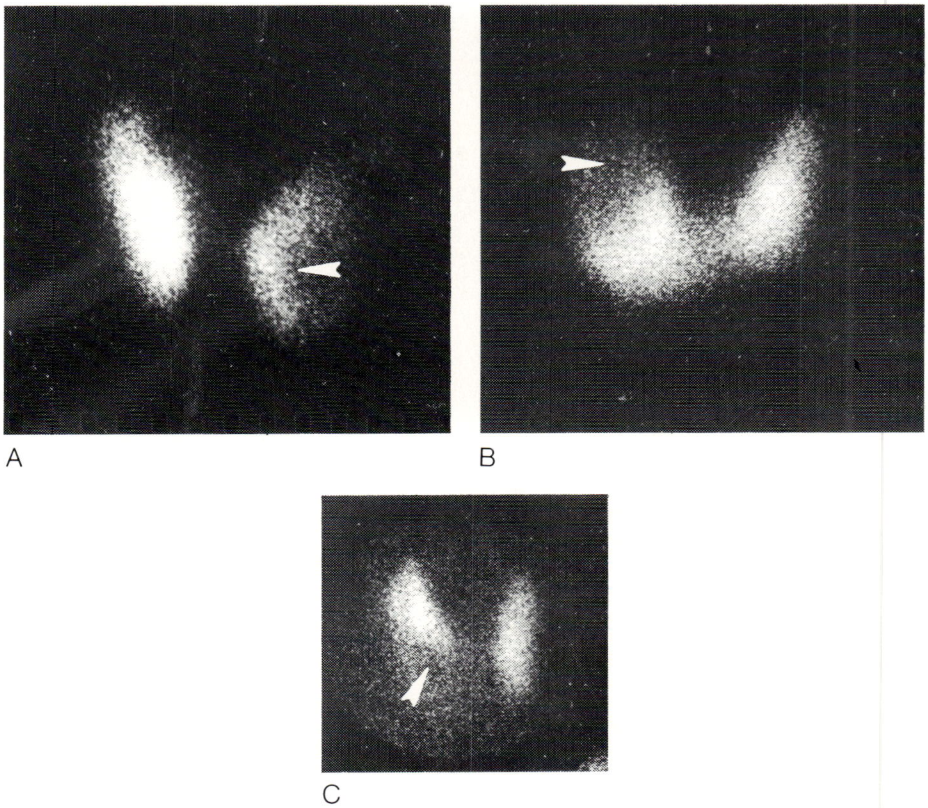


**FIG. 21. FOLLICULAR ADENOCARCINOMA.** Follicular adenocarcinoma is responsible for about 25 percent of malignant thyroid neoplasms. Like the papillary type, the follicular adenocarcinoma usually occurs as an admixture of both papillary and follicular elements, the latter predominating. Although it is not so well differentiated as the papillary type, it nevertheless has a relatively low grade of malignancy. The follicular adenocarcinoma tends to spread by the hematogenous route rather than through lymphatics. About 10 percent of the metastatic lesions from follicular adenocarcinoma contain functioning follicles, which readily take up radioactive iodine. **A.** Sharply defined tumor along lateral aspect of left lobe. As can be seen from imaging, the area of involvement (arrow) is fairly extensive and corresponds to a large, palpable nodule. This patient, a 19-year-old female, received radiation therapy to the thymus as an infant (I-123). **B.** Sharply defined at right upper pole (arrow) (I-123). **C.** Sharply defined at right lower pole (arrow) (Tc-99m).

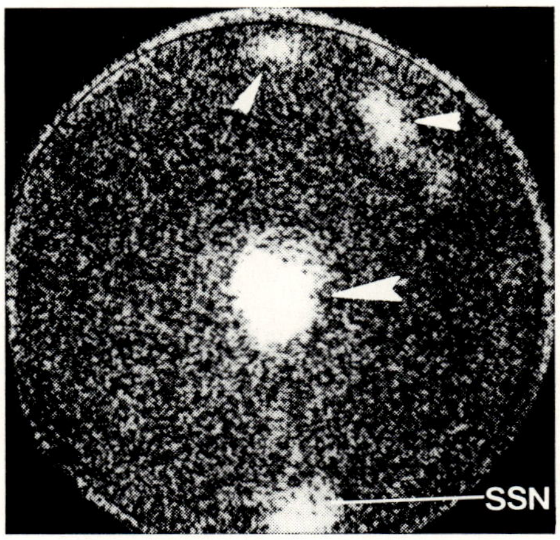


**FIG. 22.** FUNCTIONING REGIONAL METASTASES: FOLLICULAR CARCINOMA. Sites of increased radioactivity (small arrows) represent areas of nodal metastases in which radioactive iodine is taken up into the follicles. There had been an intended total thyroidectomy, and the remaining functioning thyroid glandular tissue is seen centrally (larger arrow). A marker is on the suprasternal notch (SSN) (I-123).

**FIG. 23.** THYROID METASTATIC SURVEY: NO FUNCTIONING METASTASES. Following a period of withdrawal of thyroid replacement therapy or of TSH stimulation, imaging is performed with radioiodine (I-131 or I-123) to search for possible functioning follicular metastases. The ideal time for imaging is probably 72 hours following tracer administration. **A.** 24 hours. There is no evidence of functioning thyroid metastases in a patient who has had the thyroid gland extirpated (by both surgery and I-131) and in whom there is no visualization of any remaining thyroid. Radioactivity is seen in the stomach (ST), intestinal tract (GI), and urinary bladder (UB). Note the presence of the radioactive material in submandibular glands (SG) (I-131). **B.** 48 hours. There is no evidence of functioning thyroid metastases in another patient who has had a subtotal thyroidectomy and in whom there is visualization of remaining functioning thyroid tissue (arrow). The intensity and distortion of the thyroid remnant are related to the relatively large dose of radioiodine employed (I-131). **C.** 72 hours. There is no evidence of functioning thyroid metastases in another patient in whom a subtotal thyroidectomy had been performed. There is continued visualization of the remaining thyroid as well as of the intestinal tract and bladder (I-131).

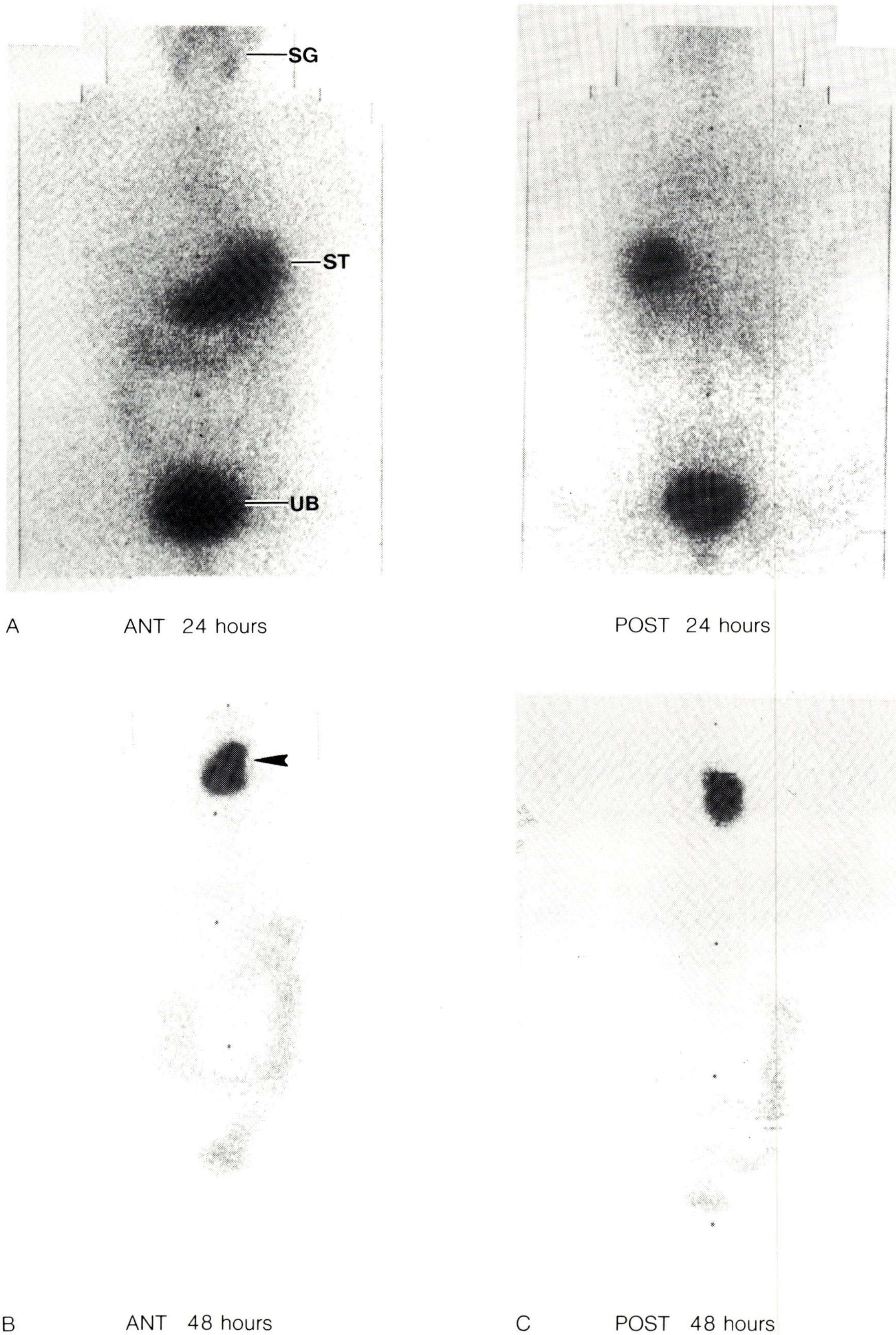


**FIG. 23.** (See legend on previous page)

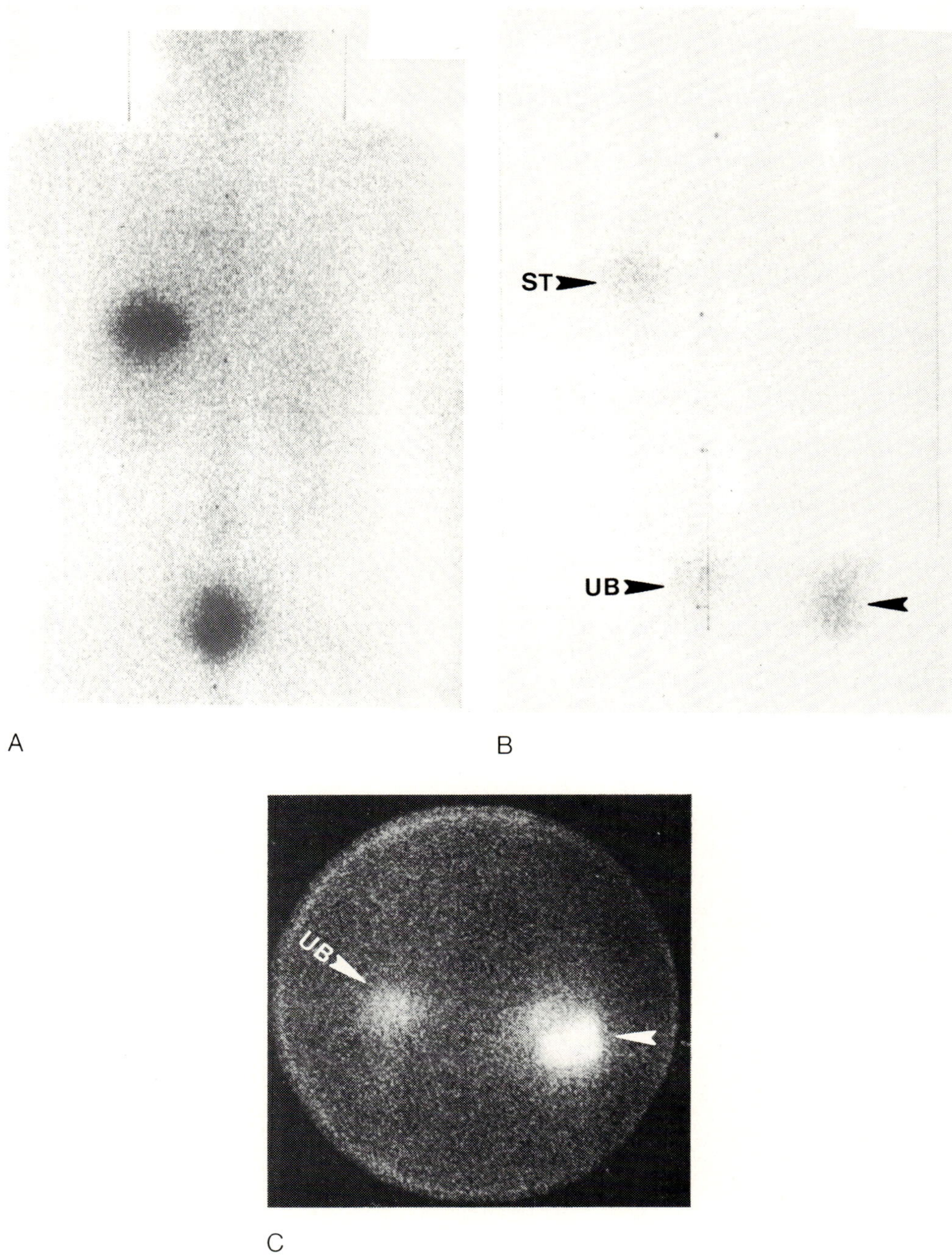


**FIG. 24. THYROID METASTATIC SURVEY: FUNCTIONING METASTASIS IN RIGHT ILIUM.** Although the 24-hour study **A** does not yet disclose the lesion, the localized area of increased radioactivity in the right ilium (arrow) is readily identifiable at 72 hours in the posterior position on both the rectilinear scan **B** and gamma camera image **C.** This is due to a functioning follicular metastasis at that site. The increased radioactivity centrally is due to the urinary bladder (UB). The thyroid gland is not visible and the stomach (ST) is visualized.

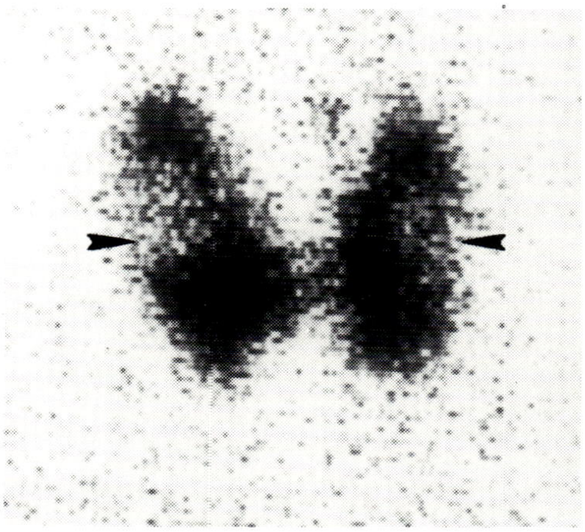

A

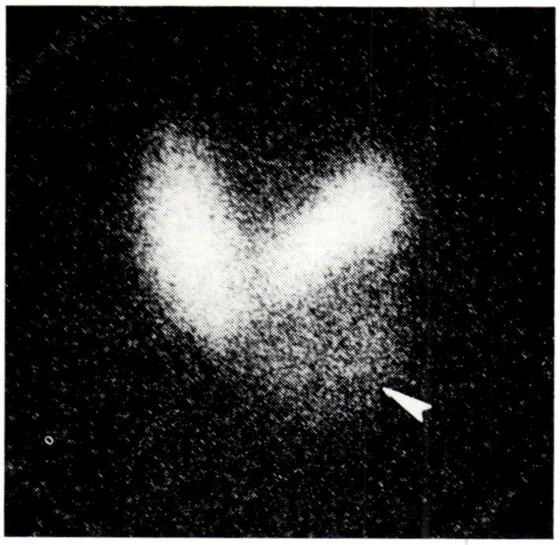

B

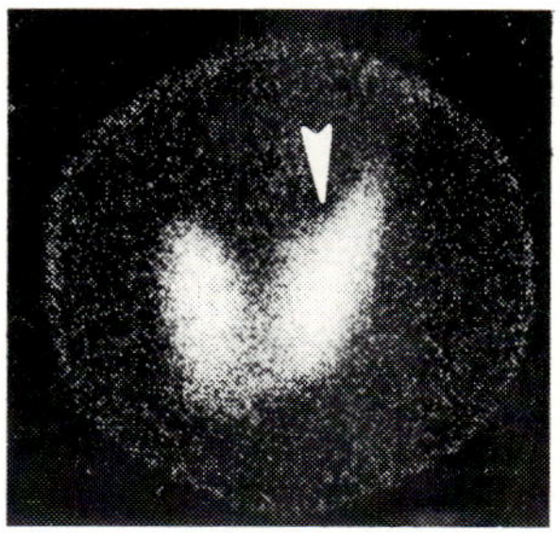

C

**FIG. 25.** LESS COMMON NEOPLASTIC INVOLVEMENT. **A.** Medullary carcinoma. Medullary carcinoma of the thyroid accounts for about 10 percent of malignant thyroid lesions. The tumor secretes calcitonin, and elevated blood or urine calcitonin levels along with palpable thyroid nodules may be a more reliable indicator of involvement than radionuclide imaging. Metastases occur through both hematogenous and lymphatic routes. In about 15 percent of patients with medullary carcinoma, the malady is familial. In these cases the thyroid involvement is often multicentric (such as that seen in the illustration) and there may be associated bilateral pheochromocytoma and parathyroid hyperplasia (Sipple's syndrome). In the nonfamilial variety, usually only one lobe of the thyroid is involved (I-131). (From Anderson RJ, Sizemore GW, Wahner HW, et al: Clin Nucl Med 3:147, 1978). **B.** Metastatic lesion to the thyroid. The area of absent radioactivity (arrow) in the left lobe is due to a metastasis from a carcinoma of the nasopharynx. About 10 percent of metastatic neoplasms involve the thyroid gland (I-123). **C.** Extrinsic compression (arrow) due to cervical metastasis from a pheochromocytoma.

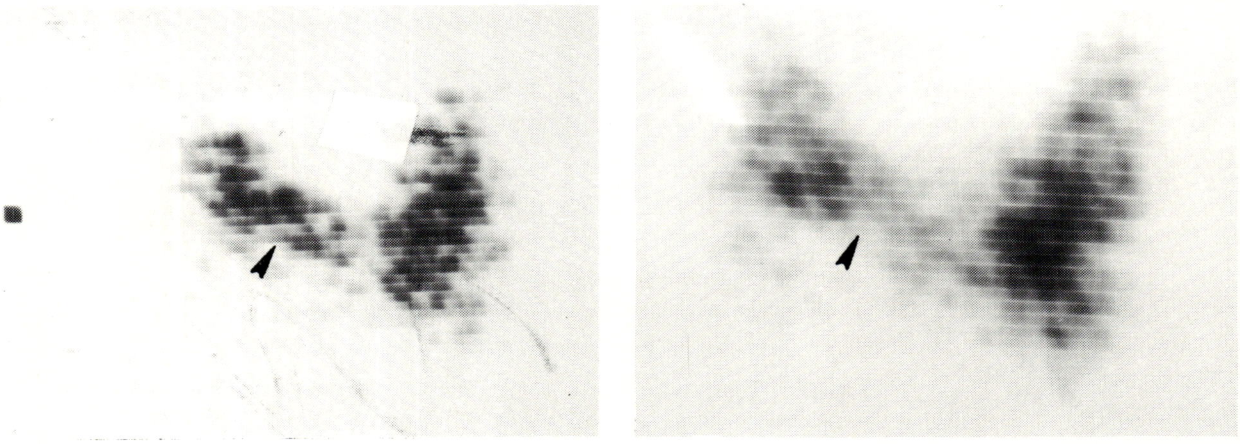

A B

**FIG. 26. UNDIFFERENTIATED OR ANAPLASTIC CARCINOMA.** Anaplastic carcinoma of the thyroid, which makes up about 15 percent of thyroid malignancies, is a highly malignant lesion and readily metastasizes. Of the two major types, small cell and giant cell, the latter carries the worse prognosis and usually occurs in patients 60 years of age or older. These tumors often cause major architectural distortions of the thyroid gland. **A.** Thyroid scan of a 52-year-old female who was found to have an irregular, hard right lower pole nodule on physical examination. Scanning shows a corresponding irregular area of absent activity at the right lower pole. For further clarification, the study was repeated following TSH stimulation and this is seen in **B.** The lesion is unchanged, although it is more sharply defined. At surgery, the neoplasm was found to be undifferentiated carcinoma, small cell type.

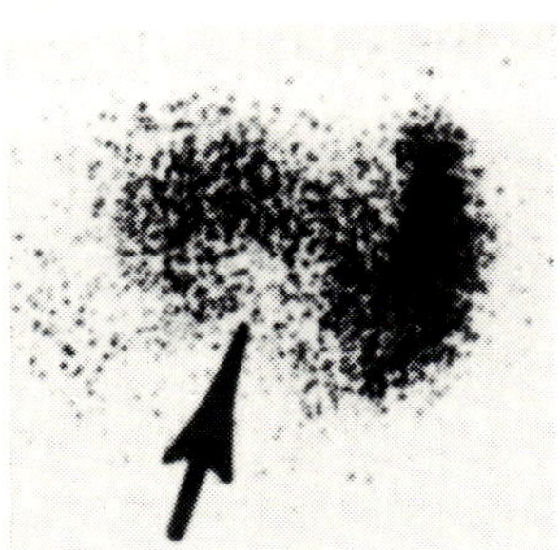

**FIG. 27. ANAPLASTIC CARCINOMA (LARGE CELL TYPE).** The figure shows thyroid imaging in a 63-year-old female who was found to have an irregular, large, stony hard mass in the region of the right lower pole on physical examination. The irregular area of absent activity at the right lower pole corresponds with the palpable lesion. Note the further involvement in the right lobe as evidenced by reduction in radioactivity on that side.

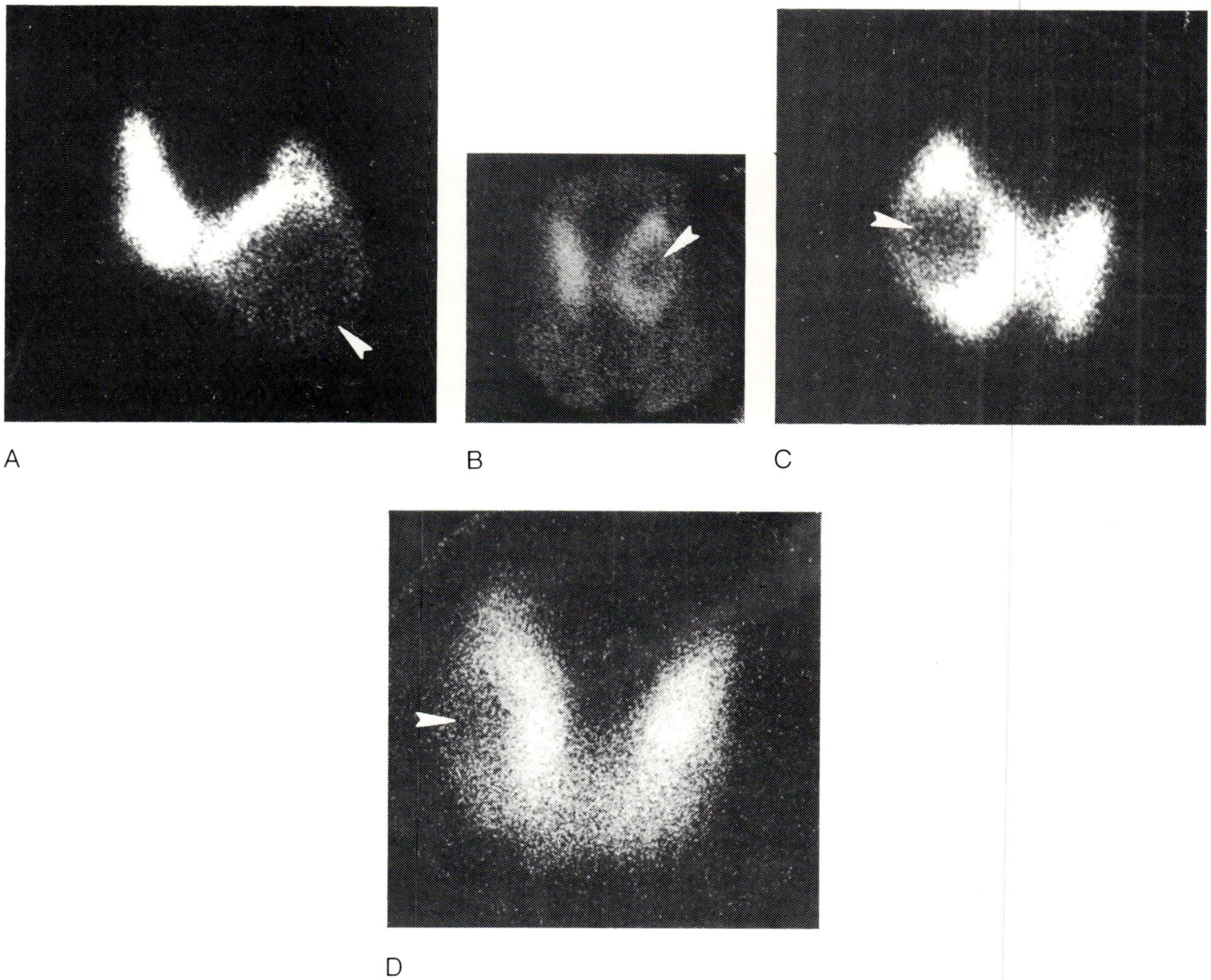


**FIG. 28.** THYROID CYST. A solitary cystic lesion is usually seen as a rounded area of absent radioactivity. Although there are no imaging characteristics to distinguish it from a solid lesion, such as tumor, such information is forthcoming from ultrasound studies. **A.** Enormous cyst in left lobe, identified as a well defined area of absent radioactivity (arrow) (I-123). Imaging with Tc-99m in **B** shows the left lobe to be largely replaced by a cyst, while in **C** the I-123 image shows similar involvement in the right lobe (arrow). **D.** Small cyst identified along the lateral aspect of the right lobe (I-123).

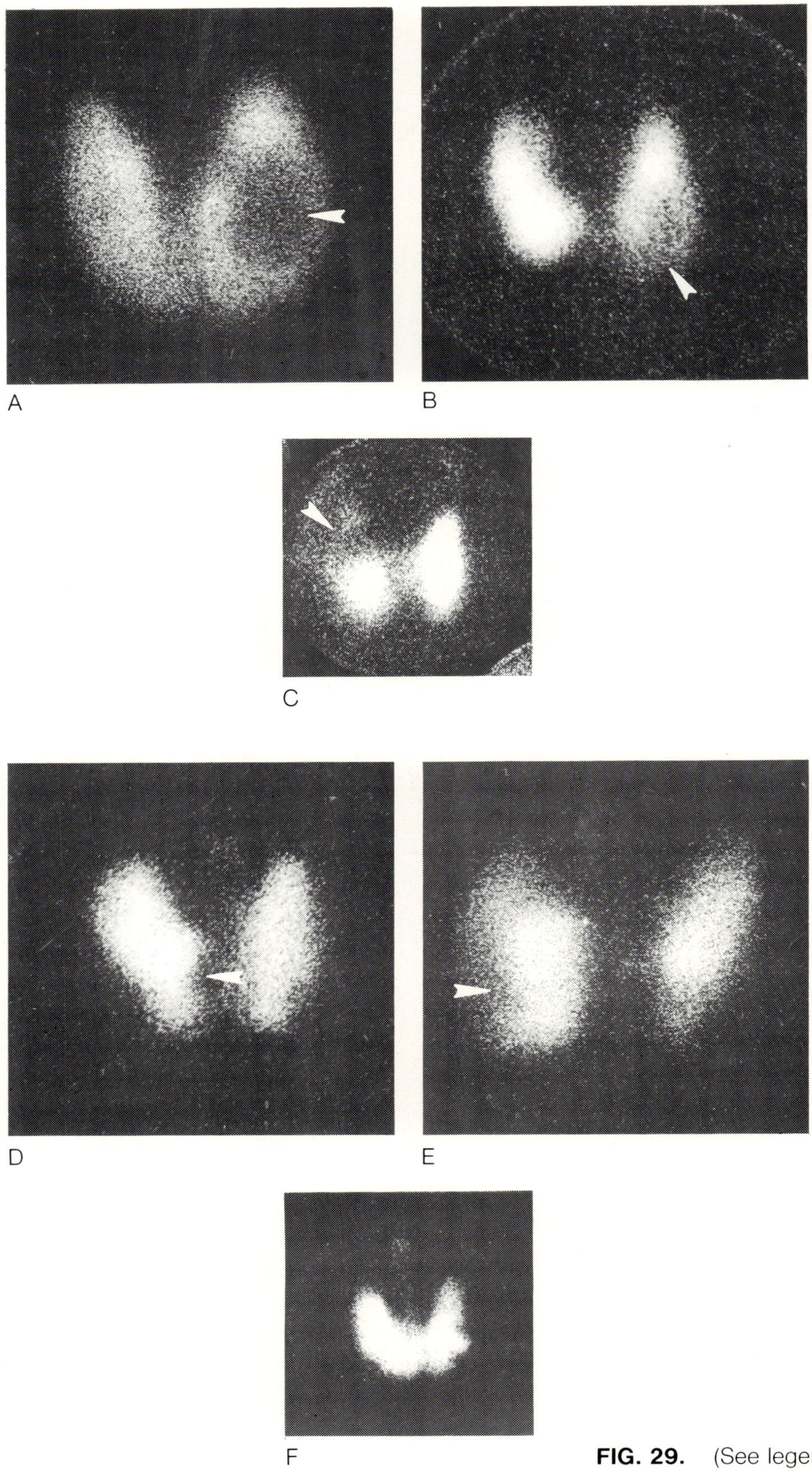


**FIG. 29.** (See legend next page)

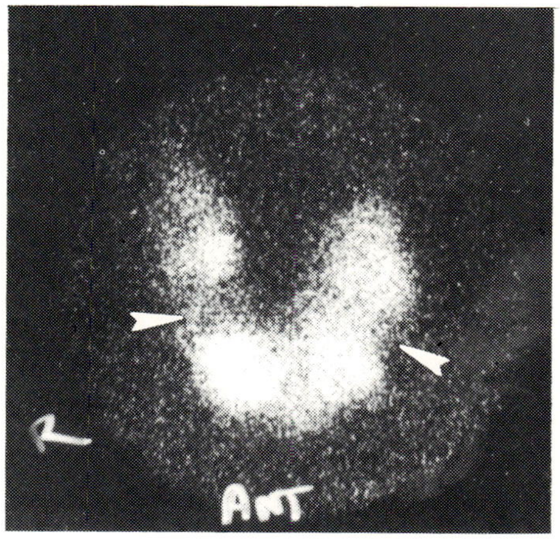


G

**FIG. 29.** **HASHIMOTO'S THYROIDITIS.** There are no distinctive imaging characteristics in chronic thyroiditis. Areas of absent and reduced radioactivity are due to fibrosis, lymphocytic infiltration and reduced RAI uptake. Such sites of absent activity may be associated with corresponding palpable nodules. Although palpable nodules detected on physical examination coincide with imaging findings of nonfunctioning or "cold" nodules, further laboratory studies (e.g., thyroid autoantibodies) and follow-up imaging may help establish the diagnosis. **A.** Hashimoto's thyroiditis masquerading as a solitary, discrete nonfunctioning nodule (arrow) in the left lobe (I-123). **B.** A solitary, firm nodule at the left lower pole corresponds to the slightly irregular area of absent radioactivity in that area (I-123). **C.** Irregularly reduced activity (arrow) at the right upper pole associated at that site with a palpable nodule that is round and firm (I-123). **D.** Palpable nodule in isthmus related to a rounded area of absent activity (arrow) due to involvement with thyroiditis (I-123). **E.** Localized area of absent radioactivity (arrow) corresponds to the site of a solitary, palpable nodule. In this case, the imaging characteristics are not unlike those that may be seen with neoplasm (I-123). **F.** Multiple areas of absent radioactivity and architectural distortion (I-123). **G.** Multiple areas of absent radioactivity (arrows) are similar to those seen in a multinodular goiter. Multiple, palpable nodules in this patient are associated with the many areas of absent radioactivity (Tc-99m).

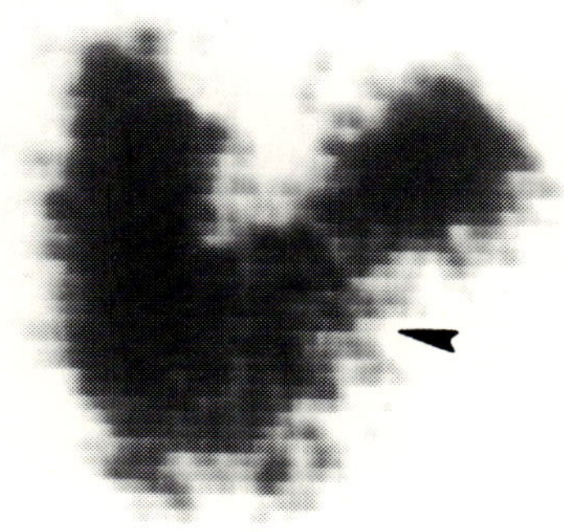

**FIG. 30.** SUBACUTE THYROIDITIS. Imaging of the patient with the enlarged, tender gland of subacute thyroiditis is often unrewarding. There is usually a failure to deliver sufficient radioiodine to the thyroid (in association with the low RAI uptake) for decent imaging. Area of absent radioactivity (arrow) corresponds to a swollen, tender, firm area in the thyroid gland. The imaging appearance may be confused with that of a large nonfunctioning or "cold" nodule (I-131).

## NODULAR GOITER

The development of nodular goiter is often the end result of continued and frustrated attempts by the thyroid gland to compensate for undersecretion of thyroid hormone. In attempting to secrete additional hormone to meet the body's requirements, greatly enlarged follicles eventually develop, which contain only small amounts of colloid and are lined by flattened endothelium. Through compression by the greatly enlarged follicle, the surrounding thyroid tissue becomes fibrotic. Subsequently, a fibrous capsule forms around the follicle; this encapsulated structure is a thyroid nodule. In addition, enlarged follicles rupture and fibrotic changes occur around several ruptured follicles or groups of follicles. The result is even larger nodules. Degenerative changes (hemorrhagic, cystic, ischemic, necrotic) commonly take place within these encapsulated nodules.

The remaining, functioning thyroid tissue is interspersed outside and between the nodules. It is this portion of the gland that takes up radioactive iodine, as seen on thyroid imaging. If the remaining functioning part of the gland becomes involved with oversecretion of thyroid hormone, resulting in a hyperthyroid state, a toxic, multinodular goiter is present. However, there are no imaging characteristics to distinguish such a gland from a nontoxic, multinodular goiter.

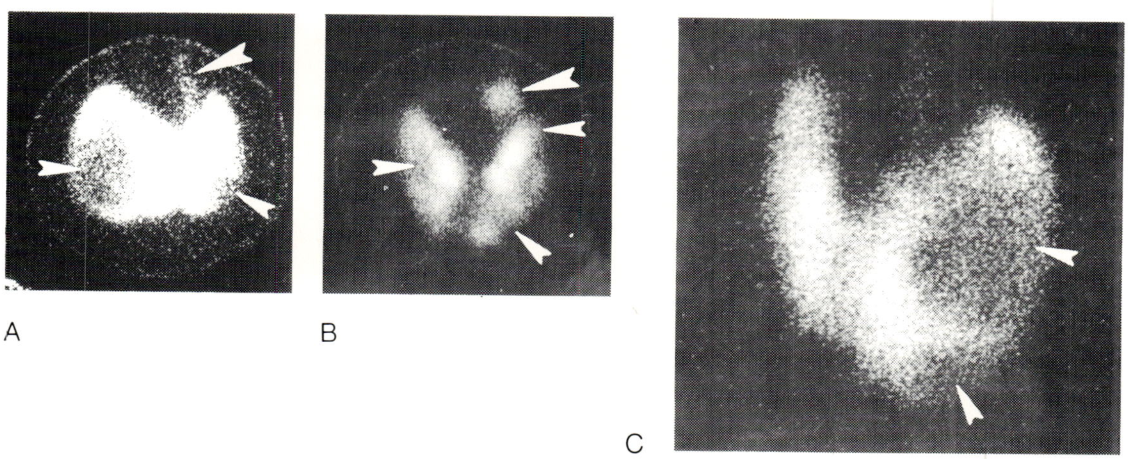


**FIG. 31.** TOXIC MULTINODULAR GOITER. Multiple areas of absent radioactivity representing multiple nodules characterize the images in each of these patients with hyperthyroidism. **A.** Bilateral involvement (small arrows) with increased production of thyroid hormone from the remaining functioning thyroid tissue. Note the visualization of the pyramidal lobe (broken arrow), undoubtedly associated with the elevated radioiodine uptake (I-123). **B.** Multiple nodules (arrows) seen bilaterally. There is a somewhat rounded pyramidal lobe ( larger arrows) related to the left upper pole (I-123). **C.** Predominant involvement of left lobe with two large nodules (arrows) clearly demonstrated. No right-sided nodules were palpable (I-123).

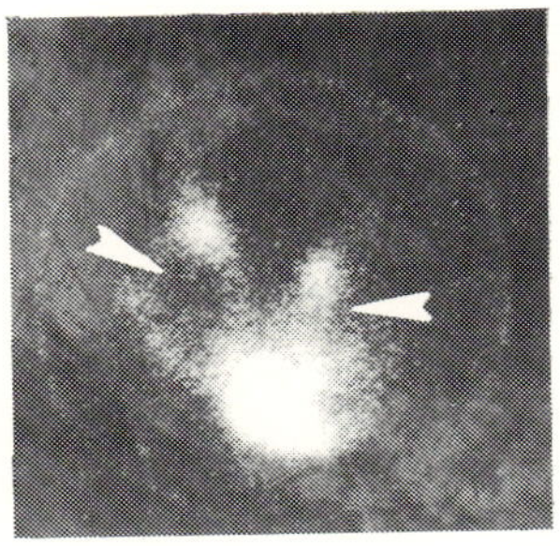

A

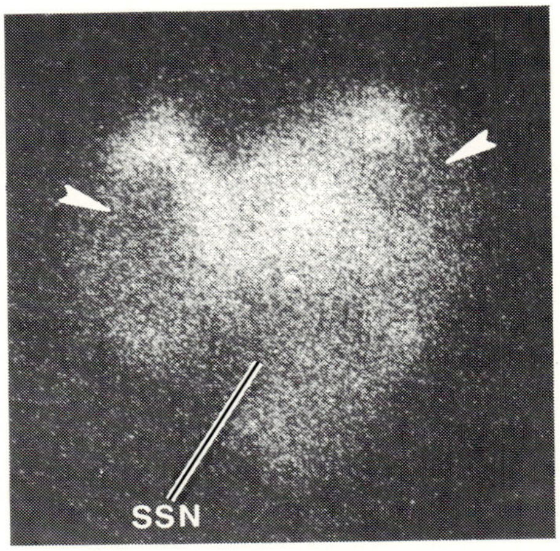


B

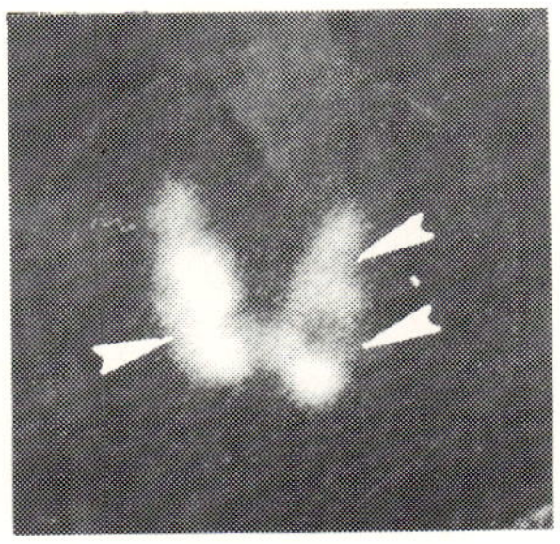

C

**FIG. 32.** NONTOXIC MULTINODULAR GOITER WITH DIFFUSE INVOLVEMENT WITH NODULES IN BOTH LOBES. **A.** Extensive nodular formation in both lobes (arrows) with functioning tissue demonstrated in region of isthmus (I-123). **B.** Diffuse nodularity (arrows) with the distorted left lobe showing evidence of substernal extension (SSN—suprasternal notch) (I-123). **C.** Although the basic architecture of the gland has been preserved, nodules (arrows) in both lobes are identified. Islands of functioning thyroid tissue remain scattered throughout (I-123).

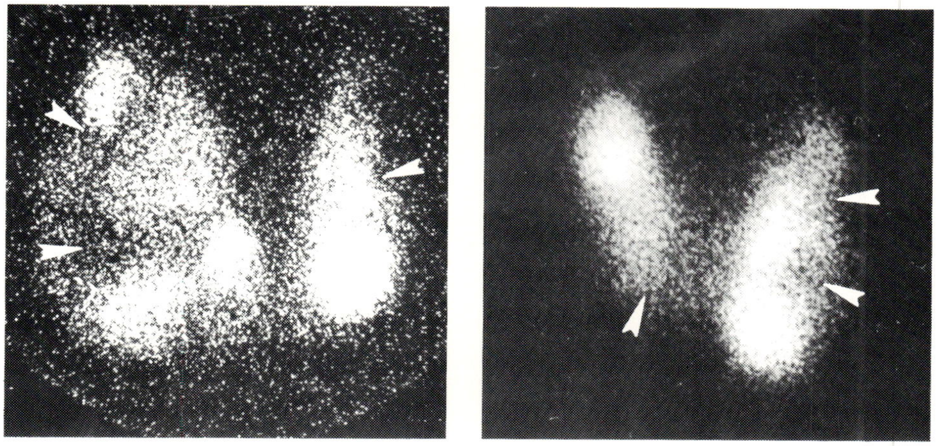

A B

**FIG. 33. NONTOXIC MULTINODULAR GOITER WITH ASYMMETRICAL INVOLVEMENT. A.** Although nodules (arrows) are seen in both lobes, distortion is predominant in the left lobe (I-123). **B.** Multiple nodules (arrows) are seen in the left lobe while only one is present (arrow) in the smaller right lobe. There is no marked enlargement of a lobe as seen in **A** (I-123).

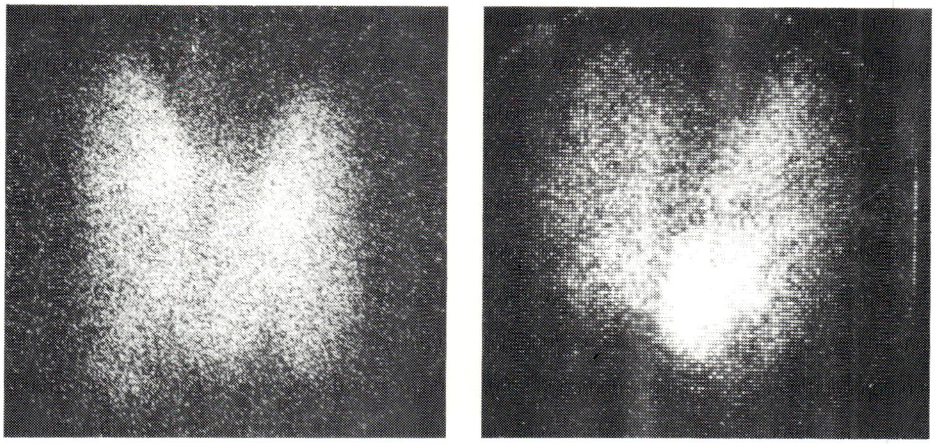

A B

**FIG. 34. NONTOXIC MULTINODULAR GOITER WITH LITTLE OR NO MANIFESTATION OF NODULES ON THYROID IMAGING.** Although multiple nodules are present on physical examination in these enlarged glands, imaging demonstrates no multiple, discrete areas of absent activity. This is related, in part, to functioning thyroid tissue anterior or posterior to regions of involvement. **A.** Markedly enlarged thyroid gland in which there is no reflection of multiple, palpable nodules (I-123). **B.** Enhanced computerized image of patient with multiple palpable nodules except at the left lower pole. The latter represents the site of greatest uptake, but the demonstration of nodules is not distinct (I-123).

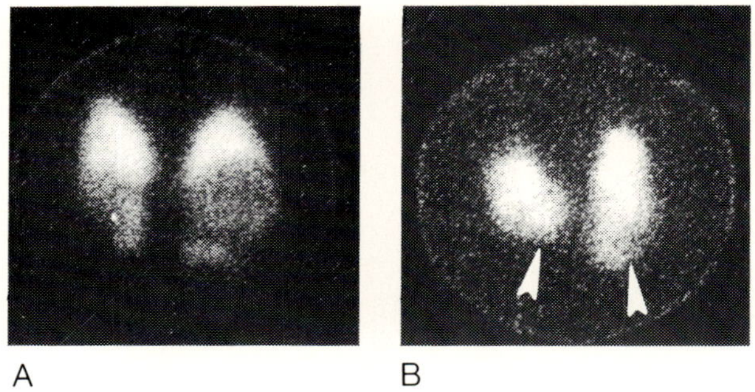


**FIG. 35. NONTOXIC MULTINODULAR GOITER WITH PREDOMINANTLY LOWER POLE INVOLVEMENT. A.** Nodule formation has resulted in reduced radioactivity in the lower half of both right and left lobes. The areas of involvement are discrete and sharply demarcated (I-123). **B.** Irregular nodule formation (arrows) at both lower poles. Although the palpable nodules were sharply defined on physical examination there is no such clear-cut identification on imaging (I-123).

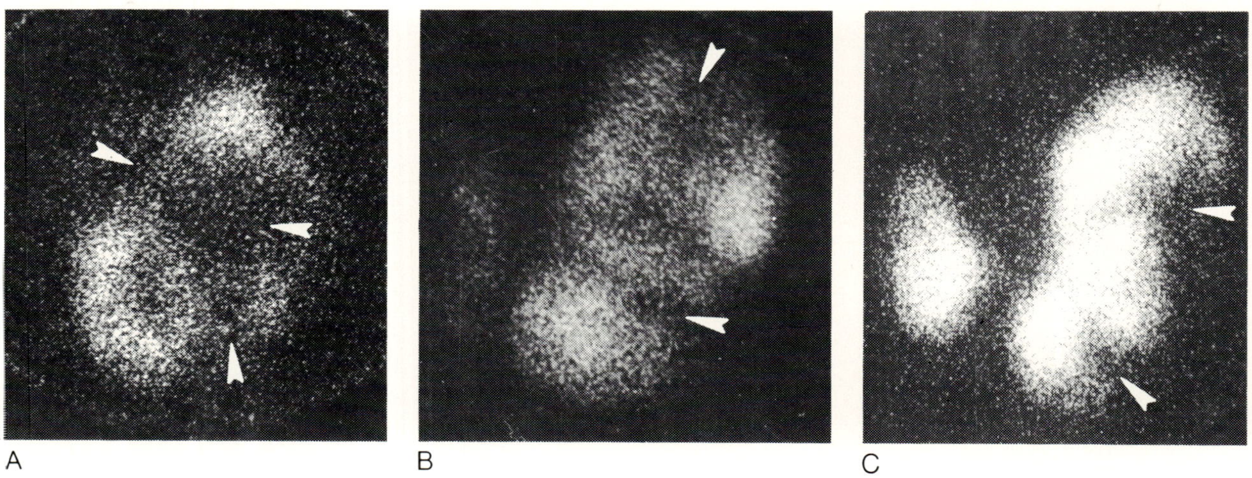


**FIG. 36. NONTOXIC MULTINODULAR GOITER WITH GROSS ARCHITECTURAL DISTORTION.** Involvement with multiple nodules has resulted in marked alteration in the usual appearance of the gland. **A.** Multiple nodules (arrows) with only a small portion of functioning thyroid tissue visible. The individual lobes cannot be identified on imaging (I-123). **B.** Multiple nodules (arrows) with almost complete replacement of the right lobe and distortion of the left lobe (I-123). **C.** Multiple nodules with replacement of the upper half of the right lobe and distortion in the configuration of the left lobe (arrows) (I-123).

## Suggested Reading

Attie JN, Moskowitz GW, Margouleff D, et al: Feasability of total thyroidectomy in the treatment of thyroid carcinoma: postoperative radioactive iodine evaluation of 140 cases. Am J Surg 138:555–560, 1979

Bar-Sella P, Front D, Hardoff R, et al: Ultrastructural basis for different pertechnetate uptake patterns by various human brain tumours. J Neurol Neurosurg Psychiatry 42:924–930, 1979

Bauman RA, Bode HH, Hayek A, et al: Technetium 99m pertechnetate scans in congenital hypothyroidism. J Pediatr 89:268–271, 1976

Blum M, Rothschild M: Improved nonoperative diagnosis of the solitary "cold" thyroid nodule. JAMA 243:242–245, 1980

Geerdsen J: Scintigraphy and clinical evaluation of nontoxic thyroid neoplasms. Acta Chir Scan 145:133–136, 1979

Grieg WR, Gray HW: Thyroid imaging. Hundeshagen H (ed): *Encyclopedia of Medical Radiology: Nuclear Medicine, Part 2.* Heidelberg, Springer-Verlag, 1978, pp 137–153

Hooper PL, Turner JR, Conway MJ, et al: Thyroid uptake of $^{123}$I in a normal population. Arch Intern Med 140:757–758, 1980

Irwin RS, Braman SS, Arvanitidis AN, et al: $^{131}$I thyroid scanning in preoperative diagnosis of mediastinal goiter. Ann Intern Med 88:73–74, 1978

Johnson PM: Thyroid and whole-body scanning. In Werner SC, Ingbar SH (eds): *The Thyroid, Ed.4.* Hagerstown, Harper and Row, 1978, pp 297–317

Massin JP, Planchon C, Perez R: Comparison of $^{99m}$Tc-pertechnetate and $^{131}$I in scanning of thyroid nodules. Clin Nucl Med 2:324–338, 1979

Olsen KJ: Scintigraphic estimation of thyroid volume and dose distribution at treatment with $^{131}$I. Acta Radiol Oncol Radiat Phys Biol 17:74–80, 1979

Potchen EJ, Adelstein SJ, Hoffer PB, James AE, Jr, McNeil BJ, Siegel BA (eds): *Nuclear Radiology Syllabus.* Chicago, American College of Radiology, 1974, pp 288–335

Quinn JL, III, Henkin RE: Scanning techniques to assess thyroid nodules. Annu Rev Med 26:193–201, 1975

Stucker FJ. Jr, Lacher AB, Hirokawa RH: The grand biopsy for the "cold" thyroid nodule. Laryngoscope 89:1524–1431, 1979

Thomas CG Jr, Buckwalter JA, Staab EV, et al: Evaluation of dominant thyroid masses. Ann Surg 183:463–469, 1976

Turner JW, Spencer RP: Thyroid carcinoma presenting as a pertechnetate "hot" nodule, but without $^{131}$I uptake: case report. J Nucl Med 17:22–23, 1976

Wiener JD, deVries AAA: On the natural history of Plummer's disease. Clin Nucl Med 4:181–190, 1980

# 4/Salivary Gland Imaging

Salivary gland imaging is best performed with Tc-99m pertechnetate. The tissue localization of pertechnetate is similar to that of iodide since it is selectively concentrated by the salivary glands, thyroid gland, choroid plexus, and gastric mucosa. For salivary gland imaging, Tc-99m pertechnetate is the agent of choice because it has a short half-life, which allows large doses to be safely used with low radiation exposure to the patient. It has excellent physical properties for use with a scintillation camera or rectilinear scanner, and it is inexpensive and readily available in sterile form for intravenous administration.

Following injection, pertechnetate is actively removed from the blood, concentrated in the salivary glands, and secreted in saliva. Normally, the parotid and submandibular gland images are well seen but the sublingual and minor salivary glands are not. An intravenous dose of 5 to 10 mCi of Tc-99m pertechnetate is administered, and after 2 to 3 minutes an anterior image is obtained showing the relative vascularity of the major salivary glands, and questionably related neck masses. After 15 minutes, static images are obtained in multiple views that show the relative function of the salivary glands and their ability to concentrate pertechnetate. The patient is instructed to eat a regular meal, including grapefruit as a stimulus to secretion of saliva. Anterior, oblique, and posterior static images are then obtained for evidence of abnormal retention in the major salivary glands or their draining ducts.

At any time during the examination, enlarged views of an individual parotid or submandibular gland may be obtained with a pinhole or convergent hole collimator. Limitations of spatial resolution prevent the detection of small cold lesions, and it is unlikely that a mass would be detected that is not clinically palpable. However, in a patient with a questionable mass or unexplained symptoms, an abnormal study showing alteration of major salivary gland size, vascularity, or ability to concentrate and excrete pertechnetate establishes the presence of salivary gland disease. Asymmetric findings are especially significant, although some diseases affect all of the salivary glands more or less uniformly.

In general, *increased* salivary gland concentration of Tc-99m pertechnetate is seen with acute sialadenitis, either bacterial or viral (mumps), following acute salivary duct obstruction, with Mikulicz's disease, and with one of the less common primary tumors, Warthin's tumor. Mass lesions that cause *cold* defects include most primary and metastatic tumors, cysts, and some abscesses.

*Decreased* function ranging from mild to absent is seen with chronic sialadenitis; certain connective tissue diseases including rheumatoid arthritis, Sjögren's syndrome, systemic lupus erythematosus, sarcoidosis, and scleroderma; and following local radiation therapy. Temporary alteration of function is caused by some drugs, including atropine and perchlorate. Serial studies in treatable diseases can be used to evaluate the effectiveness of therapy in that they supply perhaps more objective information than the patient's symptomatic response.

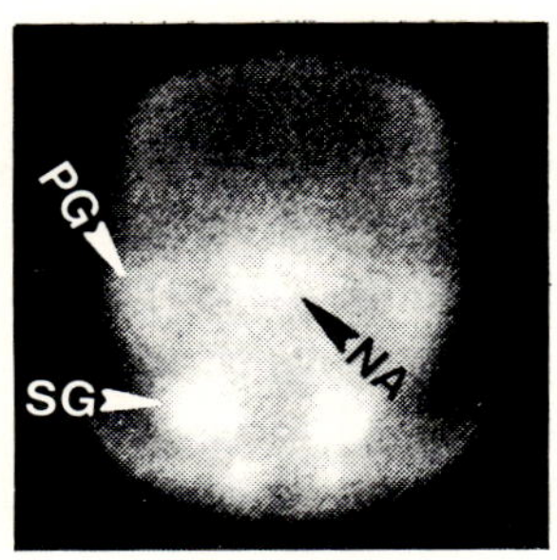


A R ANT

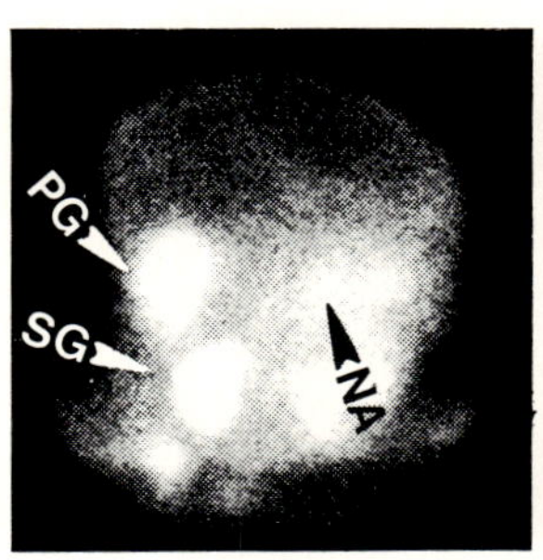


B R A O

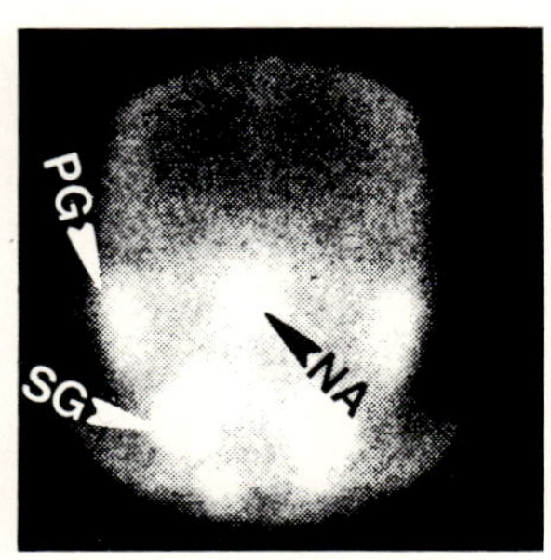


C R ANT

**FIG. 1. A–C.** (See legend next page)

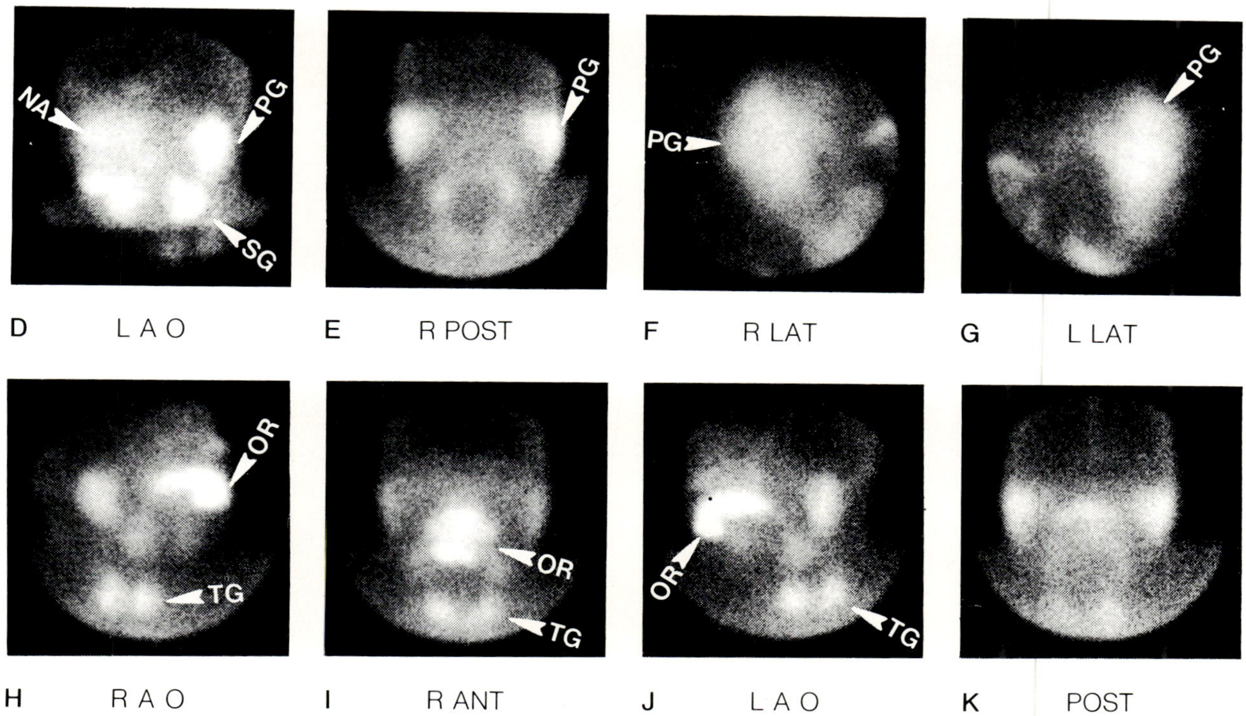


**FIG. 1. NORMAL SALIVARY GLAND STUDY.** Parotid gland (PG), submandibular gland (SG), nasal (NA), oral radioactivity (OR), thyroid gland (TG) partially obscured in some views by overlying lead sheet. Two minutes after intravenous injection of Tc-99m pertechnetate, there is symmetric vascularity of the parotid and submandibular glands (**A**). Oral activity is not yet visible. Equal concentration and uniform glandular distribution are visible at 10 to 20 minutes (**B** through **E**). Lateral views of parotid glands (**F** and **G**) are enlarged using pinhole collimator. After the patient's eating (**H** through **K**), most of the pertechnetate has been secreted in the saliva but oral activity remains intense and for the most part cannot be removed by mouthwashing, probably because of adsorption to the oral and lingual mucosa. Sublingual and minor salivary gland activity is not normally visible.

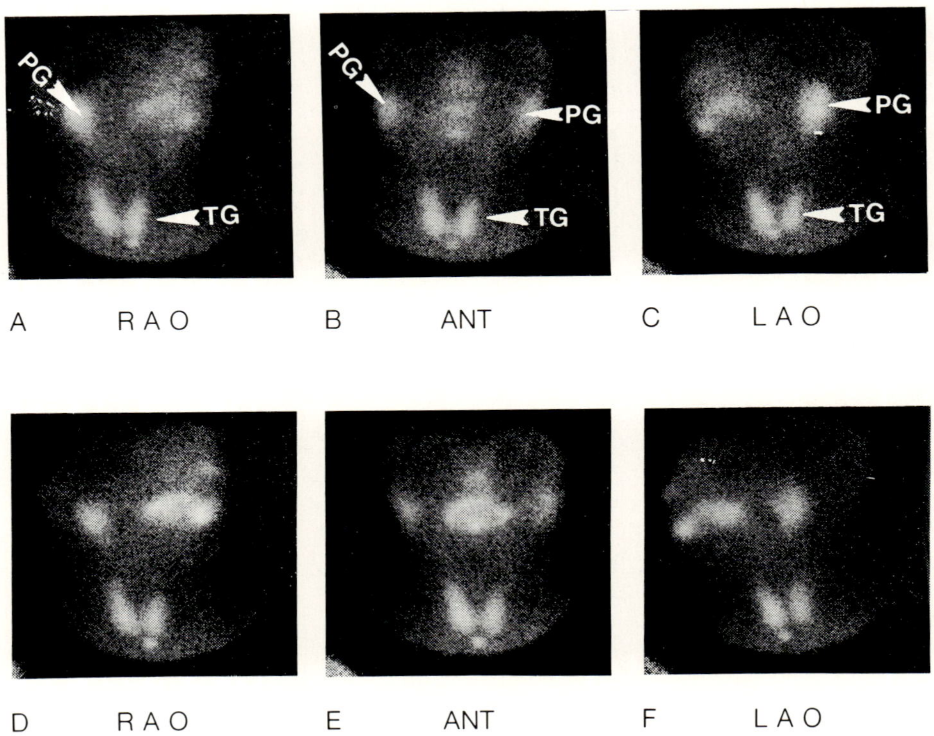


**FIG. 2. ABSENT SUBMANDIBULAR GLAND FUNCTION.** At 15 minutes (**A** through **C**) the parotid and thyroid glands are clearly visible (arrows), but there is no definite concentration of technetium pertechnetate in the submandibular glands. After the patient has eaten (**D** through **F**), secreted radioactivity is present in the mouth but lack of submandibular activity persists, because of either congenital absence or unexplained loss of function. This was an incidental finding in this study, which was performed for evaluation of a nodule overlying the left parotid gland. At surgery, a 1.2 cm mixed tumor of the left parotid was found. Mixed tumors may be pertechnetate cold or warm, but this patient's false negative parotid study probably was due to the scintillation camera's limited capability in resolving lesions smaller than 1 to 2 cm.

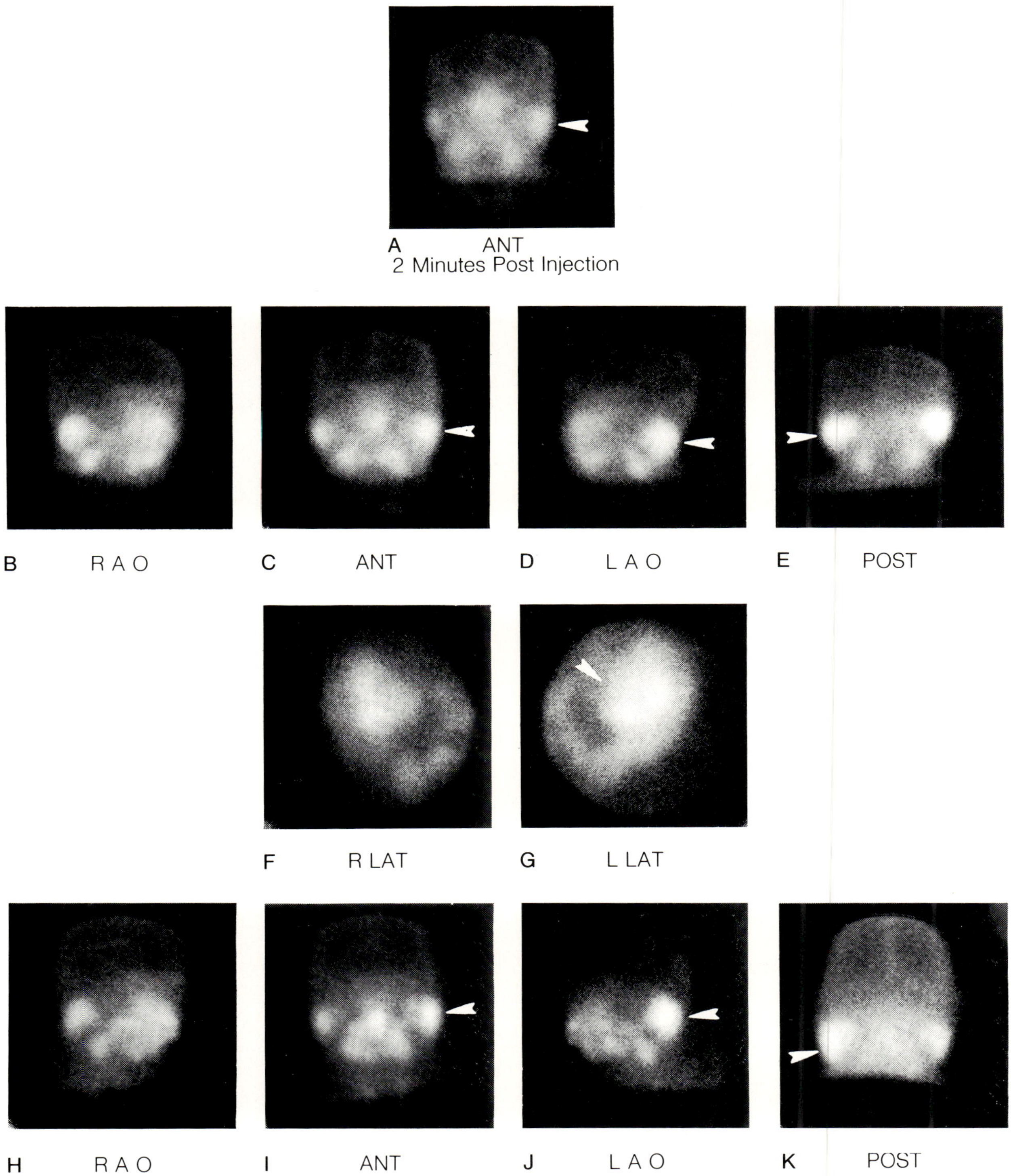


**FIG. 3. ACUTE SIALADENITIS.** The pattern of images in patients with infectious and obstructive sialadenitis is variable but seems to be related to the chronicity of the disease. A diffusely enlarged gland with increased radioactivity (arrows) throughout the study (**A** at 2 minutes, **B** through **G** at 10 to 30 minutes, **H** through **K** after meal) is usually seen with acute infec-

tions, whereas chronic infection results in decreased activity (Fig. 6). A parotid or submandibular duct that remains well visualized suggests duct obstruction. Decreased activity on one side of the tongue or mouth may be visible with impairment of function or obstruction of drainage of the ipsilateral parotid or submandibular gland.

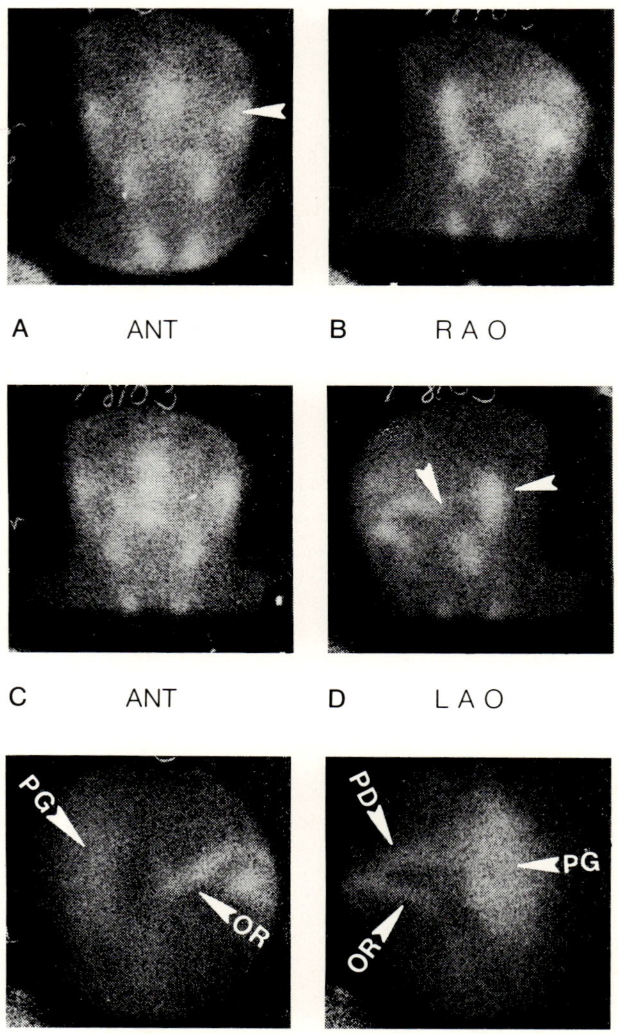


A ANT
B RAO
C ANT
D LAO
E R LAT
F L LAT

**FIG. 4.** (See legend next page)

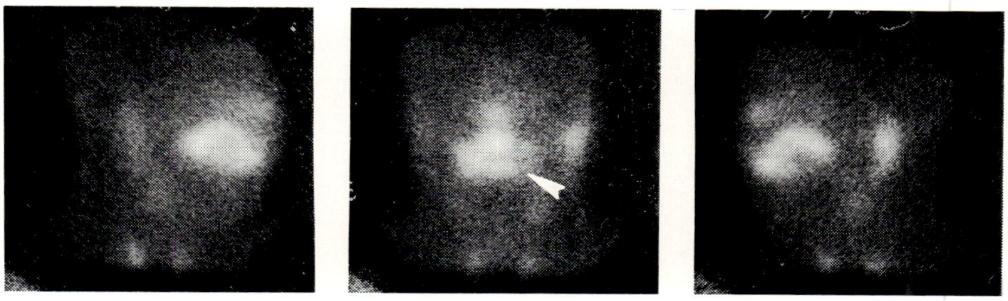

G RAO H ANT I LAO

**FIG. 4. PAROTID DUCT LIGATION.** Patient with painful swelling of the parotid gland associated with small duct calculi underwent parotid duct ligation as a minimal surgical procedure to induce gland atrophy. This study was performed several months later because of recurrent symptoms. Two minutes after intravenous injection of Tc-99m pertechnetate there is slightly increased vascularity of the left parotid (**A,** arrow) due to inflammation. At 15 minutes (**B** through **D**) radioactivity is visible in the enlarged left parotid gland and duct (**D,** arrows) but better defined in enlarged view (**F**) taken with a pinhole collimator (PG—parotid gland, PD—parotid duct, OR—oral activity). In comparison, the unobstructed right parotid gland (**E**) does not retain activity. After the patient has eaten (**G** through **I**), some activity remains in the left parotid but its duct has drained. Note less activity in left side of mouth (**H,** arrow) than in the right, probably due to impaired function of the left parotid. The overall impression is that the left parotid duct is only partially occluded by the ligation or has recanalized. The parotid has not ceased functioning, and there is probably recurrent sialadenitis. Successful ligation of the parotid duct should have resulted in an atrophic, cold gland on this imaging study.

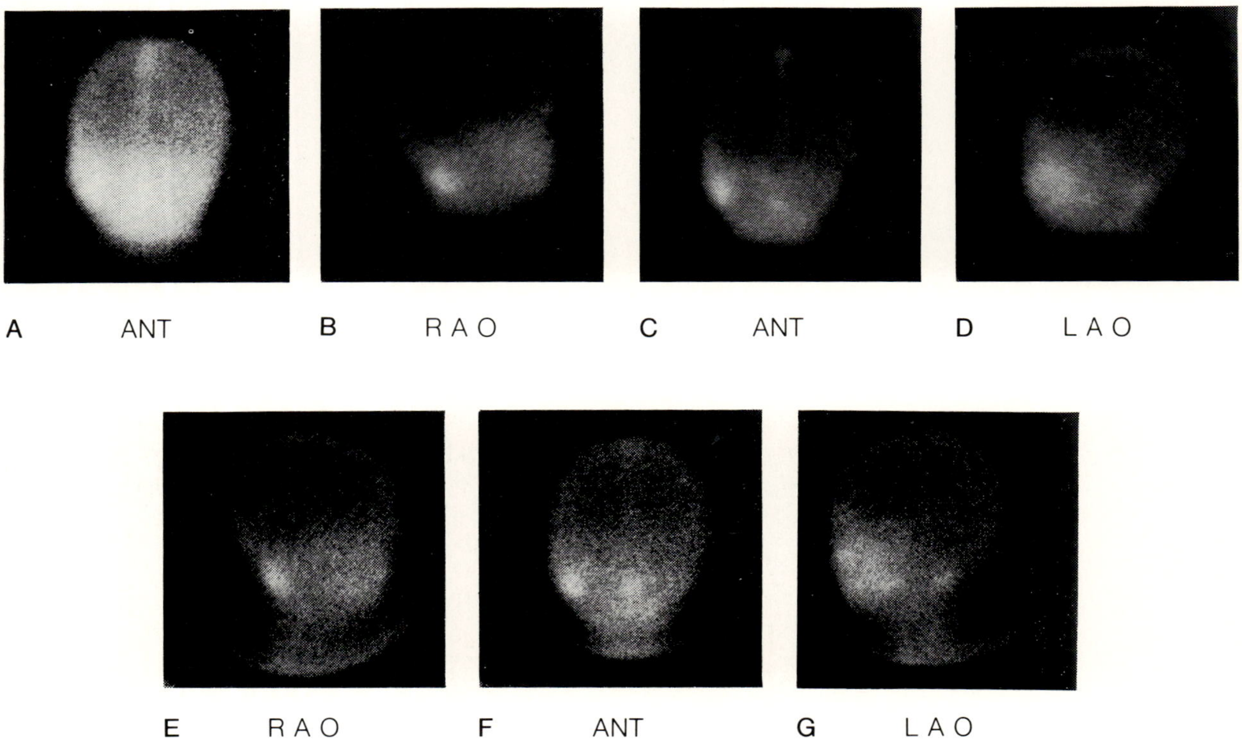


**FIG. 5. ACUTE SUPPURATIVE PAROTITIS.** A ten-day history of painful swelling of the right parotid gland in a 9-year-old girl preceded this study. At surgery, pus was drained from the right parotid space. Despite poor image resolution due to the child's agitation, the right parotid area is seen to be hot at 2 minutes (**A**), at 10 minutes (**B** through **D**), and after she has eaten (**E** through **G**). In some cases of abscess, a cold parotid defect may be visible, especially if the course is more chronic.

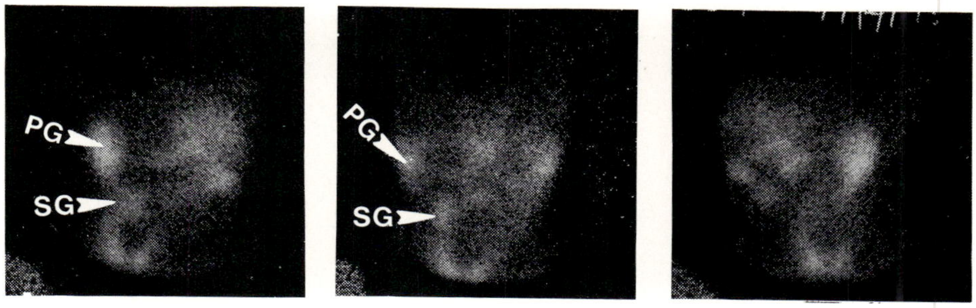


A RAO B ANT C LAO

**FIG. 6.** **CHRONIC SIALADENITIS.** Sixty-seven-year-old woman has a firm palpable mass at inferior aspect of the angle of the mandible on the left side. She had noticed the mass for several months but had no related symptoms. Salivary gland images show normal concentration in parotids and in right submandibular gland (**A** and **B**, arrows) but negligible radioactivity in the left submandibular area. The gland was resected and showed chronic sialadenitis with several small calculi in the salivary duct. Chronic sialadenitis with fibrosis, atrophy, and loss of function is accompanied by a loss of ability to concentrate pertechnetate. The gland is devoid of radioactivity and appears cold.

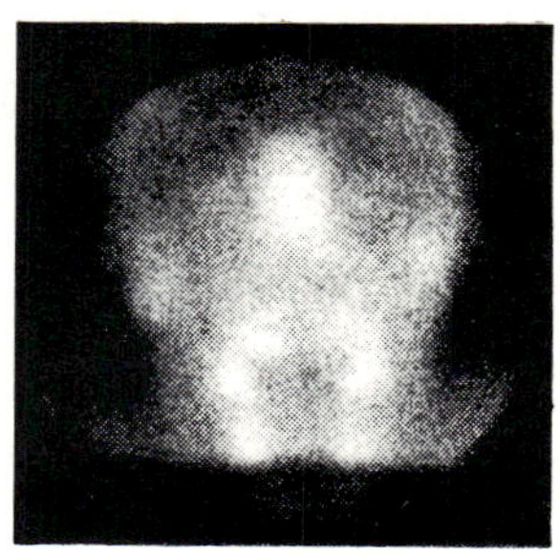

A ANT

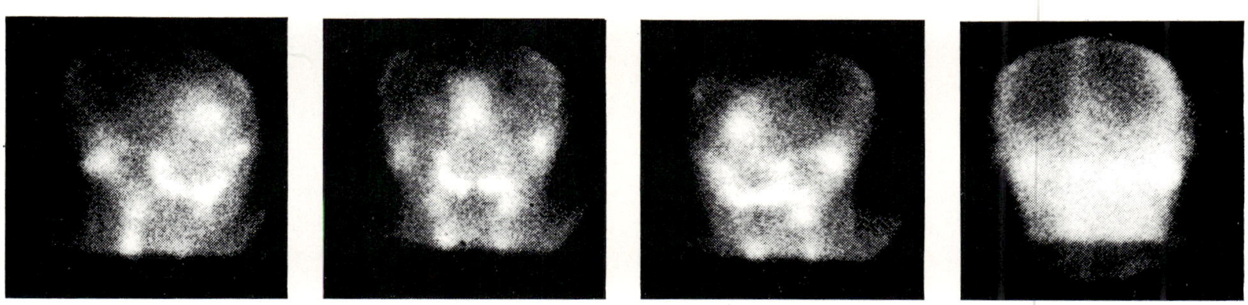

B RAO C ANT D LAO E POST

**FIG. 7. A–E.** (See legend on page 169)

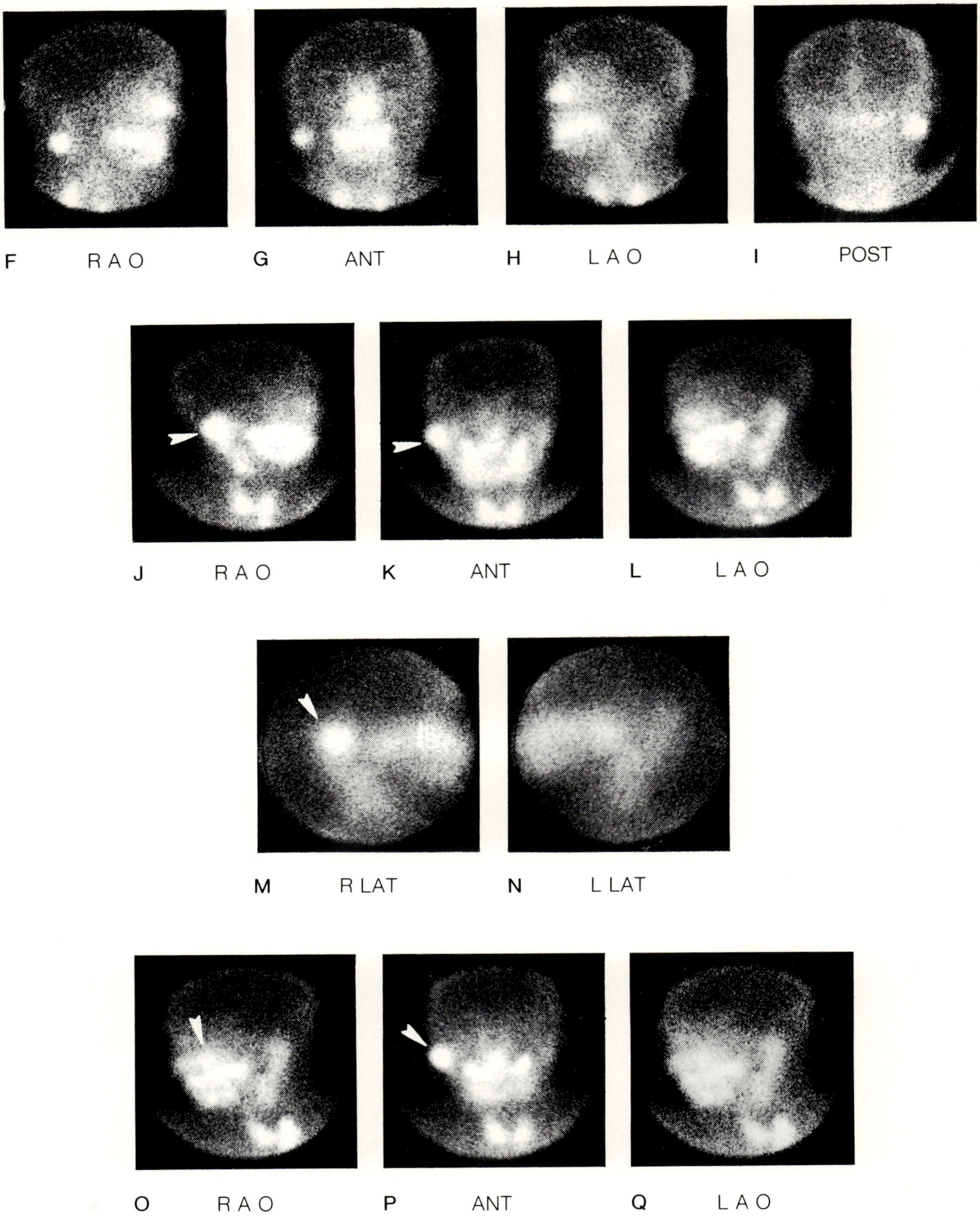


**FIG. 7. F–Q.** (See legend next page)

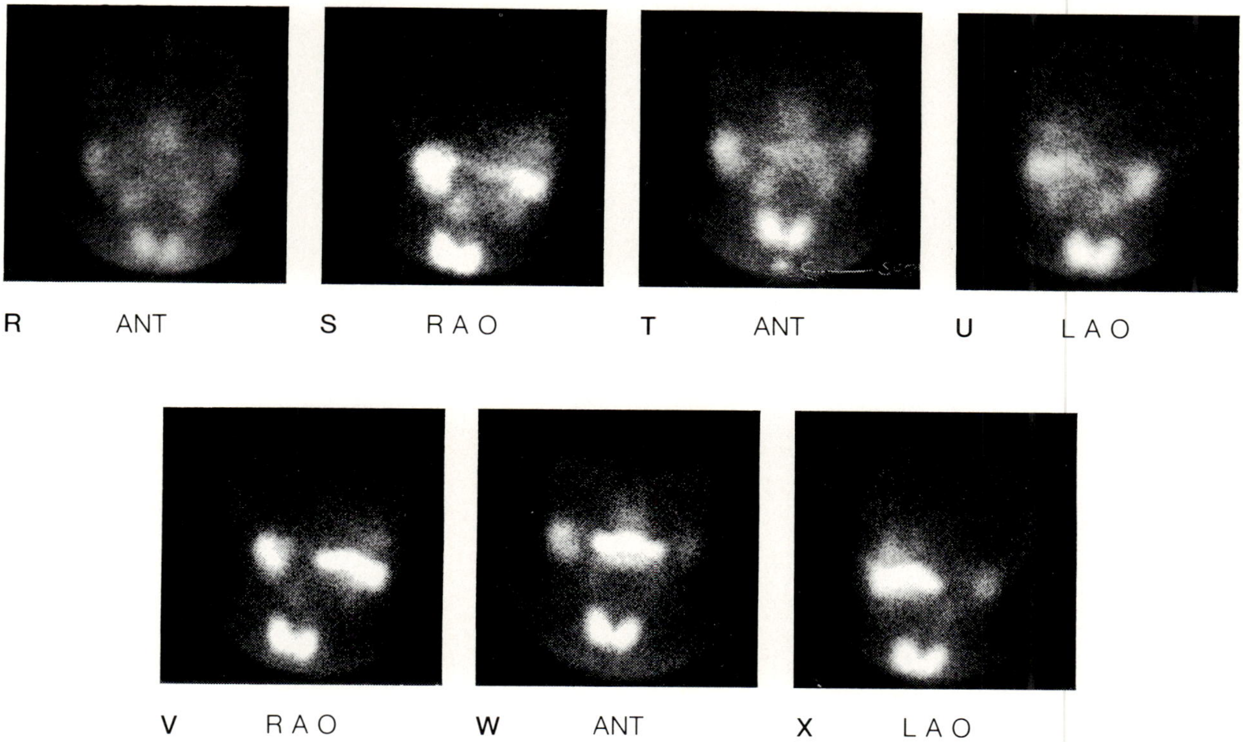


**FIG. 7. WARTHIN'S TUMOR OF THE PAROTID GLAND.** A painless mass at the angle of the mandible on the right side shows increased activity at 2 minutes (**A**), 10 to 20 minutes (**B** through **E**), and after the patient's eating (**F** through **I**). The tumor is typically located in the lower pole of the superficial lobe. In another patient (**J** through **Q**) the tumor (arrows) lies in the upper pole, appearing as an intense focus of activity most clearly visible in enlarged view (**M**) and following a meal (**O** through **Q**). The images in these two patients are characteristic of Warthin's tumor (papillary cystadenoma lymphomatosum), which contains well differentiated ductal epithelium—the cells that normally secrete pertechnetate. A large tumor in a third patient involves almost the entire superficial lobe of the right parotid gland (**R** at 2 minutes, **S** through **U** at 10 to 20 minutes, **V** through **X** after meal). Acute bacterial sialadenitis may show a similar pattern but is usually associated with pain, tenderness, more rapid enlargement of the gland, and a febrile course. There may be evidence of obstruction of the salivary duct. Acute viral parotitis, such as mumps, may occur in the adult but is usually a febrile illness accompanied by constitutional disturbance, painful swelling of one or more salivary glands, sometimes by acute inflammation of the testicle, pancreas, or ovary, and, rarely, by encephalitis. Note that the parotid gland does not have anatomically defined superficial and deep lobes, but these designations are a surgical convenience relating to the interposition of the facial nerve.

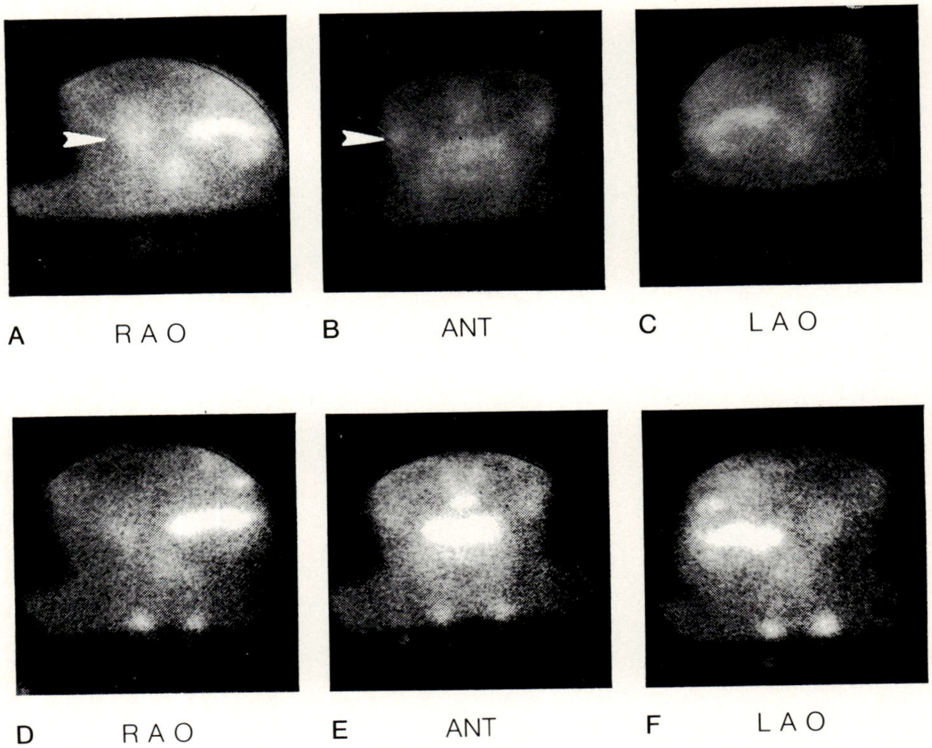


**FIG. 8. LIPOMA OF PAROTID GLAND.** A soft, nontender lump anterior to the right ear was present for one year in this 44-year-old man. Salivary gland images at 15 minutes (**A** through **C**) show decreased concentration of pertechnetate in the superior half of the right parotid gland (arrows). There is normal activity in the remainder of the right parotid, equal to the other salivary glands. A lead shield overlies the lower neck to decrease the contribution of counts from the thyroid gland. After the patient has eaten (**D** through **F**), no radioactivity is retained in any of the major salivary glands, and there is no evidence of delayed concentration in the right parotid lesion, which remains cold. The findings are nonspecific but establish that the right parotid is abnormal. A painless mass that causes a discrete cold defect in an otherwise normally functioning gland is usually due to a tumor or cyst. A 3 × 2 × 2 cm lipoma was found at surgery.

## Suggested Reading

Abdel-Dayem HM: Congenital absence of submaxillary gland detected on $^{99m}$Tc-pertechnetate thyroid imaging. Clin Nucl Med 3:442, 1978

Abramson AL, Levy LM, Goodman M, et al: Salivary gland scintiscanning with technetium 99m pertechnetate. Laryngoscope 79:1105–1117, 1969

Alarcon-Segovia D, Gonzalez-Jimenez Y, Garza LR, et al: Radioisotopic evaluation of salivary gland dysfunction in Sjögren's syndrome. AJR 112:373–379, 1971

Ausband JR, Kittrell BJ, Cowan RJ: Radioisotope scanning for parotid oncocytoma. Arch Otolaryngol 93:628–629, 1971

Boedecker RA, Sty JR, Thompson N: Salivary gland scintigraphy in atypical mycobacterial infection. Clin Nucl Med 4:202, 1979

Burt RW: Accumulation of $^{123}$I in a Warthin's tumor. Clin Nucl Med 3:155–156, 1978

Daniels TE, Powell MR, Sylvester RA, et al: An evaluation of salivary scintigraphy in Sjögren's syndrome. Arthritis Rheum 22:809–814, 1979

De Rossi G: The diagnostic value of radioiostopes and thermography in salivary gland diseases. Radiol Diagn (Berl) 19:505–511, 1978

Gates GA: Radiosialographic aspects of salivary gland disorders. Laryngoscope 82:115–130, 1972

Grove AS Jr, DiChiro G: Salivary gland scanning with technetium-99m pertechnetate. Am J Roentgenol 102:109–116, 1968

Hannum JS, Harrill JA, Maynard CD: $^{99m}$Tc-sodium pertechnetate scanning of a cystadenoma of the larynx. A case report. Clin Nucl Med 1:230–232, 1976

Jafek BW, Strife JL: Accessory lobe of the submandibular gland. Diagn Radiol 109:75–78, 1973

Karlsson G, Lind M: Salivary gland scintigraphy Diagnostic verification of parotid saliva flow through the maxillary sinus and nose. Arch Otorhino-laryngol (NY) 218:263–277, 1978

Lunia S, Chodos RB, Lunia C, et al: Oxyphilic adenoma of the patrotid gland. Identification with $^{99m}$Tc-pertechnetate. Radiology 128:690, 1978

McGuire WF, McCabe BF: Limitations of parotid scans. Ann Otol Rhinol Laryngol 86:247–250, 1977

Noyek AM, Zizmor J, Musumeci R, et al: The radiologic diagnosis of malignant tumors of the salivary glands. J Otolaryngol 6:381–385, 1977

Parret J, Peyrin JO: Radioisotopic investigations in salivary pathology. Clin Nucl Med 4:250–261, 1979

Prince JR, Dukstein WG, White WE: A radioisotopic evaluation of a salivary fistula. Clin Nucl Med 3:334, 1978

Reiskin AB, Puri S: Radiographic and radionuclide appearance of Warthin's tumors. Conn Med 42:503–506, 1978

Sagar VV, Piccone JM, Meckelnburg RL: Dynamic flow study in Warthin's tumor of parotid gland. Clin Nucl Med 2:404–405, 1977

Schall GL: The role of radionuclide scanning in the evaluation of neoplasms of the salivary glands: A review. J Surg Oncol 3:699, 1971

Shall GL, Anderson LG, Buchignani JS, et al: Investigation of major salivary duct obstruction by sequential salivary scintigraphy. AJR 113:655–659, 1971

Schall GL, Anderson LG, Wolf RO, et al: Xerostomia in Sjögren's syndrome: Evaluation by sequential salivary scintigraphy. JAMA 216:2109–2116, 1971

Schall GL, DiChiro G: Clinical usefulness of salivary gland scanning. Semin Nucl Med 2:270–277, 1972

Schall GL, Larson SM, Anderson LG, et al: Quantification of parotid gland uptake of pertechnetate using a gamma scintillation camera and a "region-of-interest" system. AJR 115:689–697, 1972

Schmitt G, Lehmann G, Strotges MW, et al: The diagnostic value of sialography and scintigraphy in salivary gland diseases. Br J Radiol 49:326–329, 1976

Sorsdahl OA, Williams CM, Bruno FP: Scintillation camera scanning of the salivary glands. AJR 92:1477–1480, 1969

Stebner FC, Byler WR, DuSault LA, et al: $^{99m}$Tc pertechnetate scanning of salivary glands. Radiology 90:583–585, 1968

Van Den Akker HP, Sokole EB, Van Der Schoot JB: Origin and location of the oral activity in sequential salivary gland scintigraphy with $^{99m}$Tc-pertechnetate. J Nucl Med 17:959–964, 1976

Van Den Akker HP, Sokole EB, Van Der Schoot JB: The influence of dental restorations on salivary gland scintigraphy with 99mTc-pertechnetate. Oral Surg 46:594–597, 1978

# 5/Bone Imaging

With the availability of fluorine-18 (F-18) and technetium-99m phosphate (Tc-99m-P) radiopharmaceuticals in recent years, bone imaging has become a valuable and often requested procedure in diagnosis of a multiplicity of bone diseases. Such a status could not previously have been attained when the only generally available bone agent was strontium-85 (Sr-85) which the (then) AEC restricted to use in cancer patients. Another strontium isotope, strontium 87m (Sr-87m) is conveniently available from a generator which can be bought and kept in the nuclear medicine department. This radionuclide has a photon energy of 0.39 MeV and a short physical half-life of 2.8 hours. Because of the rapidly dropping count rate, imaging must be performed within a few hours of injection, but blood and soft tissue background activity remain high at this time, resulting in an undesirably low bone/background ratio.

F-18 is an excellent bone-seeking agent with a very short physical half-life of 1.8 hours and an acceptably low radiation dose to the patient; however, F-18 is cyclotron-produced, and its rapid decay rate requires that the user be located close to one of the few commercial suppliers. Also, the high photon energy of 0.51 MeV is less than ideal for imaging purposes, especially for a nuclear medicine department equipped only with regular scintillation cameras, which are more suited to lower photon energy radionuclides.

Tc-99m-P radiopharmaceuticals are currently the agents of choice because of their ready availability and ease of preparation from a kit, high specificity for bone with negligible patient toxicity or side effects, and the excellent physical properties of Tc-99m. Although there are minor differences among Tc-99m polyphosphate, diphosphonate, and pyrophosphate in regard to blood, tissue, and renal clearance rates, similar diagnostic results are obtained with each of these bone agents. However, Tc-99m-methylene diphosphonate has since become available and is currently the agent of choice. Two major factors that influence the localization of these radiopharmaceuticals in bone are the regional bone blood supply and the rate of bone turnover. Images become abnormal when either or both of these interrelated processes are significantly altered by a disease.

An important application of bone imaging is in a total body survey before definitive surgery in patients with tumors that tend to metastasize to bone, especially tumors of the breast, lung, prostate, and kidney. Compared with other current methods used to detect skeletal metastases, including clinical

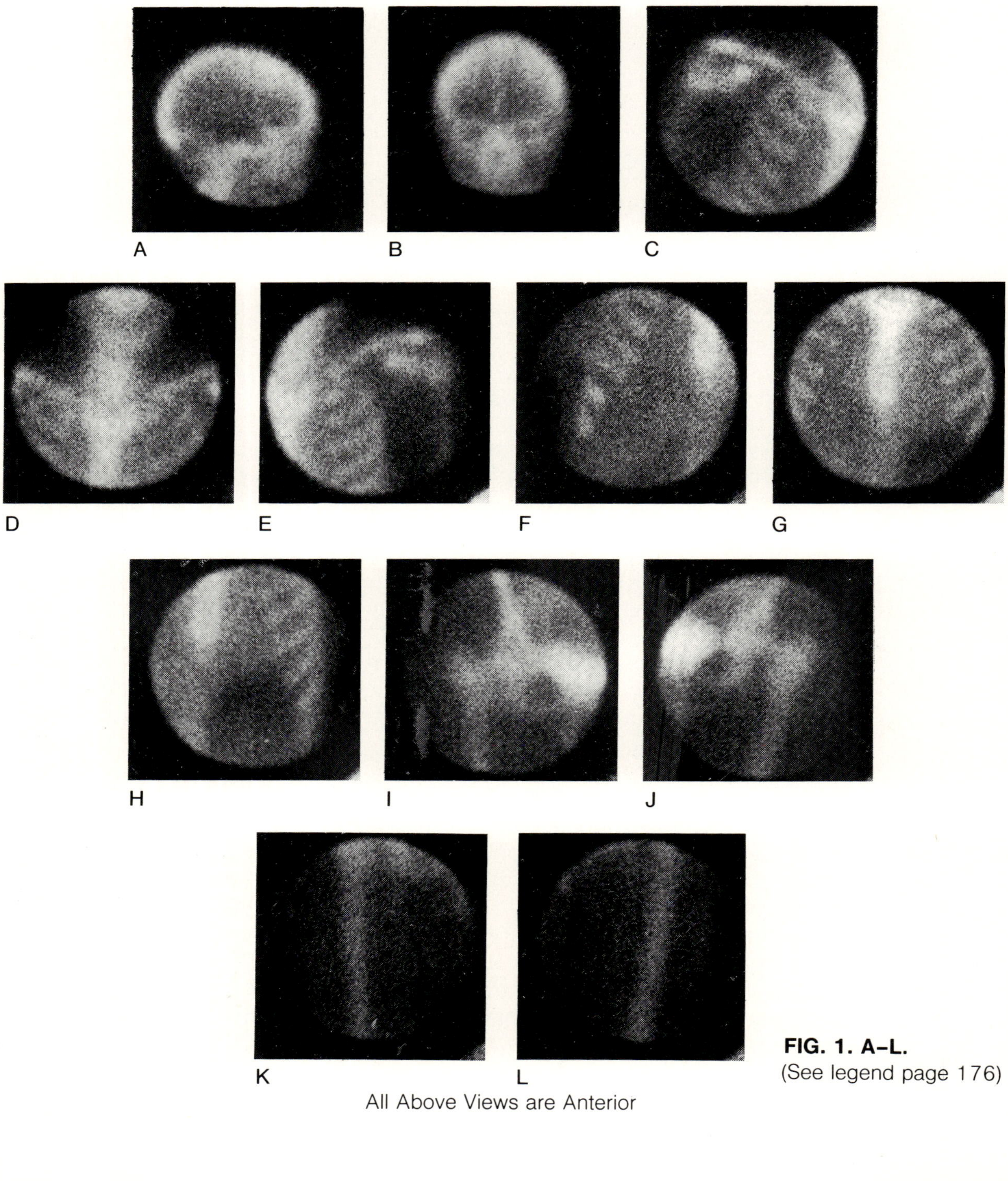

All Above Views are Anterior

**FIG. 1. A–L.**
(See legend page 176)

findings, radiographic bone survey, and serum alkaline phosphatase determination, radionuclide bone imaging is often more sensitive; and unlike the lab study, it locates the site of the lesion. Bone metastases are often detected before they cause symptoms and sometimes many months before they can be found by conventional radiographic examination.

Bone imaging is useful for patients with unexplained pain seemingly of skeletal origin. A positive study is confirmatory, and because of a low false negative rate, a negative study can often exclude underlying bone disease as the source of symptoms. Exceptions are bone marrow involvement with metastatic carcinoma (often anaplastic and widespread), lymphoma, and multiple myeloma. Bone images in these diseases may provide no significant findings unless fractures are present. In myeloma, cold focal lesions may sometimes be seen, corresponding to punched-out osteolytic defects in radiographs. Overall, cold bone lesions are much less commonly encountered than hot lesions, and in addition to myeloma may be found in a variety of conditions. In polyarthritis, a joint survey often discloses more widespread disease than is suspected clinically. In many types of benign and malignant bone disease, serial studies may provide objective evidence of response to therapy.

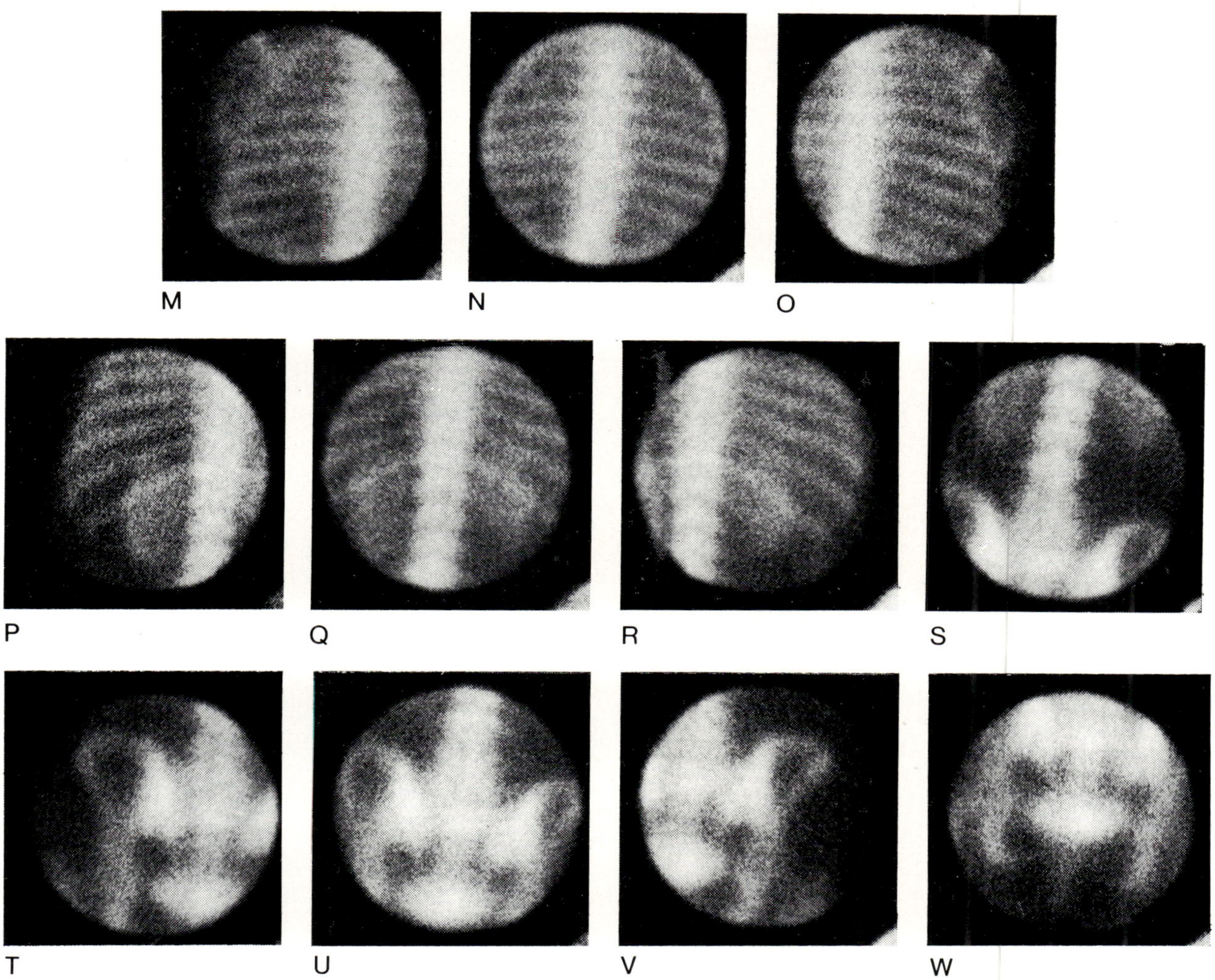


All Above Views are Posterior

**FIG. 1. M–W.** (See legend next page)

**FIG. 1. NORMAL.** Technetium-99m pyrophosphate (TcPYP) bone images taken anteriorly (**A** through **L**) and posteriorly (**M** through **W**) include the common sites of metastasis. Distal extremities may be included if symptomatic. Because asymmetric findings are usually significant, the scintillation camera factors should include preset time rather than preset count rate (usually two or three minutes per frame) to obtain mirror images. Distribution of bone agent in the skull may be patchy, but normally it is more or less symmetric. Areas of slightly increased concentration in the neck, shoulders, sterno-clavicular joints, tips of the scapulae, sacro-iliac joints and sometimes anterior ends of ribs should not be considered pathologic unless the distribution is noticeably asymmetric. In right-handed persons, slightly more radioactivity may be seen in the right shoulder than in the left shoulder. In left-handed persons the opposite is true, presumably as a consequence of dominant use of one limb. Because Tc-99m phosphate radiopharmaceuticals (TcP) are mainly excreted by the kidneys, their images are usually clearly visible (except Tc-99m methylene diphosphonate TcMDP). Normally, equal radioactivity is present in each kidney. By voiding just prior to imaging the pelvis, bladder activity can be reduced but is rarely eliminated, probably because of adsorption to the bladder mucosa.

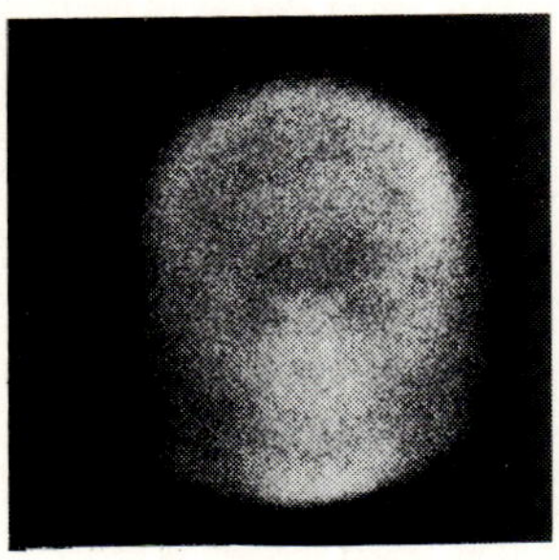

A

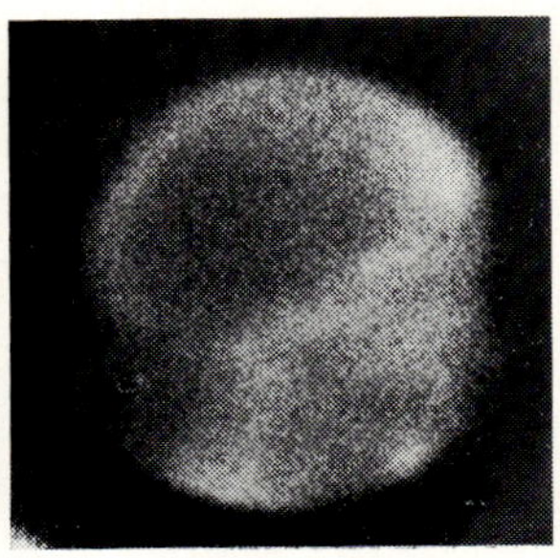

B

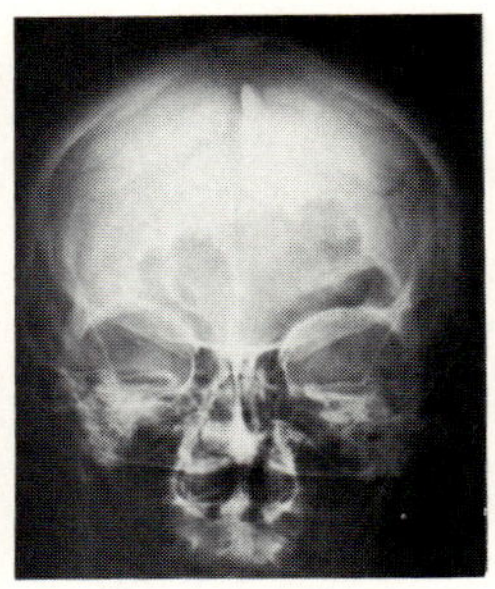

C

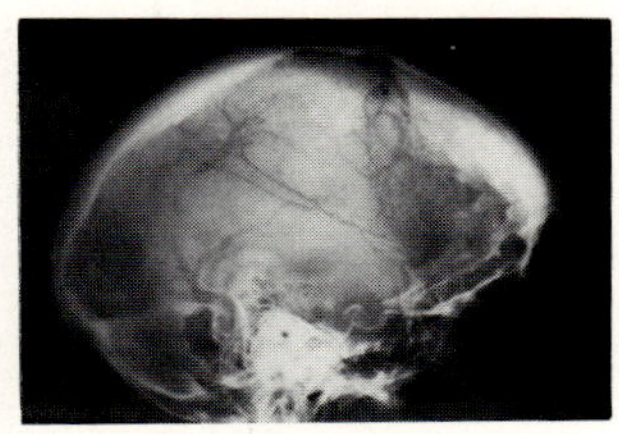

D

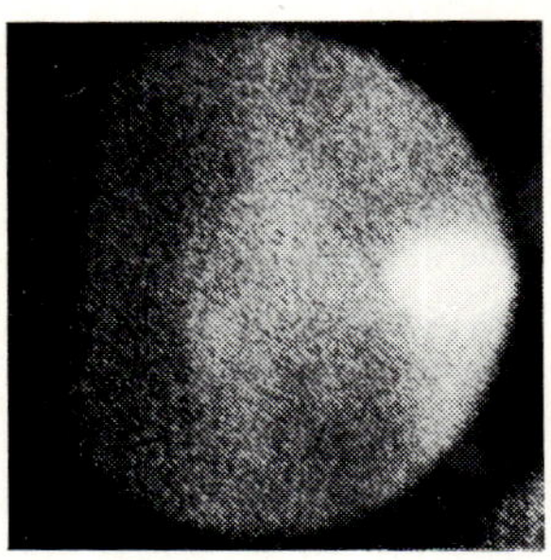

E

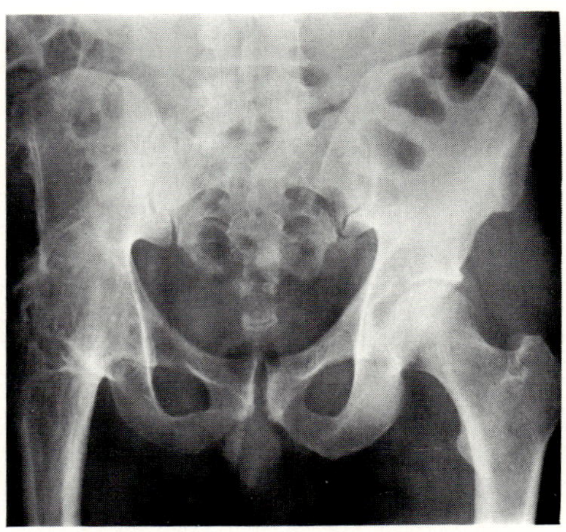

F

**FIG. 2. VARIANTS.** Whenever a bone image differs from the expected appearance, x-rays should be examined for an explanation. Some variants are fairly common (**A** through **D**, hyperostosis frontalis interna), and in other cases a condition may be unrelated to the patient's current illness (**E** and **F**, ankylosis of the right hip since 1939).

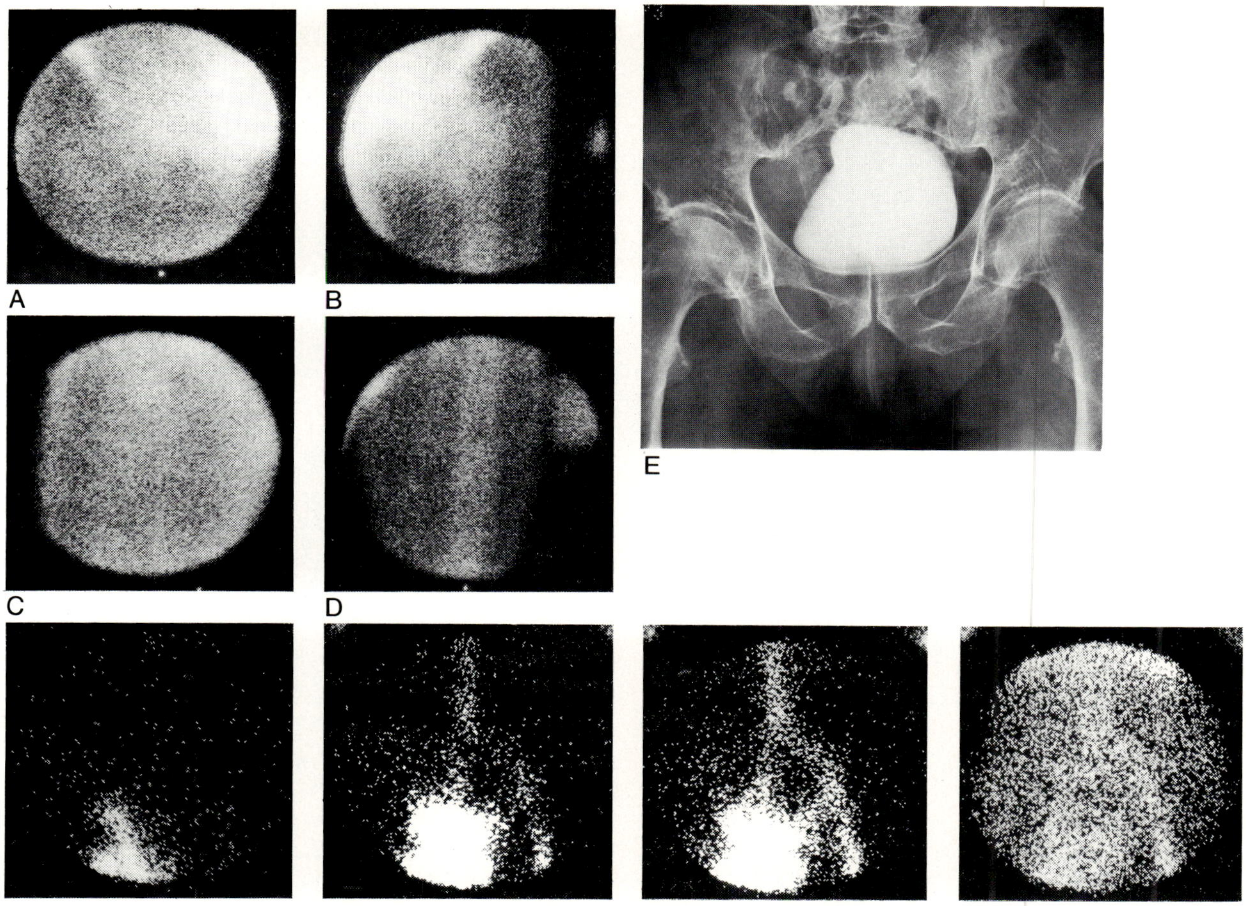

A B C D E F G H I

**FIG. 3. VASCULAR OBSTRUCTION.** A major determinant of bone localization of TcP is blood supply. Arterial, venous, or lymphatic obstruction results in a decreased amount of TcP delivered to bone and/or removed from soft tissues in the distribution of the obstructed vessels. The findings are most marked when the major vessels of an entire limb are involved. Poor localization in the femur, high level of soft-tissue activity, and enlargement of the right leg (**A** and **C**) compared to the normal left (**B** and **D**) are due to lymphoma in the right groin and pelvis, which causes vascular obstruction. Bone mineralization and architecture are normal (**E**), but a soft tissue mass is suspected because of the concave extrinsic pressure deformity on the right side of the contrast-filled bladder. A similar deformity is seen in the bladder filled with normally excreted TcP (**A**). Radionuclide venogram (**F** through **I** at 20, 30, 40, and 120 seconds) following bilateral simultaneous pedal vein injection of Tc-99m pertechnetate shows large irregular blood pool of previously radiated tumor and pelvic collateral circulation. The patient's edematous right leg is due to venous and probably lymphatic obstruction by a locally extensive lymphoma. Decreased concentration of TcP in bones of an extremity may also be seen with stenosis or occlusion of the major arterial supply. The opposite effect, increased bone agent delivered to an extremity, may follow ipsilateral sympathectomy. If an entire dose of TcP is injected directly into the brachial artery, a ''hot gauntlet'' appearance below the level of injection results from the high local concentration of bone agent as it perfuses the tissues in the first pass.

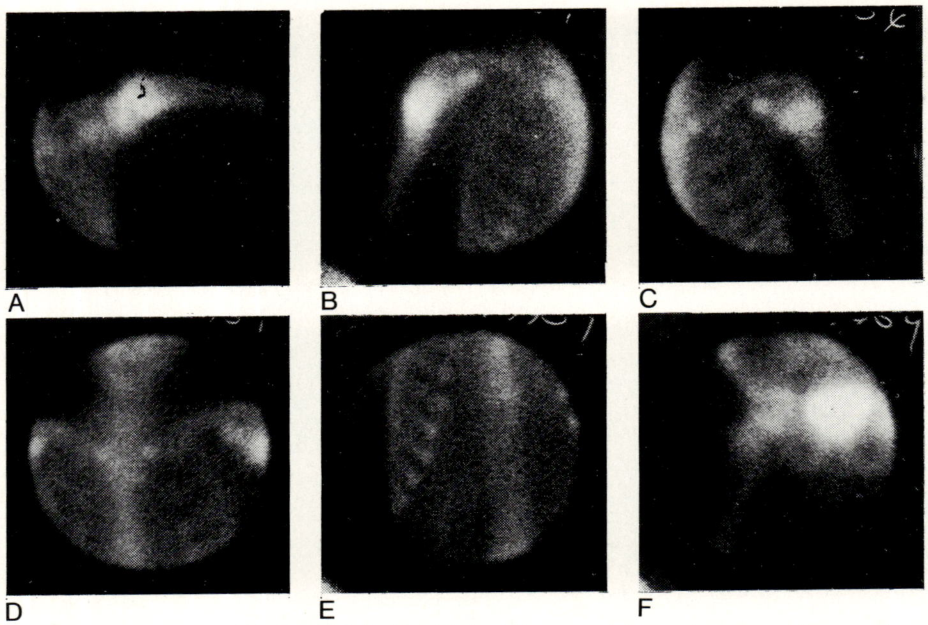


**FIG. 4. HEALING FRACTURE.** This 10-year-old boy fractured the neck of the right humerus six weeks prior to the study. Increased concentration of bone agent at the fracture site is seen in posterior (**A**) and anterior (**B**) views, compared to normal distribution in anterior view of left shoulder (**C**). Increased radioactivity may be seen as early as the first day of fracture but may be delayed for several days if a large hematoma forms at the fracture site and prevents local delivery of the blood-borne radiopharmaceutical. With clot organization and the onset of bone repair there is an increase in the local deposition of TcP, which continues throughout the healing phase, lasting for several months and sometimes for many years but usually to a lesser degree. Additional frames (**D** through **F**) in same patient are included to show normally increased concentration of bone agent in growth centers of an adolescent. Inner end of clavicles (**D**), costochondral junctions (**E**), and femoral epiphyses (**F**) are typical examples. Compare these and normal shoulder (**C**) with adult pattern in Fig. 1.

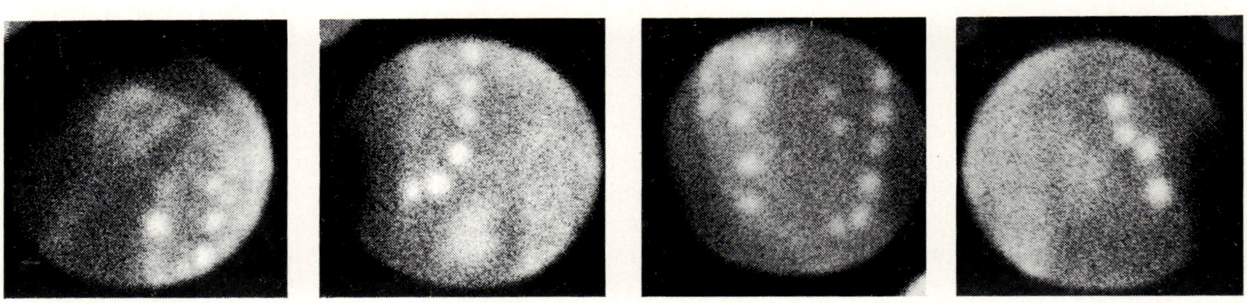

A R Upper　　B R Lower　　C R LAT　　D L Lower

**FIG. 5. MULTIPLE RIB FRACTURES.** An 83-year-old woman fell and fractured many ribs. The multiple focal lesions (**A** through **D**) have a chain-of-beads appearance. Linear distribution of rib lesions is typical of traumatic fractures. Pathological fractures due to neoplastic metastases are usually randomly distributed.

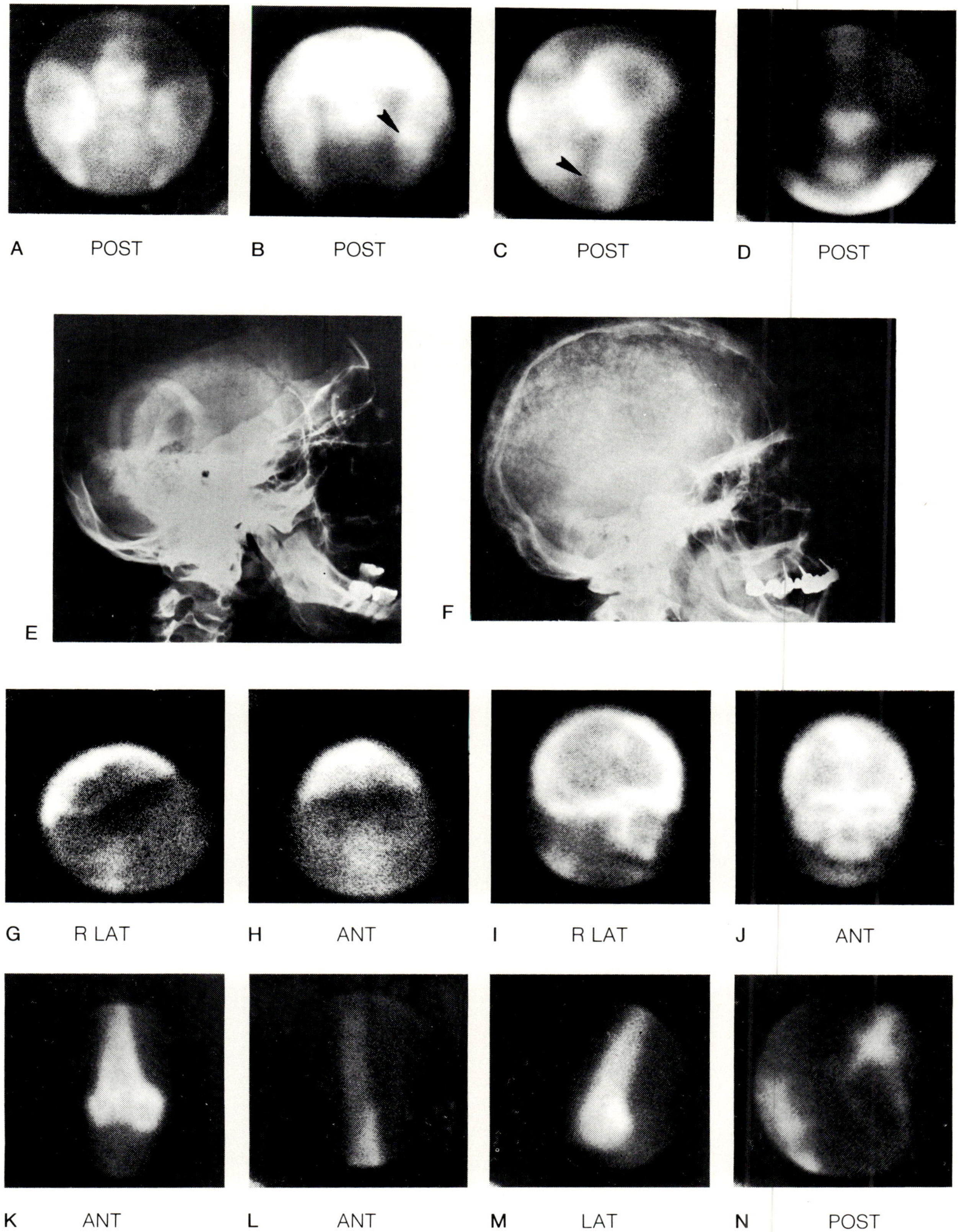


**FIG. 6. A–N.** (See legend next page)

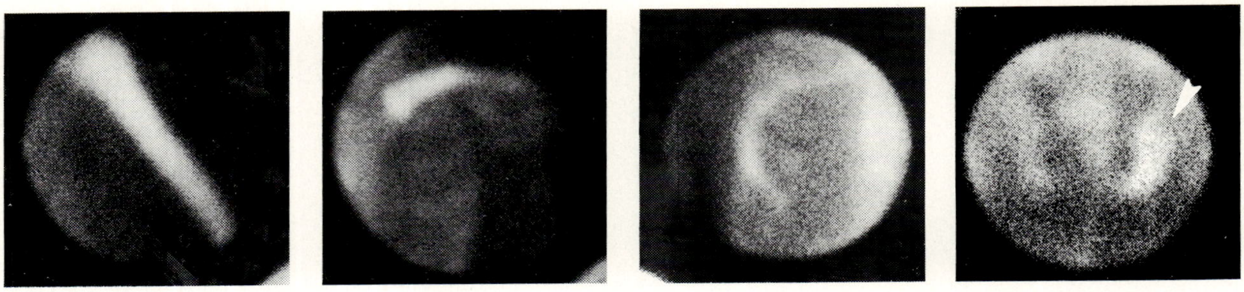

O ANT P ANT Q ANT R POST

**FIG. 6. PAGET'S DISEASE OF BONE.** Markedly increased concentration of TcP diffusely distributed throughout most of an involved bone is typical of Paget's disease. The most common sites of involvement are the pelvis and vertebrae (**A**). Lesions in another patient (**B** through **D**) are so intense that normal femurs, vertebrae, and kidneys are barely seen, yet a healing fracture of the right ischium ( arrow ) is detectable as a transverse band of even greater concentration of bone agent. Unexplained findings such as this, which do not fit the expected pattern of disease, require radiographic correlation. Skull images are abnormal in the early osteoporosis circumscripta phase (**E, G,** and **H**) and later when the entire skull and facial bones—but rarely the mandible—are involved (**F, I,** and **J**). In contradistinction, the ''hot head'' seen in secondary hyperparathyroidism (renal osteodystrophy) includes the mandible. Paget's disease starts at either end of a long bone such as the femur (**K** through **M**) or tibia and progresses lengthwise along the shaft. Enlargement, cortical thickening, and bowing of long bones may be seen, almost as well as in radiographs. Scapula, humerus, clavicle, and rib (**N** through **Q**) are less commonly involved than those bones mentioned above. In all cases the bone is easily identified. Frame **R** is part of a total body bone survey performed preoperatively in a man with a resectable mass in the lung. The only abnormal finding is increased bone agent in the right ischium ( arrow ). Radiographs showed increased bone density, but biopsy was considered necessary to exclude a metastatic lesion. Paget's disease was found. Although a metastasis may occasionally involve a bone diffusely, this distribution is more typical of Paget's disease. Note that by imaging the pelvis with the patient prone, excreted radioactivity will run cephalad into the fundus of the bladder away from the pubic bones and ischium, allowing better visualization of these structures.

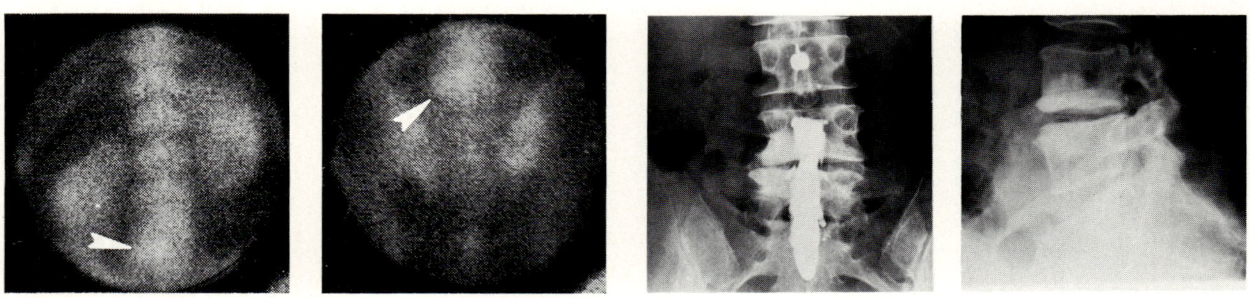

A POST B POST C L LAT D P A

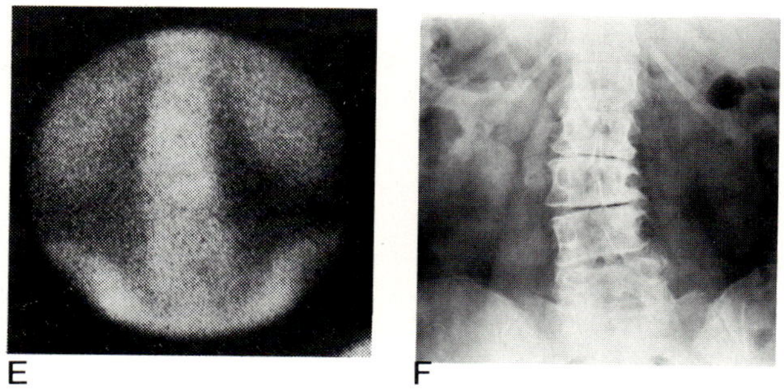

E F

**FIG. 7. DEGENERATIVE DISC DISEASE.** Subtle increased concentration of TcP is present on the left side of the fourth and fifth lumbar vertebrae (**A** and **B**, arrows). Osteophytes and bone sclerosis bordering an asymmetrically narrowed interspace at the L4-L5 level are the radiographic findings (**C** and **D**) that accompany a degenerated intervertebral disc in this patient. The myelogram shows a concave extrinsic pressure defect on the column of contrast medium due to extruded disc material. A similar finding of increased deposition of TcP may be seen in vertebrae at the apex of a scoliotic curvature and is due to abnormal weight-bearing stresses with locally increased bone turnover. Scoliosis and disc degeneration often coexist (**E** and **F**).

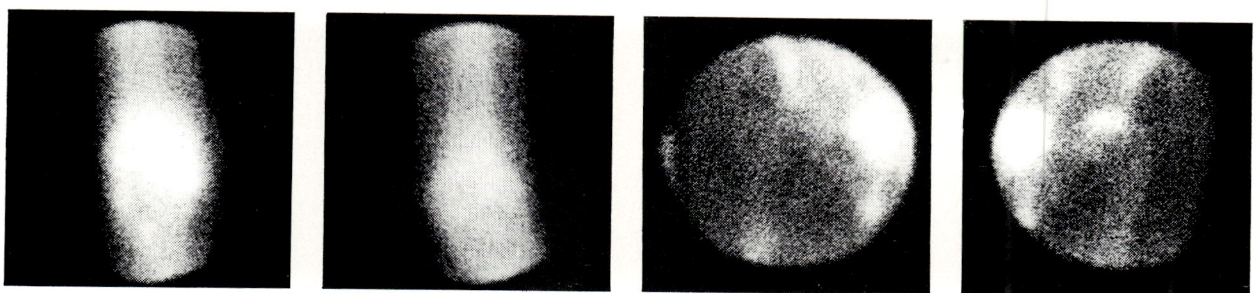

A ANT R B ANT L C ANT R D ANT L

**FIG. 8. DEGENERATIVE JOINT DISEASE.** Abnormal localization of bone agent in the region of a joint may be seen with any form of arthritis. With osteoarthritis, negligible to moderately increased activity diffusely involves the joint area (**A** and **B**, knees). In some cases, involvement may be limited to only one region of a joint, usually where the stresses are greatest. However, x-rays should be reviewed since an unsuspected cause may be present. An elderly woman with normal image of the right hip (**C**) and a lesion confined to the superior margin of the left hip joint (**D**) has had a pinned hip fracture with the pin later removed because of protrusion into the acetabulum (**E**). Joint images are function studies of bone turnover and are likely to be positive when degeneration and repair of bone are actually taking place. As such, images correlate better with symptoms than with radiographs, which show permanent, irreversible anatomical changes that have occurred up to this point and do not necessarily relate to the patient's current status.

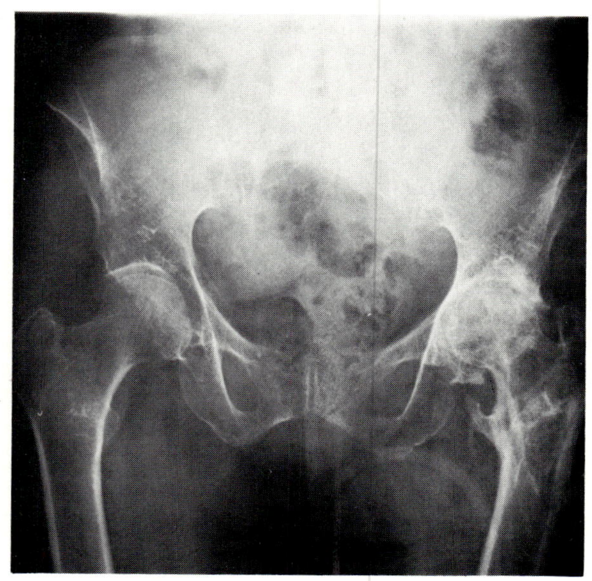

E

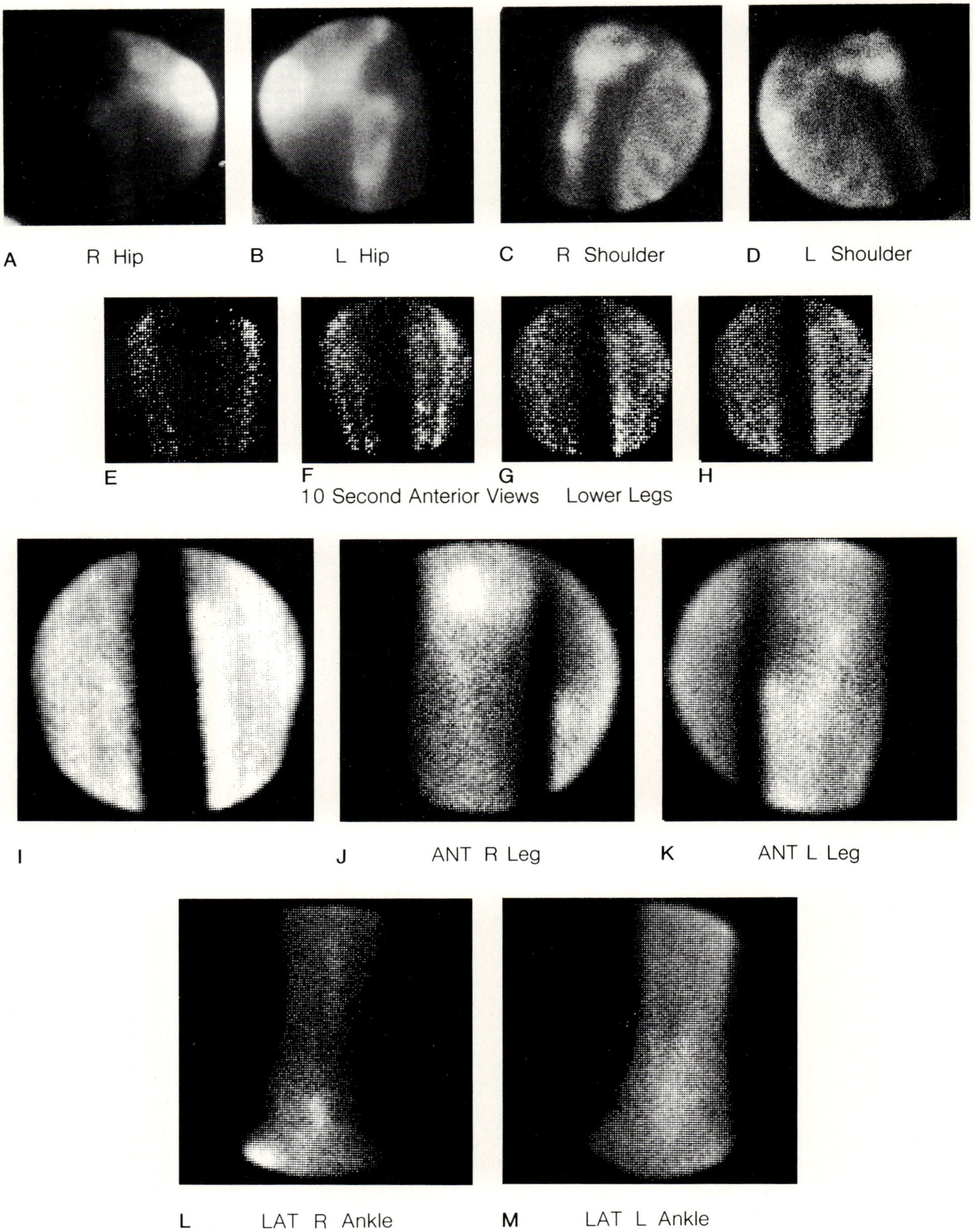


**FIG. 9. A–M.** (See legend next page)

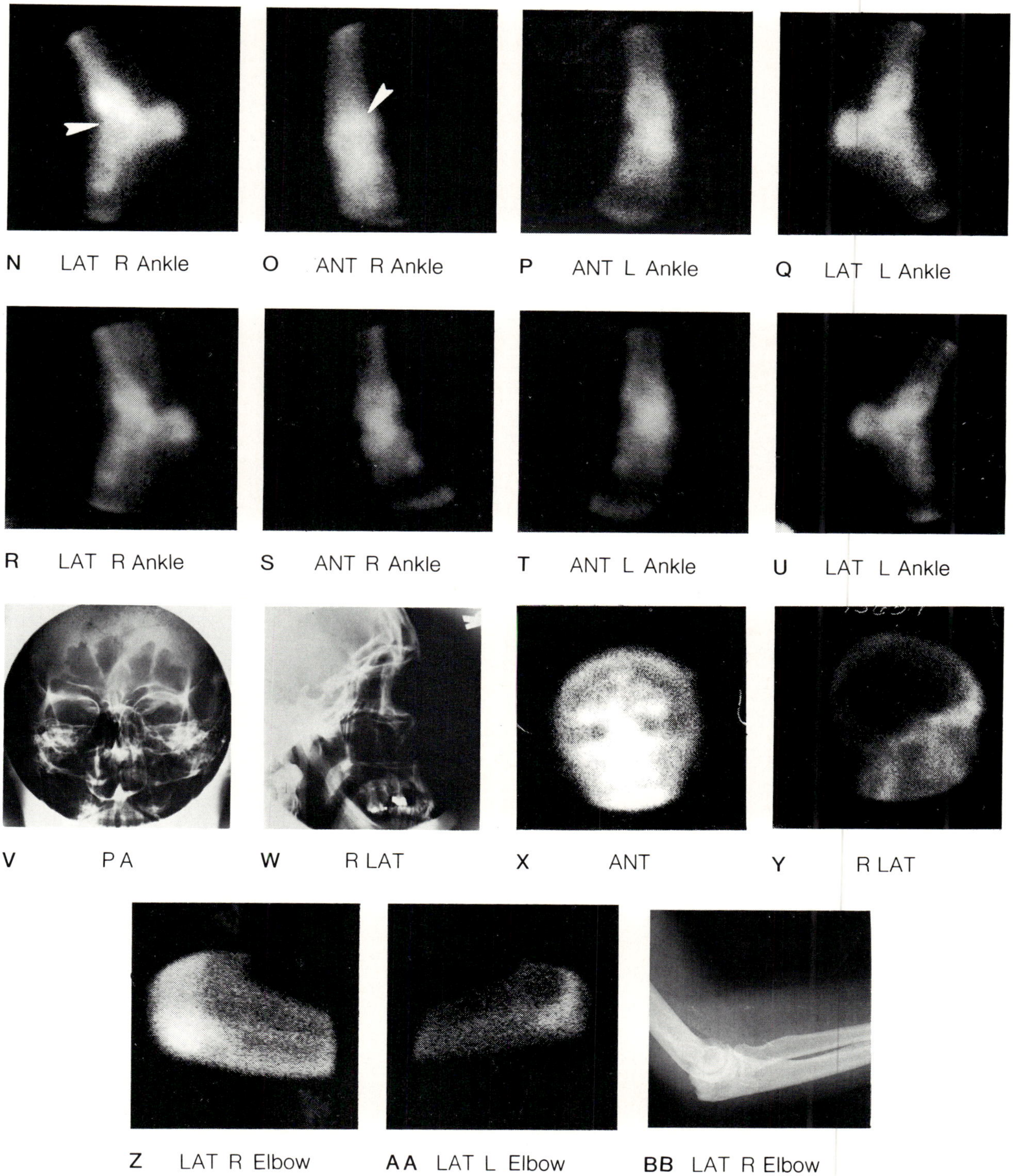


**FIG. 9. ACUTE OSTEOMYELITIS.** Osteomyelitis may result from hematogenous spread of infection, penetrating wounds, or extension from infected adjacent soft tissues. Acute hematogenous osteomyelitis commonly starts in the metaphyseal area of a long bone, especially the femur, humerus, and tibia. The earliest bone image lesion may be cold but becomes hot within several days, increasing in extent and then fading over the ensu-

ing weeks and months with effective treatment. The bone images may remain positive for years with indolent infection. Early in the disease, radiographic changes may not be seen for a week or more after the bone images are positive, or a lesion may produce no symptoms, especially at a second site of involvement. Hence, total body imaging should be performed in every case. A 15-year-old male with staphylococcal bacteremia and pain in the left thigh had total body bone imaging, which shows osteomyelitis of the proximal left femur (**A** and **B**) and also involvement of the right humerus with periostitis (**C** and **D**). The last was asymptomatic at the time of the study. Lesions in bone images are usually more extensive than in radiographs. Occasionally, false negatives occur. Blood pool images taken just after intravenous injection of TcP show increased radioactivity in an extremity with osteomyelitis, cellulitis, or other diseases which command an increased blood supply (**E** through **H**, sequential views and **I**, 300K enlarged image at 3 minutes in patient with cellulitis of the left leg). Images taken 2 hours later show diffuse soft-tissue activity with cellulitis alone (**J** through **M**, same patient), but a focal bone lesion would be present with osteomyelitis. Abnormal bone images not typical of a known disease pattern require special attention. Long bone images of a 23-year-old male show abnormally increased metaphyseal concentration of TcP (**N** through **Q**) typical of peripheral expansion of bone marrow, in this case due to sickle-thalassemia disease. In addition, a focal hot lesion in the distal right tibia (**N** and **O**, arrows) represents acute osteomyelitis, which fades after one month of intensive antibiotic therapy (**R** through **U**), correlating well with clinical improvement. Osteomyelitis by extension from contiguous soft-tissue infection is seen in a woman who has had frontal sinusitis with two episodes of right periorbital abscess requiring drainage. X-ray examination (**V** and **W**) is consistent with sinusitis with loss of cortical bone in the wall of the right frontal sinus and supraorbital rim due to osteomyelitis. Bone images (**X** and **Y**) show more extensive disease with increased concentration of TcP extending beyond the sinus walls, across the supraorbital rims and into the floor of the anterior cranial fossa. A patient with infected olecranon bursitis developed cellulitis of the arm. Bone images show an intense focus of TcP in the olecranon process of the right elbow and diffusely increased soft-tissue activity (**Z**) compared to the normal left (**AA**). Radiographs show cortical erosion of the olecranon process (**BB**) compatible with osteomyelitis by direct extension from suppuration in the olecranon bursa.

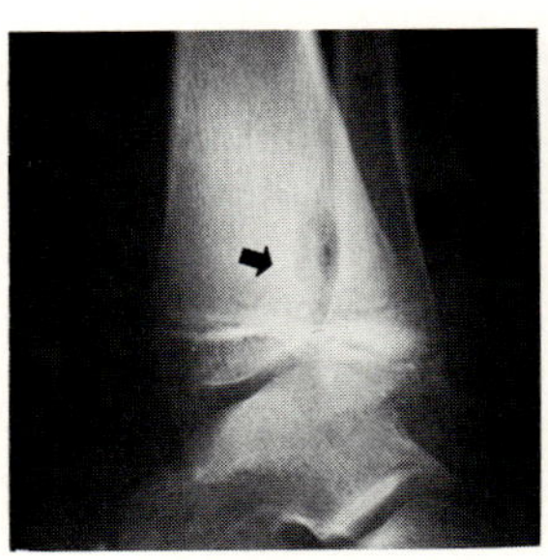

A

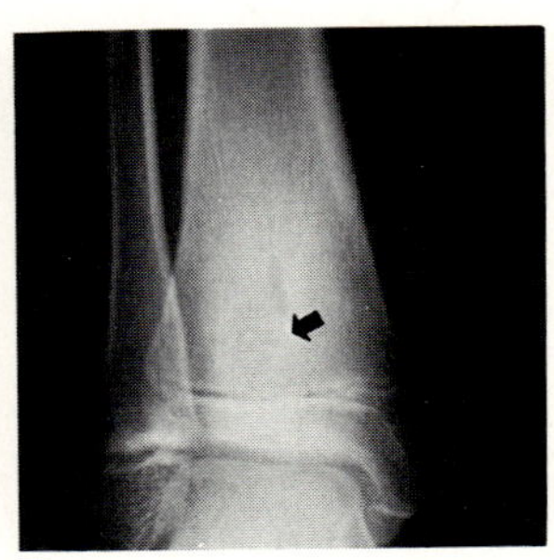

B

**FIG. 10. A,B.** (See legend next page)

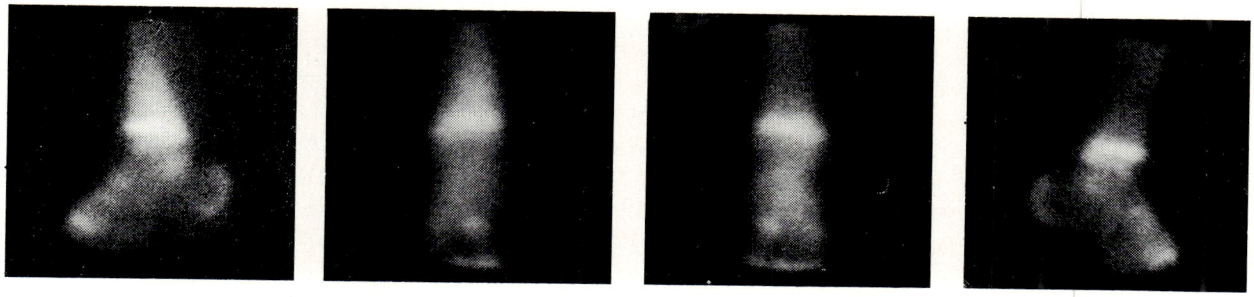


**FIG. 10. CHRONIC OSTEOMYELITIS.** X-rays of a 14-year-old-male with mild pain and tenderness over the right ankle show an area of decreased bone density surrounded by faint sclerosis (**A** and **B**, arrows). In the bone images (**C** through **F**) the lesion is a little more extensive, involving the metaphysis and slowly fading into the shaft (**C** and **D**). The transverse band of intense activity corresponding to the epiphyseal plate of the tibia is normal in actively growing bones. Surgery revealed chronic osteomyelitis (Brodie's abscess).

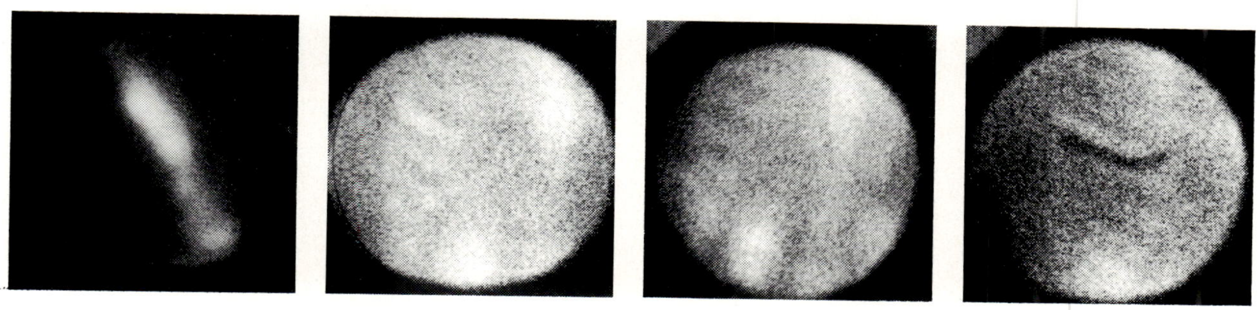


**FIG. 11. FIBROUS DYSPLASIA.** Total body imaging may show one or more bones to be involved with fibrous dysplasia, often at clinically unsuspected sites. The concentration of TcP in individual lesions tends to be intense, as in active Paget's disease. Unlike Paget's, fibrous dysplasia involves the shaft rather than starting at the end of a long bone, and the distribution of TcP is uneven to spotty, deforming the normal appearance of the bone (**A,** left humerus). However, the findings can vary. A woman treated nine years prior for ovarian carcinoma has bone images showing increased concentration of TcP in the right fifth rib (**B**), which was normal one year ago (**C**). Diffuse metastatic involvement of a rib is less common than a focal lesion, but since this was a new finding in a cancer patient with negative x-rays, an excisional biopsy was performed after careful preoperative localization. In **D** the linear dark area represents a lead strip taped in the intercostal space adjacent to the abnormal rib. Since the skin overlying the ribs is very mobile, the patient is instructed to move as little as possible while being transferred to the x-ray table for a localization film taken in the same position with the lead strip in place. If delays are expected, a portable x-ray unit could be brought to the nuclear medicine department and a radiograph taken without moving the patient. Poor bone detail is unimportant since the portable film is used only for counting the rib numbers. The sur-

geon should be supplied with a control radiograph to be viewed in the operating room, clearly marked with the side and the number of the rib, and the exact segment to be biopsied, preferably outlined and cross-hatched with a red china-marker pencil. At the time of biopsy, the surgeon estimates the desired rib, applies a clamp and has an x-ray taken. The clamped rib is counted and the segment matched with the cross-hatched rib in the control film. If necessary, the clamp is moved and repeat films are taken until the match is correct. Postbiopsy radiographs are taken to confirm that the correct segment has been removed. Whatever the method used to locate and identify the site of any lesion, the outcome must be a successful biopsy. In the above patient, no tumor was found in the removed portion of the right fifth rib. However, the bone architecture was abnormal, due to early fibrous dysplasia. The images of bone lesions are generally nonspecific, and a solitary lesion in a cancer patient with negative x-rays should not be considered metastatic unless there is supportive evidence. If further management hinges on specific identification of the solitary lesion, then biopsy is necessary.

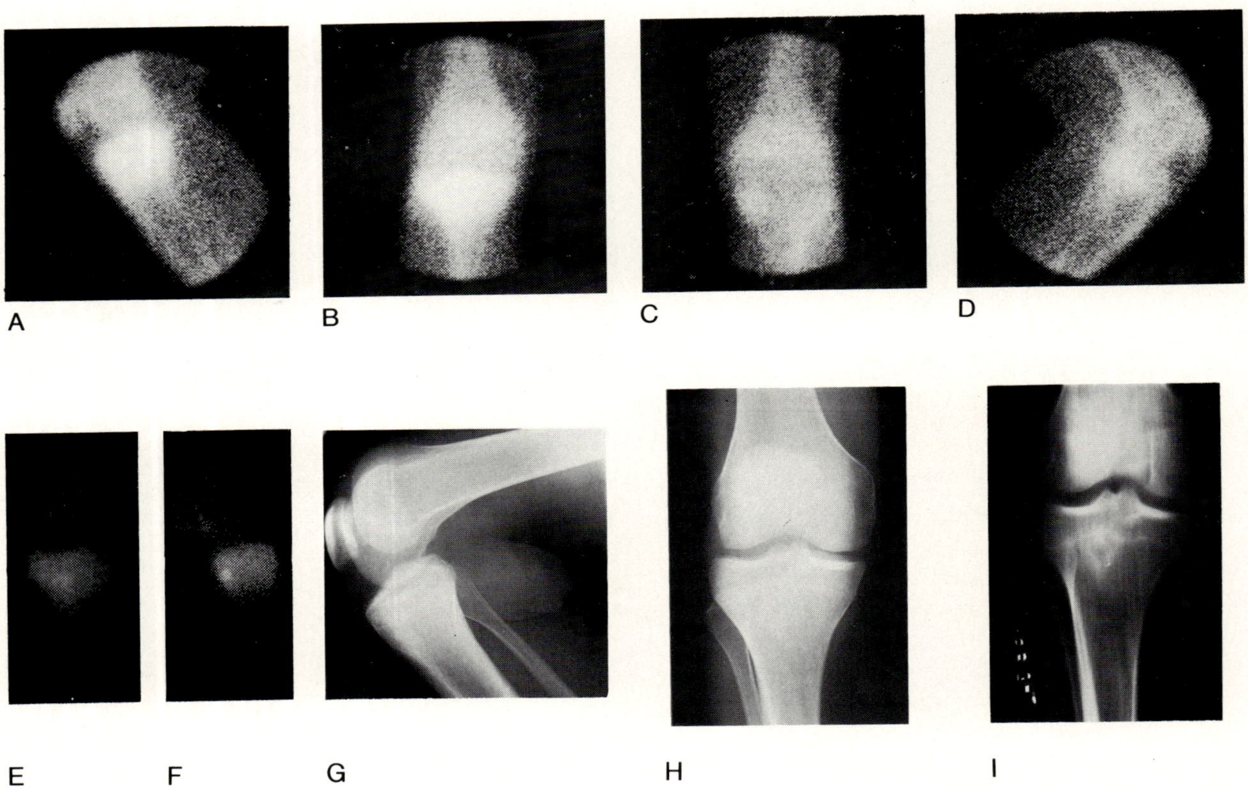


**FIG. 12.** OSTEOID OSTEOMA. In general, benign bone tumors do not produce striking blood pool or bone images but often appear relatively normal. This helps to differentiate them from inflammatory or malignant bone lesions. Among the exceptions, some cases of osteoid osteoma may show avid concentration of TcP (metaphysis in **A** and **B,** compared to normal **C** and **D**). In this 19-year-old male, the nidus lies posteriorly in the tibial metaphysis and is best appreciated in darker images (**E** and **F,** otherwise identical to **A** and **B**). The radiographic findings (**G** and **H,** very subtle in original films) are enhanced by linear tomography (**I**).

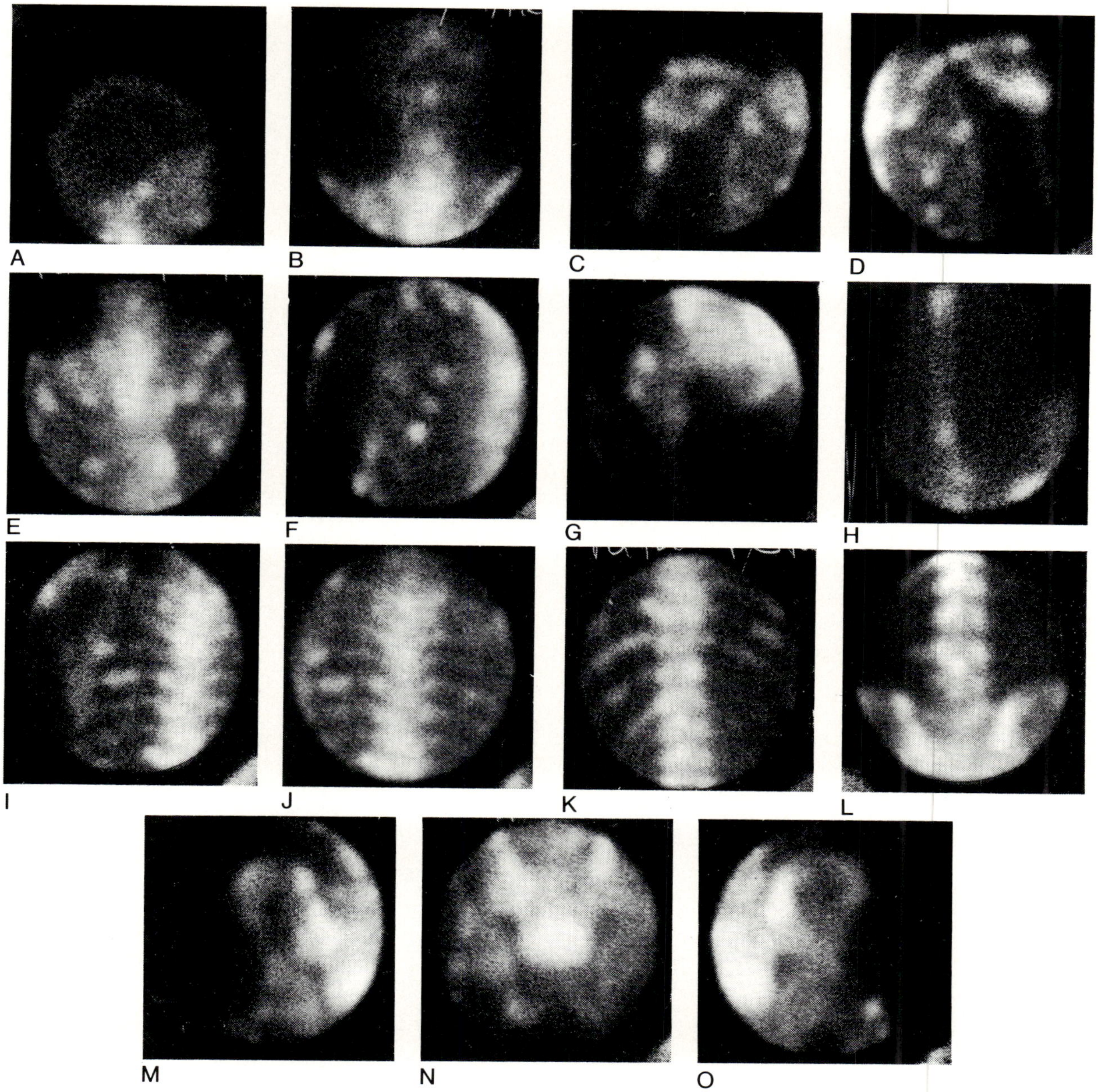


**FIG. 13.** METASTATIC CARCINOMA OF THE PROSTATE. **Multifocal Pattern.** In bone images, untreated lesions of metastatic carcinoma are hottest when they are osteoblastic, especially from prostate and breast. Widespread disease is seen in anterior (**A** through **H**) and posterior (**I** through **O**) views, which contain multiple lesions in every frame. In some bones the distribution of activity tends to be even, but the overall pattern is of multiple separate focal lesions.

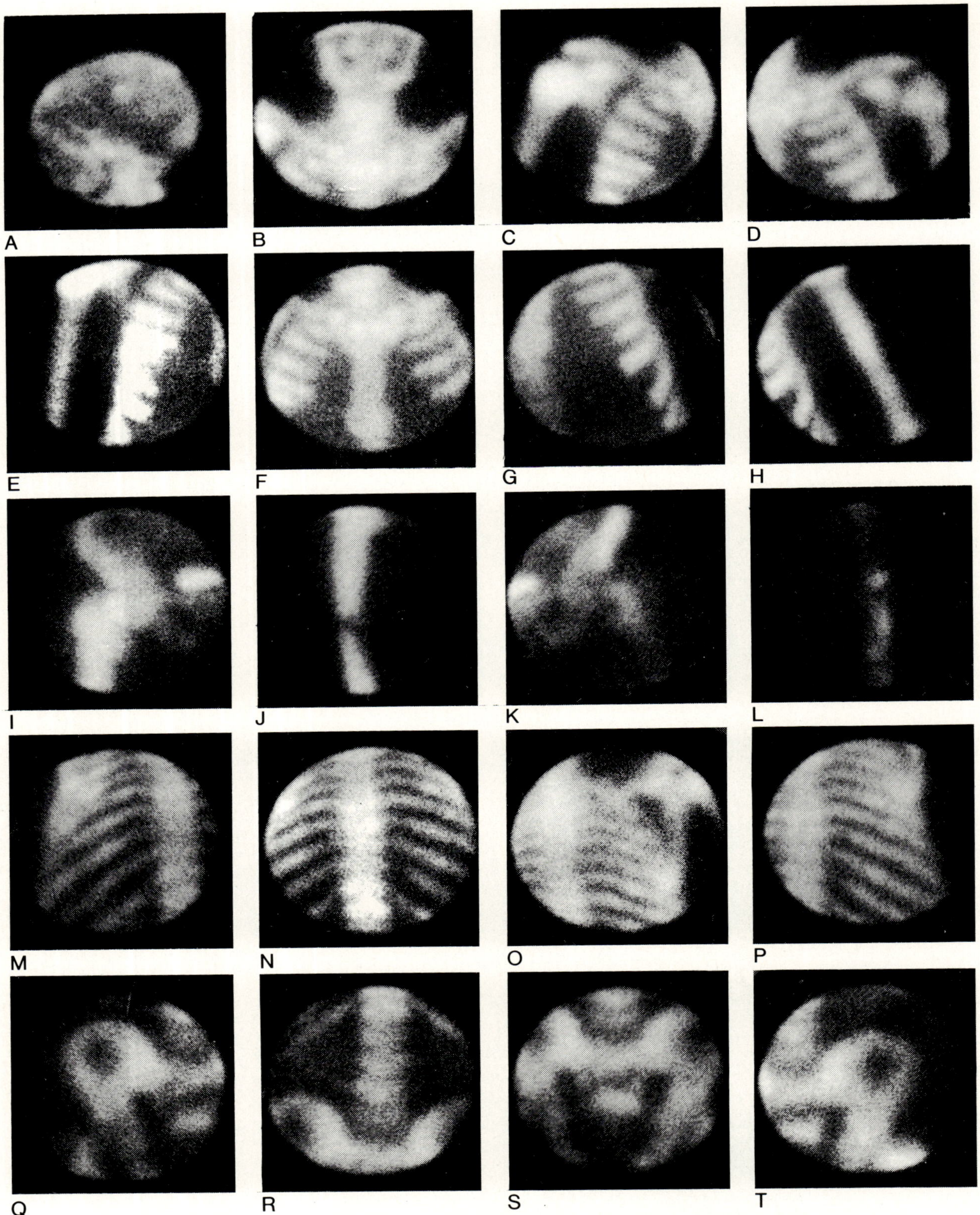


**FIG. 14.** METASTATIC CARCINOMA OF THE PROSTATE. **Diffuse Pattern.** Almost every bone is uniformly involved (**A** through **L** anterior, **M** through **T** posterior views). This could be passed as a normal, excellent detail study, especially if the technician was not alert to the high count rates

and turned the intensity down to compensate. But the background activity is less than expected, the kidneys are not seen (normally, the kidneys should be about the same intensity as the spine), the distribution of bone agent is not truly uniform, and in several areas individual lesions are seen, as in the skull (**A**) and left femur (**K** and **L**). A diffuse pattern does not establish a diagnosis of widespread carcinoma of the prostate, since it may be seen with other disseminated malignancies, especially carcinoma of the breast. Other causes include hyperthyroidism (in which activity is increased in all bones, especially the extremities), and hyperparathyroidism (usually secondary), although this pattern may sometimes be spotty as with multifocal metastatic carcinoma. Paget's disease may diffusely involve many bones but is usually accompanied by a relatively normal acid phosphatase and x-ray evidence of cortical thickening, enlargement of the involved bones, and coarse trabeculation and bowing of long bones. Diffuse bone metastasis is usually a late and grave sign indicating widespread bone marrow involvement.

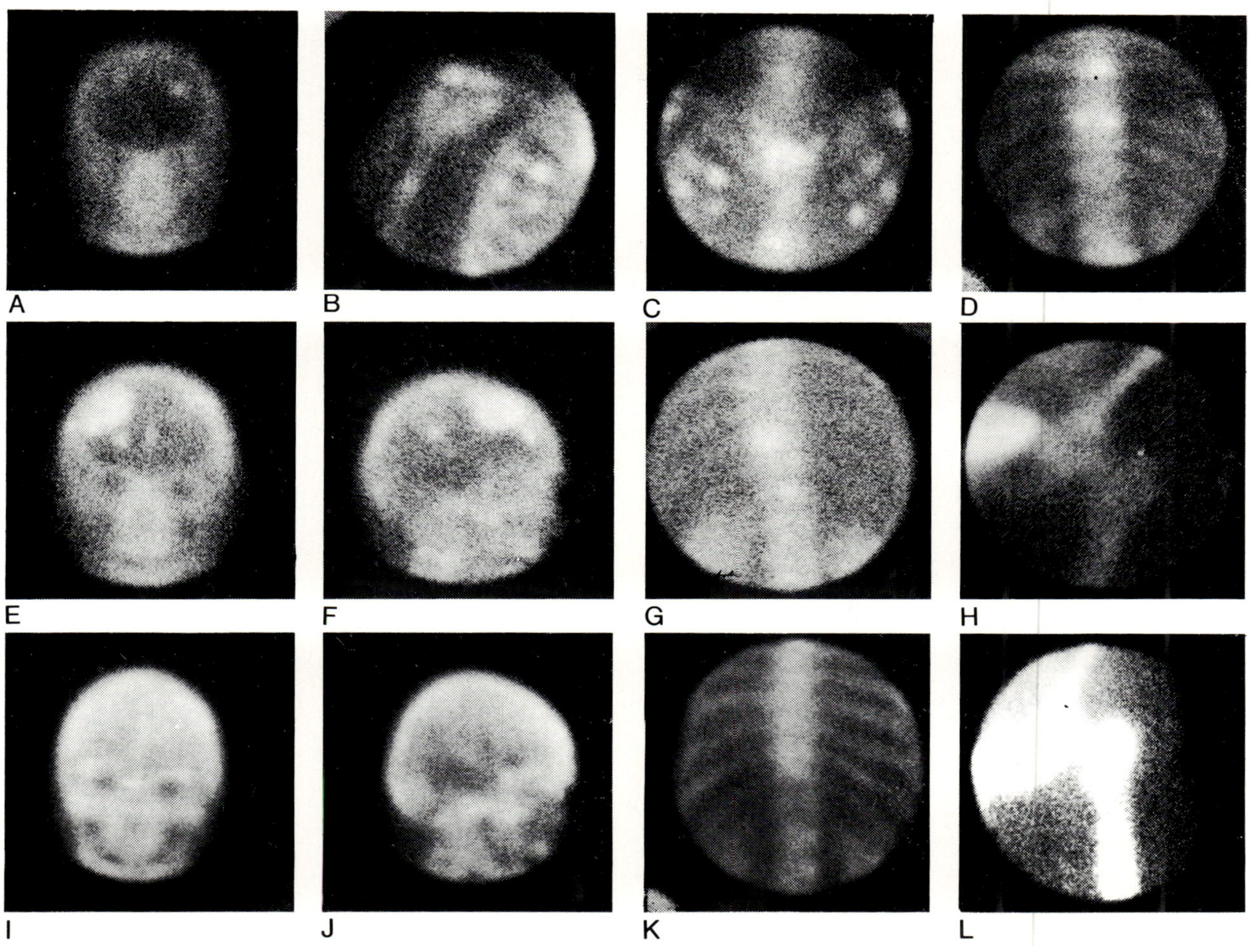

**FIG. 15. METASTATIC CARCINOMA OF THE BREAST.** Abnormal bone images are seen with both osteolytic and sclerotic metastases. A pattern of randomly scattered focal lesions (**A** through **D**) is typical but nonspecific. Another patient has focal lesions (**E** through **H**) that progress to a more diffuse pattern (in the same regions) 2½ years later (**I** through **L**). More lesions are seen and fewer missed with bone images than by radiographic examination.

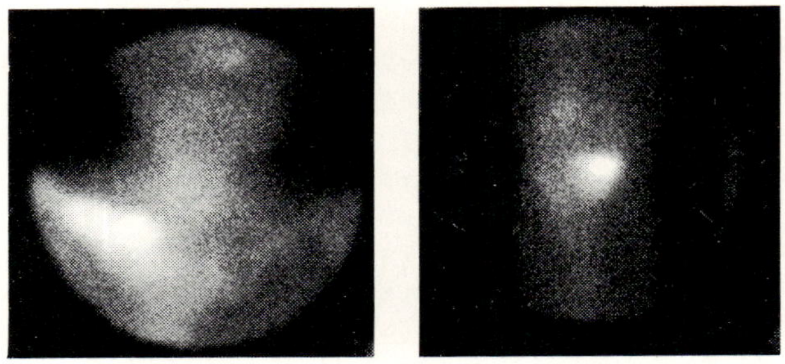

A B

**FIG. 16.** OTHER METASTASES. Unexplained bone pain, especially in cancer patients, is a common problem that may often be resolved by bone imaging, even if the primary tumor does not commonly metastasize to bone. In **A** the patient has a carcinoma of the larynx with metastasis to the right clavicle, and in **B** a patient with carcinoma of the colon has severe pain in the right knee and no significant x-ray findings. Abnormal bone images establish the presence and location of a lesion. The information is etiologically nonspecific, and biopsy may be needed as a basis for further management. On the other hand, normal bone images would make significant bone disease unlikely.

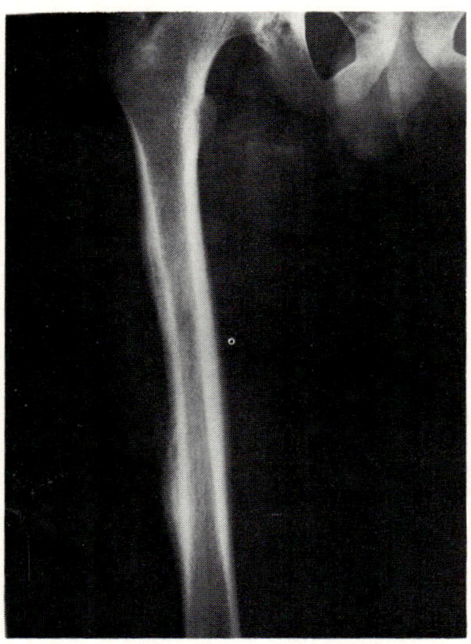

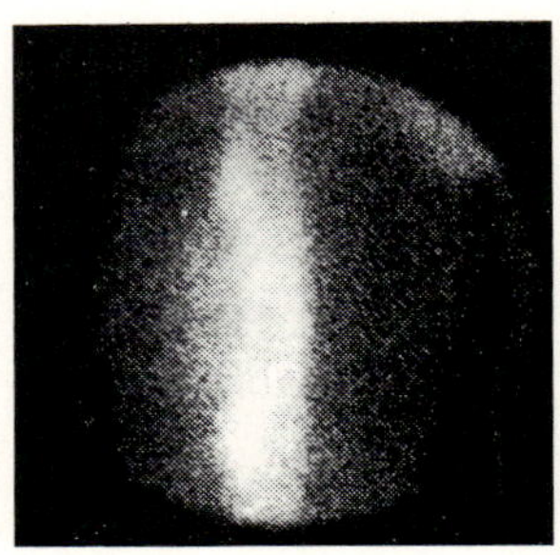

B R Femur

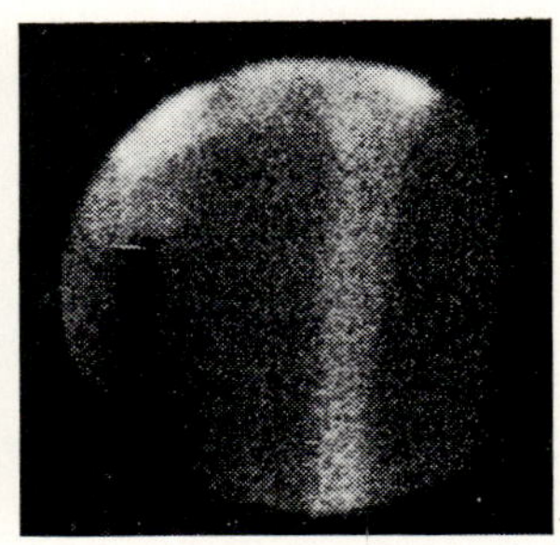

C L Femur

A

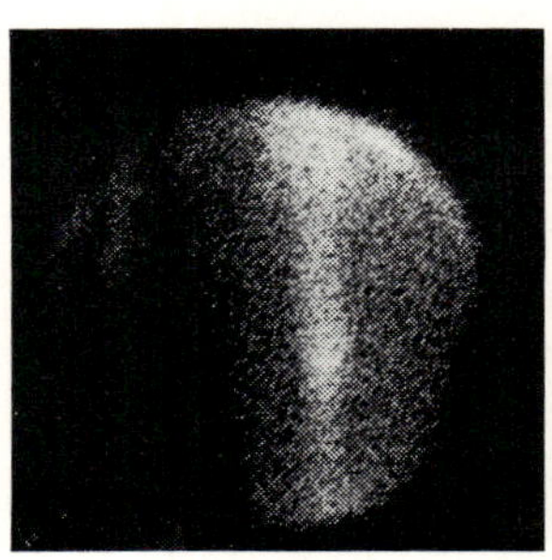

D R Femur

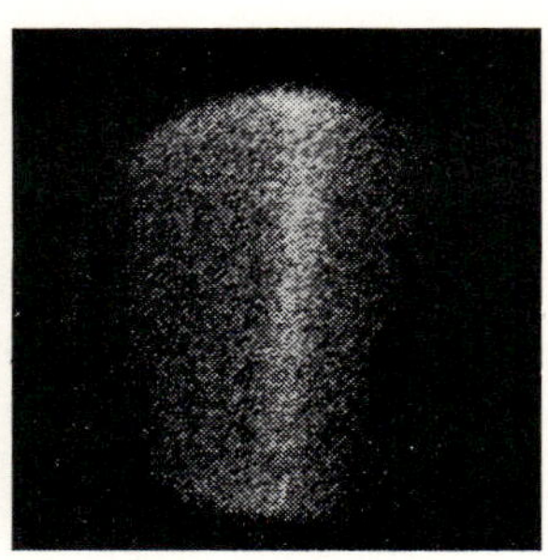

E L Femur

**FIG. 17. A–E.**
(See legend next page)

**FIG. 17. PRIMARY MALIGNANCIES INVOLVING BONE.** The malignant nature of most of the tumorous lesions is obvious from their radiographic appearance. Blood pool images obtained immediately after injection of radiopharmaceutical indicate high vascularity, and the bone images several hours later usually show intense concentration of radioactivity in the tumor which is often more extensive than suspected from the x-rays. A soft-tissue component may be seen as in patient (**A** through **C**) with Ewing's sarcoma of the right femur. (In contrast, this combination of findings is absent with most benign bone tumors.) Nevertheless, the major purpose of bone imaging is to detect lesions elsewhere. For example, about one third of patients with Ewing's sarcoma have involvement of one or more distant bones, which are generally asymptomatic when the patient is first seen. Neuroblastoma involving bone usually occurs in multiple metaphyseal sites and shows a conical area of increased activity, but very destructive lesions may be cold, especially in the spine. Bone marrow involvement by lymphoma may not be detected without biopsy, but occasionally bone imaging may reveal the only biopsy-positive site, as in **D** and **E**, a young woman with Hodgkin's disease in the superior mediastinum and asymptomatic, x-ray negative, biopsy proven lesion in the mid-shaft of the right femur. Other multicentric tumors include histiocytosis X and multiple myeloma (described later). Metastases of osteogenic tumors may be detected in the liver, lung, or other soft-tissue sites because of their ability to concentrate Tc-99m-P. This also occurs with intrathoracic and abdominal neuroblastoma. Images should be scrutinized for such extraosseous lesions.

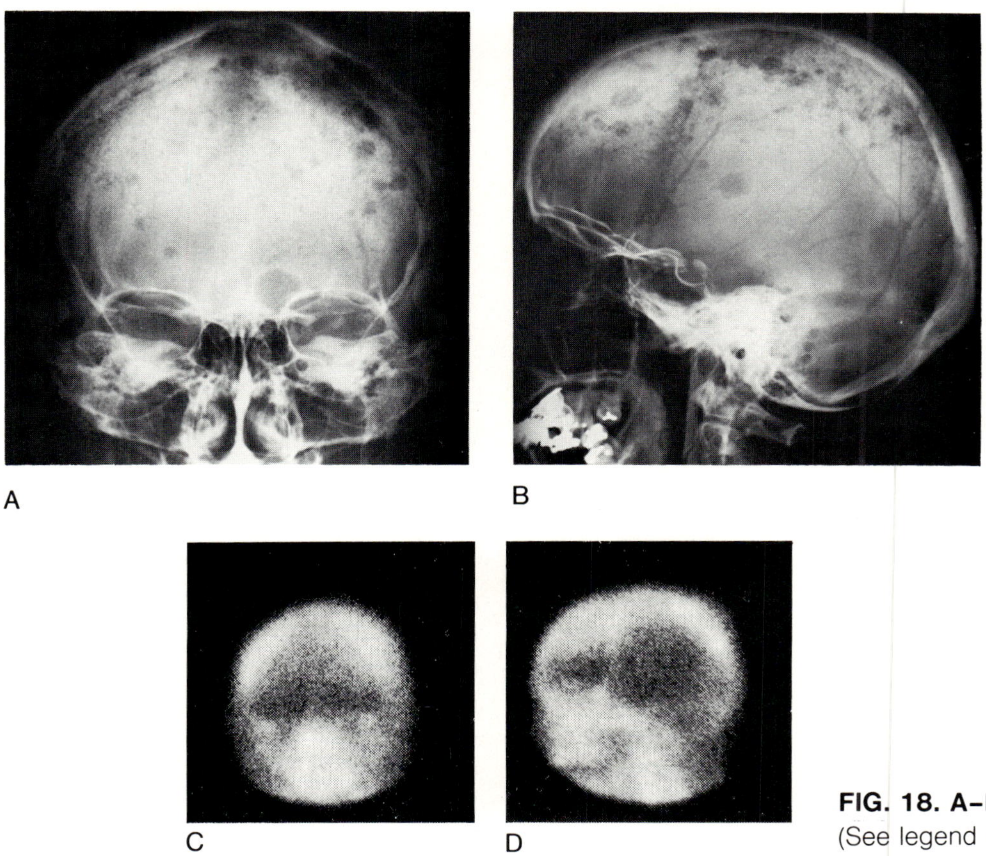


**FIG. 18. A–D.**
(See legend next page)

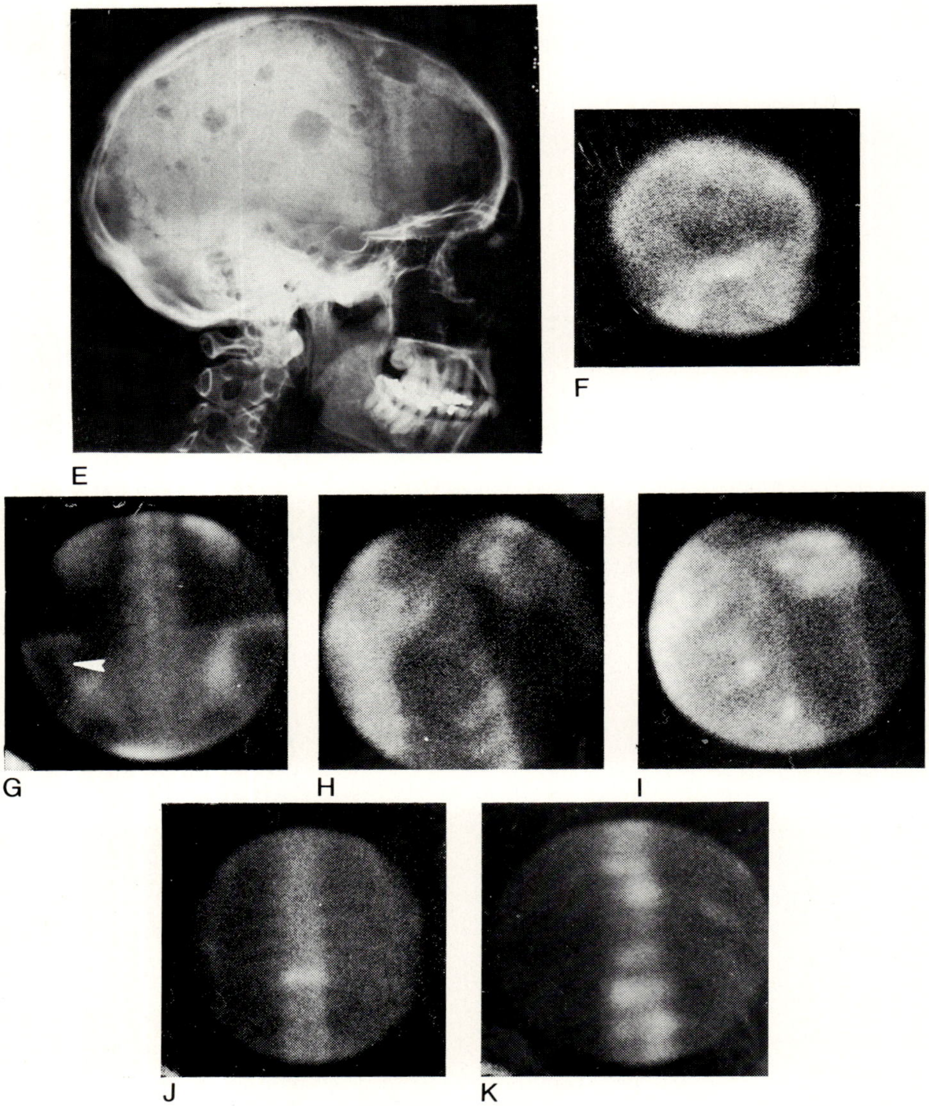


**FIG. 18.** **MULTIPLE MYELOMA.** The radiographic findings in multiple myeloma are more striking than the corresponding bone images, which are frequently normal. Occasionally a patient having multiple osteolytic lesions with areas of sclerosis (**A** and **B**) will show increased concentration of TcP (**C** and **D**), but this is very rare. The more typical radiographic appearance of purely osteolytic, punched-out lesions may sometimes be seen in bone images as focal areas devoid of radioactivity, as in the skull (**E** and **F**), the pelvis (**G,** arrow), and upper ribs (**H**). Cold areas such as these are not specific for multiple myeloma, and may be seen with other conditions (described later). In **I**, several ribs involved with multiple myeloma are poorly seen, but two focal sites of increased concentration of TcP are well defined. These are due to healing pathological fractures which show as hot spots in the same manner as simple fractures. The generalized osteoporosis that commonly accompanies multiple myeloma is usually undetected by bone imaging. In vertebral fractures, a lesion confined to the body would favor simple trauma (**J**), osteoporosis, or multiple myeloma; but involvement of one or more pedicles (**K**) is more likely due to metastatic carcinoma. However, this should not be relied on.

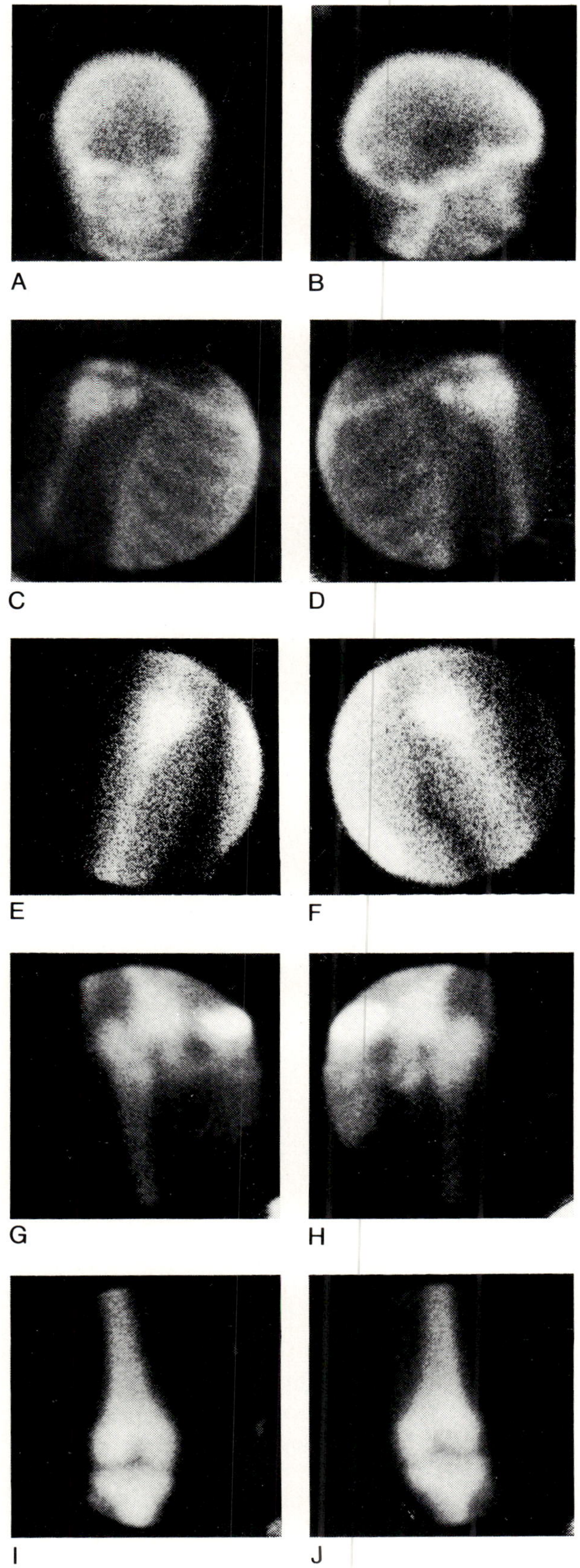


**FIG. 19.** HEMATOLOGIC DISORDERS. In diseases such as polycythemia rubra vera, myelofibrosis, sickle cell hemoglobinopathies, lymphomas, various anemias, and other hematologic disorders, the presence and extent of bone marrow abnormality can be evaluated using radiocolloids (for example, Tc-99m sulfur colloid [TcSC]) for delineating functional reticuloendothelial (RES) activity, or radioisotopes of iron such as Fe-52 for erythropoietic tissue. In most of the above disorders, the abnormal pattern of distribution of radiocolloid in any one patient is virtually identical to the abnormal pattern of distribution of radioiron. However, there are significant mismatches in some diseases such as aplastic anemia, in which erythropoiesis is absent but the RES is abundant. These studies are not discussed here since they should include the liver and spleen. Nonetheless, altered bone marrow activity may result in TcP bone image abnormalities, which should be recognized. For example, diffusely increased concentration of TcP in the ends of long bones and probably in the skull is shown in two patients (**A** through **J**) with sickle SS hemoglobinopathy. (**E** and **F**, elbows of a woman aged 28, remaining frames of a male aged 23. The available x-rays are normal.) These findings are not specific for sickle cell disease but may be seen with peripheral expansion of bone marrow from any cause.

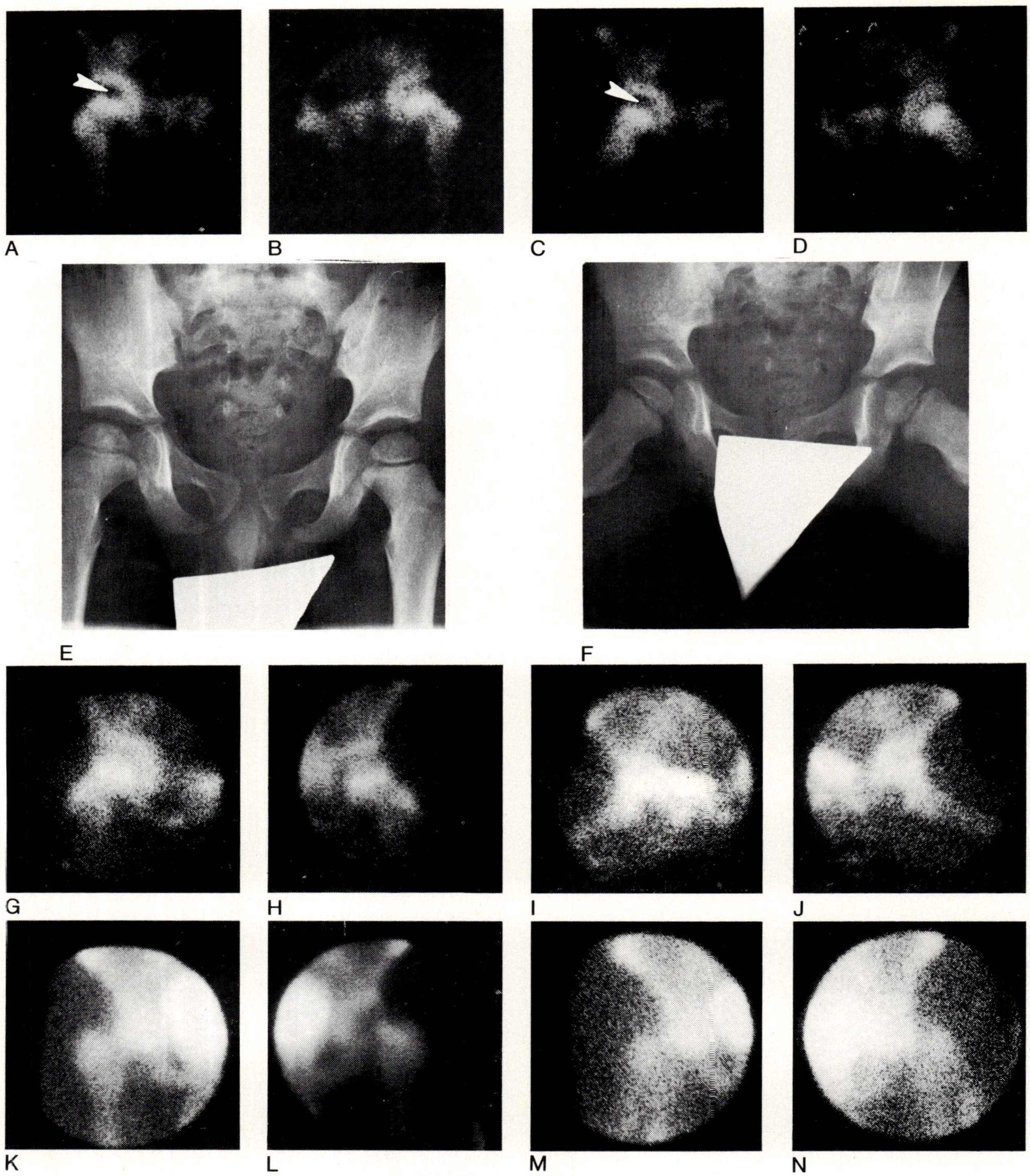


**FIG. 20. ASEPTIC NECROSIS OF THE FEMORAL HEAD.** In Legg-Perthes diseases, the earliest abnormality in bone images is a cold defect in the area of the epiphysis for the femoral head (**A** through **D,** arrows). In the ensuing weeks, this defect is slowly replaced or obscured by increased activity in the metaphysis, epiphyseal plate and/or femoral head, relating to repair and revascularization. X-rays taken early in the course are often negative when the bone images are abnormal. Mottling, subarticular radiolucency, and subsequent structural changes are seen weeks to months

later (**E** and **F**, one month from onset of symptoms). Normal bone images are seen in hip synovitis (**G** through **J**) and effectively exclude Legg-Perthe disease, provided that good resolution images are obtained. In sickle hemoglobinopathies, bone infarcts are recognized early as cold defects often contrasted by adjacent diffusely increased activity, which accompanies peripherally expanded bone marrow (**K** and **L**, 5 days after onset of pain in left hip, and **M** and **N**, 6 months later). Bone imaging should also provide clinically useful information in diagnosis and perhaps prognosis of other conditions relating to the integrity of the femoral head before or after treatment, including intracapsular fractures, slipped capital femoral epiphysis, necrosis associated with alcoholism, pancreatitis, or use of adrenal corticosteroids, etc. (Figs. **A** through **F**, courtesy of Dr. Alexander Gottschalk, Yale-New Haven Hospital, CT)

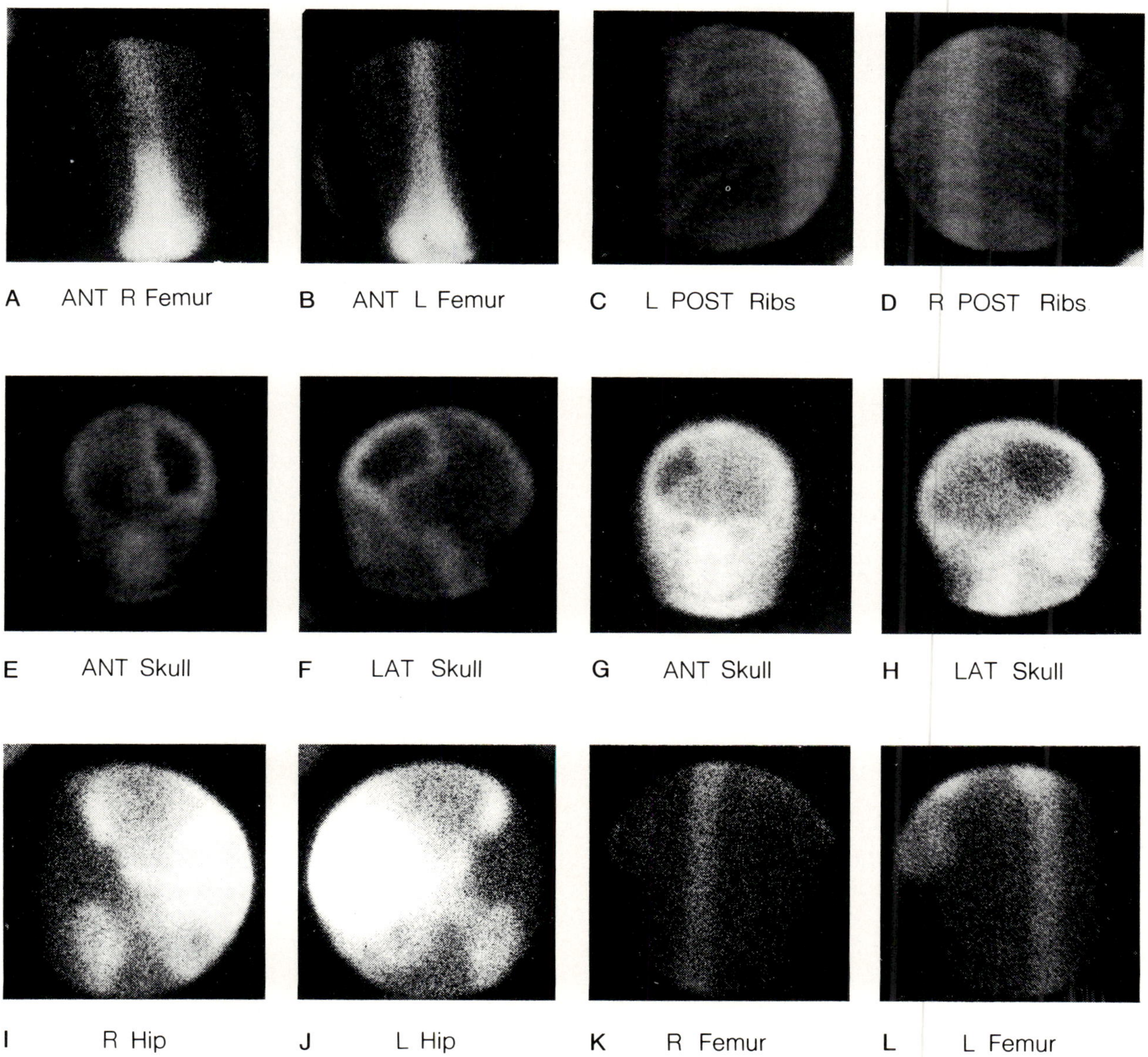


**FIG. 21. A–L.** (See legend next page)

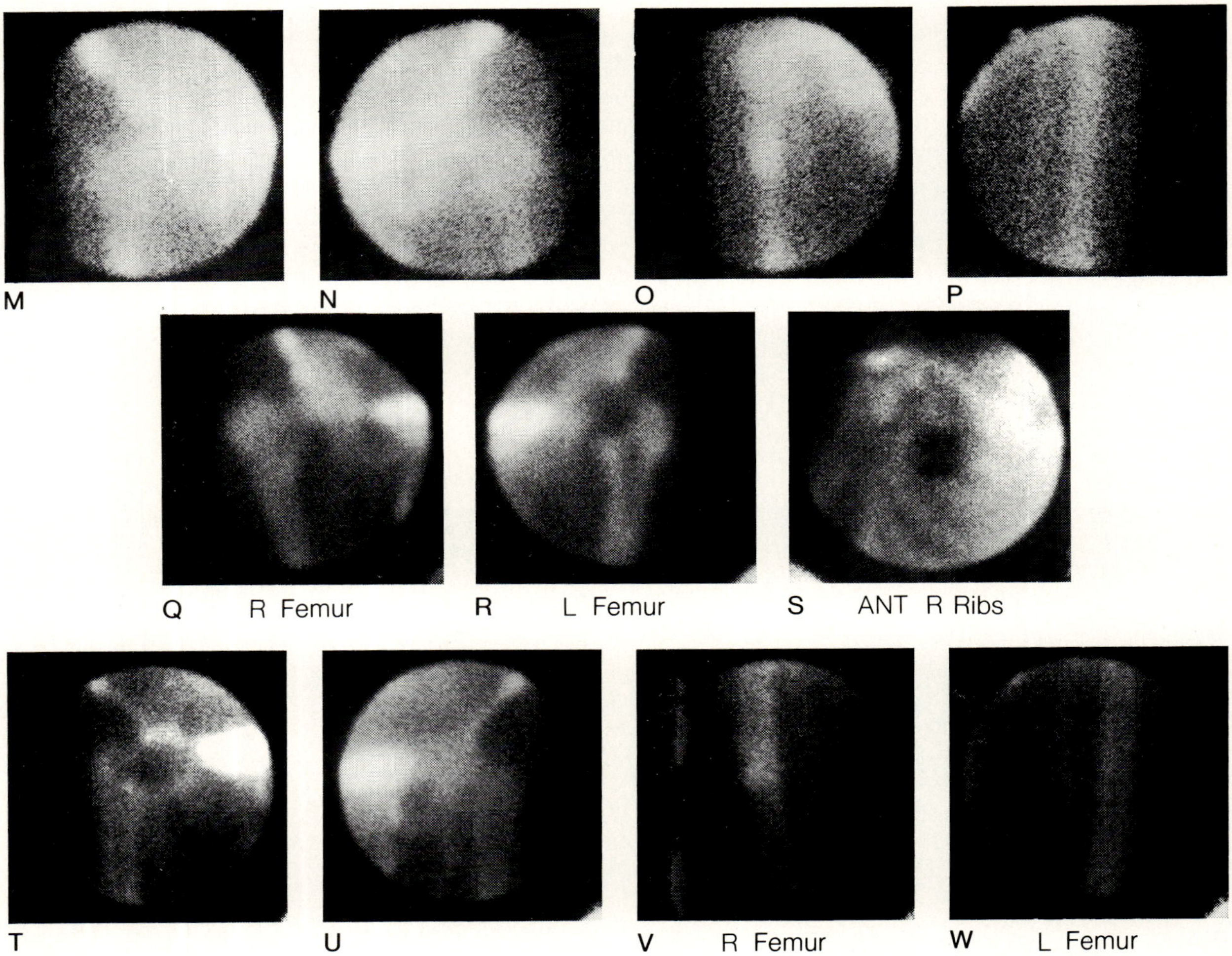


**FIG. 21.** COLD LESIONS. Photon-deficient (cold) lesions are grouped here for emphasis since the more subtle lesions could be overlooked. Several causes of cold defects are described early in this chapter and include the early phase of osteomyelitis, early aseptic necrosis of the femoral head, multiple myeloma, and some cases of metastatic malignancy. Other possibilities are simple bone cysts, histiocytosis X, sickle cell anemia with acute bone infarction (**A** and **B**, arrow, in a 24-year-old male with normal x-rays), old healed surgical defects (**C** and **D**, posterior ribs with arrow, seventh rib resected), craniotomy defects, devitalized bone flaps (**E** and **F**, 2 weeks postop, and **G** and **H**, another patient 10 months postop), and bone grafts destined for rejection. In some cases, cold defects will be obscured or replaced by increased activity as the disease progresses (**I** through **L**, oat cell carcinoma of lung metastatic to the right hip, and **M** through **P**, 6 months later) and when repair and healing occur with or without pathological fracture or therapy. Cold defects in Tc-99m-P bone images are far from subtle when produced by metallic prostheses (**Q** and **R**, replacement left hip prosthesis), fixation plates, and pacemakers (**S**), which markedly attenuate photons and result in an area colder than soft-tissue background activity. In this regard, note that increased activity at the lower margin of a hip prosthesis (**T** through **W**, arrow) is the most consistent evidence of loosening of the prosthesis. Incidentally, pathology in bone images is far less obscured by plaster casts and splints than in radiographs.

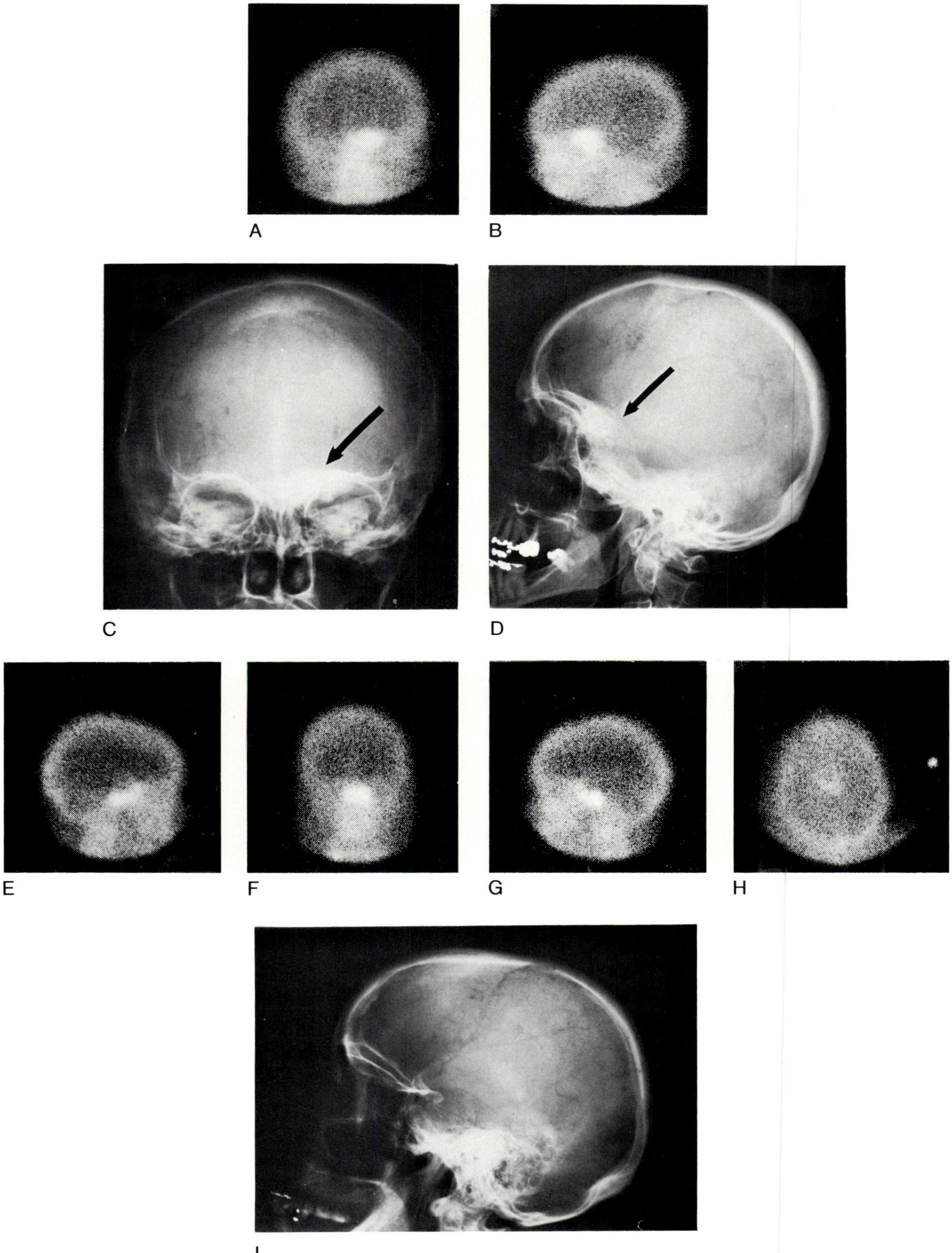


**FIG. 22. A–I.** (See legend next page)

**FIG. 22. MISCELLANEOUS BONE LESIONS.** A survey of the literature and one's experience could provide a catalog of many disorders in which the accompanying bone images are interesting if not of value in diagnosis, treatment, or prognosis. For example, a patient with a meningioma has skull images (**A** and **B**) showing intense concentration of TcP corresponding to an area of hyperostosis along the left sphenoid ridge (**C** and **D**, arrows). Meningiomas may be seen on plain skull x-rays because of their calcium content (not seen in this patient), or may be suspected if they cause hyperostosis of underlying bone, here detected by gamma imaging. In another patient, a diagnosis of pituitary chromophobe adenoma was made five years ago, and she was treated using external beam radiation therapy, clinically resulting in arrest of the tumor. TcP bone images (**E** through **H**) show increased activity in the walls of the sella turcica, indicating bone repair in response to pressure erosion and enlargement of the sella (**I**). In the workup of a patient with suspected early enlargement of the sella turcica due to pressure erosion by a tumor, aneurysm, or other cause, positive bone images may support the diagnosis, but the value of this study is yet to be shown.

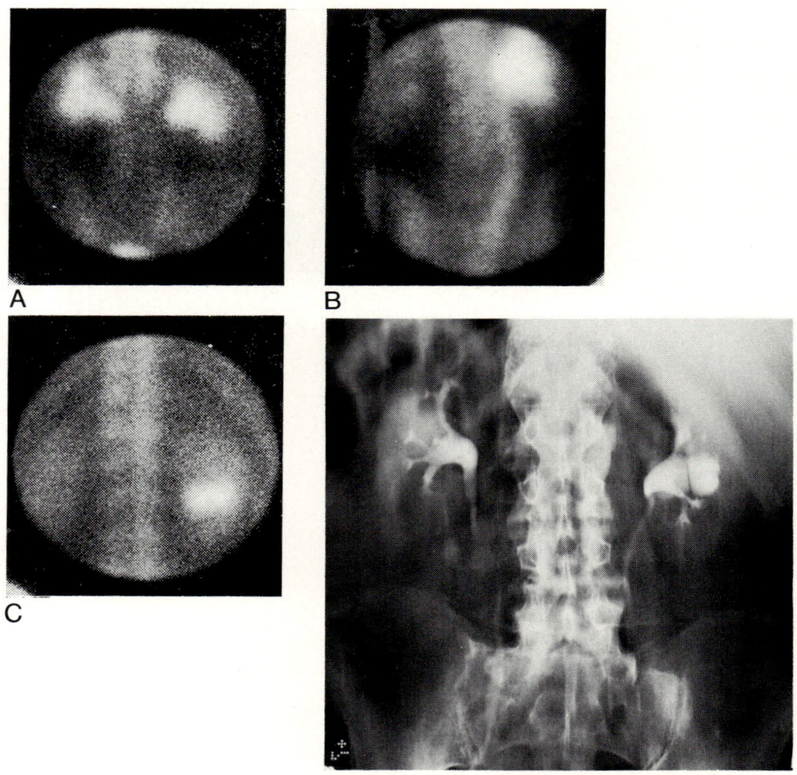


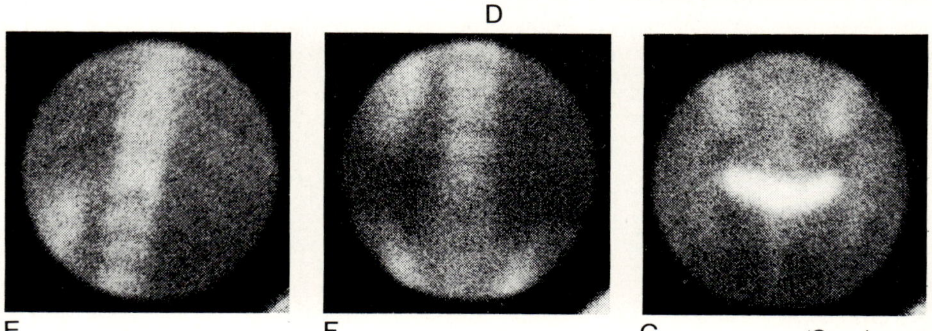


**FIG. 23. A–G.**
(See legend on page 200)

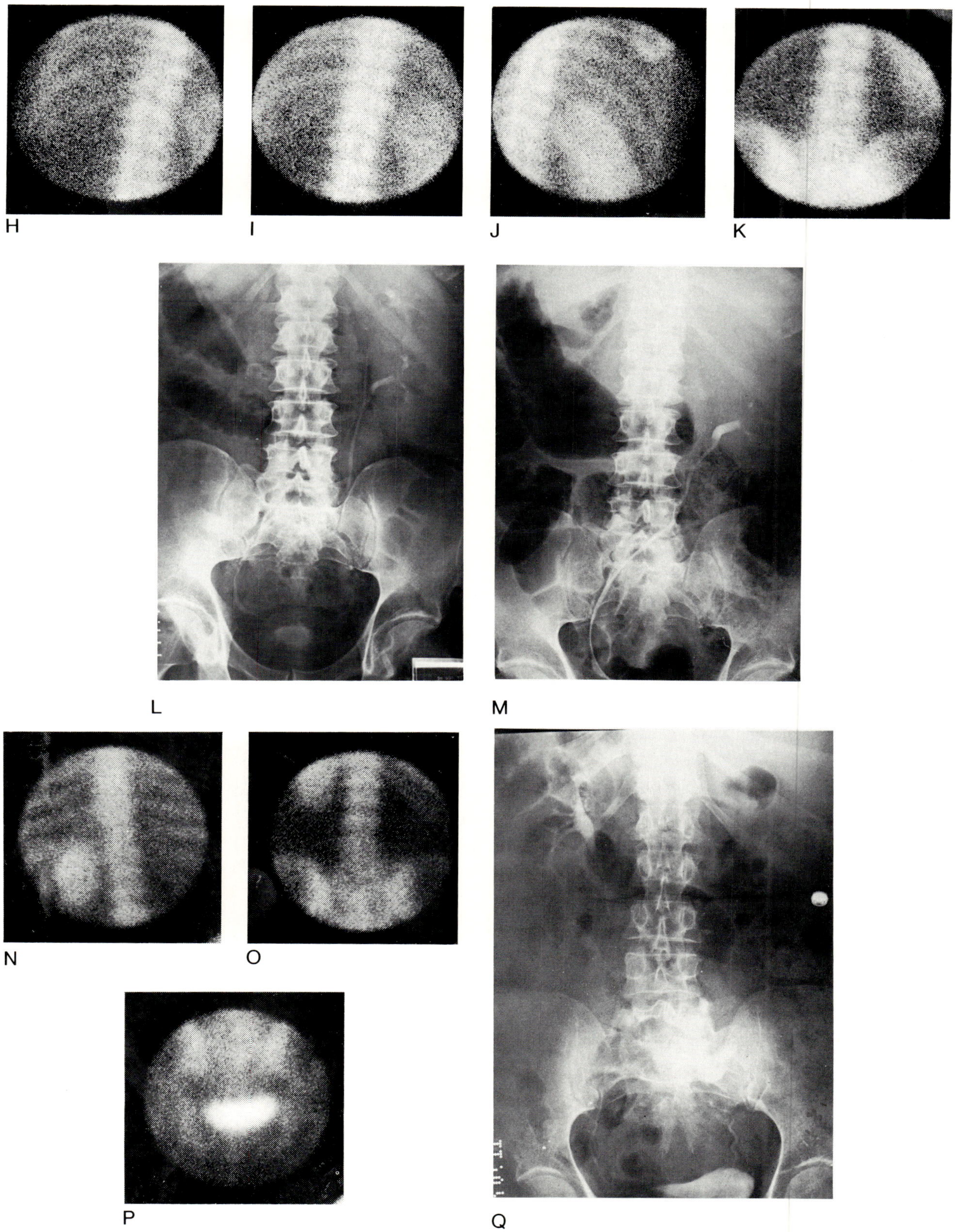


**FIG. 23. H–Q.** (See legend next page)

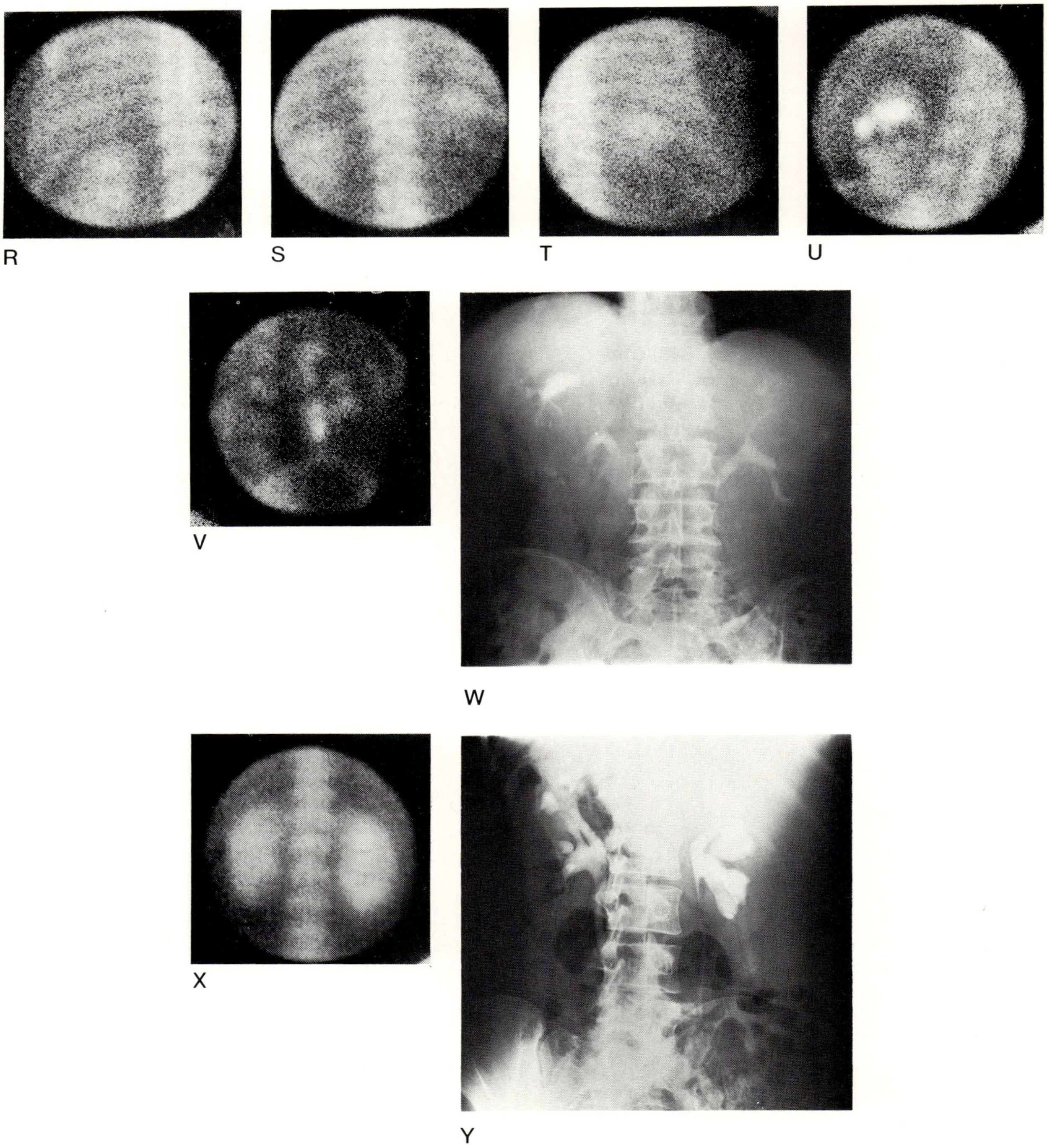


**FIG. 23. UROLOGIC SIDE-BENEFITS.** Because of renal excretion of TcP, urinary tract lesions are detectable, quite often as incidental findings. For this reason and because different indications and agents are used for renal imaging alone, several cases are described here. Bilateral hydronephrosis with retention of TcP in both kidneys and ureters (**A**: This, and all subsequent images in this section are posterior views) supports a clinical diagnosis of obstruction by a carcinoma of the bladder, but unilateral obstruction (**B**) was not suspected in a patient with carcinoma of the colon. A dumbbell-shaped collection of TcP overlying the middle pole of the right

kidney (**C**) represents two large diverticula communicating with the collecting system of the kidney (**D,** tomogram from intravenous pyelogram: This and subsequent x-rays are reversed to match the gamma images). A nonfunctioning or absent kidney (**E** through **G**) is readily detected. In another patient, absent left kidney activity and homogeneously enlarged right kidney (**H** through **K**) could also be due to left nephrectomy with compensatory hypertrophy of the remaining kidney, but this patient had a congenital anomaly with crossed renal ectopia and fusion of both renal elements on the right side. Intravenous pyelogram (**L**) and retrograde pyelogram (**M**) show a large unilateral kidney shadow with two separate collecting systems and ureters. One of the ureters crosses the midline and inserts into the contralateral side of the bladder. Failure to visualize the right kidney (**N** through **P**) in a woman with carcinoma of the uterus could be interpreted as fairly long-standing obstruction of the ureter by locally extensive tumor. However, an IVP shows an ectopic but otherwise normal kidney (**Q,** arrow), which was obscured by the sacrum. These cases are presented to show that when one kidney is not seen in bone images, further evaluation is required, since this does not necessarily mean that the kidney is absent or nonfunctioning. A renal mass, such as a cyst or neoplasm displacing and destroying normal renal tissue, may be seen as an area in the kidney devoid of activity (**R** through **T**). In this patient only the upper pole of the right kidney is seen, compared to the normal left kidney. Inflammatory lesions and infarction may cause a similar appearance. A large cyst may appear as a cold defect with less than background activity, but with left-sided lesions care should be taken to exclude a similar appearance caused by a fluid-filled stomach (gas or liquid). Enlarged kidneys containing hot areas of pooling of excreted TcP and cold areas due to cysts are well defined in a patient with polycystic kidneys (**U** and **V,** and **W** from IVP). A patient with sickle cell anemia has enlarged kidneys, which are known to occur in this disease (**X**). The right kidney is larger than the left and shows retained activity, which is pooled in enlarged calyces. Obstructive uropathy is unlikely since the pelvis or ureter are not dilated. With chronic pyelonephritis the kidney should be normal size or shrunken, not enlarged. This patient has renal papillary necrosis (**Y,** from IVP), which occurs with a significant incidence in cases of sickle hemoglobinopathy with or without renal symptoms. These cases exemplify some of the various renal disorders that may be encountered in bone imaging. As in diagnostic radiology, all the information provided by an examination should be utilized and evaluated.

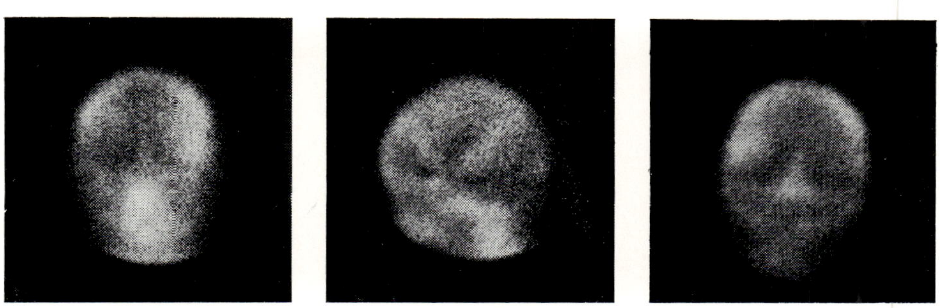

A ANT Skull B LAT Skull C POST Skull

**FIG. 24. A–C.** (See legend on page 203)

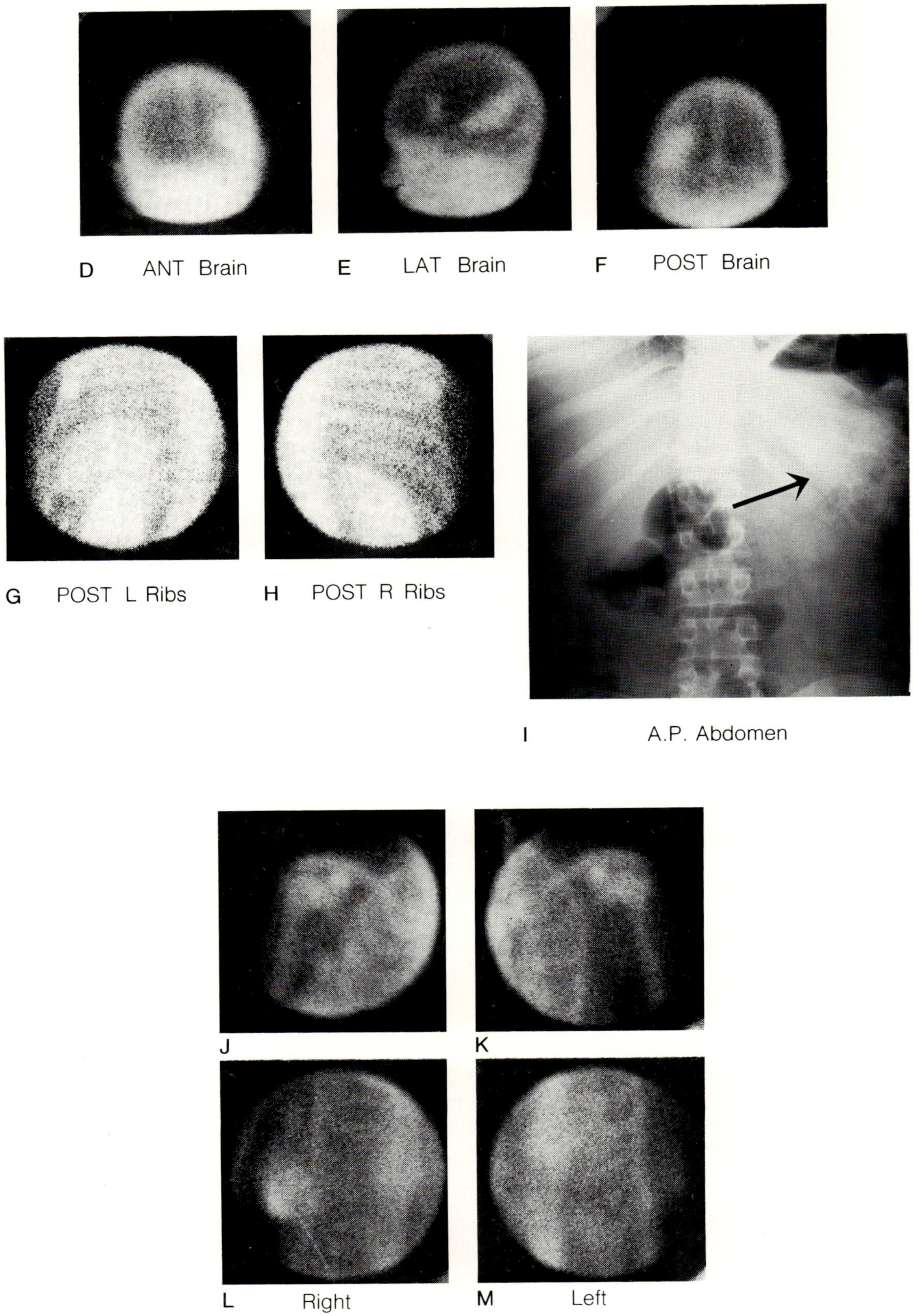


**FIG. 24. D–M.** (See legend next page)

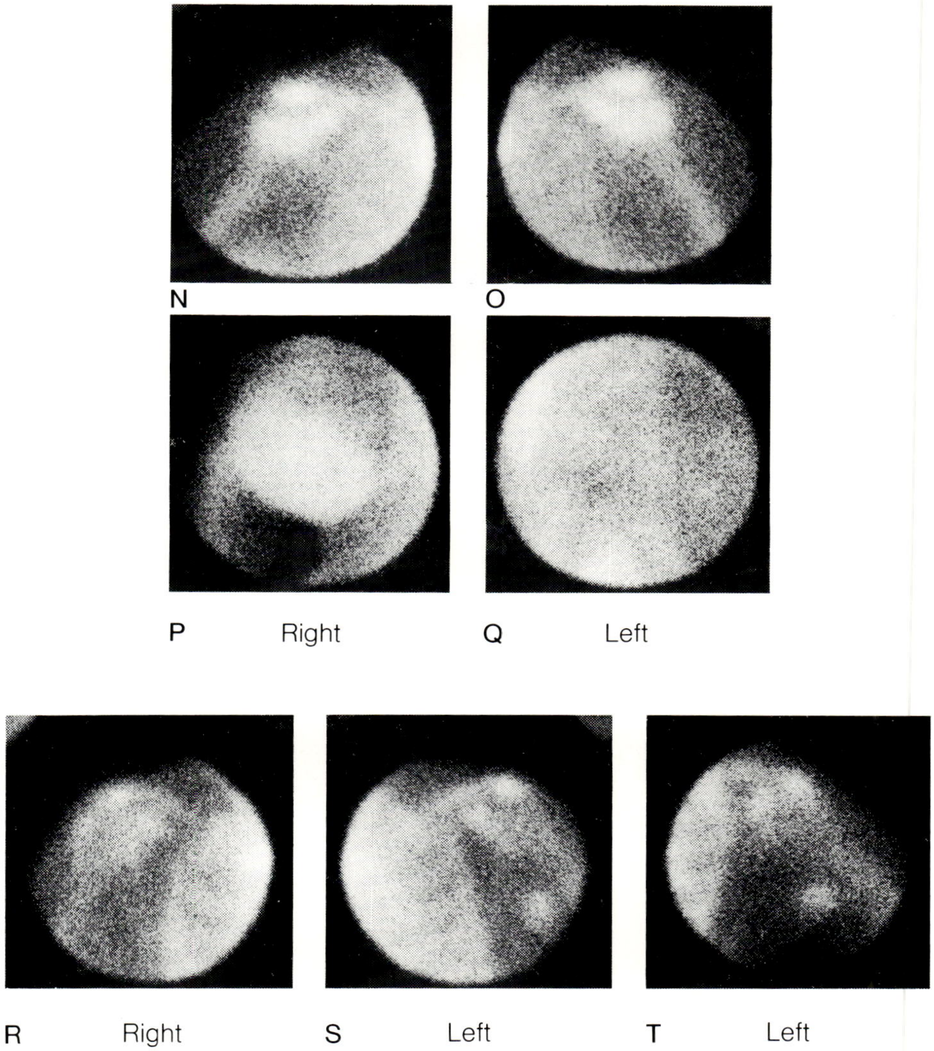


**FIG. 24. EXTRAOSSEOUS LESIONS.** Although TcP concentrates mainly in bones, it may accumulate in extraosseous lesions in sufficient amounts to be detected by imaging. Increased local blood supply, calcification, necrosis, or deposition of collagen may be contributing factors; but the mechanism remains obscure and possibly differs among the various types of lesions. Acute infarcts of myocardium or bone are detected using TcP, as described elsewhere. Acute cerebral infarction [**A** through **C** using TcP; **D** through **F,** same patient 2 days later using Tc-99m diethylenetriaminepentaacetic acid (DTPA)] and possibly infarcted, calcified spleen (**G** through **I,** arrows, an 18-year-old male with sickle SS hemoglobinopathy) are also noted during bone imaging studies. Intense activity is present in a carcinoma of the right breast (**J** and **L**) compared to normal left (**K** and **M**). The bulky tumor was necrotic and involved the axillary lymph nodes. A huge tumor of the right breast (**N** through **Q,** with breast tumor, **P,** overlying the right humerus), cystosarcoma phyllodes, was considered histologically benign and had no evidence of calcification, necrosis, or significantly increased vascularity. Abnormal images may occur in a variety of benign and malignant breast lesions and are suspicious if the distribution of activity is clearly asymmetric. Local concentration of TcP has been reported in

primary tumors including carcinoma of the kidney, ovary, and lung, in extraosseous metastases such as liver, involved with colorectal adenocarcinoma (with or without calcification), and is seen here, for example, in skin metastasis to the left anterior axillary fold from a carcinoma of the lung (**R** through **T**). Other reported cases include malignant pleural effusion; fibrothorax; healing surgical wounds; radiated soft tissues; the site of IM iron dextran injections; skeletal muscle following ischemia, trauma, or cardioversion; metastatic calcification in the lungs and in other organs with uremia and hypercalcemia; tumoral calcinosis; and skin contamination with saliva, urine, feces, or sweat. To these might also be added aortic aneurysm, massive hepatic necrosis, polymyositis, myositis ossificans, dermatomyositis, pseudoxanthoma elasticum, and calcinosis universalis. Other lesions occur, and the list will surely continue to grow. Unfortunately, very few of these findings have any clinical value.

## Suggested Reading


Bergstedt HF, Carenfelt C, Lind MG: Facial bone scintigraphy. IV. Diagnosis of bone involvement by purulent sinusitis. Acta Radiol Diagn 20:379–384, 1979

Clark, WD, Fann TR, McCrea JD, et al: Uses of bone scanning in podiatric medicine. J Am Podiatry Assoc 68:621–630, 1978

Collins JD, Bassett L, Main GD, et al: Percutaneous biopsy following positive bone scans. Radiology 132:439–442, 1979

Conway JJ: Radionuclide bone imaging in pediatrics. Pediatr Clin North Am 24:701–712, 1977

D'Ambrosia RD, Shoji H, Riggins RS, et al: Scintigraphy in the diagnosis of osteonecrosis. Clin Orthop 130:139–143, 1978

De Graaf P, Schicht IM, Pauwels EK, et al: Bone scintigraphy in renal osteodystrophy. J Nucl Med 19:1289–1296, 1978

De Rossi G, Focacci C, Maini CL, et al: The particular usefulness of radioisotope methods in some benign bone diseases. Eur J Nucl Med 4:203–206, 1979

Donato AT, Ammerman EG, Sullesta O: Bone scanning in the evaluation of patients with lung cancer. Ann Thorac Surg 27:300–304, 1979

Esdaile J, Hawkins D, Rosenthall L: Radionuclide joint imaging in the seronegative spondyloarthropathies. Clin Orthop 143:46–52, 1979

Fasting OJ, Langeland N, Bjerkreim P, et al: Bone scintigraphy in early diagnosis of erthes' disease. Acta Orthop Scand 49:169–174, 1978

Fogelman I, Citrin DL, Turner JG, et al: Semi-quantitative interpretation of the bone scan in metabolic bone disease: definition and validation of the metabolic index. Eur J Nucl Med 4:287–289, 1979

Fogelman I, McKillop JH, Bessent RG, et al: The role of bone scanning in osteomalacia. J Nucl Med 19:245–248, 1978

Front D, Hardoff R, Robinson E: Bone scintigraphy in primary tumors of the head and neck. Cancer 42:111–117, 1978

Garcia DA, Tow DE, Sullivan TM, et al: The appearances of common dental diseases on radionuclide bone images of the jaws. J Dent Res 58:1040–1046, 1979

Hardoff R, Front D: The value of delayed (24-hour) bone scintigraphy. Clin Nucl Med 3:39–42, 1978

Howman-Giles RB, Gilday DL, Ash JM: Radionuclide skeletal survey in neuroblastoma. Radiology 131:497–502, 1979

Humphreys RP, Gilday DL, Ash JM, et al: Radiopharmaceutical bone scanning in pediatric neurosurgery. Childs Brain 5:249–262, 1979

Kelly RJ, Cowan RJ, Ferree CB, et al: Efficacy of radionuclide scanning in patients with lung cancer. JAMA 242:2855–2857, 1979

McNeil BJ: Rationale for the use of bone scans in selected metastatic and primary bone tumors. Semin Nucl Med 8:336–345, 1978

Noyek AM: Bone scanning in otolaryngology. Laryngoscope 89:1–87, 1979

Pabst HW, Langhammer H: Detection and differential diagnosis of bone lesions by scintigraphy. Eur J Nucl Med 2:261–268, 1977

Pilbrow WJ: The urinary tract image obtained during $^{99m}$Tc bone scanning. Clin Radiol 30:71–77, 1979

Proceedings of the British Institute of Radiology. Benign bone disease—role of radioisotope techniques. Abstracts. Br J Radiol 52:246–252, 1979

Rosenthall L, Hawkins D: Radionuclide joint imaging in the diagnosis of synovial disease. Semin Arthritis Rheum 7:49–61, 1977

Roub LW, Gumerman LW, Hanley EN; et al: Bone stress: a radionuclide perspective. Radiology 132:431–438, 1979

Sain A, Sham R, Silver L: Bone scan in sickle cell crisis. Clin Nucl Med 3:85–90, 1978

Smith AJ Jr, Sy W, Lao R: Bone scan evidence of renal osteodystrophy in undialyzed uremic patients. Proc Clin Dial Transplant Forum 8:130–136, 1978

Sty JR, Babbitt DP, Kun L: Atlas of $^{99m}$Tc-methylene diphosphonate renal images in pediatric oncology. Clin Nucl Med 4:122–127, 1979

Tait MV, Gilday DL, Ash JM, et al: Craniosynostosis: correlation of bone scans, radiographs, and surgical findings. Radiology 133:615–621, 1979

Treves S: Skeletal scintigraphy in the diagnosis of acute ostemyelitis. Hosp Pract 14:66–73, 1979

Webber MM, Wagner J, Cragin MD: Radionuclide patterns of femoral head disease. Int J Nucl Med Biol 4:167–177, 1977

Weiss PE, Mall JC, Hoffer PB, et al: $^{99m}$Tc-methylene diphosphonate bone imaging in the evaluation of total hip prostheses. Radiology 133:727–729, 1979

Wenger DR, Bobechko WP, Gilday DL: The spectrum of intervertebral disc-space infection in children. J Bone Joint Surg Am 60:100–108, 1978

Williamson BR, McLaughlin RM, Wang GW, et al: Radionuclide bone imaging as a means of differentiating loosening and infection in patients with a painful total hip prosthesis. Radiology 133:723–725, 1979

# 6/Brain Imaging

The radioactive materials that are employed in radionuclide brain imaging all show evidence of accumulation or localization at sites of structural abnormalities within the brain. This is associated with alterations in the blood-brain barrier in the areas of involvement, which allow the radionuclides to enter these regions. This property of tracer entry at sites of disease or injury is shared by all of the radionuclides that are commonly employed in brain imaging—Tc-99m sodium pertechnetate, Tc-99m DTPA,and Tc-99m glucoheptonate. The imaging characteristics of an intracranial lesion are determined, in part, by the rate and quantity of accumulation of radioactive material in the region of involvement. Some lesions may show maximum radionuclide localization within 15 minutes following intravenous administration of the tracer (e.g., meningiomas), while others may not show evidence of maximum accumulation until 2 or 3 hours have elapsed (e.g., some astrocytomas).

Virtually all static imaging is preceded by a blood flow study in which the carotid and major cerebral arteries may be visualized. Some entities may be seen best during this portion of the study (e.g., AV malformation), while if only static imaging was employed in such cases, the abnormality might escape detection. Findings noted on the blood flow studies often serve to direct attention to forthcoming imaging of specific pathological changes on the static studies (e.g., carotid artery stenosis and cerebral infarction, vascular lesion and meningioma).

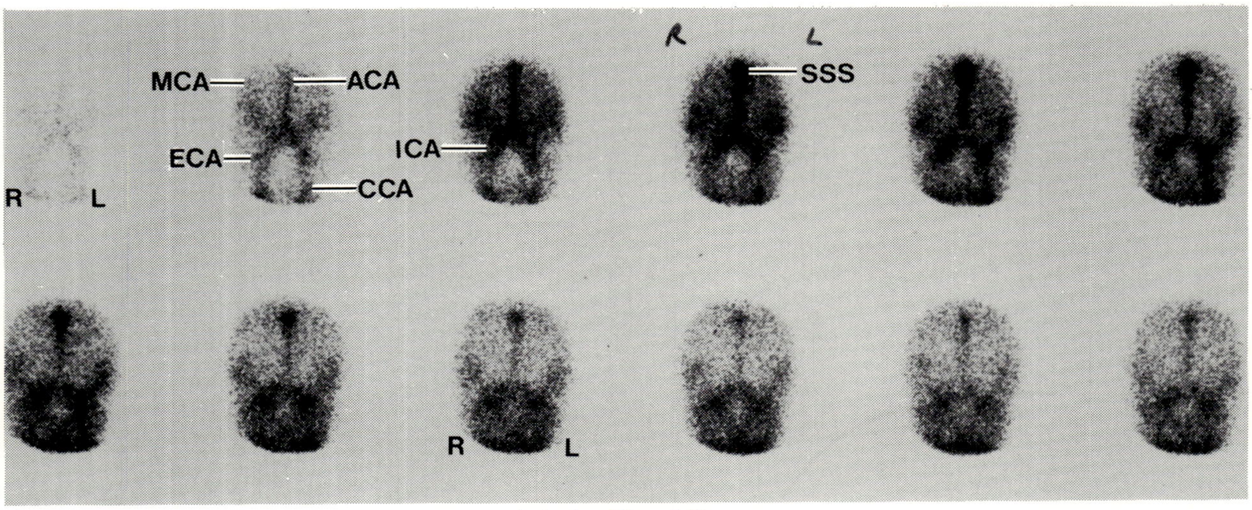


A

Anterior Blood Flow

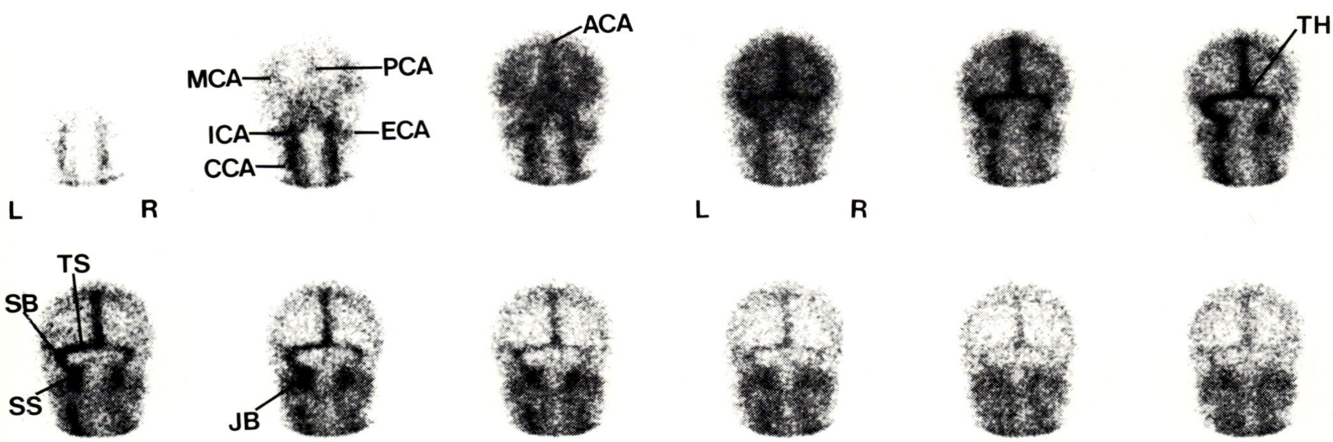


B

Posterior Blood Flow

**FIG. 1.** NORMAL BLOOD FLOW STUDIES. **A. Normal Anterior Blood Flow Study.** Frames are taken at intervals of 2 seconds and imaging commences with the appearance of the radioactive material in the carotid arteries. The common (CCA), internal (ICA), and external (ECA) carotid arteries are identified early in the arterial phase (frames 1 and 2). The distribution of the anterior cerebral (ACA) and middle cerebral (MCA) arteries are easily recognized. The duration of the arterial phase is brief and the start of the venous phase is heralded by the appearance of the radionuclide in the superior sagittal sinus (SSS). Thereafter, drainage into the jugular system obscures carotid radioactivity. **B. Normal Posterior Blood Flow Study.** As in the anterior study, the major vessels are identified during the arterial phase. In addition, the distribution of the posterior cerebral arteries (PCA) is demonstrated. During the venous phase, the superior sagittal sinus, torcular Herophili (TH), transverse sinus (TS), sigmoid bend (SB), sigmoid sinus (SS), and jugular bulb (JB) are visible.

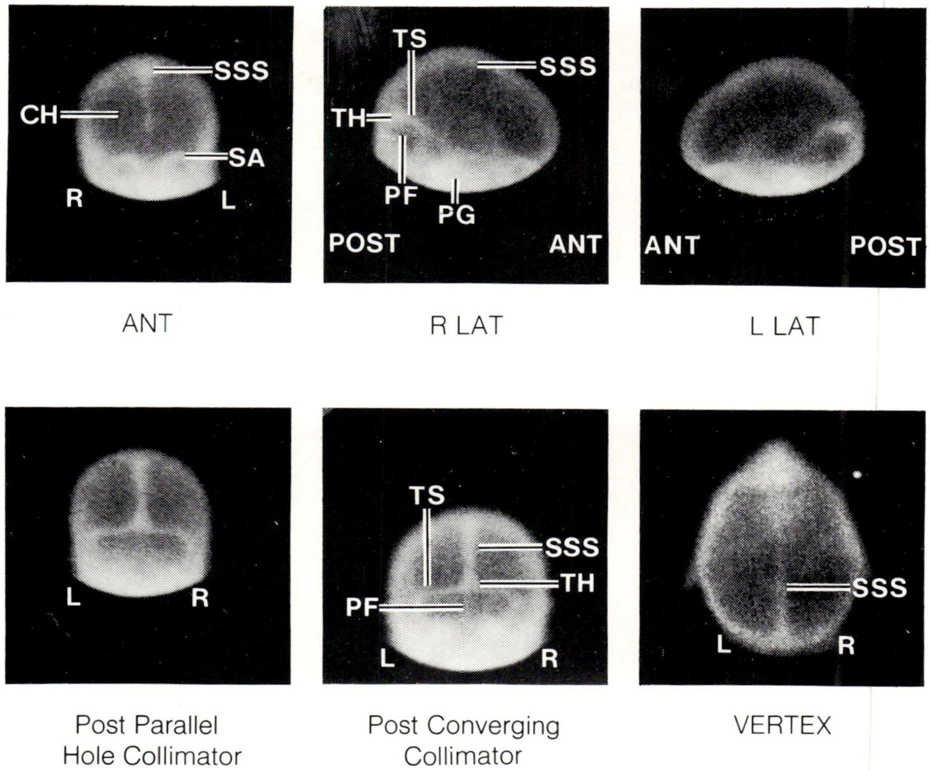


**FIG. 2.** NORMAL STATIC BRAIN IMAGING. Imaging is usually performed in the anterior, posterior, right lateral, left lateral, and vertex positions. In the anterior position, the superior sagittal sinus (SSS) and supraorbital ridges (SA) are commonly identified landmarks. The large areas of relatively absent radioactivity are the cerebral hemispheres (CH). The peripheral radioactivity is associated with vascular radioactivity in the calvarium, scalp, and draining venous lacunae.

In the lateral position, the transverse sinus (TS) is identified posteriorly and serves as a landmark for the separation of posterior fossa (PF) and supratentorial regions. With pertechnetate, the parotid gland (PG) is visible. Anteriorly, the orbit, nasal mucosa, and sphenoid sinus areas are seen. The peripheral activity visible superiorly is the superior sagittal sinus (SSS); it can be followed into the confluence of the sinuses, or torcular Herophili (TH).

Posteriorly, the superior sagittal sinus is identified along with the torcular Herophili and transverse sinuses. The posterior fossa area inferior to the transverse sinuses is well defined. Inferior to the latter, the increased radioactivity is due to the vascular posterior neck muscles. Note the improved imaging of the posterior fossa when a converging collimator is used as compared to that seen when a parallel hole collimator is employed.

The superior portion of the brain is visible in the vertex position. The midline superior sagittal sinus is a commonly identified landmark (Tc-99m sodium pertechnetate).

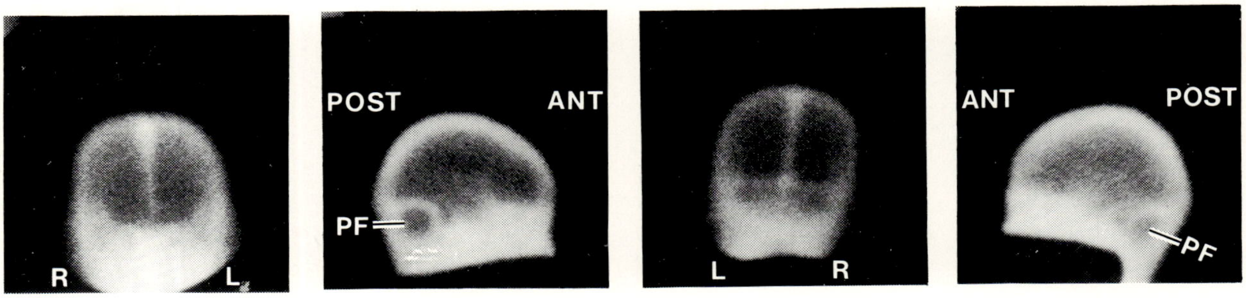


ANT R LAT POST L LAT

**FIG. 3. BRAIN IMAGING WITH Tc-99m DTPA.** There is no radionuclide uptake in the choroid plexus or salivary glands. Note the absence of parotid activity compared to that seen with pertechnetate imaging. The posterior fossa (PF) is sharply identified in the lateral positions in this 7-year-old boy.

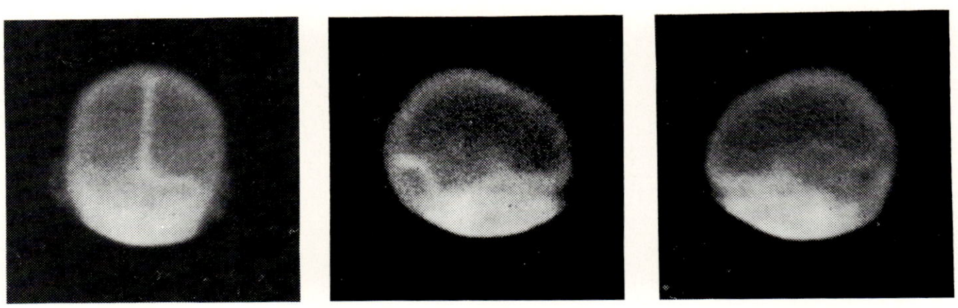

POST R LAT L LAT

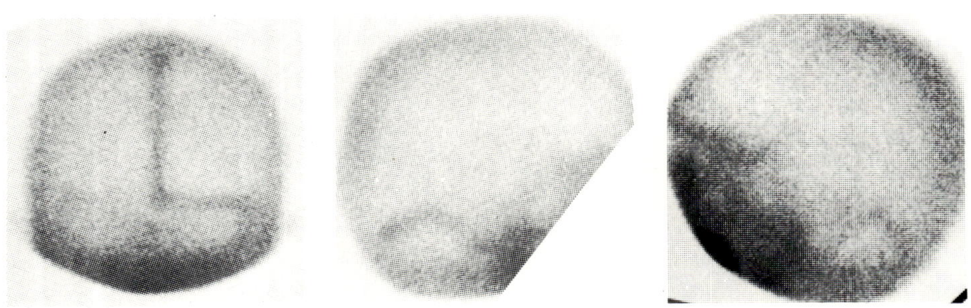

POST R LAT L LAT

**FIG. 4. UNDERDEVELOPED LEFT TRANSVERSE SINUS.** Nonvisualization of a transverse sinus occurs in approximately 20 percent of patients. Its absence is much more frequent on the left side. In each of these patients, the right transverse sinus is sharply demonstrated.

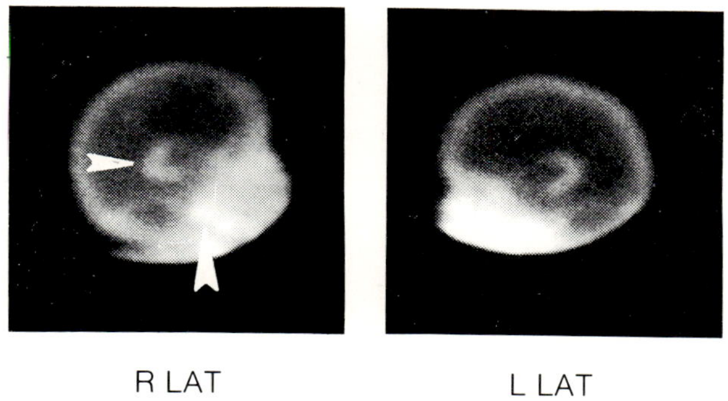


**FIG. 5. CHOROID PLEXUS VISUALIZATION WITH Tc-99m SODIUM PERTECHNETATE IMAGING.** Prior to pertechnetate injection, it is necessary to administer potassium perchlorate to block the uptake of Tc-99m sodium pertechnetate in the choroid plexus. An oral dose of 200 mg of $KClO_4$ 1 to 3 hours prior to radionuclide injection is sufficient. If the blocking dose of $KClO_4$ is not given, there will be visualization of the choroid plexus (arrows), and such visualization may be mistaken for an intracranial lesion. Tc-99m sodium pertechnetate is also taken up in the salivary glands, and ready identification of the parotid gland (open arrow) and radioactivity in the oral and buccal mucosa due to salivary secretion are common.

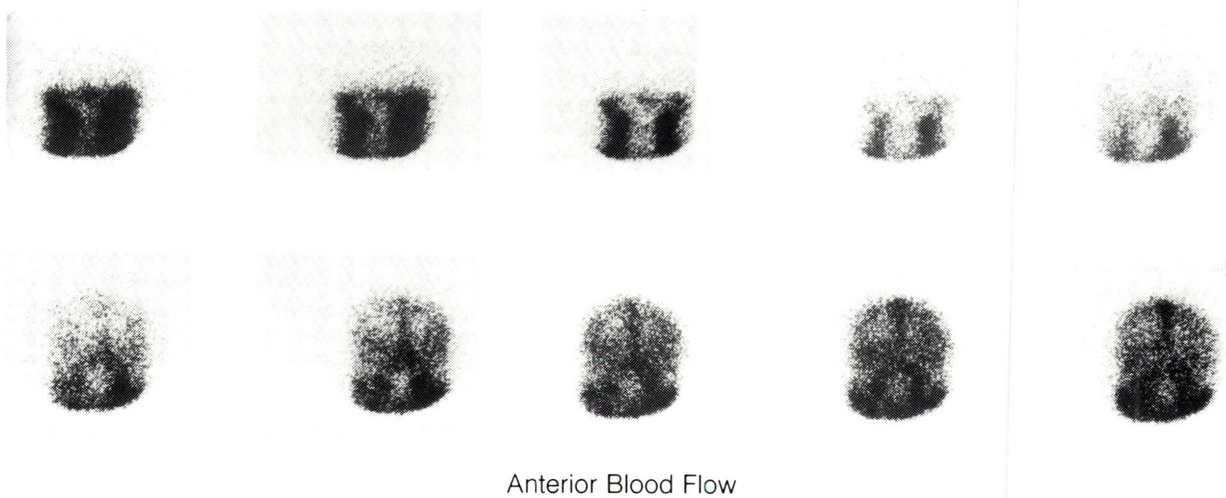


**FIG. 6. VENOUS REFLUX DUE TO SUPERIOR VENA CAVA OBSTRUCTION.** The sudden appearance of radioactivity in the cervical region immediately following radionuclide administration in an upper extremity vein is due to activity in the jugular system and *not in the carotid arteries*. In this patient with superior vena cava obstruction, both jugulars are seen 2 seconds following Tc-99m injection. This is simply a reflection of the obstruction to venous drainage and may be seen in other situations in which there is marked elevation of venous pressure. Following venous drainage through collateral vessels into the right heart, carotid artery activity superimposed on jugular activity begins to be visible at 10 seconds (frame 4), and there is tracer activity in the anterior and middle cerebral arteries at 12 seconds (frame 5).

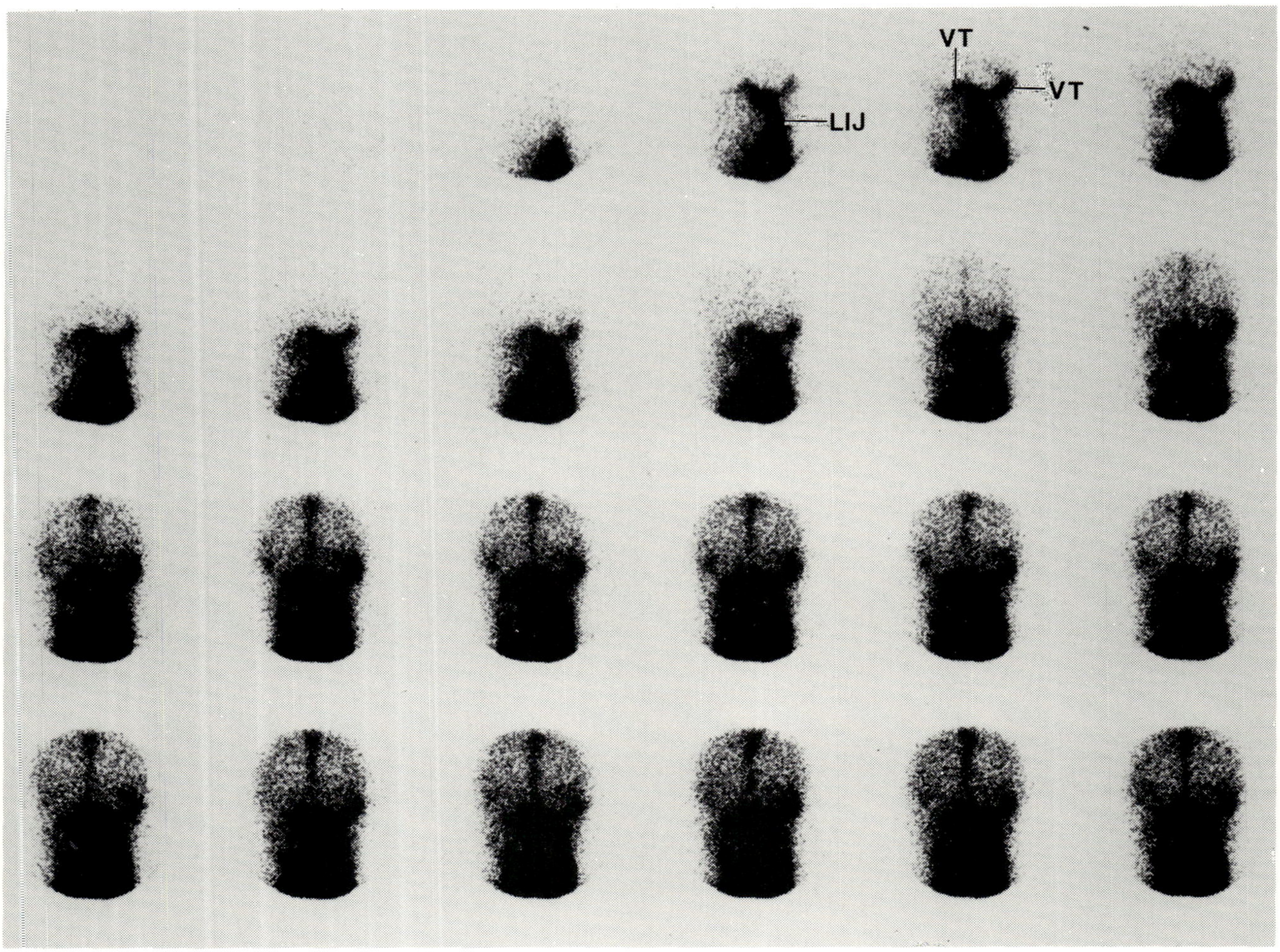


Anterior Blood Flow

**FIG. 7** (See legend next page)

**FIG. 7. VENOUS REFLUX DUE TO LEFT INNOMINATE VEIN OBSTRUCTION.** Following injection of Tc-99m in a left upper extremity vein, reflux into the left internal jugular (LIJ) system and venous tributaries (VT) is visible almost immediately. Since the obstruction is marked, entry of radioactive material into the heart via collateral veins is greatly reduced and tracer appearance during the arterial phase is difficult to demonstrate. The late arterial phase is seen at 18 seconds when middle cerebral artery distribution (arrow) is visualized.

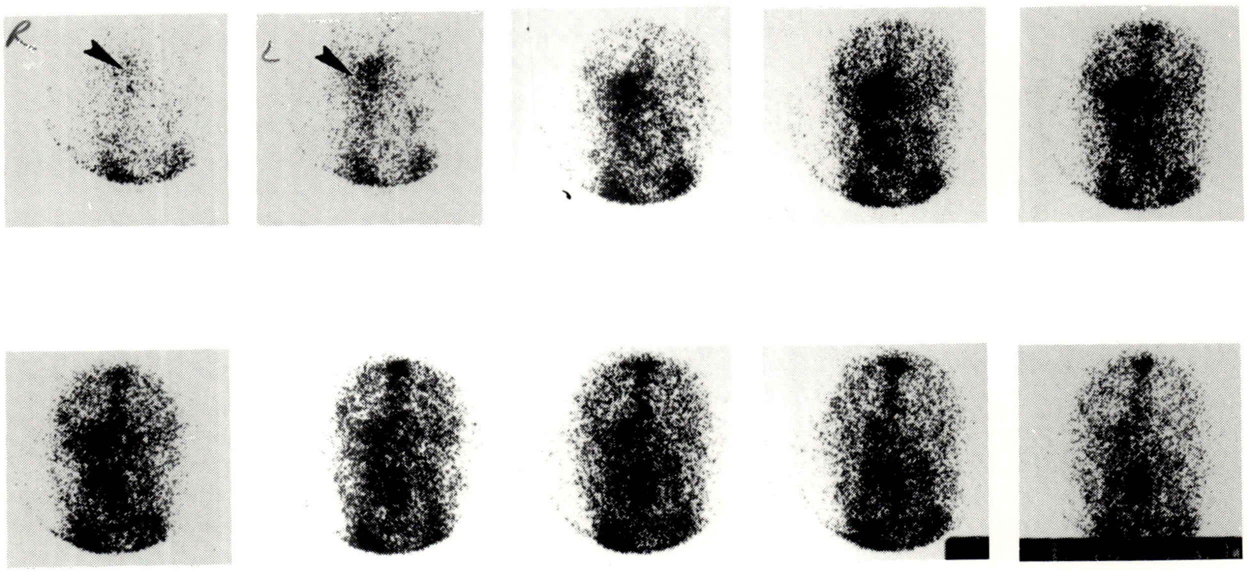

A.1.

Anterior Blood Flow

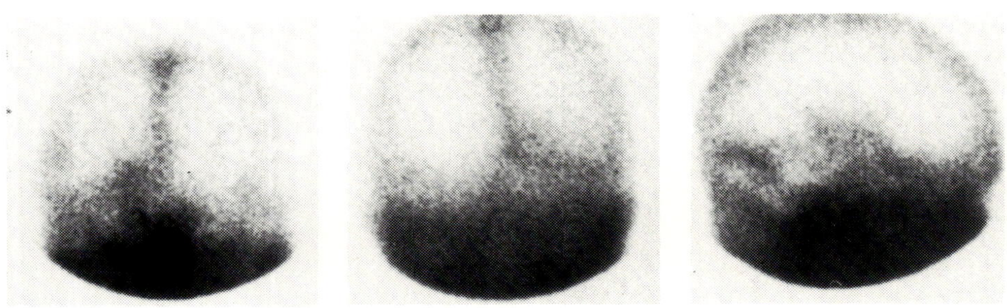

ANT POST R LAT

A.2.

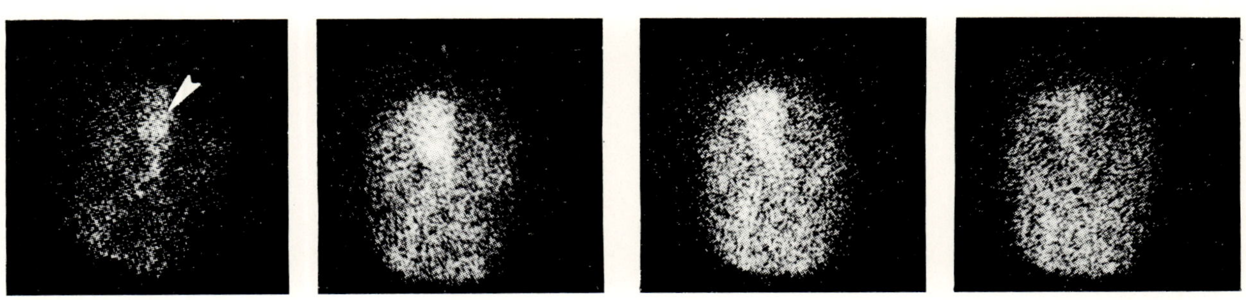

B.1. ANT R LAT POST L LAT

Anterior Blood Flow

**FIG. 8. A.1, A.2, B.1.** (See legend next page)

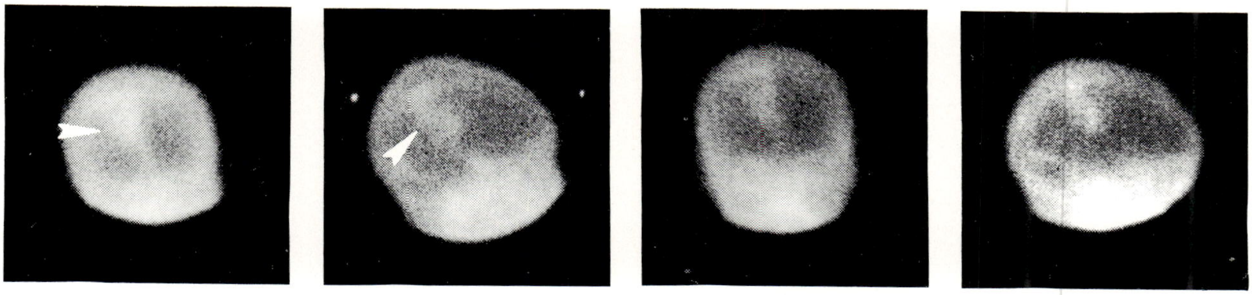

B. 2. ANT R LAT ANT R LAT

5 minutes 1 hour

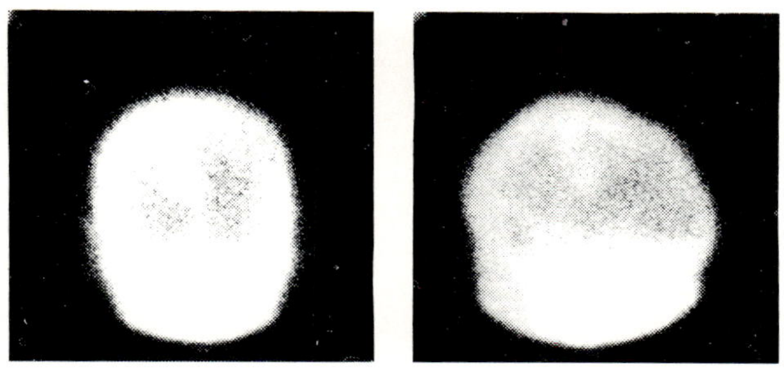

ANT R LAT

2 hours

**FIG. 8. ARTERIOVENOUS MALFORMATION.** An AV malformation (AVM) is usually seen almost immediately after the radionuclide can be seen entering the carotid arteries on the blood flow study. The sudden increase in radioactivity seen in the initial frames rapidly diminishes as the tracer leaves the site of the abnormality in the venous drainage (this is in contrast to the persistence in radioactivity seen on the blood flow study of a meningioma in Fig. 11). Although during static imaging the abnormality may be seen because of vascular radioactivity, the etiology of the lesion may be more clearly determined during the blood flow study: rapid appearance followed by rapid diminution in radioactivity. **A.** Localized area of increased radioactivity demonstrated on blood flow study . **1.** The site of the AVM is indicated on the initial blood flow image (arrow), and continues to be clearly visualized up to the frame at intervals 10 to 12 seconds and shows diminished activity thereafter. **2.** Static imaging at one hour demonstrates the site of the lesion (arrow), but it is not nearly so prominent now (Tc-99m DTPA). (Courtesy of Dr. Emmett M. Cooper, Lancaster General Hospital, Lancaster, PA) **B.** AV malformation in another patient. **1.** Blood flow study. The site of the AVM (arrow) is imaged almost immediately but can no longer be discerned with clarity during the 8- to 10-second interval. **2.** Static imaging. Although the site of the AVM (arrow) can be seen in the anterior and right lateral positions at 5 minutes, there is progressive diminution in radioactivity by 2 hours (Tc-99m sodium pertechnetate).

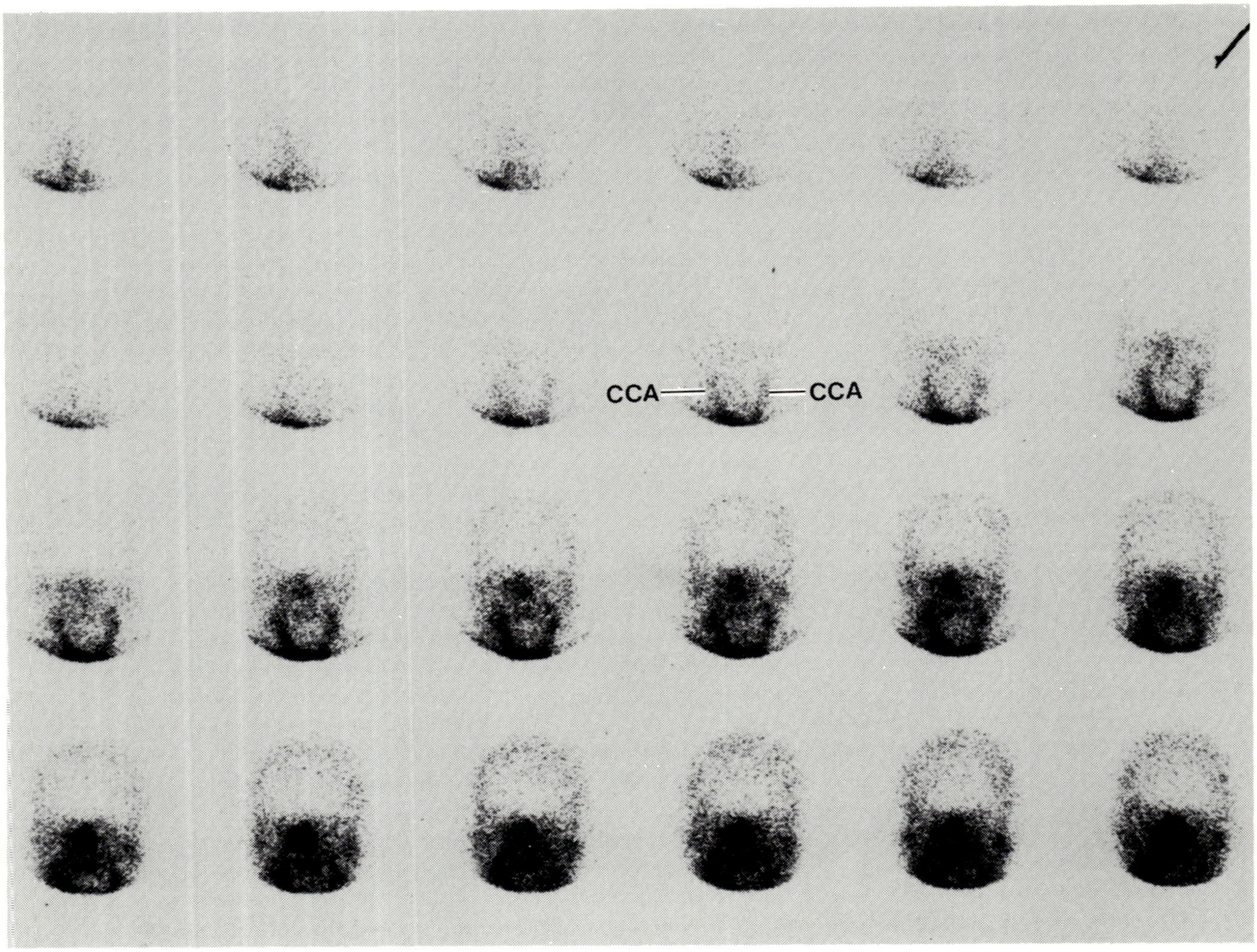


**FIG. 9.** (See legend next page)

**FIG. 9. RADIONUCLIDE BLOOD FLOW STUDIES IN CEREBRAL DEATH.** In those patients in whom further objective evidence, in addition to a flattened electroencephalogram, is sought to support a diagnosis of cerebral death, radionuclide blood flow studies may be helpful. Although the common carotid arteries (CCA) are demonstrated, there is a failure to visualize the anterior and middle cerebral arteries and there is no identification of the superior sagittal sinus. The lack of visualization of these vascular structures is related to increased intracranial pressure, cerebral edema, and thrombosis. Vascular supply to the scalp and skull help outline these areas but there is no evidence of intracerebral arterial supply or venous drainage.

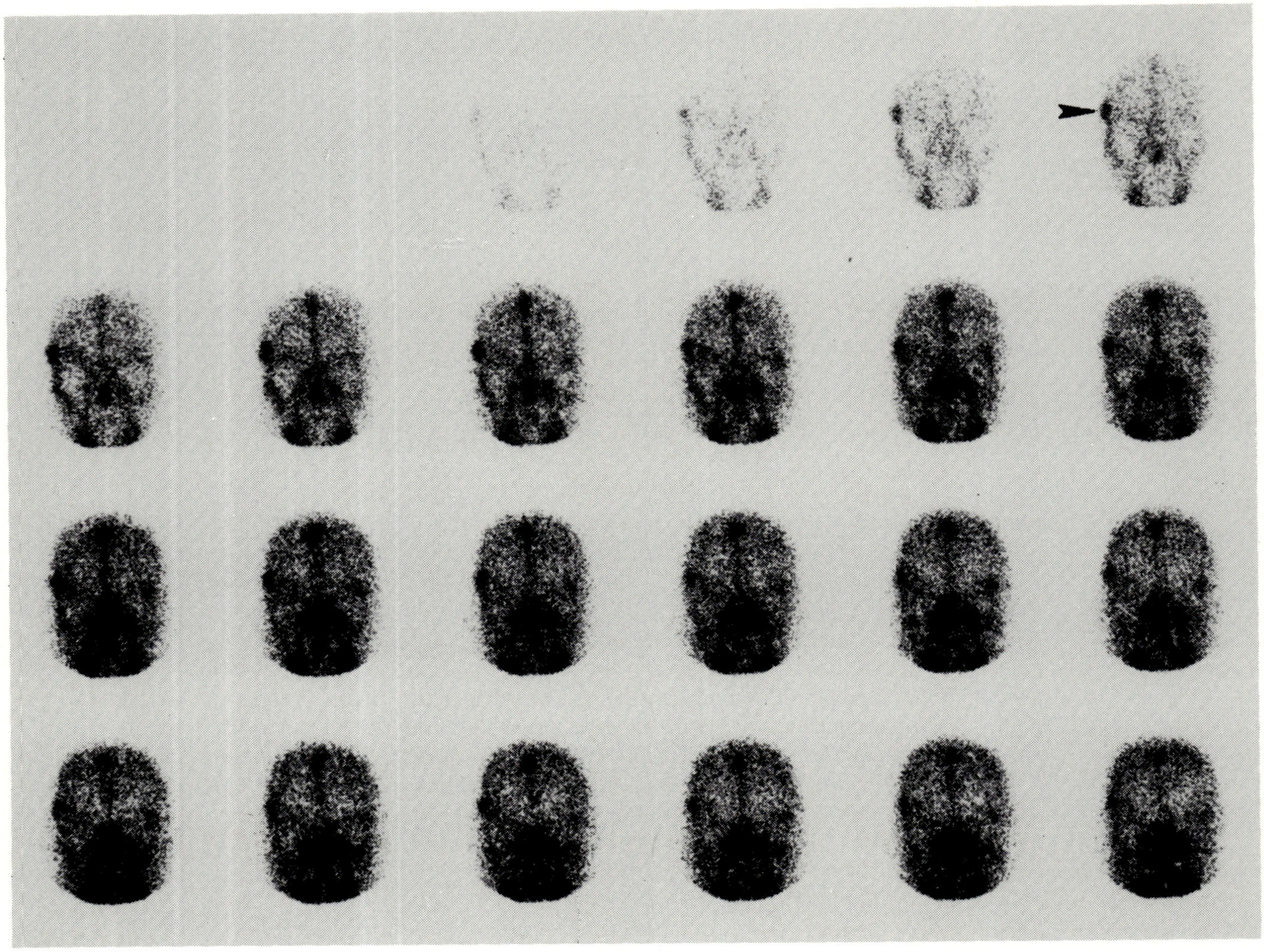

A Anterior Blood Flow

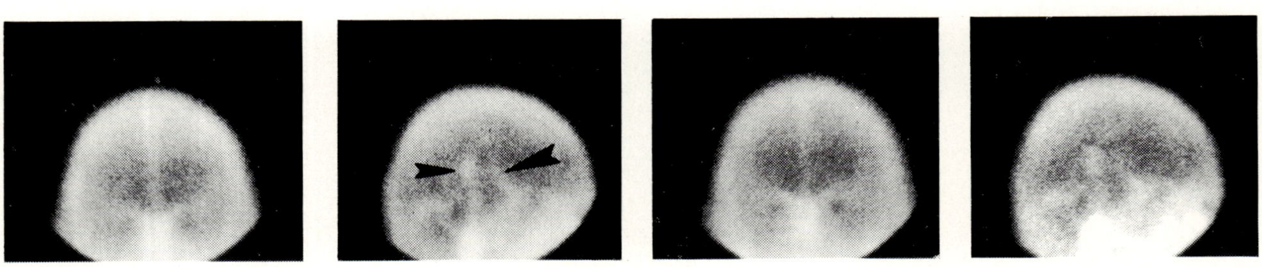

B ANT 5 minutes R LAT 5 minutes ANT 20 minutes R LAT 20 minutes

**FIG. 10. A, B.** (See legend next page)

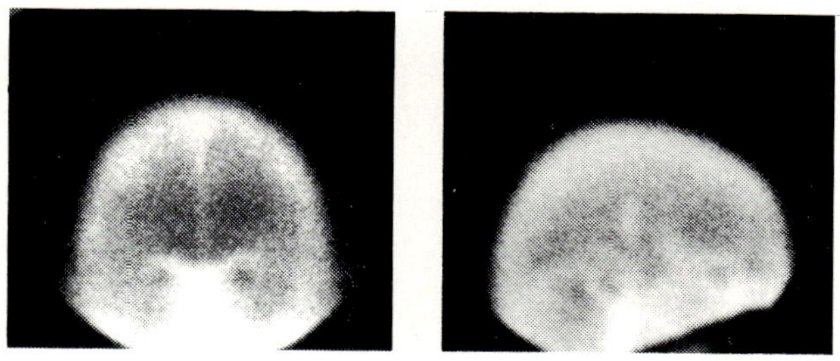


**FIG. 10. ARTERIOVENOUS MALFORMATION IN SCALP. A. Blood Flow Study.** The AVM (arrow) is identified early in the arterial phase. It is supplied by a temporal branch of the right external carotid artery (arrow). This is an unusual and rare delineation of an external carotid artery by radionuclide angiography. The duration of precise visualization of the AVM is longer than that usually observed with an intracranial AVM. **B. Static Imaging.** Static imaging in the anterior position at intervals never demonstrates the abnormality, because of its location. In the right lateral position, the AVM (arrow) is seen on the 5-minute study and diminishes in intensity thereafter. Note the draining vein ( larger arrow) anterior to the AVM. The visualization on static imaging of a localized area of increased radioactivity with even a suggestion of a draining vein should alert one to the possibility of an AVM and the necessity for performing a blood flow study, or repeating it if it already has been done (Tc-99m sodium pertechnetate).

## BRAIN TUMORS

Meningiomas are probably visualized with radionuclide brain imaging because of the localization of radioactive material in the large endothelial sinuses or spaces in these tumors. Approximately 70 percent of intracranial meningiomas may be first recognized on the blood flow study. Since static imaging is associated with the presence of radionuclide in the vascular spaces of the tumor, maximum radionuclide localization is seen about 15 minutes following tracer administration, and this is probably the optimum time for static imaging. Imaging at one hour may demonstrate the lesion with the clarity similar to that seen at 15 minutes, but it is defined less clearly with continued imaging at 2 and 3 hours.

Tumors involving the brain parenchyma, both primary and metastatic, and those of nerve sheath origin, such as acoustic neuromas, are probably visualized on static imaging because of the entry of radionuclide into the tumor cells themselves. This radionuclide accumulation in the tumor cells occurs gradually over a period of time, and the time of maximum tracer accumulation is variable. Thus, the optimum time for imaging some tumors may be 30 minutes following injection of the radioactive material while for others it may be 3 or more hours. This is, in part, the reason for doing delayed imaging for brain tumor detection. Those tumors that can be seen best only at late times (3 or 4 hours) are usually visualized with far less clarity than those that can be imaged early, because of tracer decay and excretion. Depending on the blood supply, tumors of the brain parenchyma and those of nerve sheath origin may or may not be seen on the blood flow study.

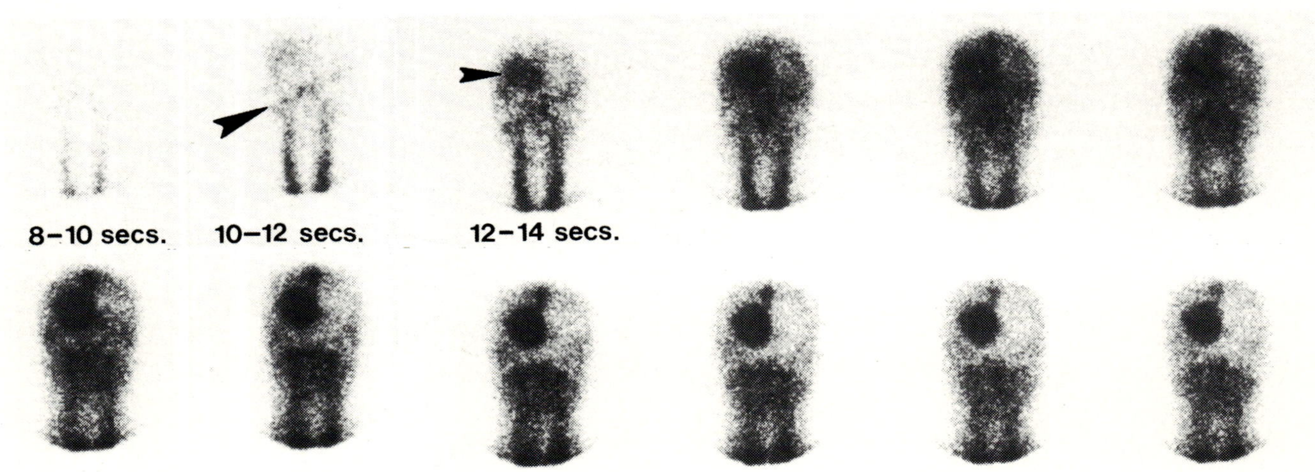


A

Blood Flow Study

**FIG. 11. A.** (See legend next page)

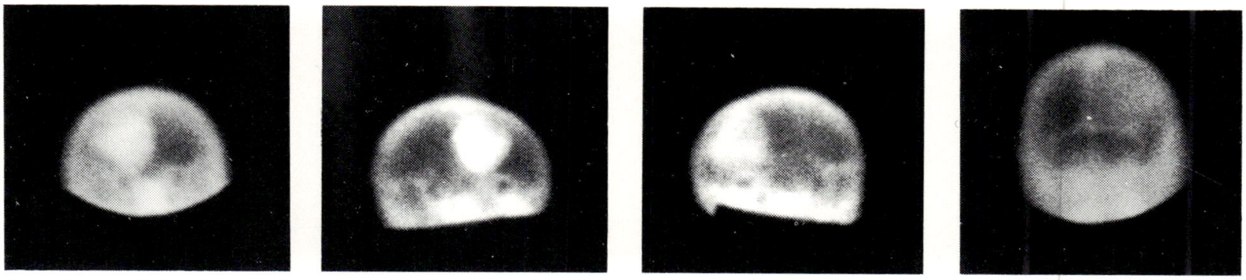

B Static Imaging

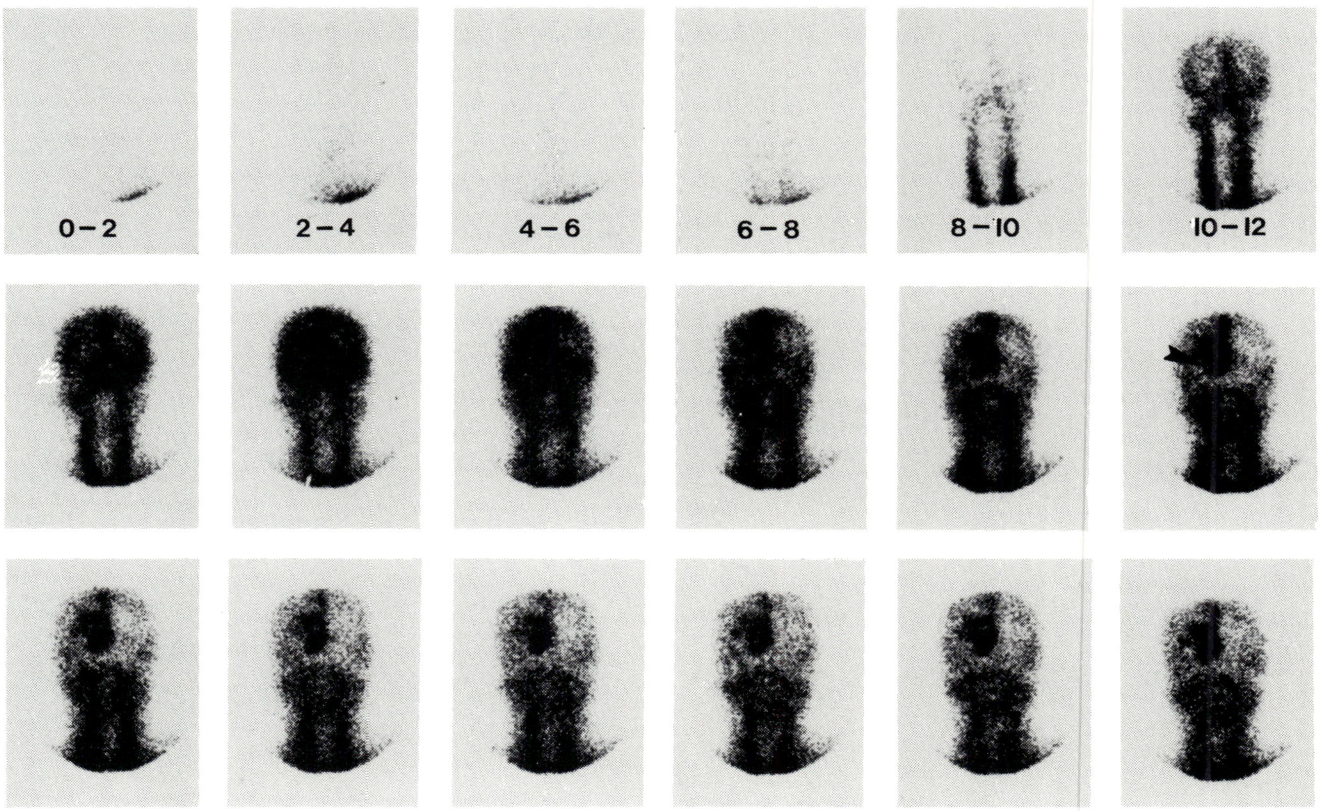


C Blood Flow Study

**FIG. 11.** RIGHT FRONTOPARIETAL MENINGIOMA. **A. Blood Flow Study.** The tumor begins to be visible on the blood flow study at 10 seconds and is clearly identified at 12 seconds (arrow) during the arterial phase. The tumor is supplied by branches from the external carotid artery ( larger arrows). Following the venous phase, there is continued persistence in excellent visualization. **B. Static Imaging.** The lesion with its intense radioactive uptake is clearly identified on this 15-minute study, which was performed with a large field of view camera and a converging collimator. **C.** Blood flow study after gelfoam embolism. Prior to surgery, gelfoam emboli were inserted into the arteries supplying the tumor, and a blood flow study was obtained immediately following the embolization procedure. There is no evidence of tumor as seen during the arterial phase at 8 and 10 seconds. However, during the venous phase and thereafter, the venous drainage from the tumor is seen (arrow) (Tc-99m sodium pertechnetate).

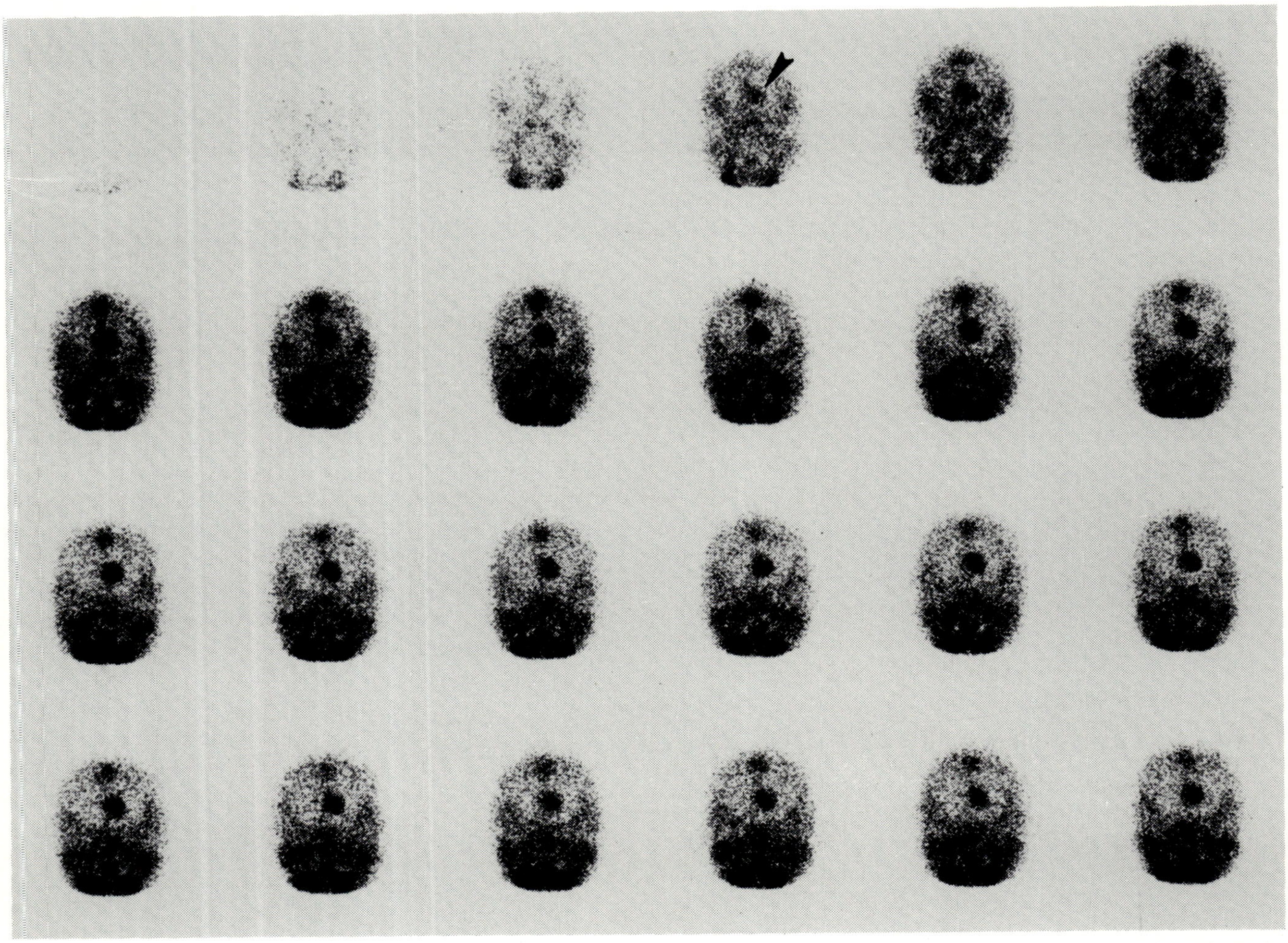

A

Anterior Blood Flow

**Fig. 12. A.** (See legend next page)

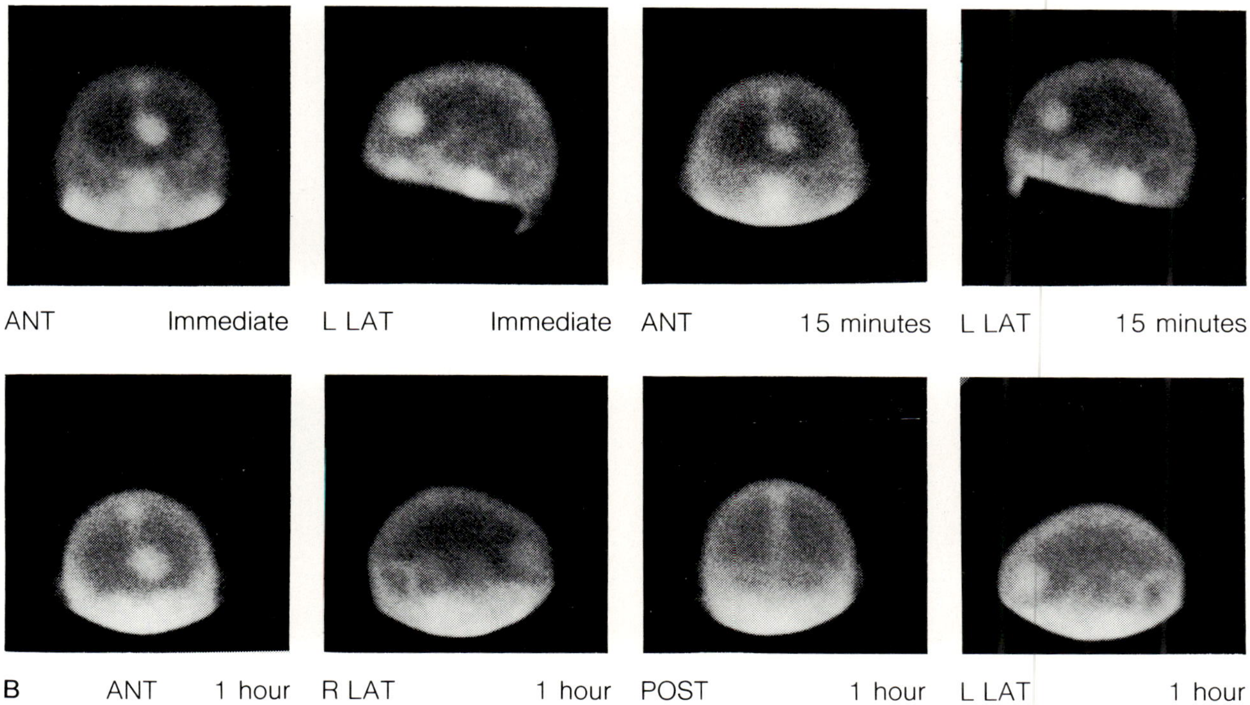


**FIG. 12.** PARASAGITTAL MENINGIOMA. A. **Blood Flow Study.** The tumor is identified (arrow) during the late arterial phase. Once the tumor is imaged on the blood flow study, it continues to be imaged thereafter. This is in contrast to the AVM seen in Fig. 8, in which the duration of imaging of the lesion is only transitory during the blood flow study. **B. Static Imaging.** The meningioma is clearly identified in the imaging performed immediately after injection, at 15 minutes, and at one hour. The immediate and 15-minute imaging were performed with a large field of view camera and a conveying collimator, while that done at one hour was performed with a 10-inch diameter crystal with a parallel hole collimator. There is similar, satisfactory tumor identification in each of the static studies.

Its location next to the midline in the anterior position assists in its diagnosis as a parasagittal lesion. The intensity as seen in the left lateral position is characteristic for meningiomas (Tc-99m sodium pertechnetate).

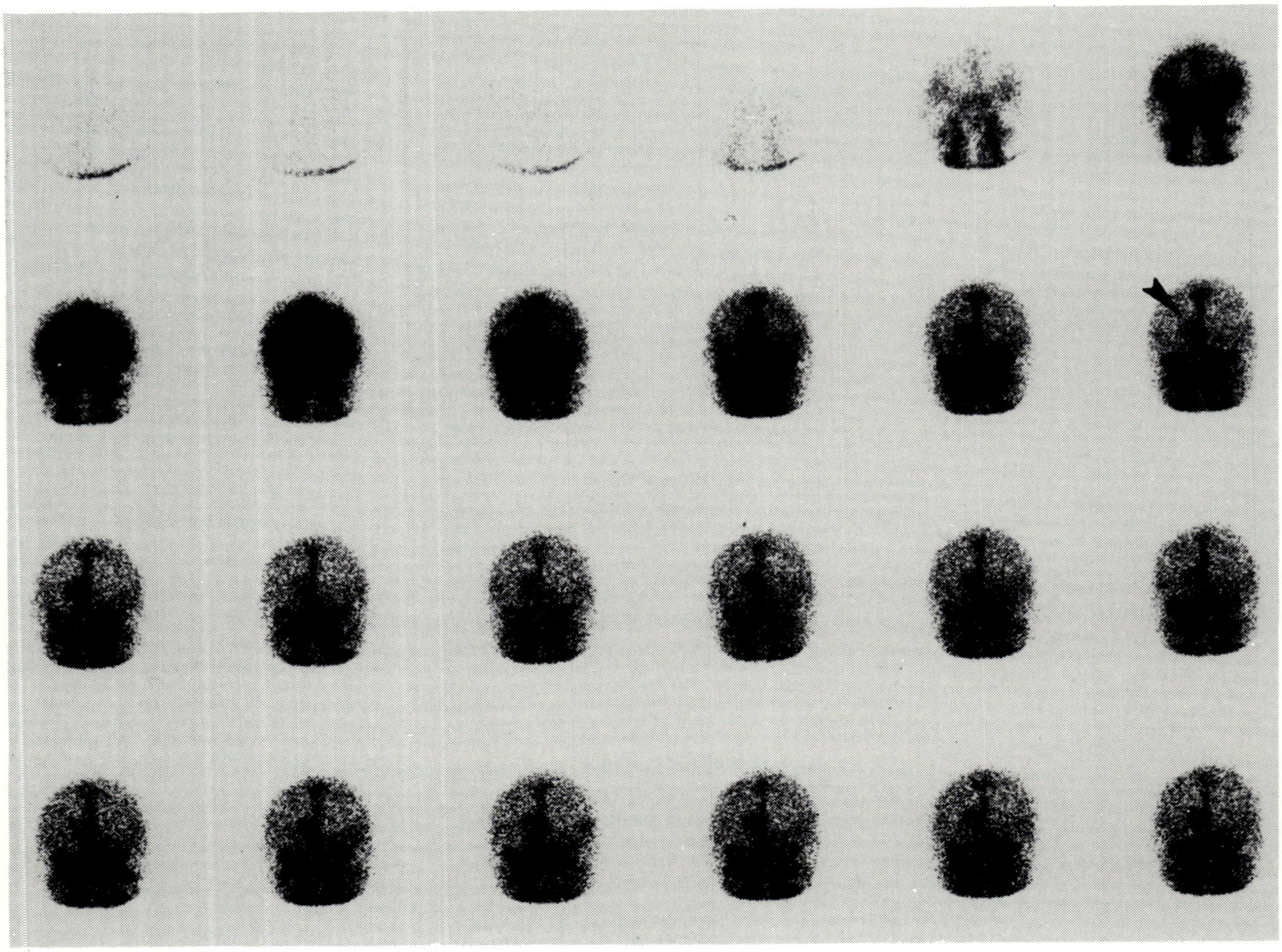

A

Posterior Blood Flow

**FIG. 13.** **LEFT PARASAGITTAL MENINGIOMA. A. Blood Flow Study.** The lesion is seen (arrow) during the late venous phase and thereafter. **B. Static Imaging.** Studies performed immediately following injection clearly identify the meningioma. Although the subsequent studies at 15 minutes and at 1 and 3.5 hours show the lesion clearly, the tumor's visualization is not improved on delayed imaging. This sequence is characteristic of most meningiomas as seen on static imaging (Tc-99m sodium pertechnetate).

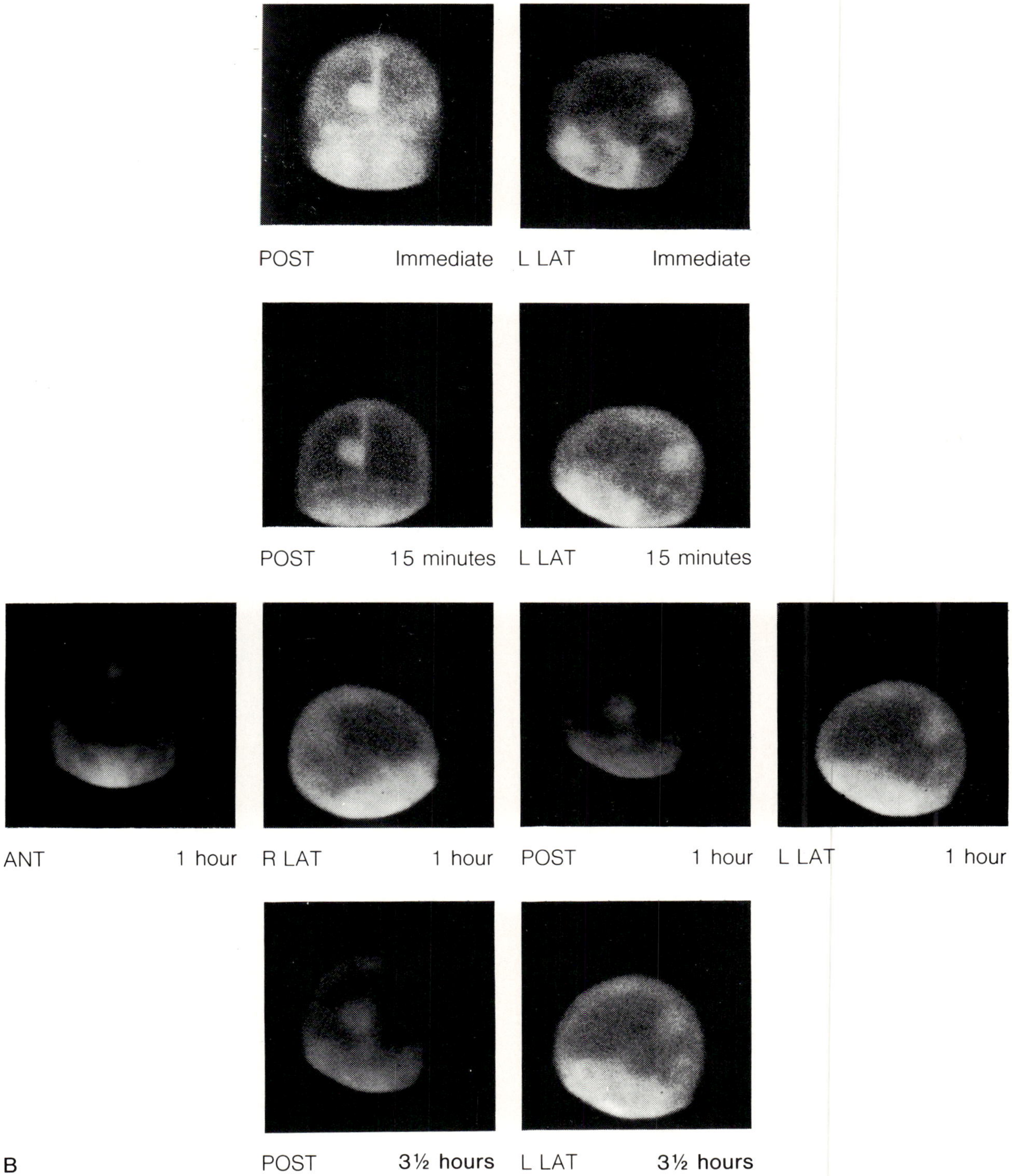


**FIG. 13. B.** (See legend on previous page)

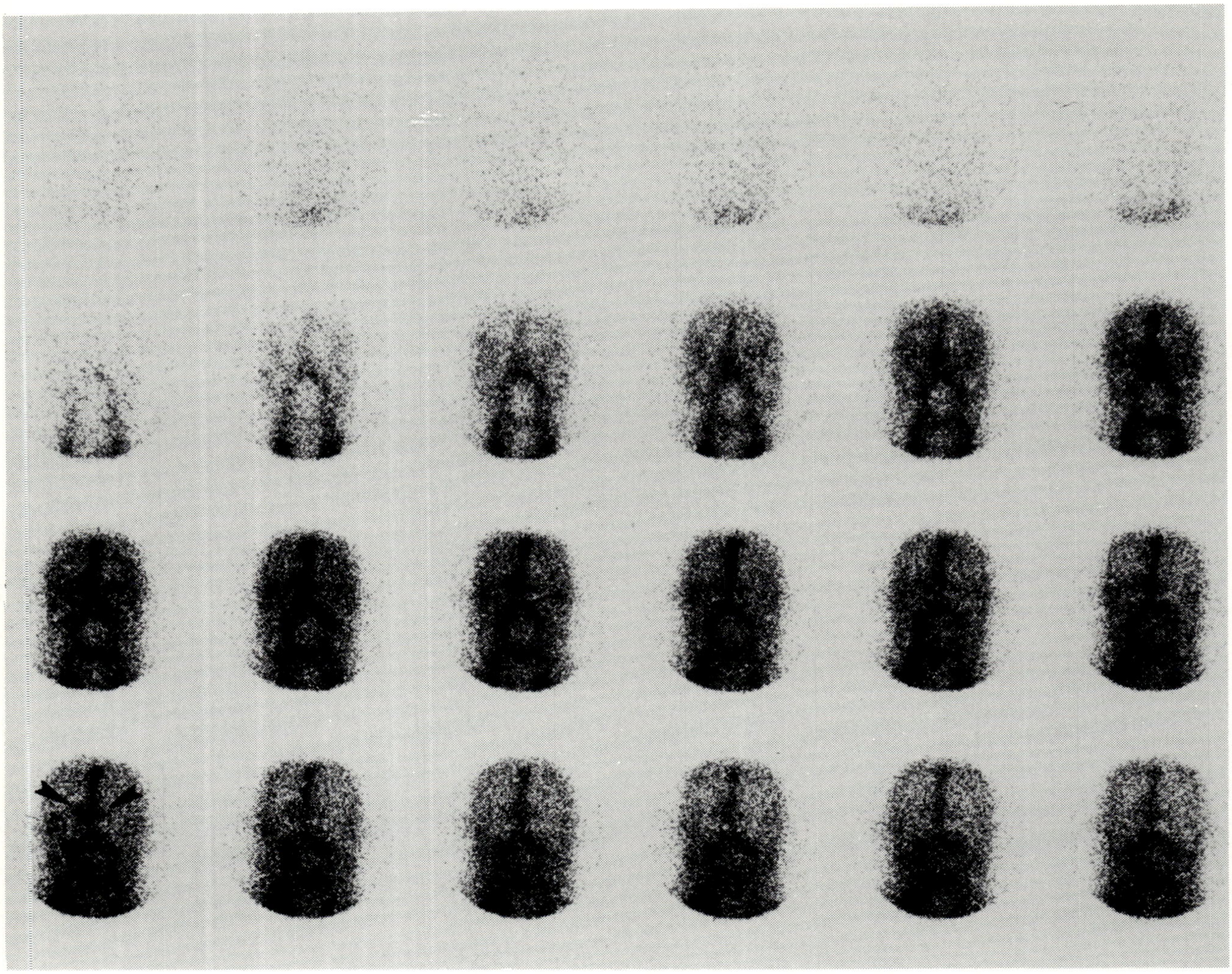

A

Anterior Blood Flow

**FIG. 14. A.** (See legend next page)

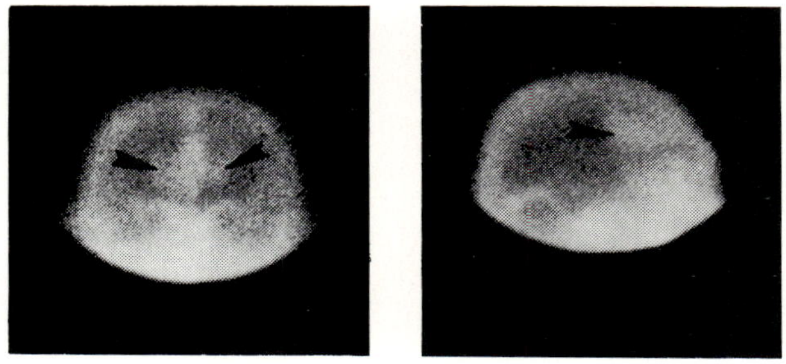

ANT 15 minutes R LAT 15 minutes

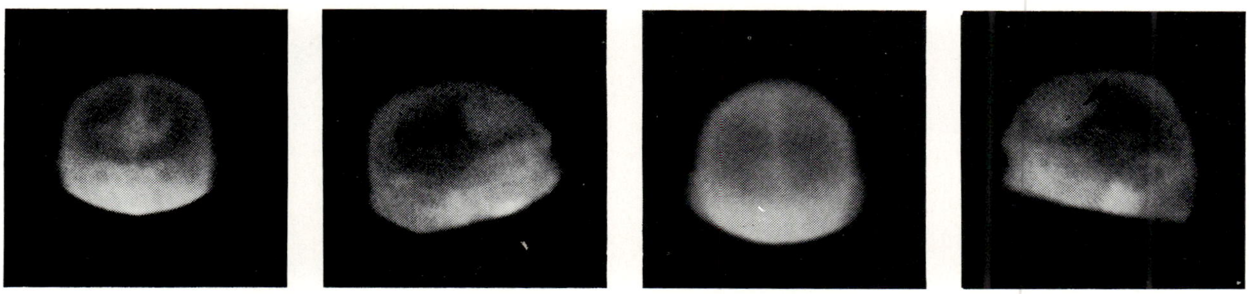

B ANT 1 hour R LAT 1 hour POST 1 hour L LAT 1 hour

**FIG. 14.** BILATERAL FALCINE MENINGIOMA. A. Blood Flow Study. The areas of increased radioactivity (arrows) can be seen late in the venous phase. **B. Static Imaging.** This dumbbell-shaped falx meningioma envelops the brain in both the right and left frontal regions. It is clearly visible at 15 minutes, and subsequent imaging does not improve its identification (Tc-99m sodium pertechnetate). A converging collimator was used for both the blood flow and static imaging.

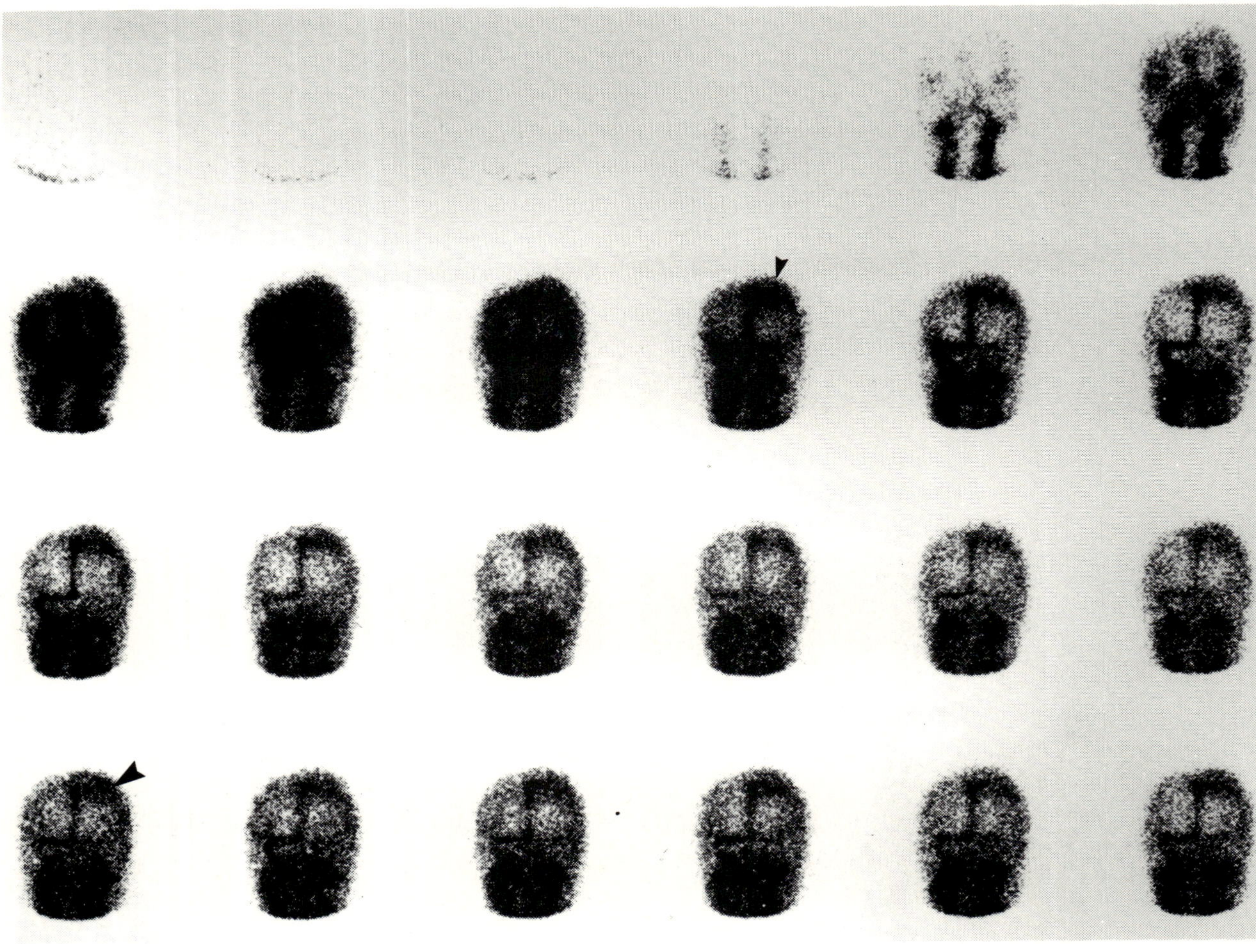

A Posterior Blood Flow

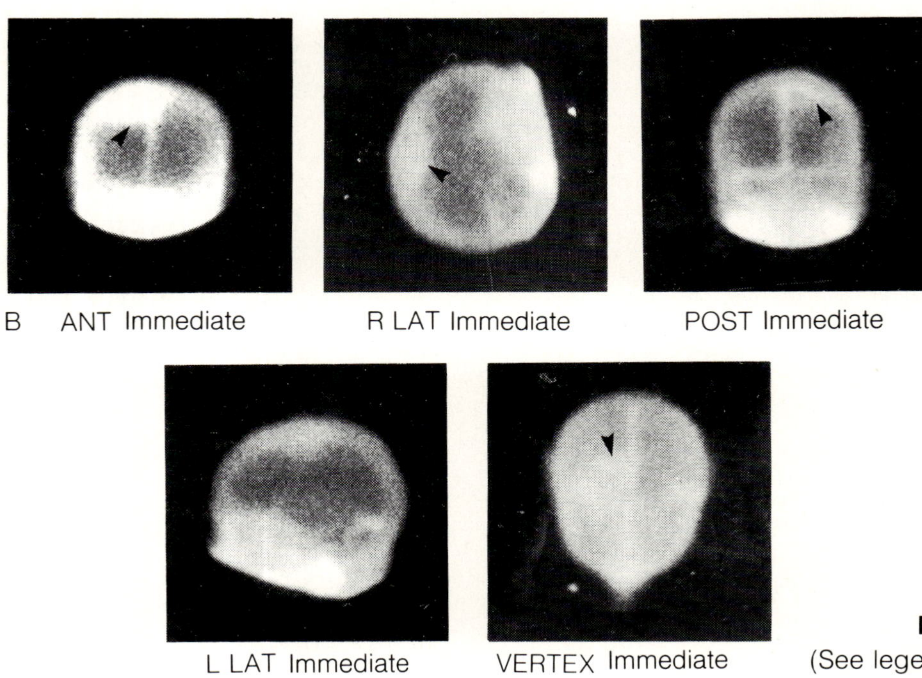


**FIG. 15. A, B.**
(See legend next page)

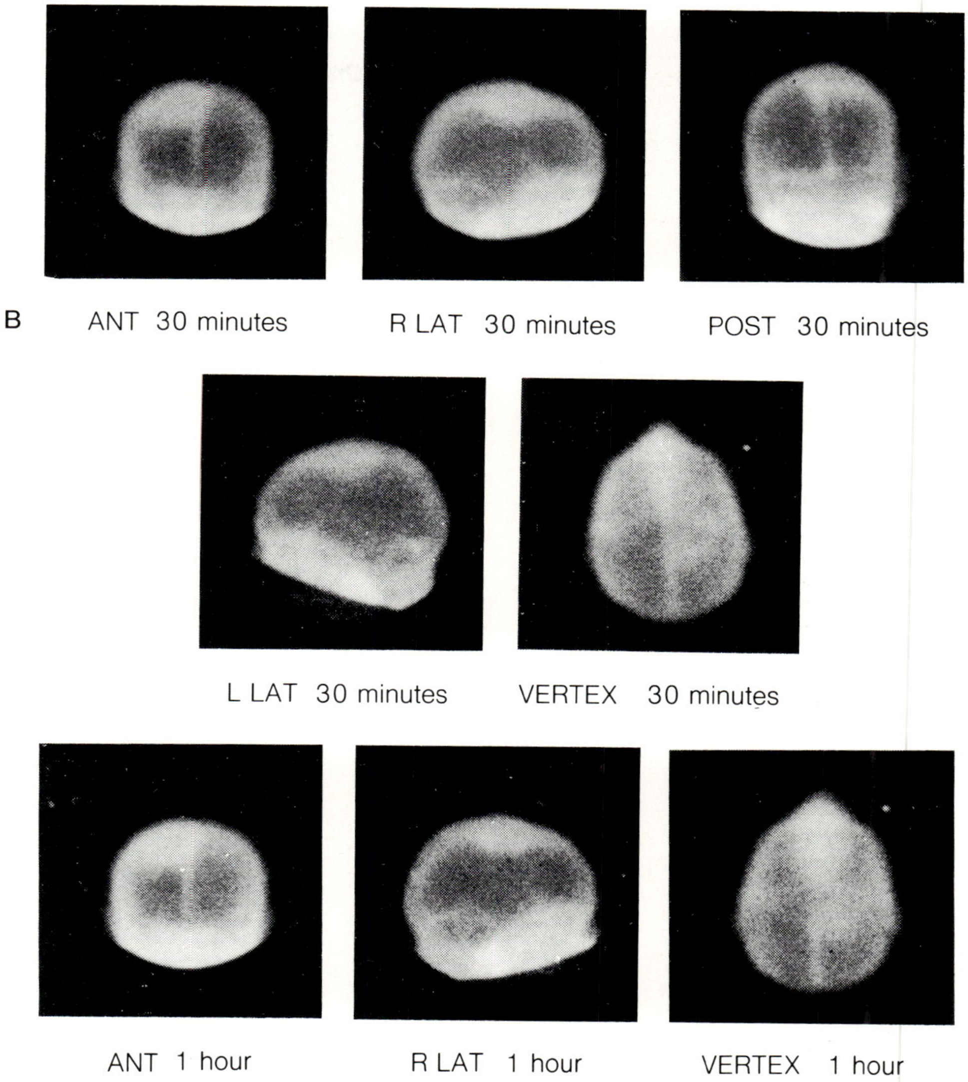


FIG. 15. MENINGIOMA WITH HYPEROSTOSIS. A. Blood Flow Study. During this blood flow study in the posterior position, increased radioactivity (arrow) is visible outside the intracranial contents and represents the area of hyperostosis in the skull. This is seen early in the arterial phase. During the venous phase, and thereafter, increased radioactivity demonstrates the site of the meningioma (larger arrow). **B. Static Imaging.** Static imaging performed immediately following the blood flow study, at 30 minutes, and at one hour clearly defines the right frontoparietal meningioma (Tc-99m sodium pertechnetate).

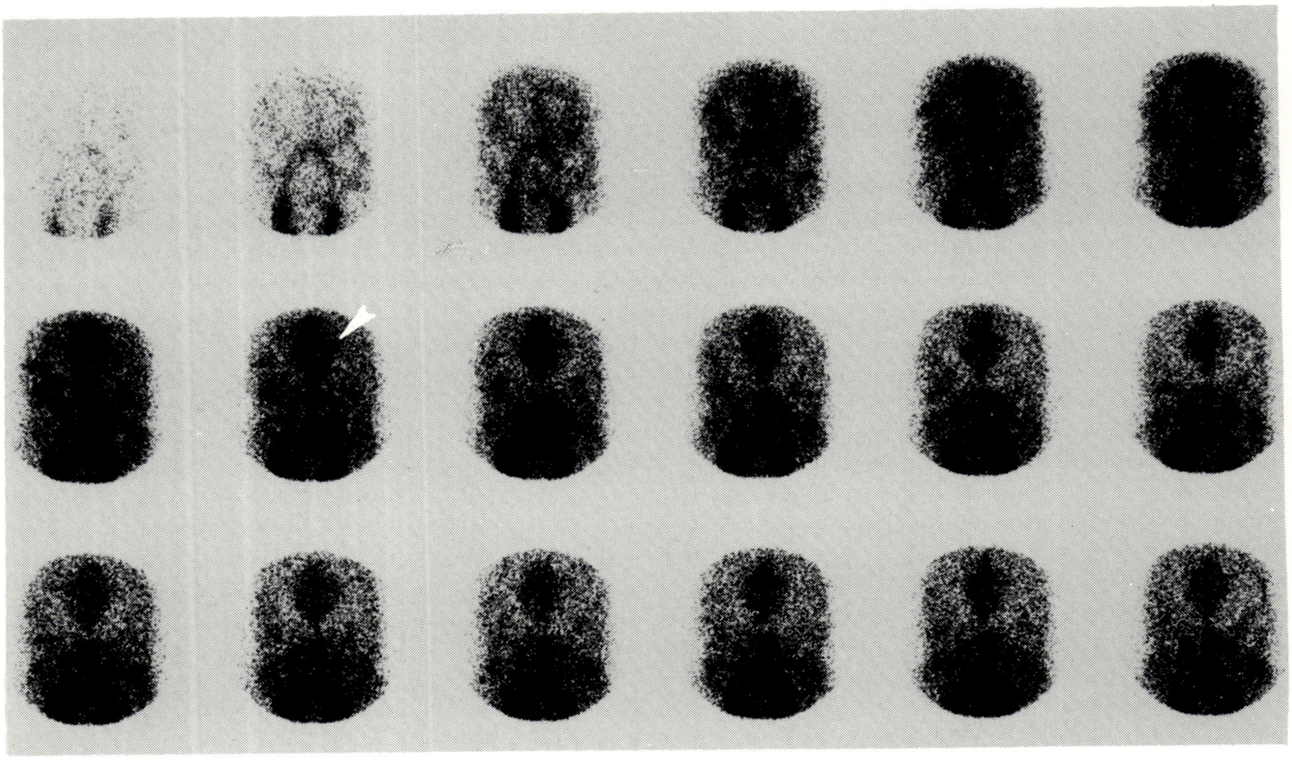

A Anterior Blood Flow

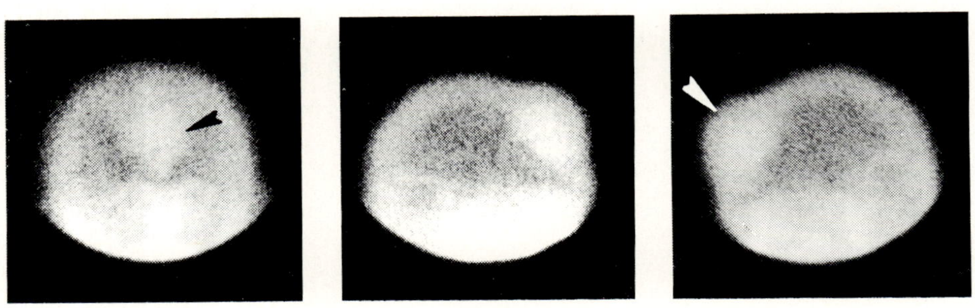

B ANT R LAT L LAT

**FIG. 16. FRONTAL MENINGIOMA WITH MARKED HYPEROSTOSIS.** All studies were performed with a converging collimator. **A. Blood Flow Study.** The site of the frontal meningioma and associated hyperostosis frontalis is depicted during the venous phase and thereafter (arrow). **B. Static Imaging.** Studies performed one hour following radionuclide administration show the anterior extension of the hyperostosis (along with the tumor). It is only in the lateral positions that the degree of bone reaction can be well appreciated (Tc-99m sodium pertechnetate).

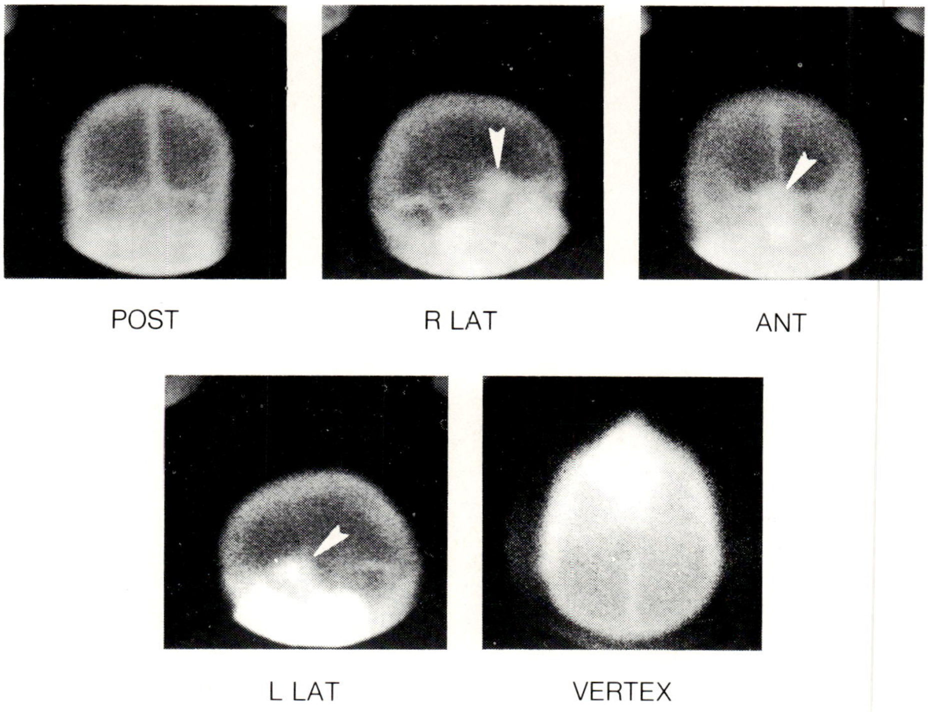


**FIG. 17. TUBERCULUM SELLAE MENINGIOMA.** These tumors are easily identified when they are large. Smaller tuberculum sellae meningiomas are not so easily demonstrated and this is due, in part, to their relatively deep location when imaging in the anterior, posterior, and lateral positions. The midline location of the lesion is seen in the anterior position (arrow). Although it is detected in the other positions (arrows), the relatively long distance from the tumor to the collimator precludes sharp visualization (Tc-99m sodium pertechnetate).

### Glioblastomas and Astrocytomas

The imaging characteristics of these tumors are similar. The optimum time for static imaging is usually between 1 and 4 hours. Radionuclide uptake may be relatively low and delineation may sometimes be considered poor. In most cases, the blood flow study does not contribute to the etiologic diagnosis.

Care must be exercised not to attempt static imaging too early following radionuclide injection, since there may have been insufficient time for the tracer to accumulate in the tumor. Thus, imaging for glioblastomas and astrocytomas at 15 minutes is often unrewarding. A more judicious approach is not to attempt static imaging until *at least* one hour has elapsed following radionuclide administration. Imaging at 2 or 3 hours may be the only time the tumor is clearly visible.

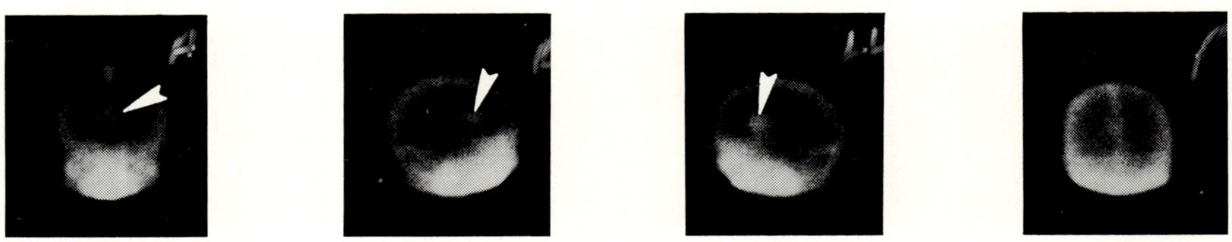

A ANT R LAT POST L LAT

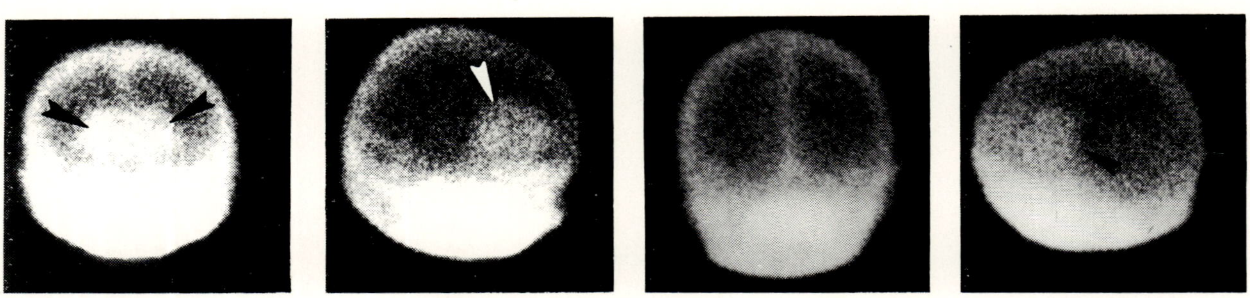

B ANT R LAT POST L LAT

**FIG. 18. TUMORS CLOSELY RELATED TO THE MIDLINE. A. Glioblastoma of Septum Pellucidum.** Static imaging. One-hour studies identify this deep-seated midline lesion. Its location far from the collimator surface may make detection difficult (Tc-99m sodium pertechnetate). **B. Glioma of the Corpus Callosum.** This butterfly-shaped tumor (arrows) extends into both the right and left cerebral hemispheres. Identification is similar in both the right and left lateral positions. Imaging was performed 2.5 hours following radionuclide injection (Tc-99m sodium pertechnetate).

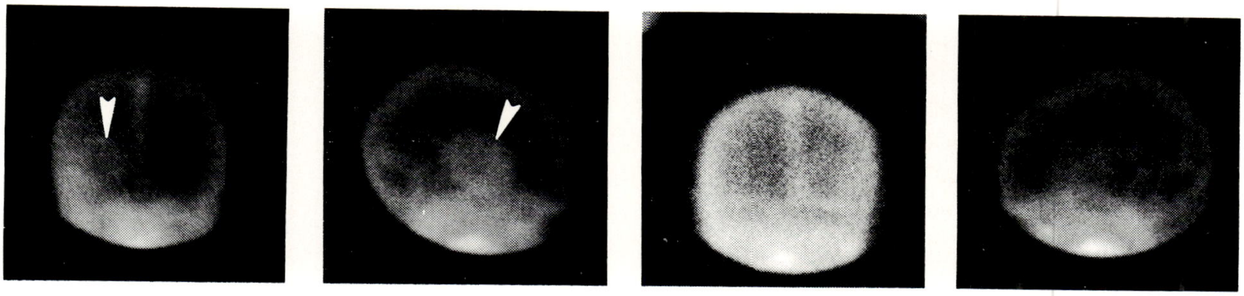

ANT R LAT POST L LAT

**FIG. 19.** GLIOBLASTOMA. The large lesion in the right frontotemporal area is easily seen in the right lateral position. It is deeply situated, and its location makes imaging somewhat more difficult in the anterior and posterior positions. These static images were performed at 1 hour. Further imaging at 2 hours would probably result in relatively increased radionuclide uptake in the tumor. Meningioma seems unlikely because of the relatively poor visualization in the anterior and posterior positions. In the imaged glioblastoma, areas of reduced uptake in the central portion of the lesion are a result of tumor necrosis; when these areas are confluent, a "doughnut" lesion may be seen (Tc-99m sodium pertechnetate).

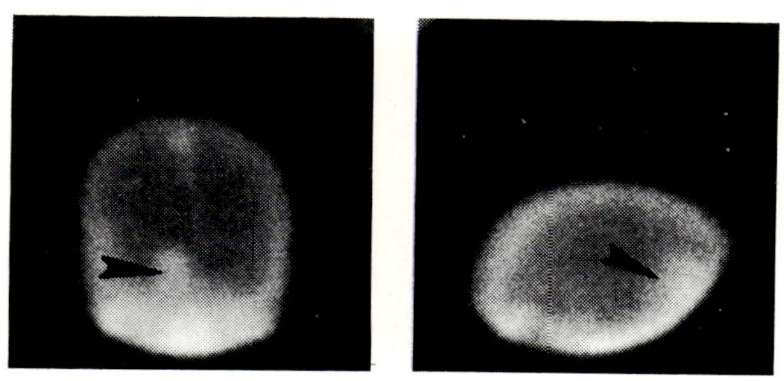

ANT R LAT

**FIG. 20.** RIGHT FRONTAL POLE GLIOBLASTOMA. This inferiorly located frontal glioblastoma (arrow) is almost at the limit of accurate brain imaging for lesions situated in a far inferior site in a cerebral hemisphere. Although the image in the right lateral position is of poor quality, its far anterior location can be seen in this position (Tc-99m sodium pertechnetate).

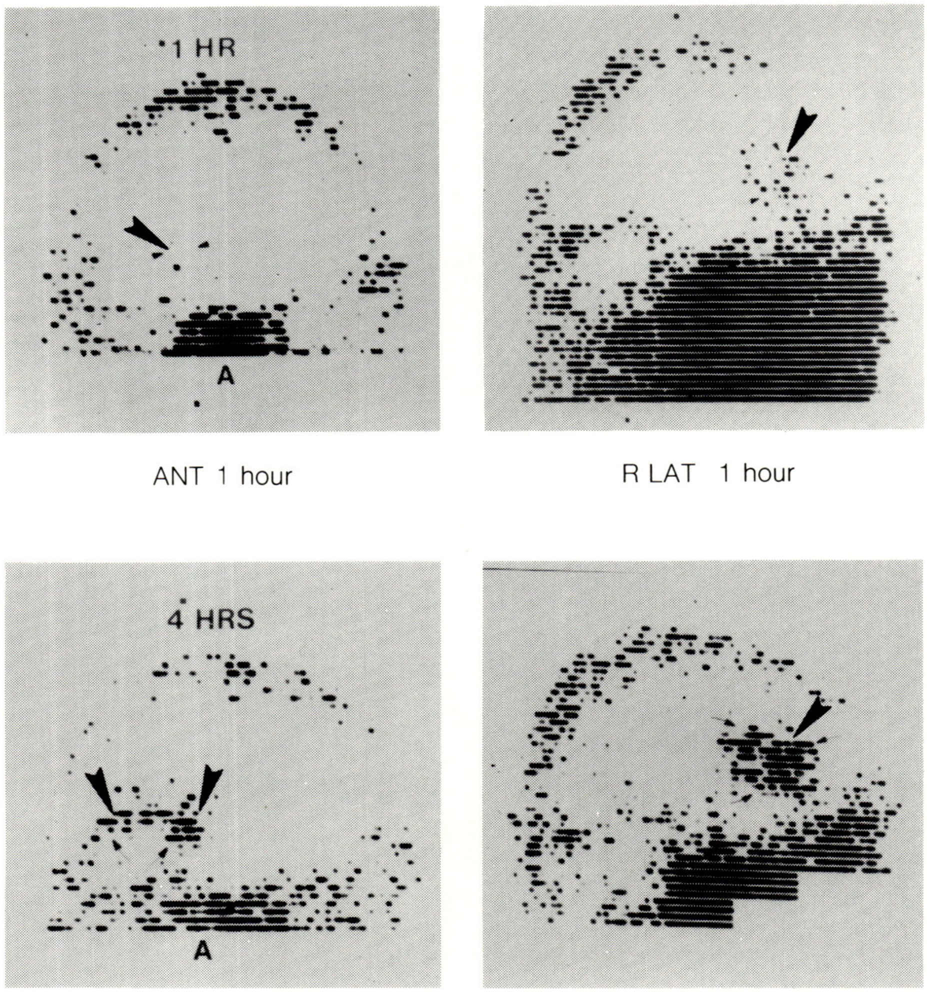


ANT 1 hour | R LAT 1 hour

ANT 3 hours | R LAT 3 hours

**FIG. 21. ASTROCYTOMA SEEN ON DELAYED IMAGING.** Initial imaging in the anterior position shows scant increase in radioactivity in the region of the tumor (arrow). The study done in the right lateral position also shows only slightly increased activity (arrow). During the ensuing period, there is continued accumulation of pertechnetate in the tumor, and at 4 hours this dumbbell-shaped astrocytoma becomes more clearly defined in the anterior and right lateral positions (Tc-99m sodium pertechnetate).

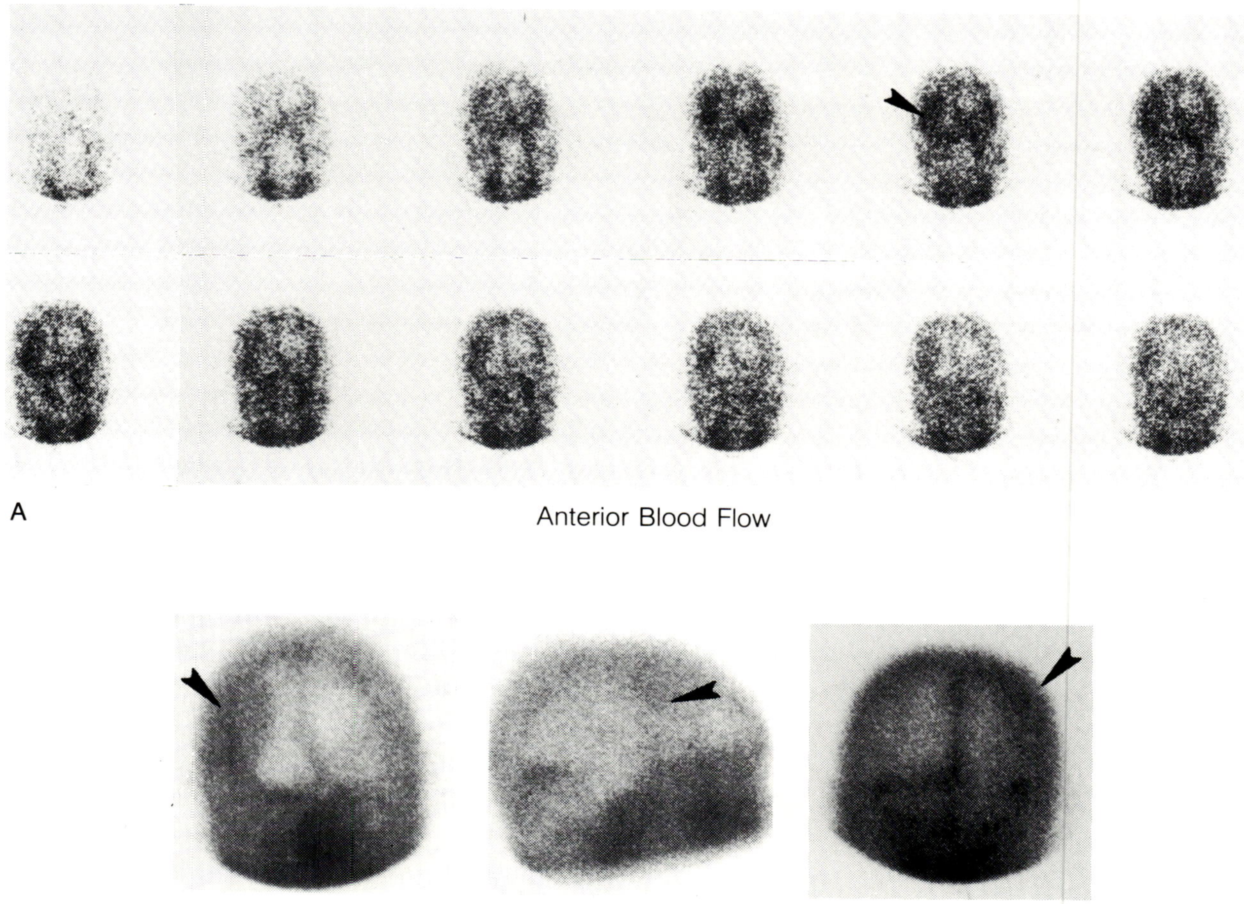

A Anterior Blood Flow

B ANT R LAT POST

**FIG. 22.** CRANIOTOMY CHANGES. Once a craniotomy has been performed, increased radioactivity is visible because of associated changes (granulation tissue, proliferation of blood vessels, bone repair). This increased activity is related to increased vascularity in the region and is clearly seen as long as the blood radioactivity is high; as the blood level falls, the changes secondary to the craniotomy became less clearly identified. Since the increased radioactivity due to craniotomy changes is a vascular phenomenon and the good visualization persists as long as the blood radioactivity is elevated, imaging at delayed times following radionuclide injection has been utilized to help distinguish craniotomy changes from recurrence of a tumor of the brain parenchyma. Presumably, as the blood level falls at the craniotomy site, increased activity will be visible at prolonged intervals if there has been tumor recurrence. This approach is occasionally successful, as seen in Fig. 22. However, in many instances the degree of tumor uptake is not sufficient to sharply distinguish it from craniotomy site uptake. In this patient with changes due to a right frontal craniotomy, the areas of increased radioactivity (arrows) are seen on both the blood flow (**A**) and static studies (**B**).

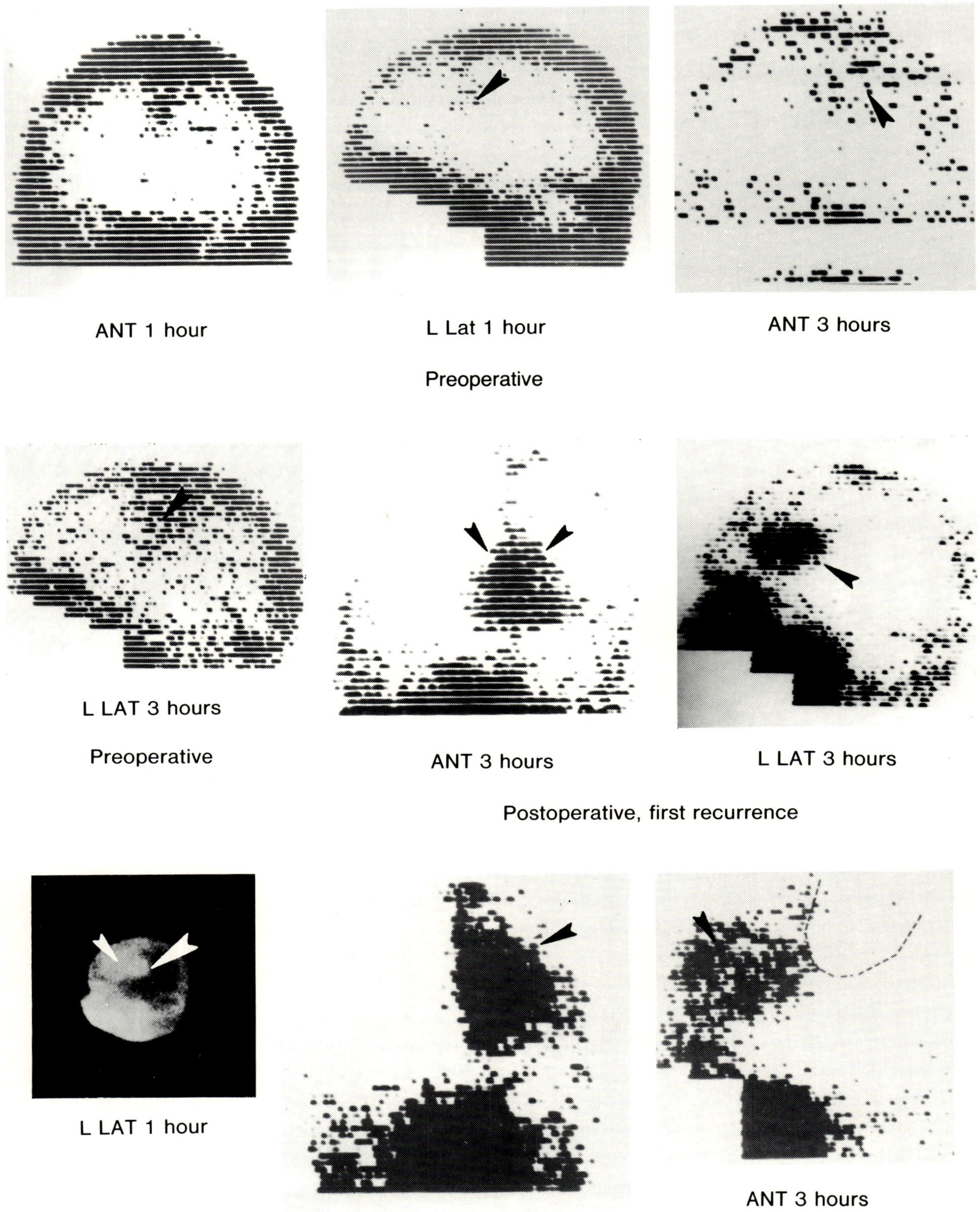


**FIG. 23.**
(See legend next page)

**FIG. 23. DISTINGUISHING CRANIOTOMY CHANGES FROM TUMOR RECURRENCE.** The preoperative study at 1 hour shows no discrete evidence of a large tumor, although the localized areas of increased radioactivity are noted. Scanning performed in the anterior and left lateral positions 3 hours after technetium injection demonstrates a fairly extensive lesion in the left frontoparietal region (arrow). Although there is far more radioactive accumulation in the tumor at this time, the lesion is not visualized with great clarity because by this time much of the radioactive material has been excreted and there has been radioactive decay. At surgery, the tumor was found to be a glioblastoma. The first postoperative scan was performed 1 year after tumor removal. At this time, the delayed study shows a somewhat rounded area of increased radioactivity, as seen in the left lateral position, just anterior to the craniotomy site through which the initial lesion had been excised. In the anterior position, there appears to be tumor extension to the midline. The recurrence was removed by utilizing the original craniotomy site. The second postoperative study was performed 2 years after surgery. Initial imaging with the scintillation camera at 1 hour shows two areas of increased radioactivity: the posterior increase ( larger arrow) is related to the craniotomy site; the larger anterior area of increased radioactivity but lower intensity indicates tumor recurrence (arrow). Delayed studies at 3 hours show the remaining radioactivity to be situated somewhat anteriorly, and at this time the craniotomy site (broken line) is no longer visible on the scan. This is because the radioactive material continues to accumulate in the tumor, but as the blood level falls, the radioactivity in the craniotomy region falls, too. Note the extension of the tumor in the anterior position. Thus, tumor recurrence and changes due to craniotomy may be distinguished through delayed scanning, the latter showing reduced activity over a number of hours and the former showing the increase so characteristic of parenchymatous lesions.

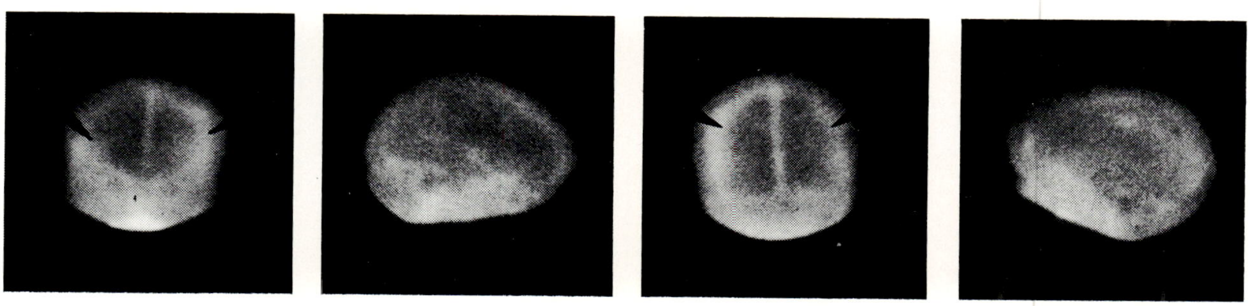

Anterior | R LAT | Posterior | L LAT

**FIG. 24. POSTOPERATIVE CHANGES.** Increased radioactivity (arrow) associated with changes secondary to prior evacuation of bilateral subdural hematoma.

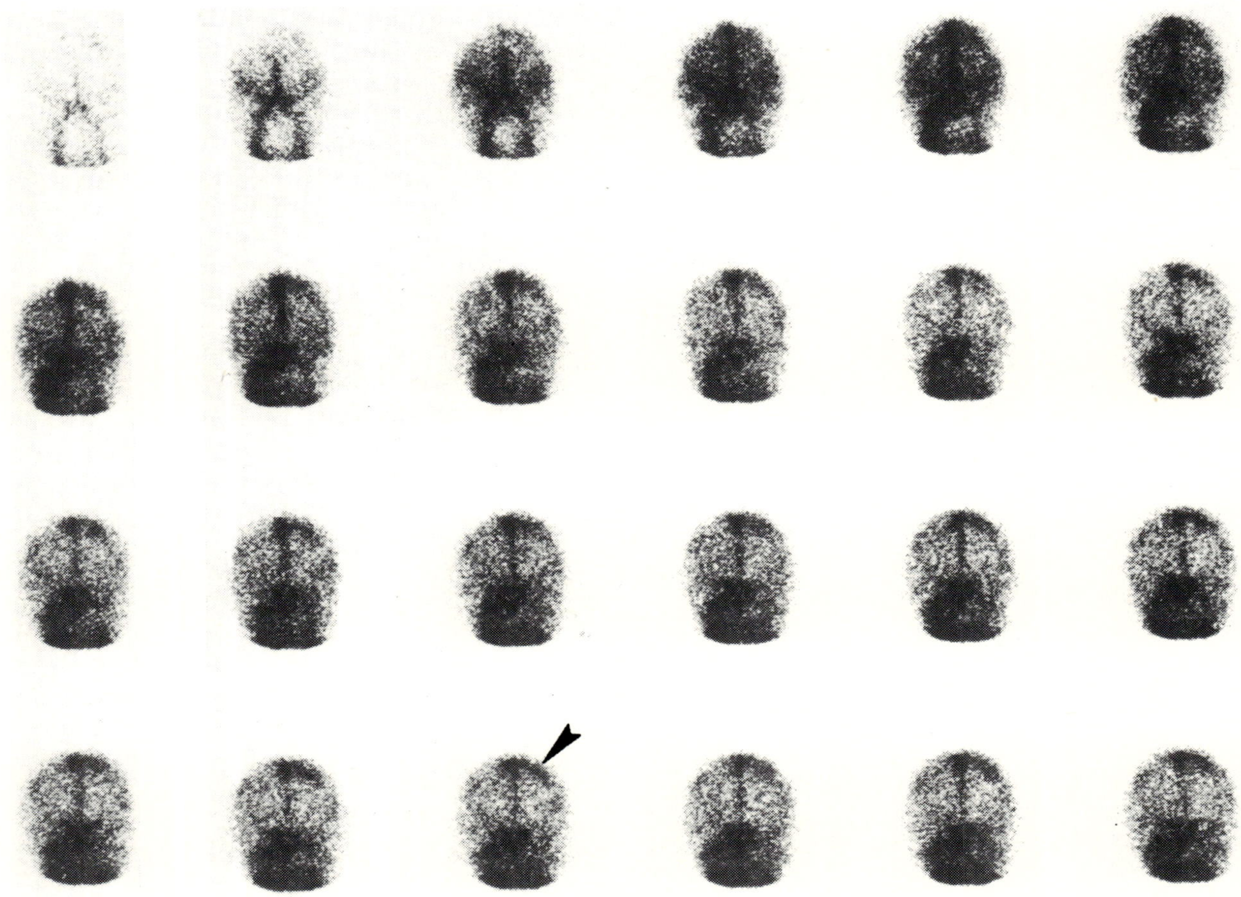

A.I

Anterior Blood Flow

**FIG. 25. A.I.** (See legend on page 241)

Brain Imaging

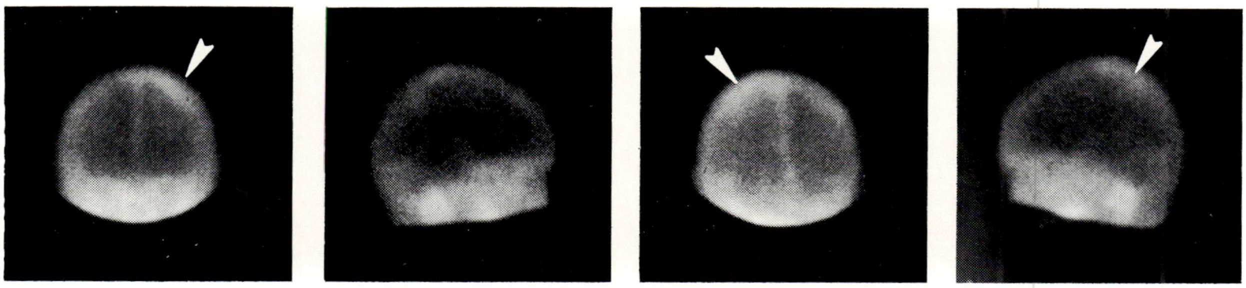

A.II ANT R LAT POST L LAT

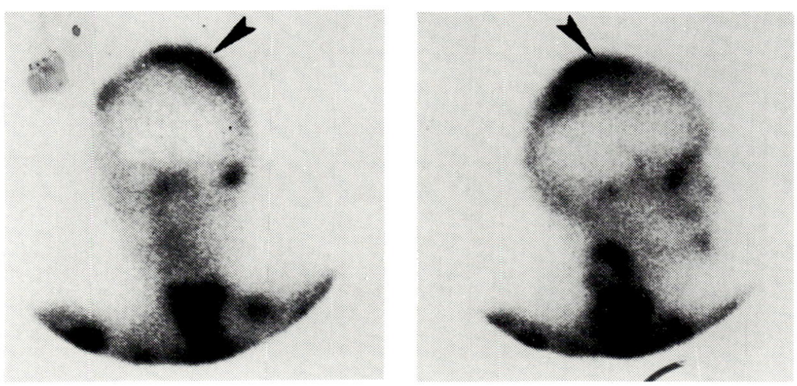

A.III ANT R LAT

Bone Imaging

**FIG. 25. A.**II, **A.**III. (See legend on page 241)

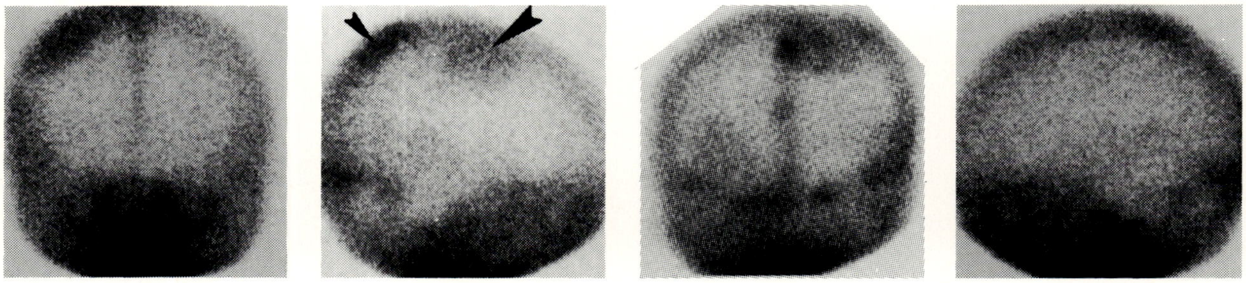

B.I ANT R LAT POST L LAT

Brain Imaging

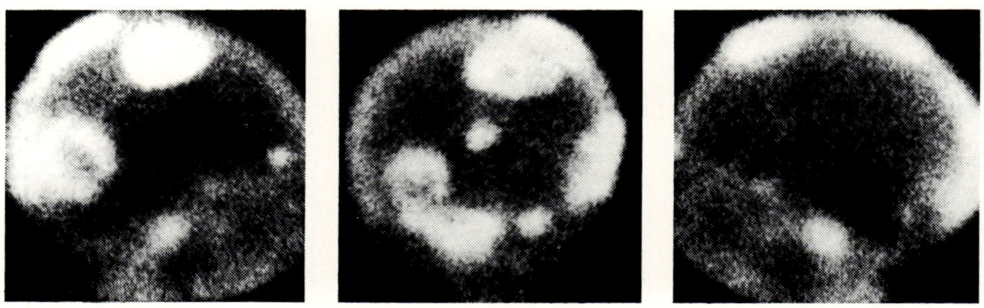

B.II R LAT POST L LAT

Bone Imaging

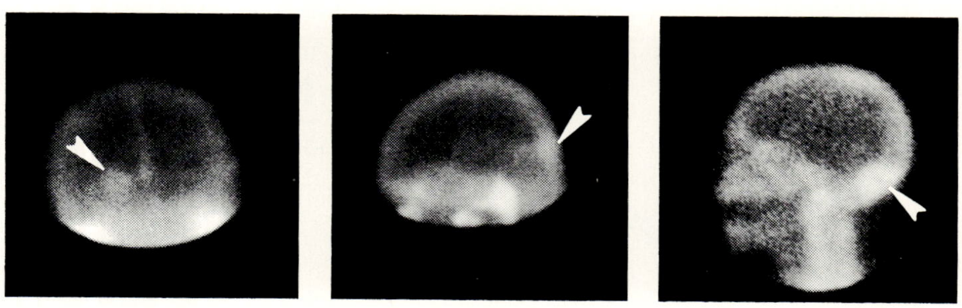

C POST L LAT L LAT

Brain Imaging Brain Imaging Bone Imaging

**FIG. 25. B.I, B.II, C.** (See legend next page)

**FIG. 25. SKULL INVOLVEMENT.** Localized areas of increased radioactivity at sites of skull metastases may sometimes be seen on brain imaging. The peripheral location of the abnormality in the calvarium is consistent with bone involvement. The increased radioactivity is often of low intensity. Confirmation should be obtained by skull x-ray or bone imaging. Occasionally, a skull metastasis may extend into the meninges, and there will be brain involvement, too. **A. Metastases from Carcinoma of Breast. I.** Blood flow study shows increased activity (arrow) at site of involvement in left parietal bone. **II.** Static brain imaging shows areas of increased activity (arrows) overlying the calvarium (Tc-99m sodium pertechnetate). **III.** Bone imaging clearly identifies the sites of skull involvement (Tc-99m diphosphonate). **B. Extension into the Meninges (Primary: Carcinoma of Breast). I.** Static brain imaging shows multiple areas of increased activity associated with skull involvement. The right posterior parietal lesion (solid arrows) is undoubtedly in the calvarium, as seen on brain imaging. The lesion in the right frontoparietal area ( large arrow) has extended from bone into the meninges (Tc-99m sodium pertechnetate). **II.** Bone imaging shows that the areas of involvement are indeed in the skull. Relatively few of the skull metastases visible on bone imaging were detected on the pertechnetate study (Tc-99m diphosphonate). **C. Patient with Oat Cell Carcinoma of Lung with Metastatic Lesion to Left Occipital Bone.** Brain imaging in the posterior position shows a localized area of increased radioactivity (arrow), which appears to overlie the left transverse sinus. However, in the left lateral position the area of increased radioactivity (arrow) is seen to be in the calvarium (Tc-99m sodium pertechnetate). Bone imaging performed with Tc-99m diphosphonate identifies the abnormality more clearly in the left occipital bone (arrow).

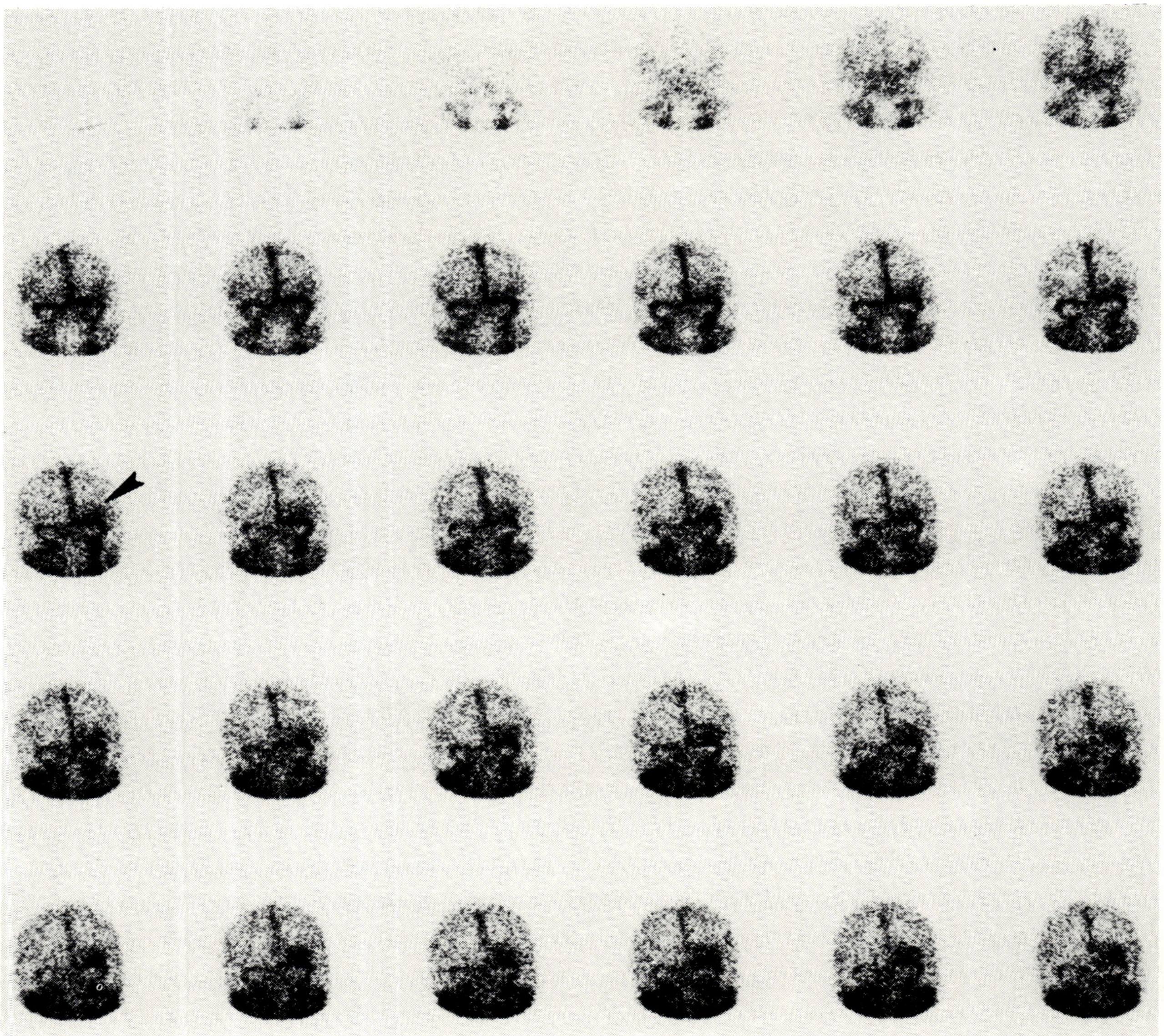

A Posterior Blood Flow

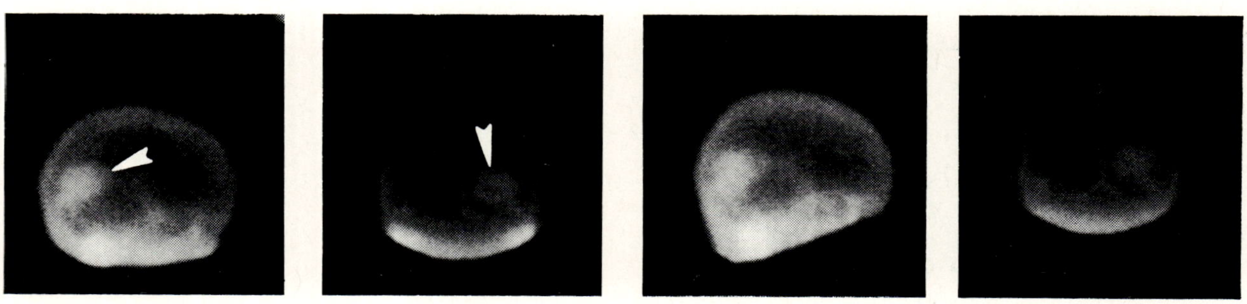

B R LAT 15 minutes POST 15 minutes R LAT 1 hour POST 1 hour

**FIG. 26. A, B.** (See legend next page)

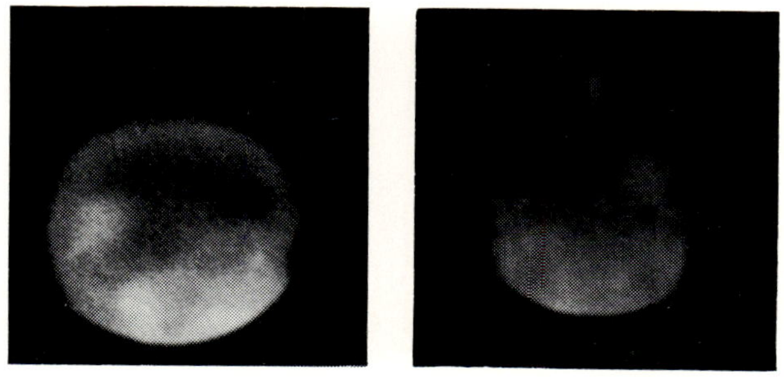

B R LAT 3½ hours POST 3½ hours

**FIG. 26.** GLIOSARCOMA. **A. Blood Flow Study.** The site of the tumor (arrow) is identified late in the venous phase on this posterior blood flow study. Note the persistence of the area of increased activity. The relation of the lesion to the transverse sinus (TS) demonstrates that it is supratentorial. **B. Static Imaging.** There is excellent radionuclide visualization of the tumor at 15 minutes following tracer injection. There is also good visualization (arrow) at 1 hour and 3.5 hours. It is interesting that this tumor, which is characterized histologically by endothelial proliferation, has imaging characteristics similar to those observed with meningiomas (see Fig. 11) (Tc-99m sodium pertechnetate).

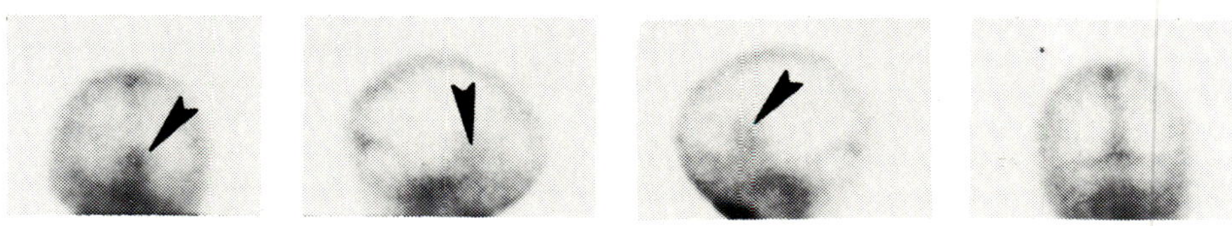

ANT 1 hour R LAT 1 hour L LAT 1 hour POST 1 hour

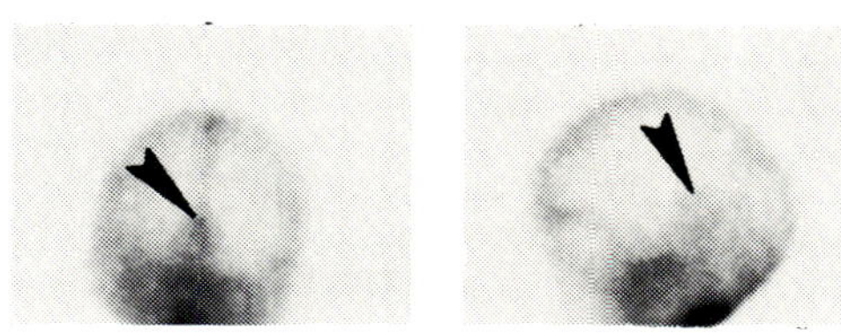

ANT 2 hours R LAT 2 hours

**FIG. 27.** CRANIOPHARYNGIOMA. A sellar or parasellar tumor is characteristically recognized on the brain scan as a localized area of increased radioactivity in the anterior position, closely related to the midline and inferiorly placed. The normal brain scan usually shows no evidence of increased radioactivity in this area. Although the lesion in this case is large, its relatively deep location is responsible in part for its less than excellent imaging. Notice how the space-occupying lesion appears to extend from the region of the sella in both lateral positions. Delayed scanning usually does not improve imaging in such patients, and in this case, imaging at 2 hours shows no improvement over that obtained on the 1-hour study.

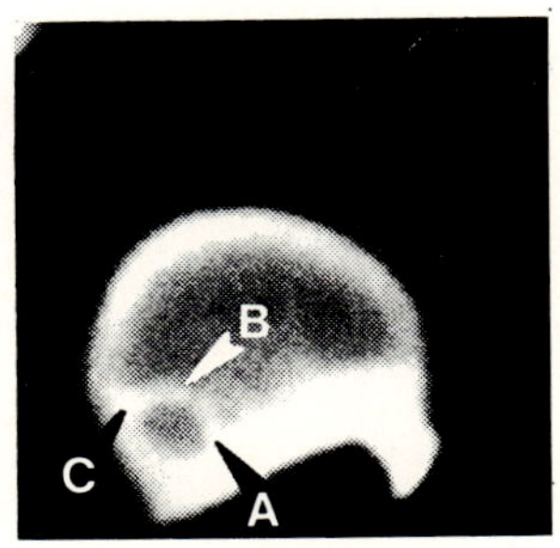


R LAT

**FIG. 28. LOCATION OF POSTERIOR FOSSA TUMORS.** A great deal of information may be gleaned from imaging in a lateral position in regard to location of a posterior fossa lesion. **A. Cerebellopontine Angle Tumors.** This area is related to the site in which the anterior portion of the transverse sinus (and sigmoid bend) may be seen on the image. This is the location in which acoustic neuromas are seen. **B. Tumors of the Cerebellum, Including the Vermis.** This region is related to the imaging projection of the mid-portion of the transverse sinus. **C. Tumors of the Cerebellum That Extend Far Posteriorly.** This area is related to the region of the torcular Herophili.

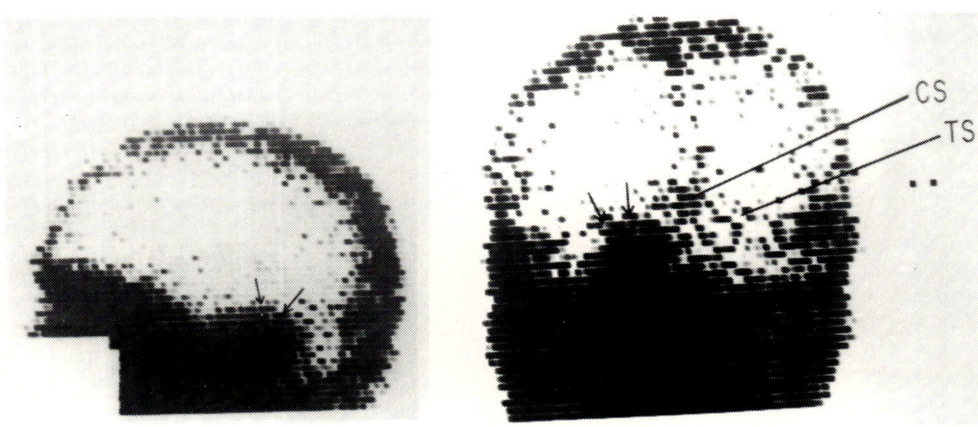


A R LAT POST

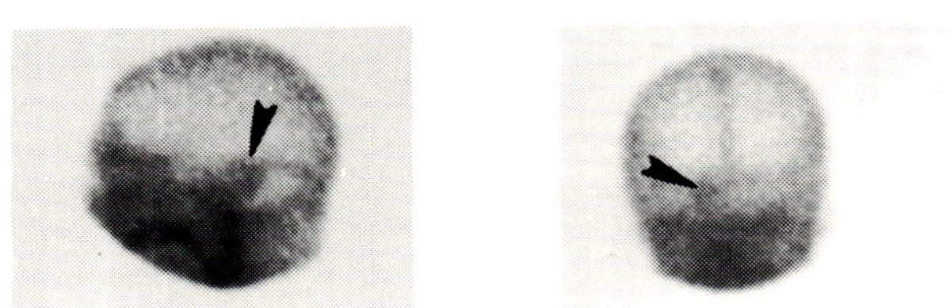

B L LAT POST

**FIG. 29. ACOUSTIC NEUROMA. A.** The area of increased radioactivity (arrow) is readily identified in the left lateral position. Its relative anterior location suggests that it is in the cerebellopontine angle region. In the posterior position, it is seen to lie in the posterior fossa region and to the left of the midline. Note the relationship to the transverse sinus (TS) and the confluence of the sinuses (CS). The optimum time for imaging acoustic neuromas is between 2 and 2.5 hours following pertechnetate injection. The visualized findings are characteristic for this tumor (Tc-99m sodium pertechnetate). **B.** Another patient with a left-sided acoustic neuroma as seen on camera imaging (Tc-99m sodium pertechnetate).

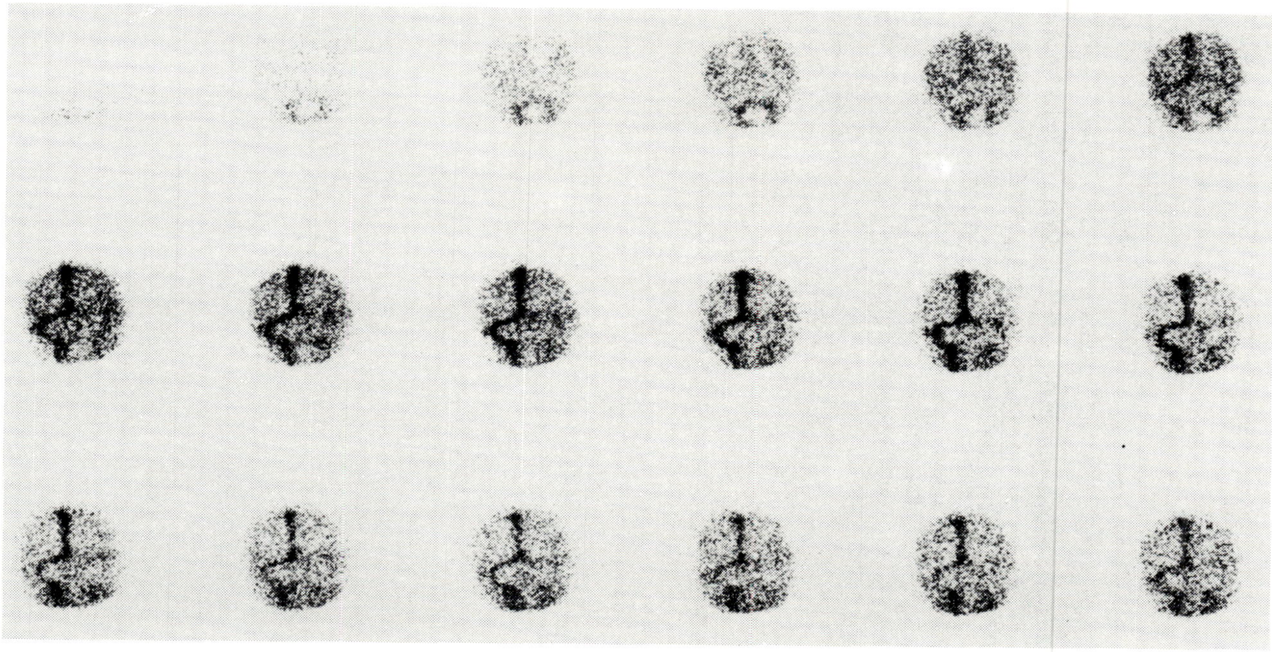

A Posterior Blood Flow

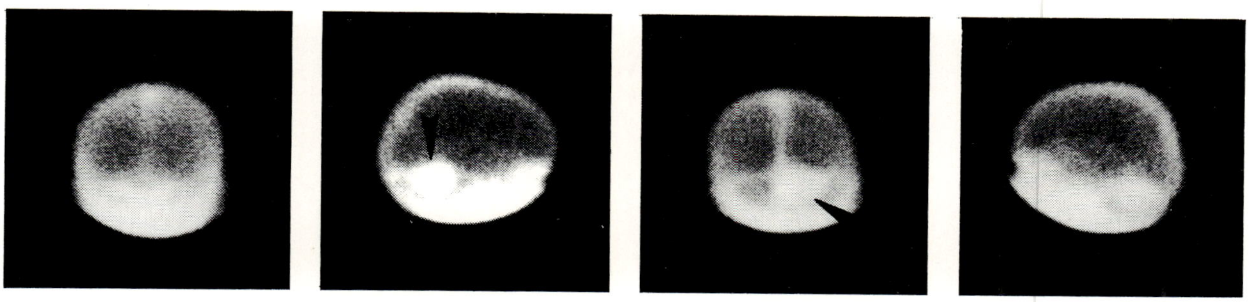

B ANT R LAT POST L LAT

**FIG. 30. ASTROCYTOMA INVOLVING LEFT CEREBELLAR HEMISPHERE AND VERMIS. A. Blood Flow Study.** The blood flow study performed in the posterior position fails to show increased radioactivity at the site of involvement subsequently identified on static imaging in this 3-year-old child. Note the failure of the right transverse sinus to be imaged on this portion of the study. **B. Static Imaging.** As seen in the right lateral position, the rounded area of increased radioactivity (arrow) appears to be related to the mid-portion of the right transverse sinus. This helps define its location in the right cerebellar hemisphere, possibly including the vermis. In the posterior position, the tumor is identified in the right posterior fossa area, and its extension to the midline confirms the suspicion of involvement of the vermis.

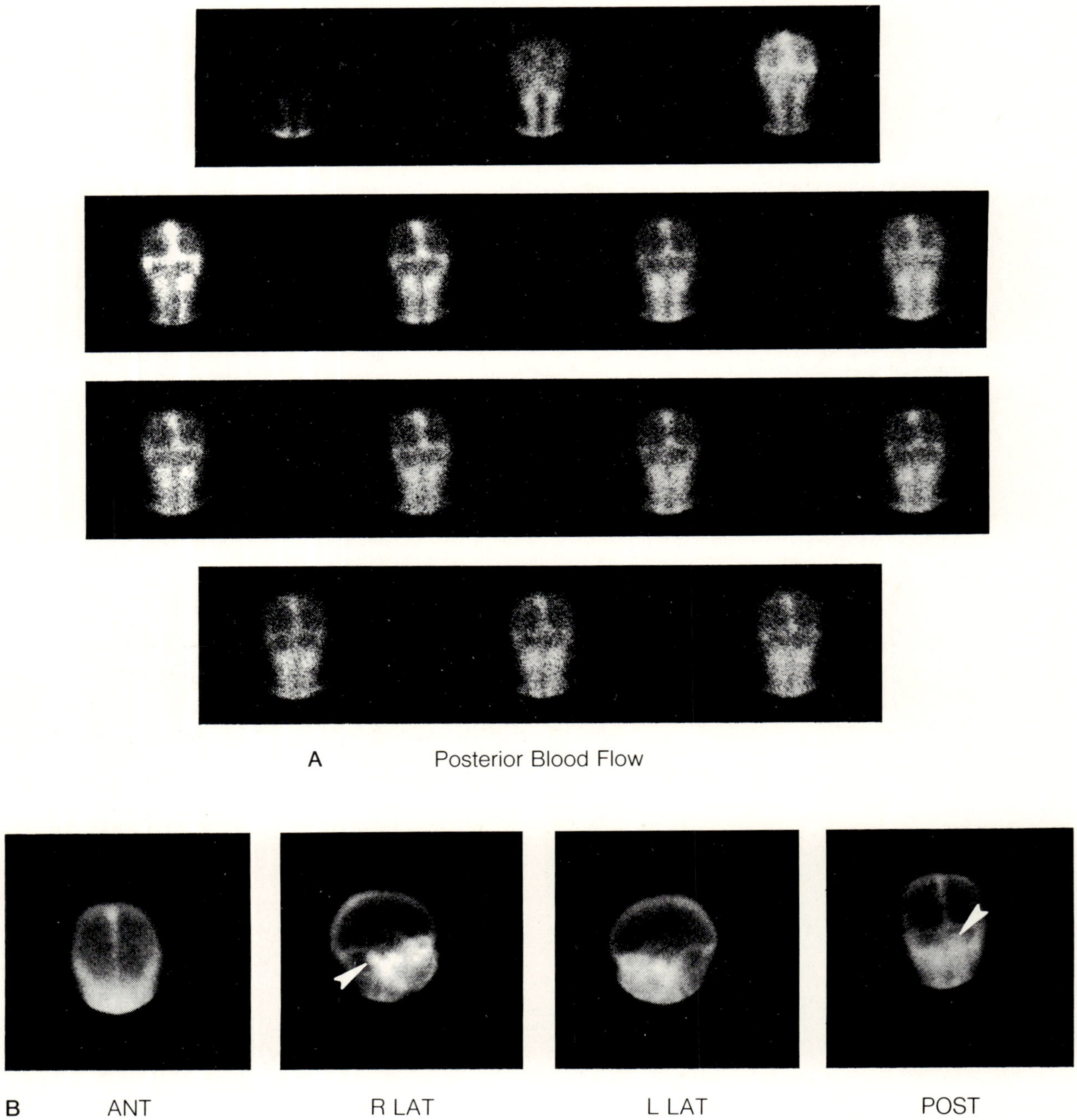


**FIG. 31. ASTROCYTOMA OF CEREBELLUM NOT VISIBLE ON BLOOD FLOW STUDY. A. Blood Flow Study**. The blood flow study performed in the posterior position fails to identify the site of the tumor. **B. Static Imaging.** Although the right lateral image shows the tumor (arrow) to have a relatively anterior location, it was found to be situated in the right cerebellar hemisphere. It is clearly visible in the right posterior fossa in the posterior position (Tc-99m sodium pertechnetate).

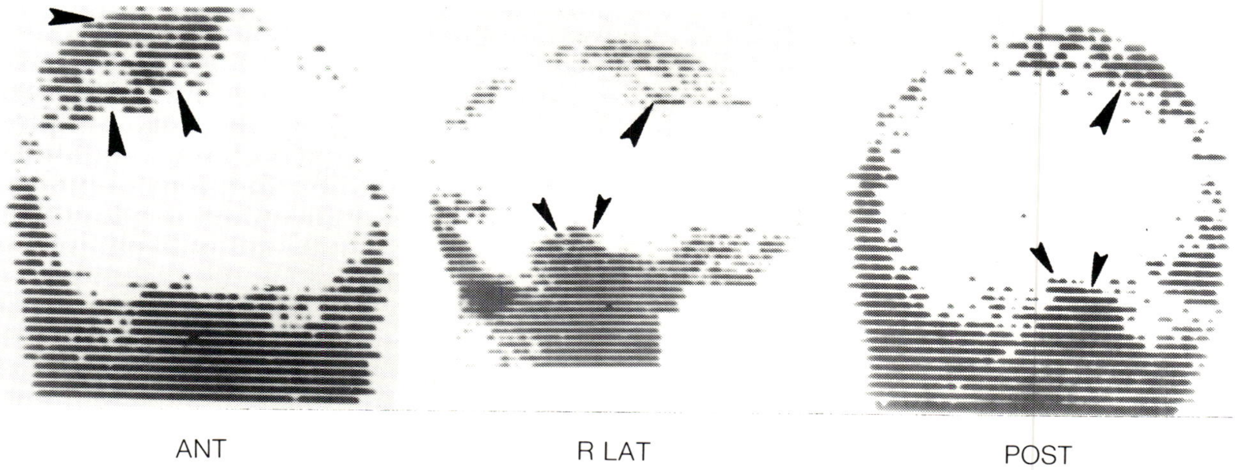


**FIG. 32.** **MULTIPLE INTRACRANIAL TUMORS IN VON RECKLING-HAUSEN'S DISEASE.** This patient with an acoustic neuroma (arrows) later developed a right frontal meningioma ( larger arrows). The site of the acoustic neuroma is defined from its anterior location in the right lateral position (in the area of the cerebellopontine angle [CPA]) and its somewhat eccentric location in the posterior fossa, as seen in the posterior position.

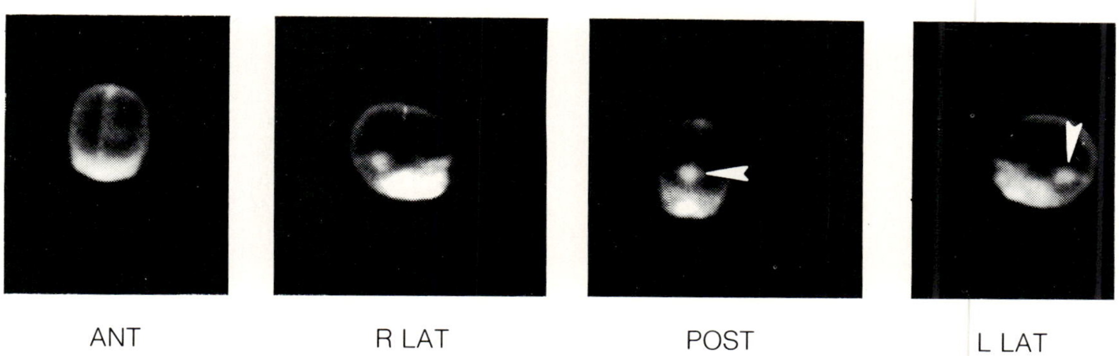


**FIG. 33.** **CEREBELLAR ASTROCYTOMA INVOLVING BOTH HEMI-SPHERES AND VERMIS.** From the location of the tumor (arrow) in the left lateral position, its mid-position location as related to the transverse sinus image is noted. Its extension to the midline is depicted in the posterior position (Tc-99m sodium pertechnetate).

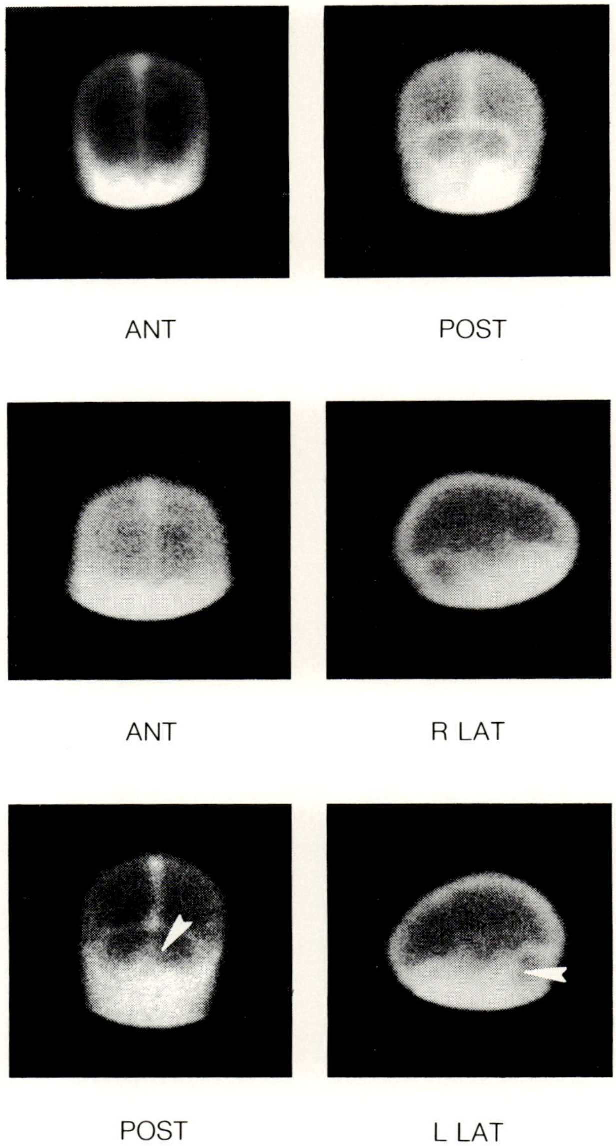


**FIG. 34.** (See legend next page)

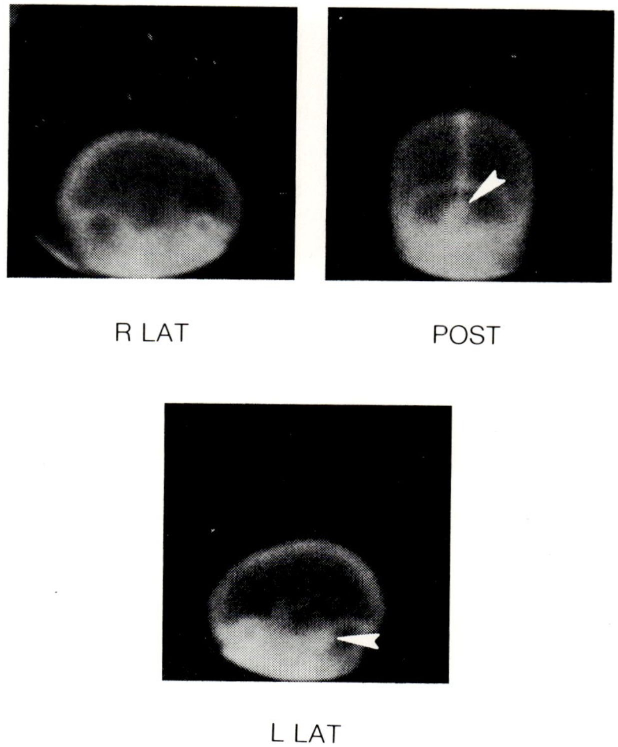


**FIG. 34. EPENDYMOMA OF FOURTH VENTRICLE.** The demonstration of the tumor in this 3-year-old boy seems clearest on delayed imaging. Initial anterior and posterior imaging, following the completion of the blood flow study, showed no evidence of the lesion. Tumor identification (arrow) seems best at 4 hours. Its visualization in the left lateral position is similar to the location seen with tumors of the cerebellopontine angle, such as acoustic neuromas. However, in the posterior position, it is demonstrated to be practically midline (Tc-99m DTPA).

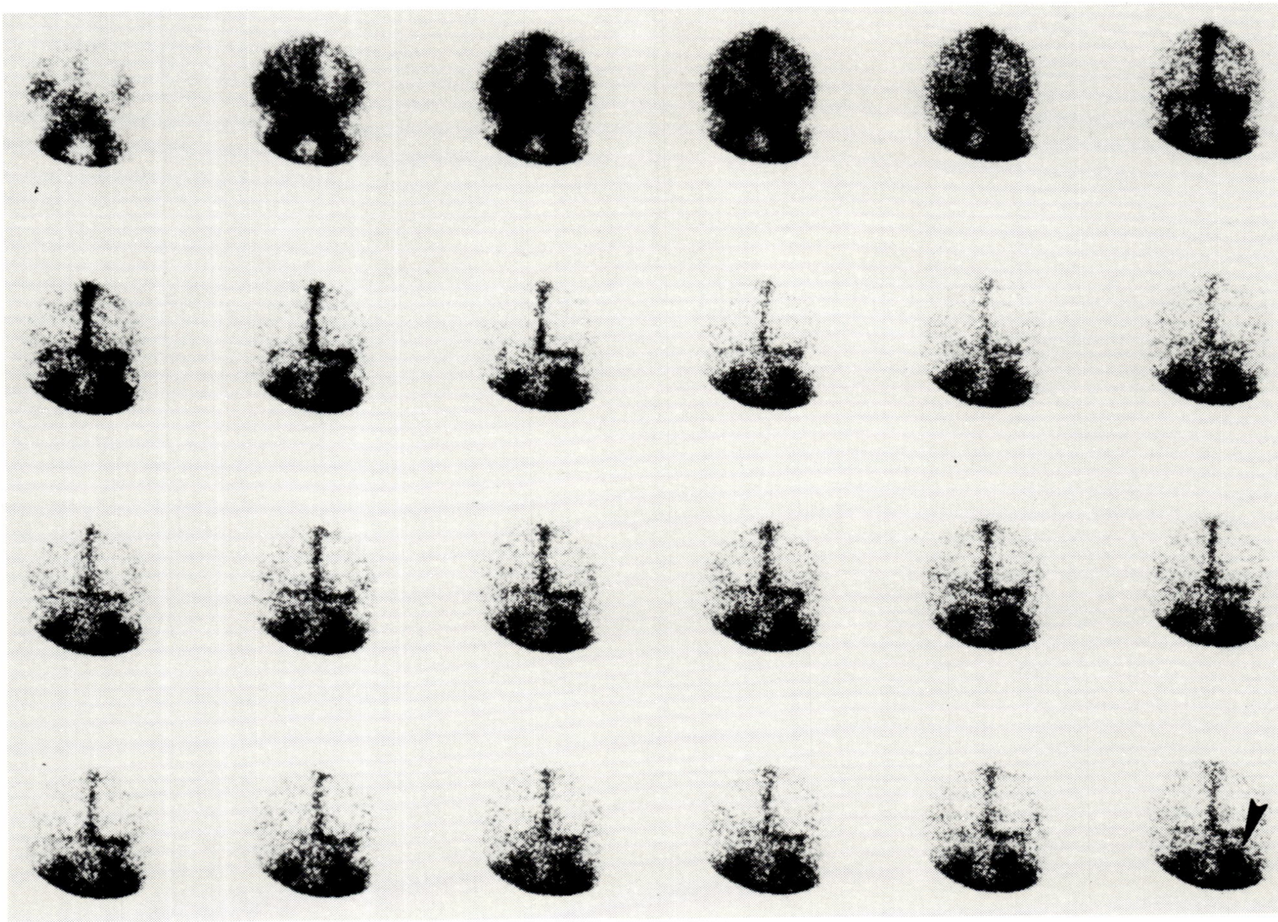

A Posterior Blood Flow

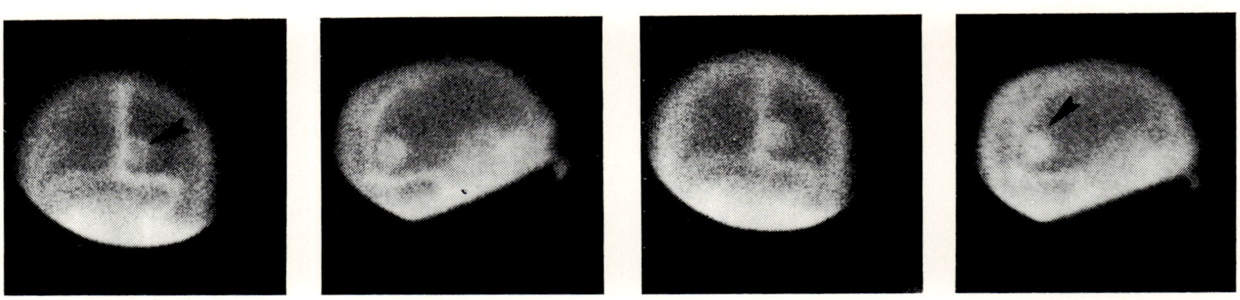

B POST Immediate    R LAT Immediate    POST 15 minutes    R LAT 15 minutes

**FIG. 35. A, B.** (See legend next page)

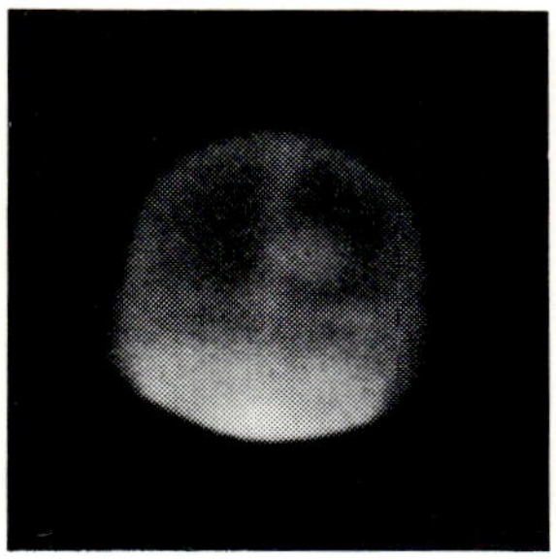

POST 60 minutes

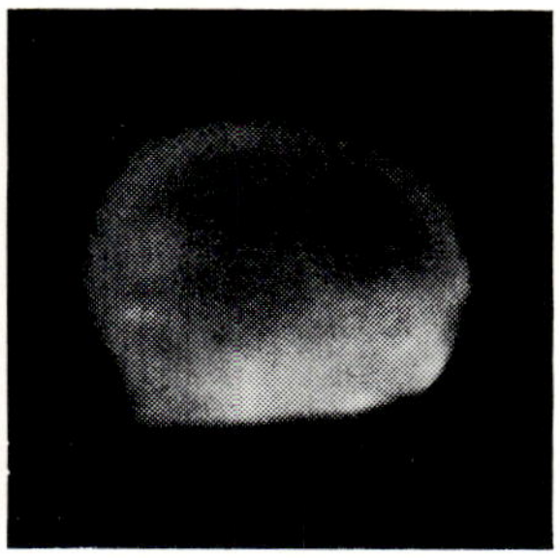

R LAT 60 minutes

**FIG. 35.** SOLITARY METASTASIS TO RIGHT OCCIPITAL LOBE. A. **Blood Flow Study.** The blood flow study in the posterior position shows no evidence of a vascular lesion during the arterial phase or early venous phase. Very late in the blood flow study an area of increased radioactivity is seen (arrow). This is probably due to retention of a small amount of radioactive material that has accumulated with recirculation. **B. Static Imaging.** The static studies performed immediately following the blood flow study, at 15 minutes, and at one hour help distinguish the lesion from a meningioma. Although the rounded area of increased activity that abuts on the midline is clearly demonstrated in the immediate posterior image, the uptake and imaging intensity increase at 15 minutes and increase still further at one hour. The continued increased uptake suggests that this is a tumor of the brain parenchyma rather than a meningioma, but whether it is a primary or metastatic tumor cannot be determined from this study. This turned out to be a metastasis from a bronchogenic carcinoma (Tc-99m sodium pertechnetate).

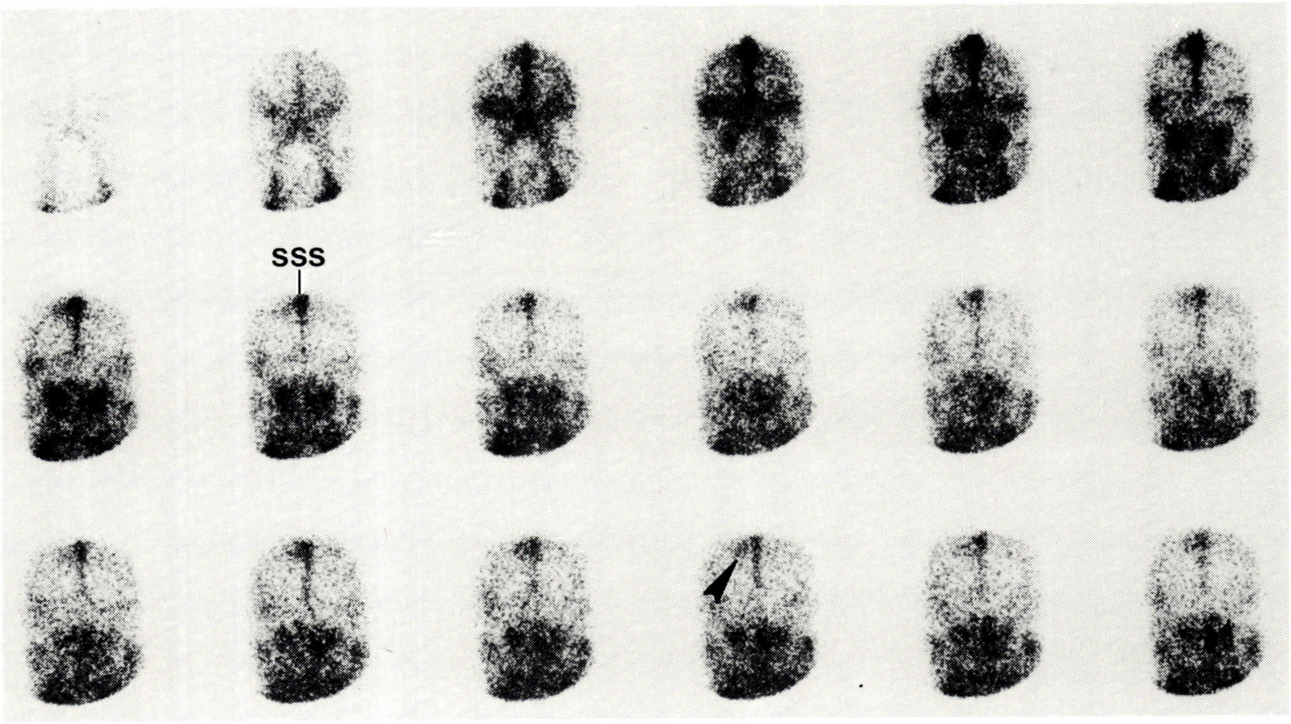


A.1. Anterior Blood Flow

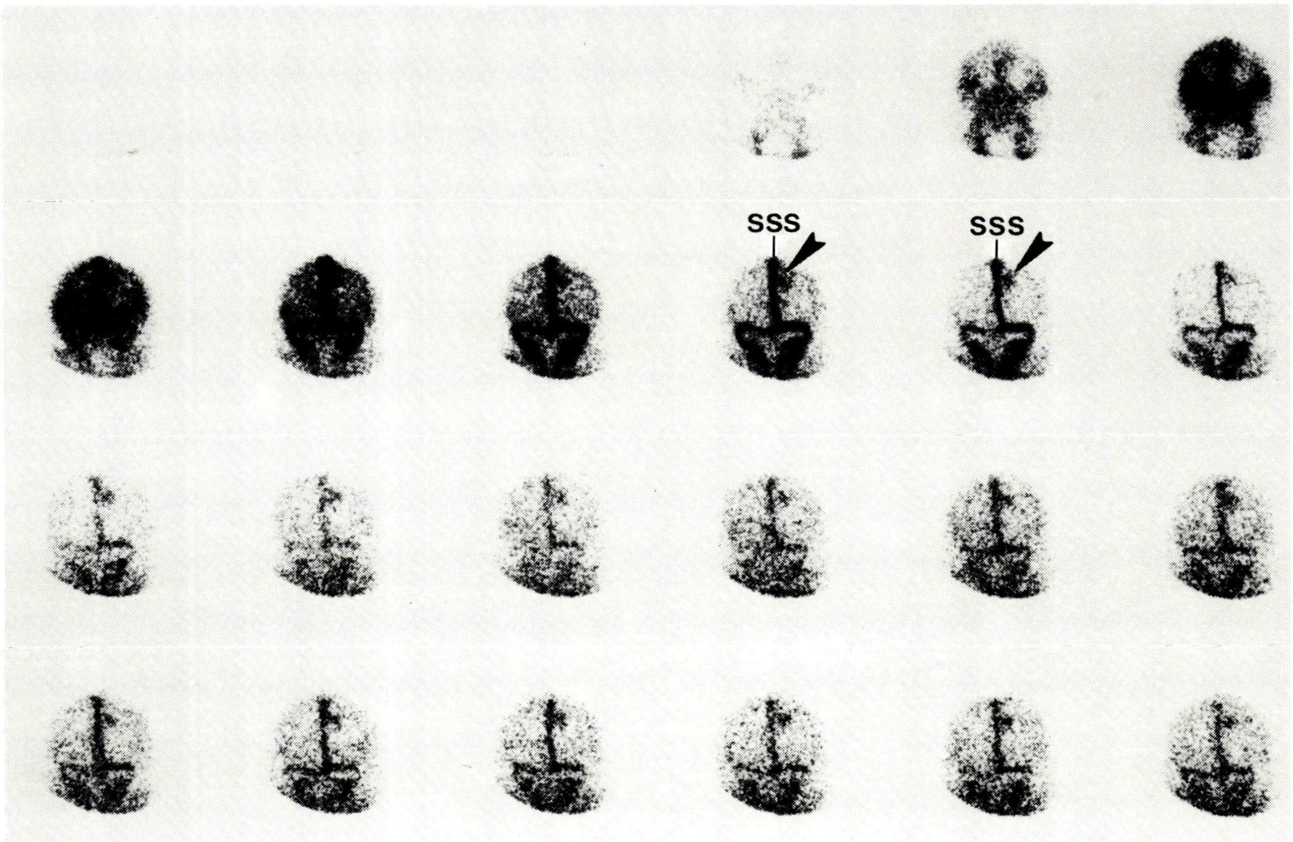


A.2. Posterior Blood Flow

**FIG. 36. A.1, A.2** (See legend next page)

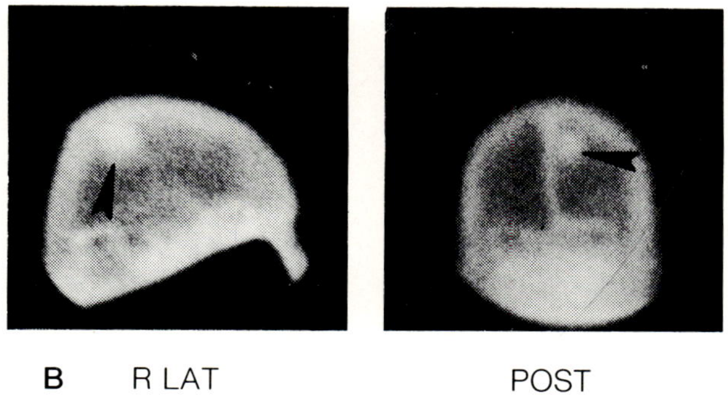


**FIG. 36.** SOLITARY METASTASIS SEEN ON BLOOD FLOW AND STATIC IMAGING. A. **Blood Flow Studies.** 1. Anterior blood flow study identifies the site of the tumor (arrow) during the venous phase only after the superior sagittal sinus (SSS) has become visible. The appearance of the latter signifies the initial portion of the venous phase. 2. Posterior blood flow study again demonstrates the metastasis (arrow), and in this position, its distinction from the superior sagittal sinus (SSS) is more clearly defined. **B. Static Imaging.** Posterior parietal metastasis from a primary in the lung is easily identified one hour after radionuclide administration (Tc-99m-DTPA).

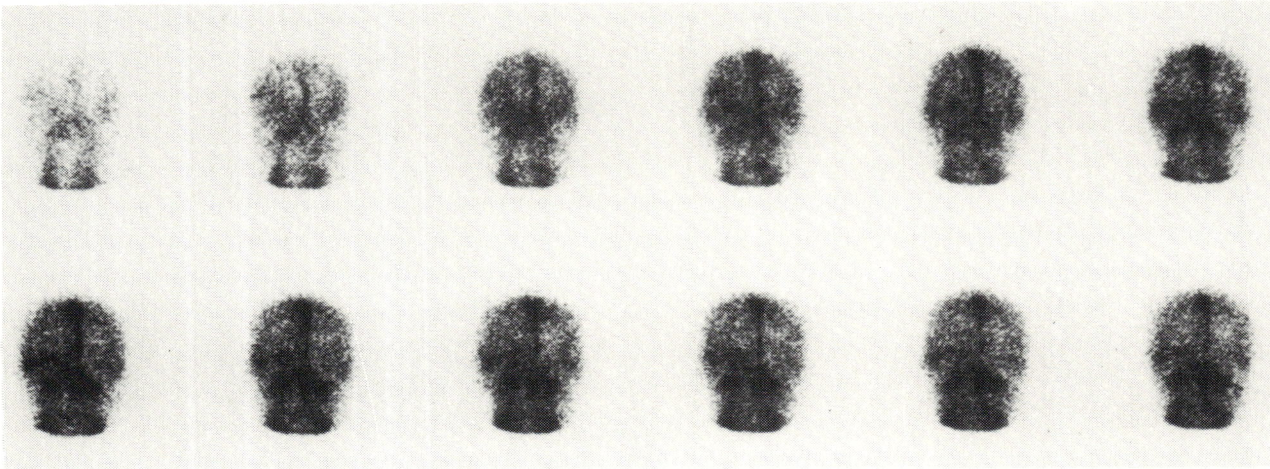

A.1.

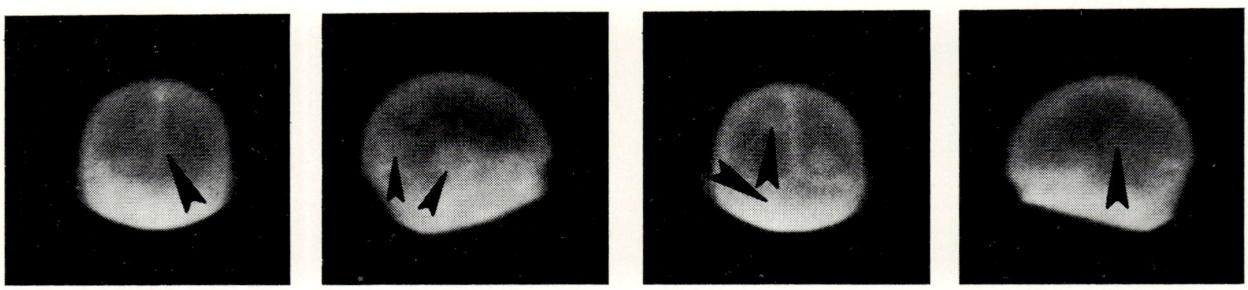

A.2 ANT R LAT POST L LAT

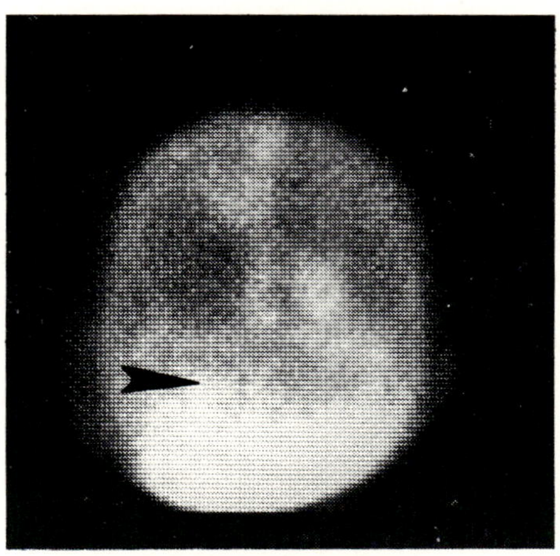

A.3. POST Computerized Enhancement

**FIG. 37. A.1, A.2, A.3** (See legend next page)

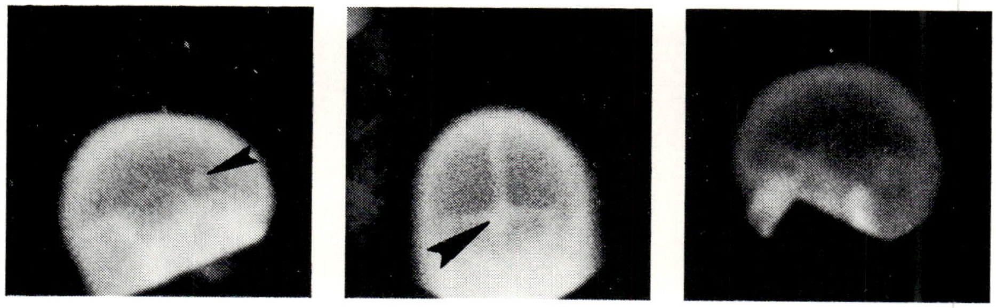

B R LAT POST L LAT

**FIG. 37. MULTIPLE METASTASES.** In those cases in which there are multiple metastases in the brain, failure to identify *all* the metastatic foci is not uncommon. Small size and the amount of increased radioactivity contributed by adjacent lesions are factors limiting the possibility of demonstrating all such lesions. **A.** Cerebral and cerebellar involvement in a patient with carcinoma of the lung. **1.** Blood flow study fails to clearly identify any of the metastases subsequently seen on static imaging. **2.** Static imaging identifies sites of involvement in the right temporal and occipital areas (small arrows) in the right lateral position, while in the posterior position the images of these lesions are superimposed and only a single area of increased radioactivity related to them is visible. A left parietooccipital metastasis situated close to the midline is demonstrated most clearly in the posterior position ( large arrows) but is also visible in the left lateral and anterior positions. A single cerebellar metastasis ( large arrows)is well seen in the posterior position only. **3.** However, computerized enhancement assists in its identification. **B.** Metastatic involvement in the right frontal lobe (small arrow) and left cerebellar hemisphere and vermis ( large arrow) in a patient with cancer of the endometrium (Tc-99m sodium pertechnetate).

## VASCULAR-TYPE LESIONS

Vascular-type lesions are associated with structural changes in the areas of involvement in the brain and alterations in the blood-brain barrier. Because of these alterations, radioactive materials may gain entry to those regions that are involved with these structural changes, and the vascular-type lesions can be detected on static imaging.

Thus, a subdural hematoma can be visualized on static imaging after a subdural membrane has formed. This usually occurs 7 to 10 days after the shearing of cortical veins as they traverse the subdural space, usually as a result of trauma, which caused the initial subdural hemorrhage. After formation of the membrane, early static imaging will show increased activity in the vascular subdural membrane while delayed imaging will show even greater radioactivity as the radionuclide gains entry to the confines within the membrane as well. Thus, the optimum time for the imaging of a subdural hematoma on static studies is about 2 hours following tracer injection.

Static imaging of cerebral infarctions is associated with the visualization of radioactivity both in the periphery of the infarction and also in the area within the zone of infarction in which there is ischemia or necrosis. Immediately following arterial occlusion, static imaging will usually show no area of increased radioactivity because no structural alteration has yet occurred to allow radionuclide entry. After 7 to 10 days, the ischemic area distal to the occluded artery will have become well demarcated and be surrounded by a proliferative zone (capillaries, fibroblasts, fibrous tissue). At this time, static imaging will show increased activity as the radioactive material accumulates in the infarcted zone. Such imaging is most clearly visible about 3 weeks after the onset of the arterial occlusion. Resolution (as the ischemic zone shrinks) is usually demonstrated by 3 months after onset.

Blood flow studies *may* detect these vascular-type lesions long before they can be seen on static imaging. Thus, blood flow studies in a subdural hematoma may demonstrate a crescentic displacement of a middle cerebral artery due to compression by the hematoma, in a manner similar to that seen with contrast angiography. In the case of a cerebral infarction, the blood flow study may identify absent flow in the involved cerebral or carotid vessel. Care must be exercised so that the subtle changes that might be detected in these blood flow studies are not overemphasized and misinterpreted.

Anterior Blood Flow

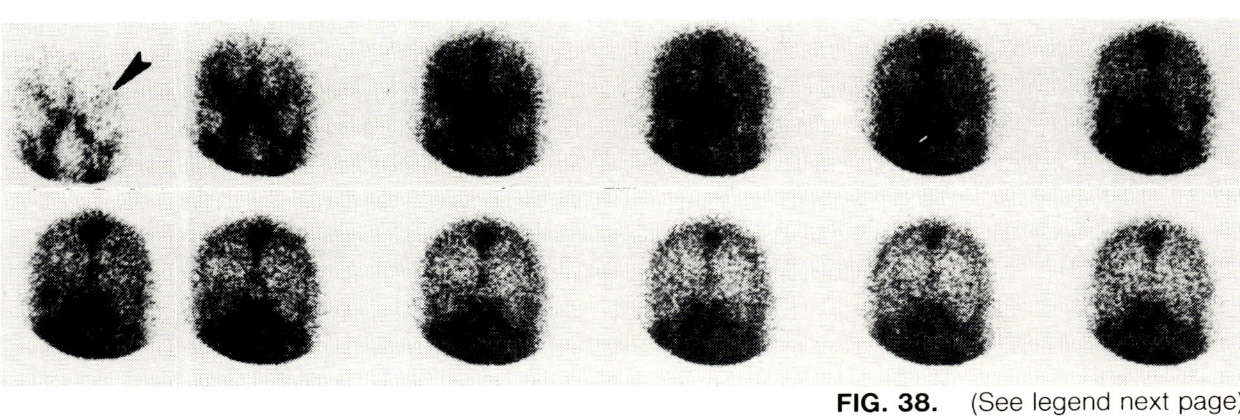

**FIG. 38.** (See legend next page)

**FIG. 38. LEFT MIDDLE CEREBRAL ARTERY OCCLUSION VISIBLE ON ANTERIOR BLOOD FLOW STUDY.** Occlusion of the left middle cerebral artery (arrow) is visible with the accompanying absence of radioactivity. Compare to contralateral side. There is perfusion from collaterals, late in the arterial phase, and delayed blood flow is indicated in the distribution of the left middle cerebral artery (Tc-99m sodium pertechnetate).

A Posterior Blood Flow

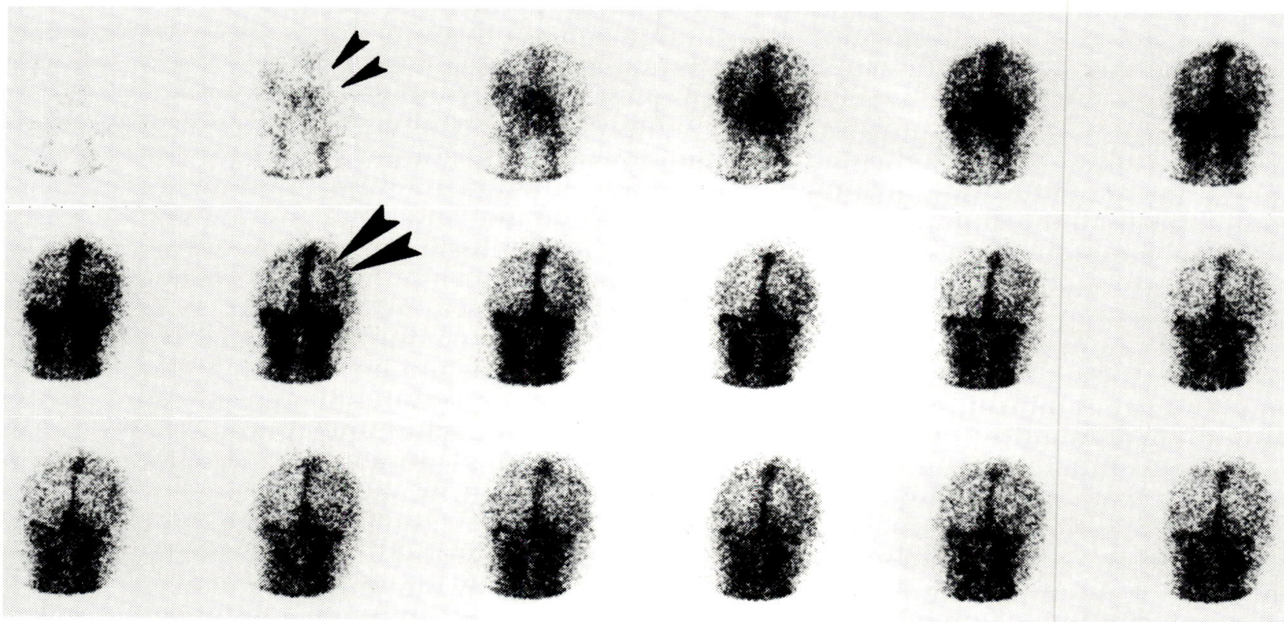

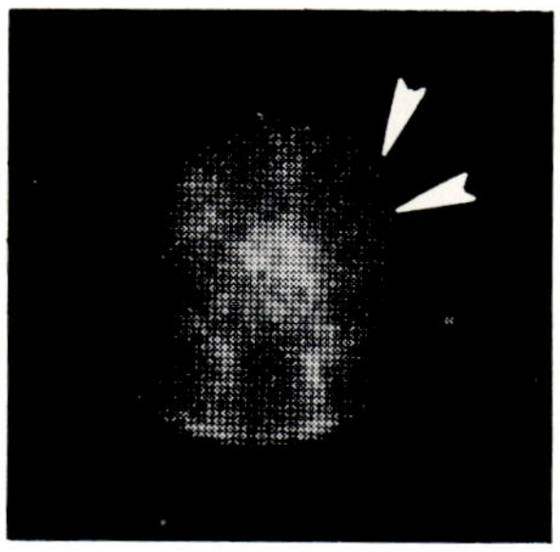

B Composite Posterior Blood Flow

**FIG. 39. RIGHT MIDDLE CEREBRAL ARTERY OCCLUSION SEEN ON POSTERIOR BLOOD FLOW STUDY. A.** Absent radioactivity (small arrows) early in the arterial phase is seen in the area of distribution of the left middle cerebral artery. "Luxury perfusion" is visible on the affected side (larger arrows) due to late filling from collateral arteries. **B.** Composite arterial blood flow image was obtained by the total blood flow imaging during the arterial phase. This defines even more clearly the absent arterial perfusion in the distribution of the left middle cerebral artery (Tc-99m sodium pertechnetate).

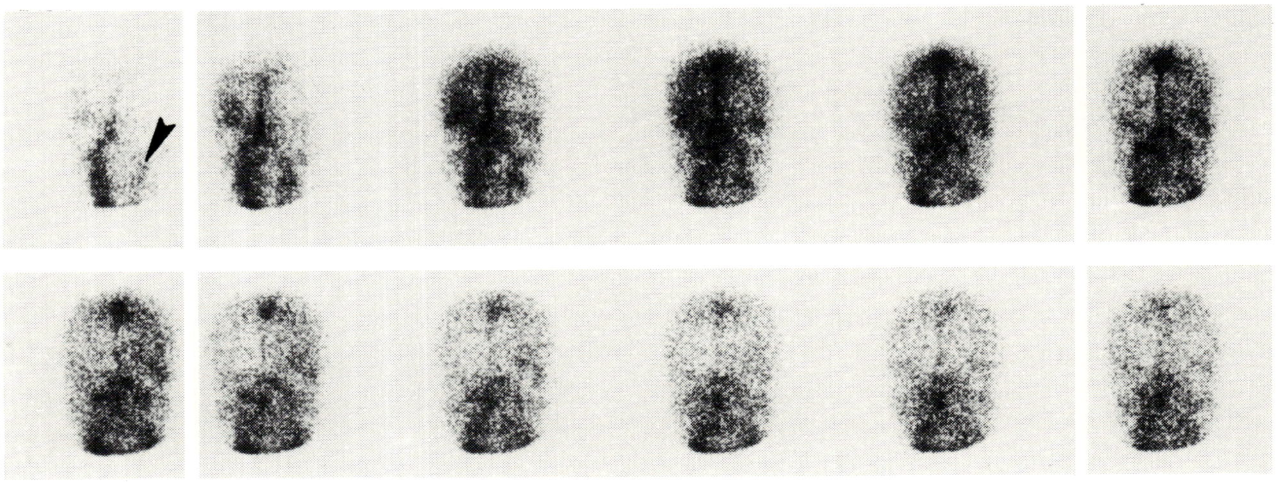

Anterior Blood Flow

**FIG. 40. LIGATION OF LEFT COMMON CAROTID ARTERY.** The site of ligation is indicated by the arrow. Only meager collateral filling in the distribution of both the left anterior and middle cerebral arteries can be seen. Note the prominence of the right common carotid artery (Tc-99m sodium pertechnetate).

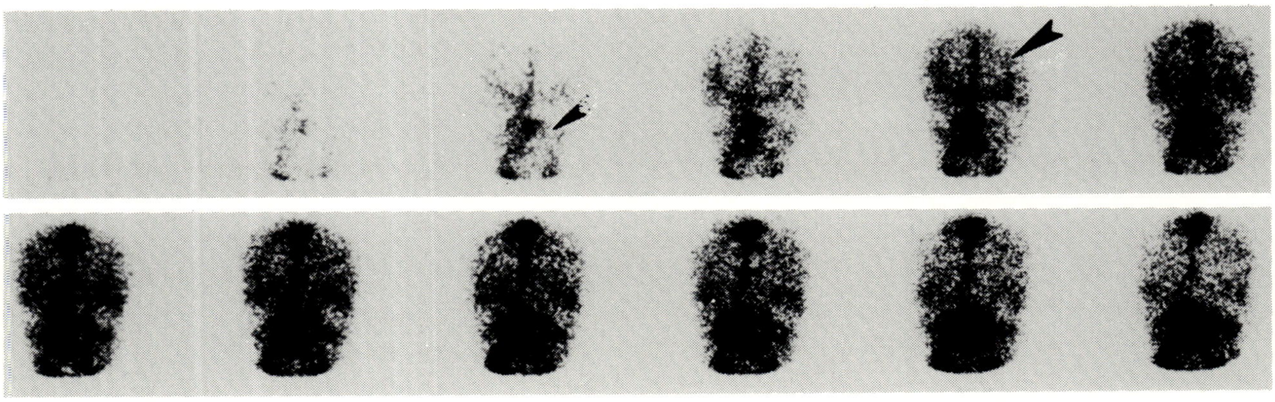

Anterior Blood Flow

**FIG. 41. LEFT INTERNAL CAROTID ARTERY OCCLUSION.** The left internal carotid artery is occluded at its origin (arrow). As may also be seen with contrast angiography, there is collateral filling of the anterior communicating artery, and blood flow in the left middle cerebral artery ( large arrow ), although reduced and delayed compared to the contralateral side, is maintained (Tc-99m DTPA).

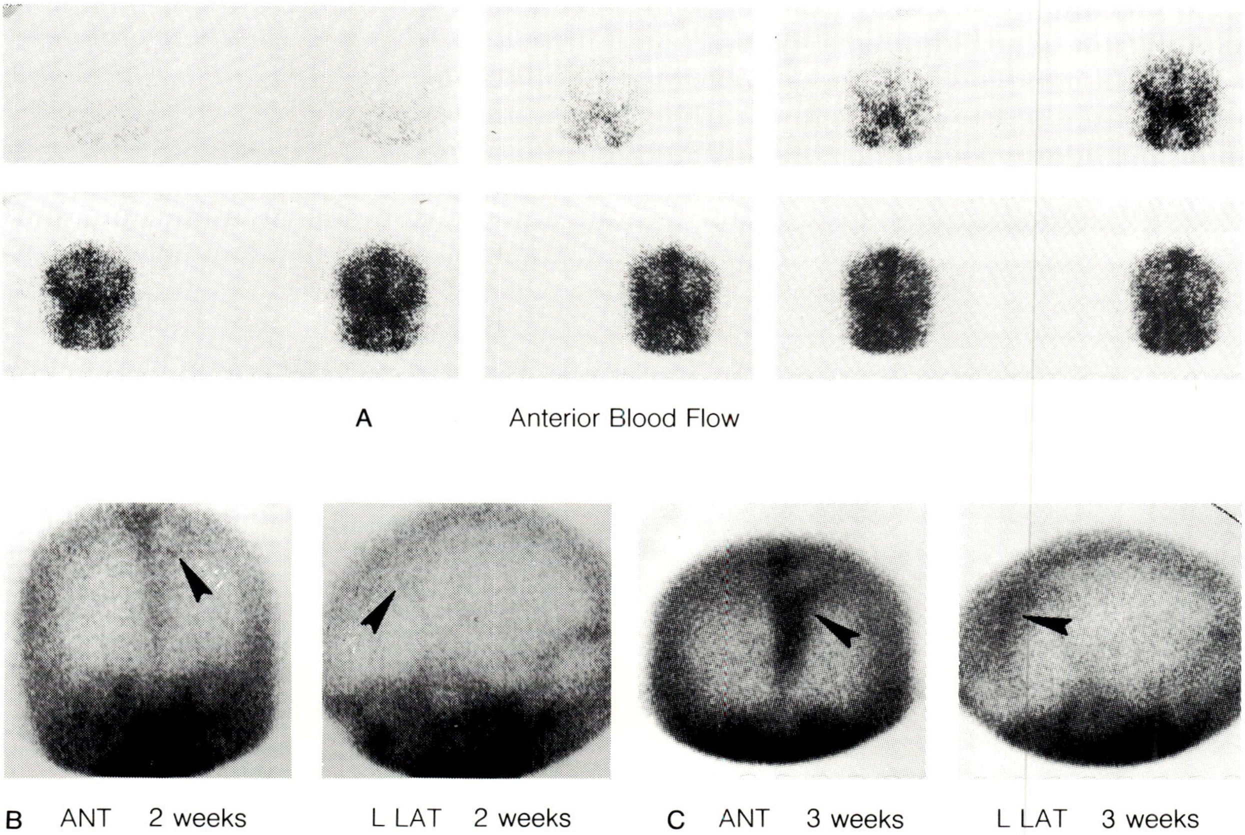


**FIG. 42. INFARCTION IN DISTRIBUTION OF LEFT ANTERIOR CEREBRAL ARTERY AND ITS EVOLUTION. A. Blood Flow Study.** The occlusion of the left anterior cerebral artery, or one of its branches, cannot be identified on the dynamic study in this patient. Demonstration of such an arterial occlusion is difficult with radionuclide methods, especially when the occlusion is unilateral. **B. Static Imaging.** Static imaging 2 weeks after the onset of symptoms shows slightly increased radioactivity (arrows) in the anterior and left lateral positions in the region of the infarction. However, the intensity is far, far less than that visible on imaging 1 week later (or 3 weeks after the onset of symptoms). **C.** Static imaging at 3 weeks clearly identifies the cerebral infarction in the left frontal region in the distribution of the left anterior cerebral artery (arrows). Imaging about 3 weeks after the arterial occlusion has occurred is usually the time of best visualization of an area of infarction (Tc-99m sodium pertechnetate).

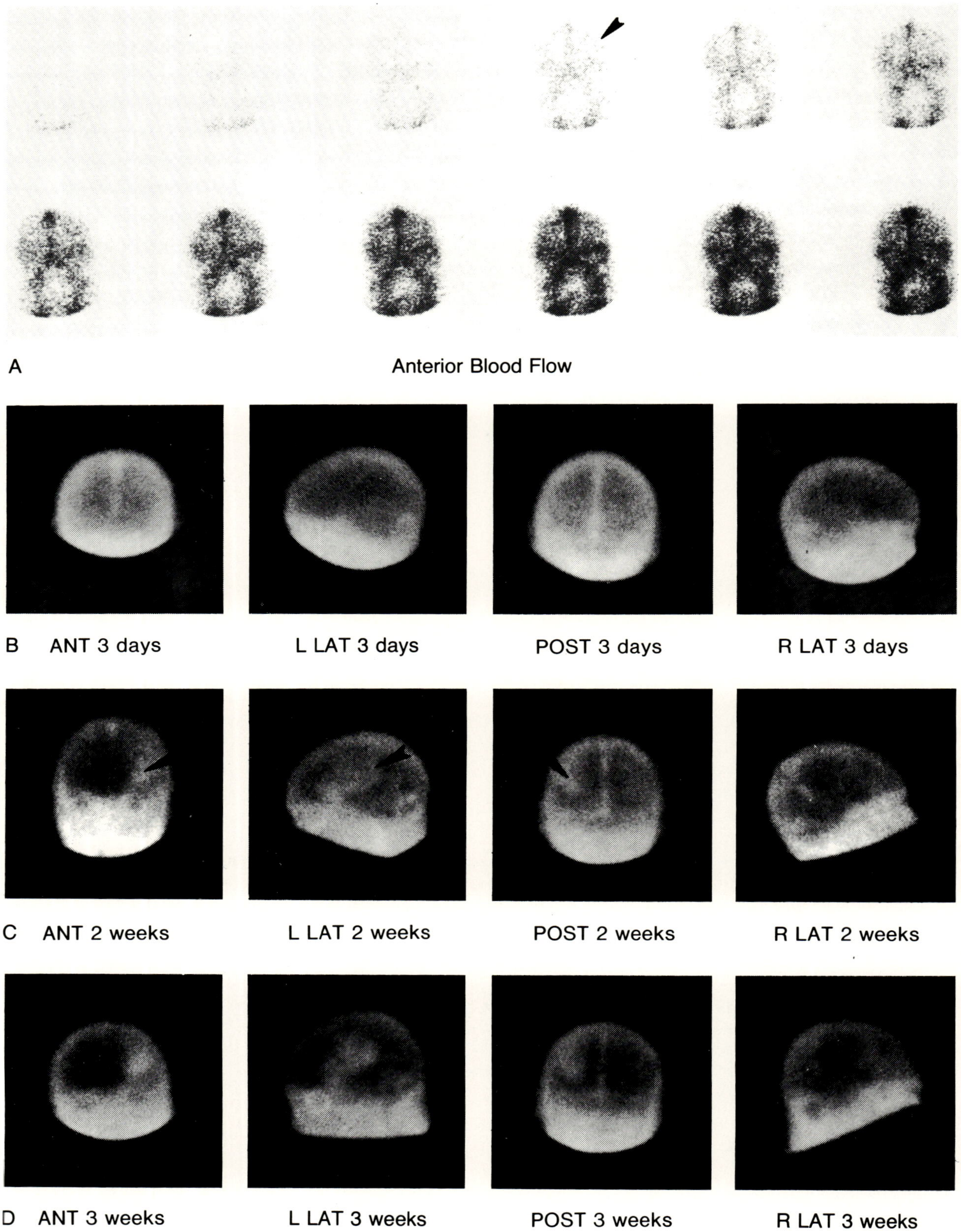


**FIG. 43.** (See legend next page)

**FIG. 43. INFARCTION IN DISTRIBUTION OF LEFT MIDDLE CEREBRAL ARTERY AND ITS RESOLUTION. A. Blood Flow Study.** This anterior blood flow study performed 3 days following the sudden onset of a right hemiplegia shows only slightly reduced radioactivity (arrow), during the arterial phase, of the area supplied by the left middle cerebral artery. This change is so subtle that, in itself, it might be considered of only questionable significance. **B. Static Imaging.** Static imaging done the same day as the blood flow study shows no evidence of a cerebral infarction. **C.** Static imaging 2 weeks after the onset of symptoms shows increased activity (arrows) in the distribution of the left middle cerebral artery, findings clearly visible in the anterior, posterior, and left lateral positions. The area of infarction was not seen at 3 days because insufficient time had elapsed for the development of a structural alteration to provide an avenue of entry for the tracer. However, at 2 weeks, the ischemic area has become surrounded by a proliferative zone and the infarction is now clearly identified as the Tc-99m gains access to it. **D.** Static imaging at 3 weeks defines the infarcted area even more sharply and with increased tracer accumulation. It is at about 3 weeks after the onset of symptoms that a cerebral infarction is most clearly visible on imaging (Tc-99m-DTPA).

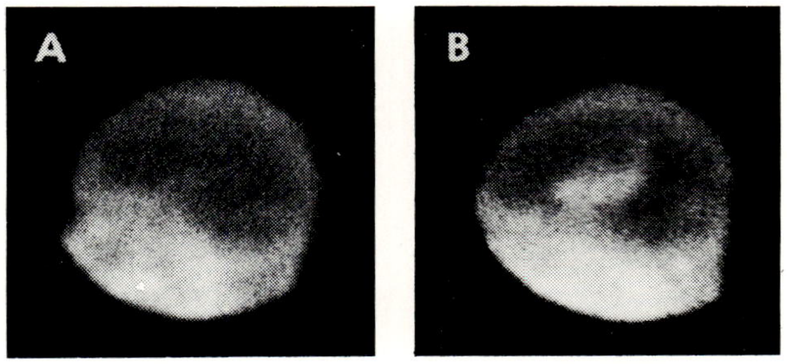


**FIG. 44. CEREBRAL INFARCTION, EVOLUTION.** Static imaging performed in the left lateral position two days following the sudden onset of a right hemiplegia shows no abnormalities. Two weeks following the episode, imaging in the same position shows a somewhat irregular area of increased radioactivity in the distribution of the left middle cerebral artery. In the interval between the first and the second studies, a structural alteration had developed within the brain allowing a tracer to enter the involved region. The sequence of normal imaging at the time of the onset of symptoms followed by demonstration of the abnormality two weeks later helped establish the presence of a vascular-type lesion, such as cerebral infarction, rather than tumor. With the latter, the area of the increased radioactivity could probably have been identified at the time of the first scan (Tc-99m sodium pertechnetate).

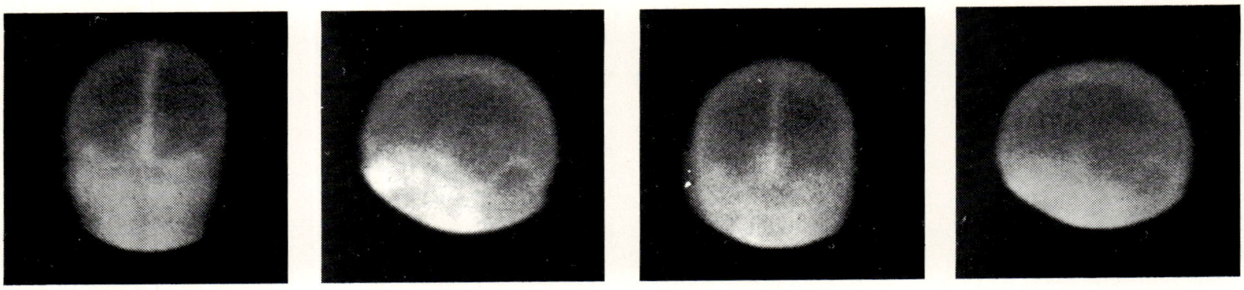

A POST Immediate | L LAT Immediate | B POST 15 minutes | L LAT 15 minutes

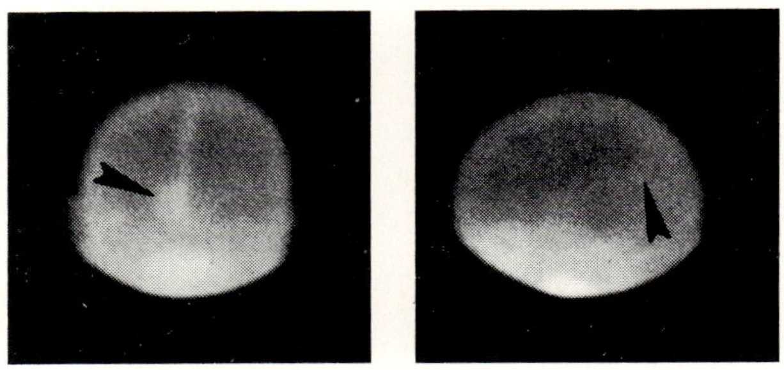

C POST 2 hours | L LAT 2 hours

**FIG. 45. INFARCTION IN DISTRIBUTION OF POSTERIOR CEREBRAL ARTERY RESEMBLING A SPACE-OCCUPYING LESION.** A cerebral infarction has no characteristic shape. In this patient, the infarcted area is round and hardly resembles the wedge-shaped area sometimes considered diagnostic of infarction. The lesion is poorly defined immediately following radionuclide administration (**A**) and at 15 minutes (**B**). However, it becomes sharply defined at 2 hours (**C**). It is barely visible in the left lateral position (Tc-99m sodium pertechnetate).

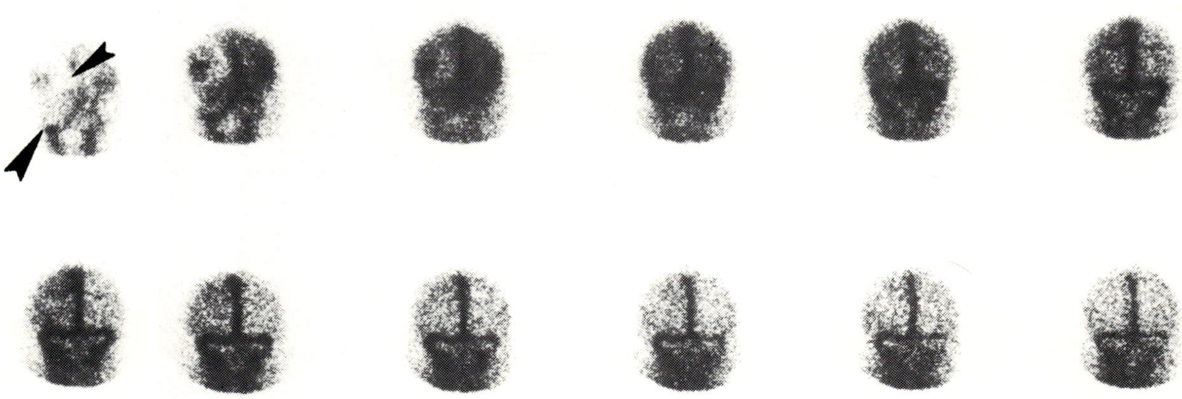

A Posterior Blood Flow

**FIG. 46. A.** (See legend next page)

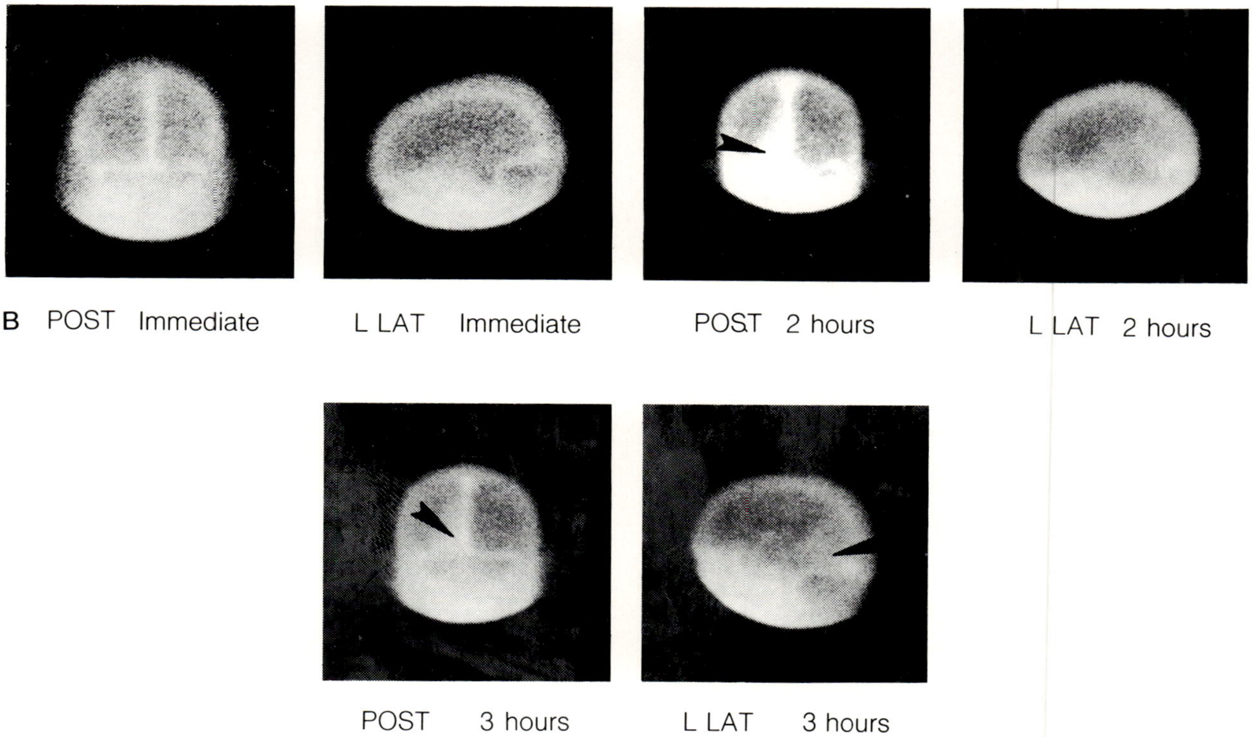


**FIG. 46. CEREBRAL INFARCTION IN THE DISTRIBUTION OF THE LEFT POSTERIOR CEREBRAL ARTERY. A. Blood Flow Study.** There is absent radioactivity in the distribution of the left posterior cerebral artery (arrow) in association with the lodging of an embolus in that vessel. In addition, there has been complete occlusion of the left common carotid artery and internal carotid artery ( larger arrow) to the carotid siphon. There is associated reduction in the distribution of the middle cerebral artery. **B. Static Imaging.** Imaging performed immediately following the blood flow study shows no clear-cut evidence of an infarction. Imaging at 2 hours shows the area of increased radioactivity of low intensity (arrows) in the distribution of the left posterior cerebral artery. On the earlier study, insufficient time had elapsed following injection to allow the tracer to gain entry to the ischemic area. However, at 2 hours, the accumulation of radionuclide in the infarcted area is visible. There is still retention of radioactive material in the region of infarction at 3 hours (Tc-99m sodium pertechnetate).

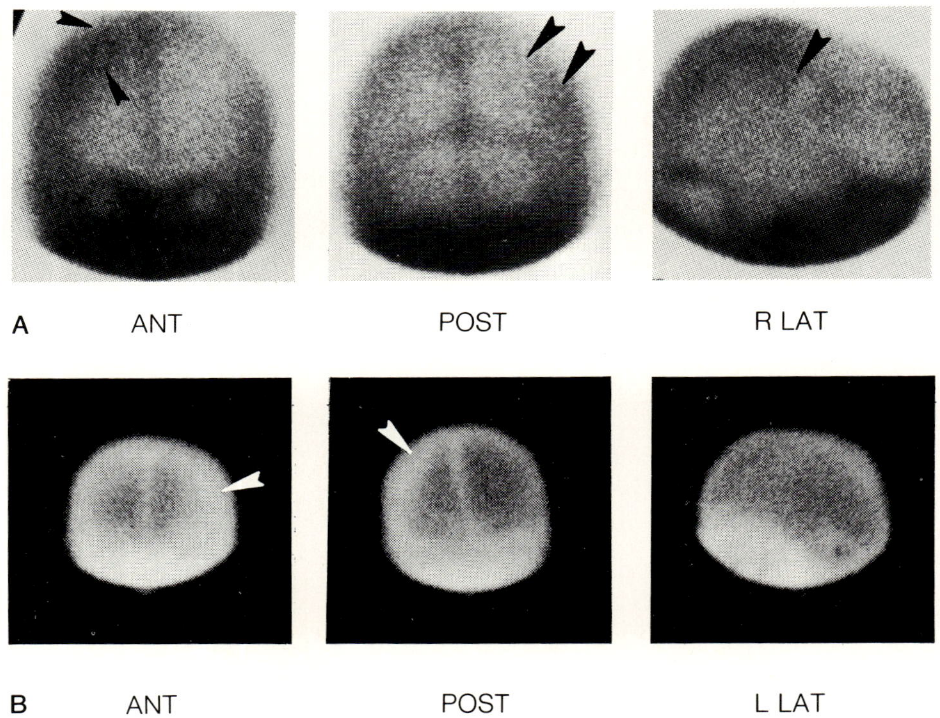


**FIG. 47.** **SUBDURAL HEMATOMA. A.** Static imaging of this right-sided subdural hematoma shows the characteristic crescentic area of increased radioactivity (arrows), most clearly visible in this case in the anterior position. The increased radioactivity is due to localization of radioactive material in the subdural membrane and within its confines. It is seen best in the anterior (or posterior) position because in this view one is visualizing the abnormality in its entire depth, from front to back. In the lateral position, imaging is disappointing because of unrewarding attempts to image a lesion that may be only a few millimeters in depth. A portion is identified, however, in the right lateral position (Tc-99m sodium pertechnetate). **B.** Left-sided subdural hematoma is seen in the anterior and posterior positions.

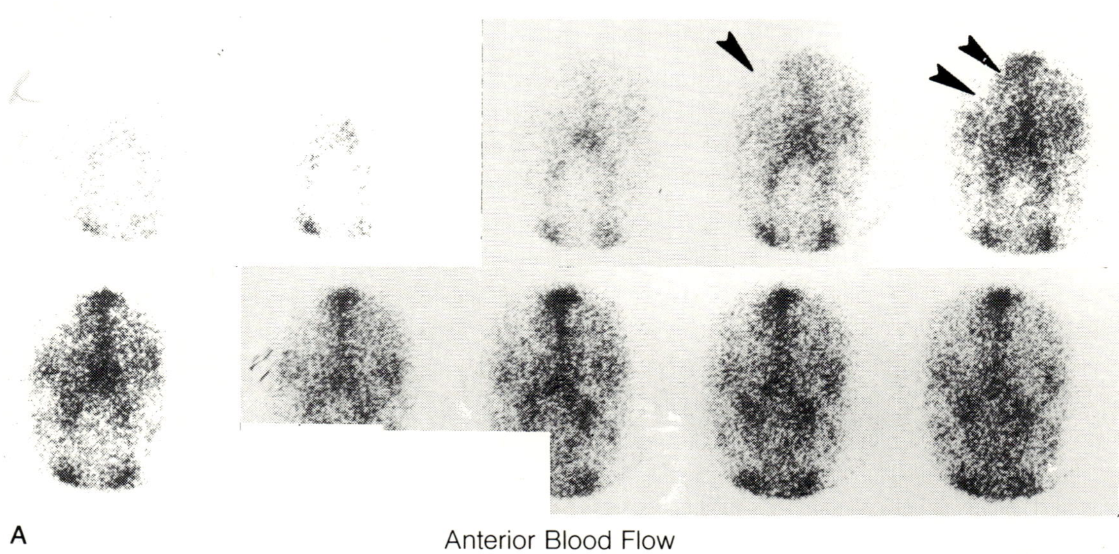


**FIG. 48.** (See legend next page)

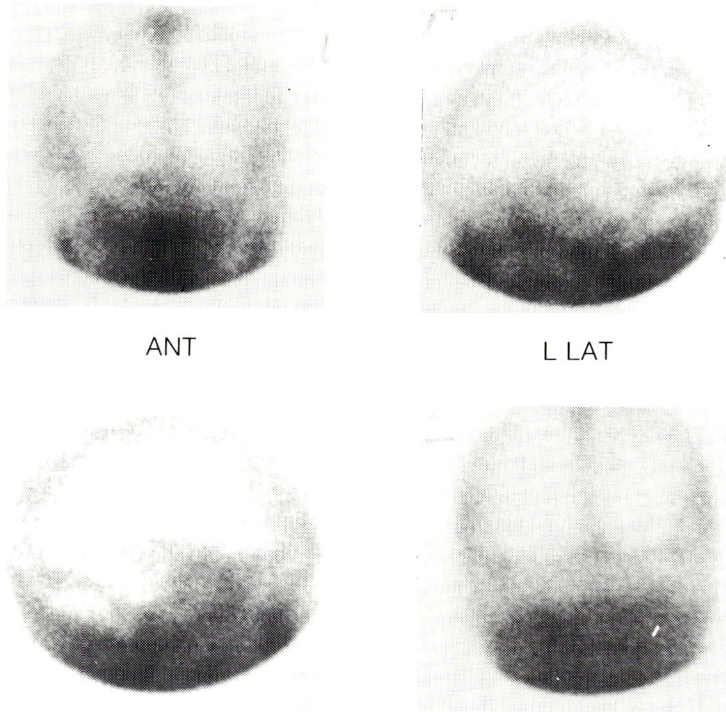


B

1 hour

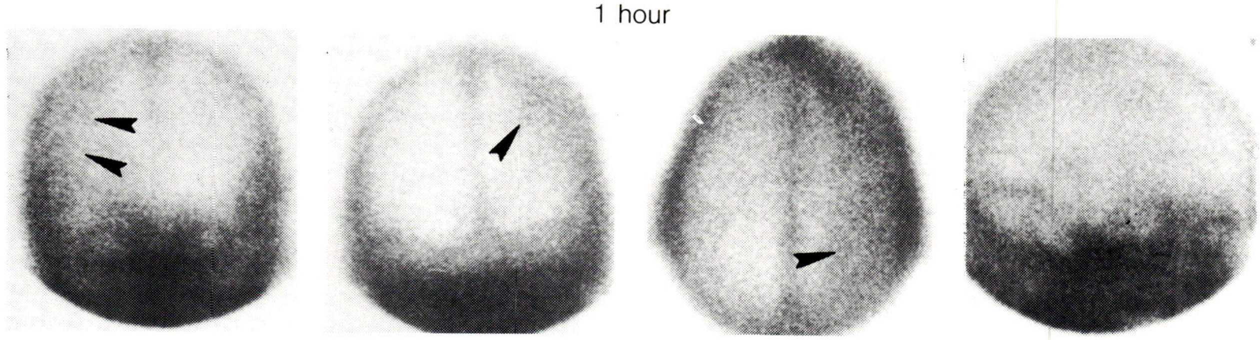


C

2 hours

**FIG. 48. SUBDURAL HEMATOMA. A. Blood Flow Study.** As with contrast angiography, the subdural hematoma is seen as an avascular area (arrows) that is compressing cortical vessels.Such a clear-cut demonstration of a subdural hematoma is rarely seen on a radionuclide blood flow study, and caution must be exercised in not overinterpreting such images when the possibility of a subdural hematoma is considered. **B. Static Imaging.** At 1 hour static imaging shows slightly increased radioactivity, peripherally, in the anterior position. **C.** However, imaging at 2 hours shows clear-cut evidence of increased radioactivity (arrows) in the anterior, posterior, and vertex positions. Since the subdural hematoma is seen on static imaging in both the subdural membrane and within the membrane's confines, accumulation of sufficient radionuclide for imaging did not occur in these areas until 2 hours had elapsed (Tc-99m DTPA). (Courtesy of Dr. Emmett M. Cooper, Lancaster General Hospital, Lancaster, PA)

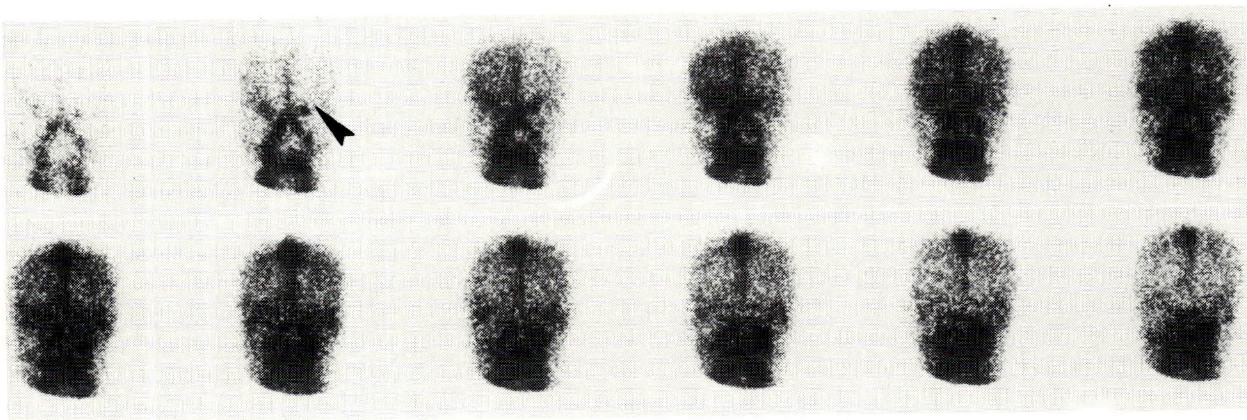

A Anterior Blood Flow

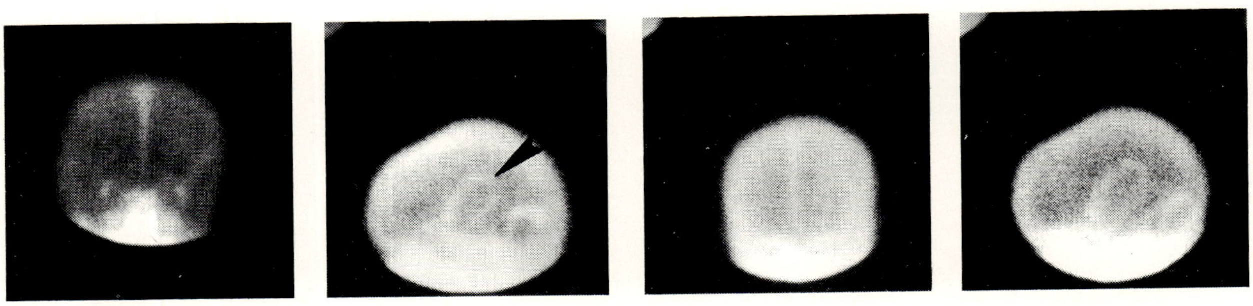

B ANT Immediate | L LAT Immediate | ANT 1 hour | L LAT 1 hour

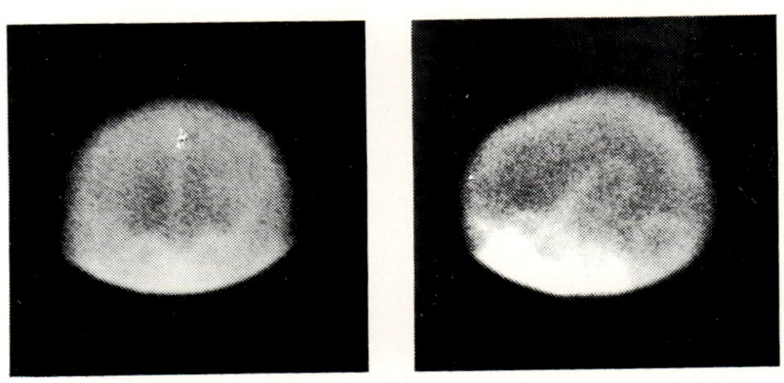

ANT 3 hours | L LAT 3 hours

**FIG. 49. A, B.** (See legend next page)

**FIG. 49. RUPTURED ANEURYSM OF LEFT MIDDLE CEREBRAL ARTERY AND INTRACEREBRAL HEMATOMA. A. Blood Flow Study.** During the arterial phase, there appears to be abrupt cessation of flow in the left middle cerebral artery (arrow). This is due to a ruptured aneurysm of the left middle cerebral artery with subsequent subarachnoid hemorrhage and left temporal intracerebral hematoma. **B. Static Imaging.** Imaging immediately following the blood flow study and at 1 hour outlines the periphery of the large temporal intracerebral hematoma as seen in the left lateral position. The reactive tissue formation is the only area visualized in the hematoma, and the radionuclide does not extend within the lesion, even on delayed imaging at 2 hours. The abnormality is identified in both the anterior and L LAT positions by the increased radioactivity of low intensity (arrow). The definition is not nearly so sharp as the definition in the left lateral position. Since imaging of the hematoma is related to its vascular perimeter, identification is easily made in the left lateral position during the immediate and 1-hour studies. As the blood radioactivity diminishes, the hematoma is imaged with far less intensity at 2 hours (Tc-99m sodium pertechnetate).

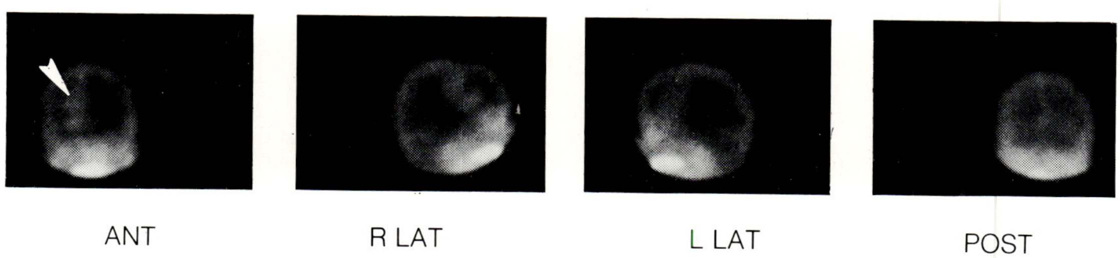


**FIG. 50. INTRACEREBRAL HEMATOMA.** After sufficient time has elapsed for the intracerebral hemorrhage to become organized and be walled off, static imaging discloses an area of increased radioactivity, usually irregular in configuration. In most cases, only a portion of the abnormality is identified with radionuclide imaging. In this patient with a large left frontal intracerebral hematoma, the irregularity of the abnormality is best seen in the left lateral position ( arrow ) (Tc-99m sodium pertechnetate).

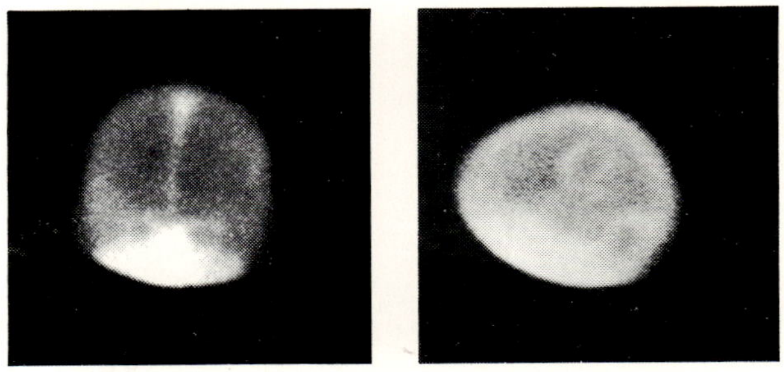

ANT Immediate L LAT

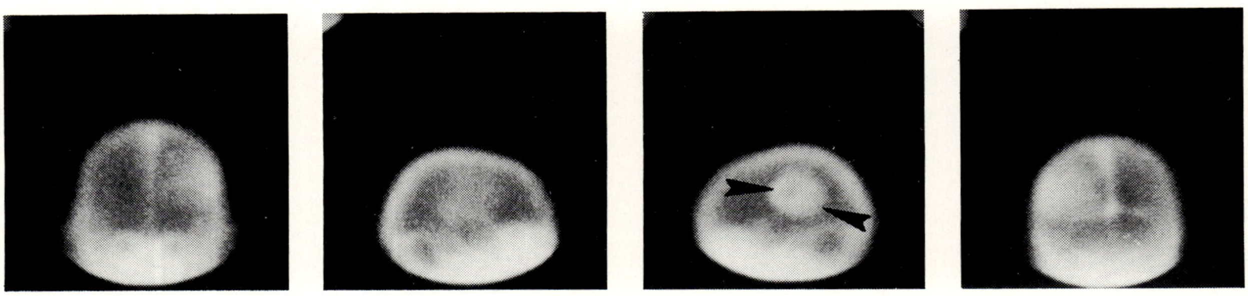

ANT R LAT L LAT POST

**FIG. 51. INTRACEREBRAL HEMATOMA.** Initial imaging immediately following tracer injection shows a peripheral area of increased radioactivity (arrows)surrounding a zone of absent radioactivity—findings obtained only in the left lateral position. Imaging at 30 minutes defines more fully the depth of the lesion as seen in the anterior and posterior positions. In the left lateral position at 30 minutes there has been continued radionuclide accumulation in the central portion of the abnormality. The imaging findings are almost identical to those that might be seen with an abscess at this site. The patient is a 10-year-old child who had suffered head trauma 3 weeks earlier (Tc-99m DTPA).

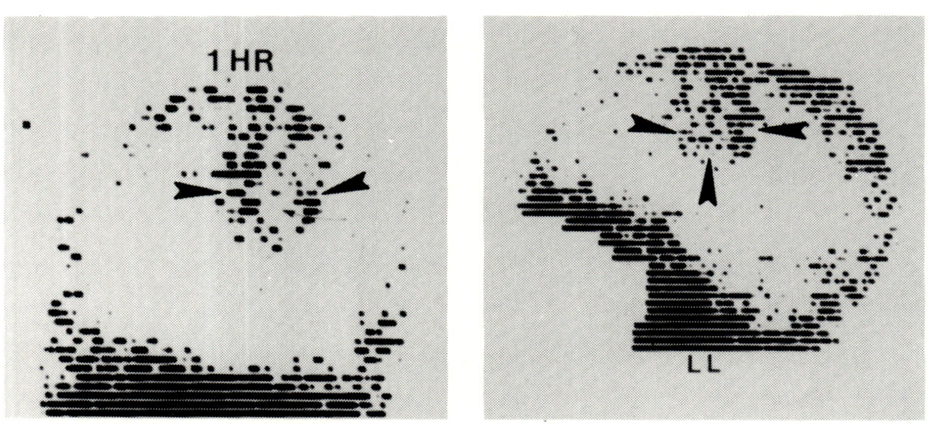


ANT 1 hour L LAT

**FIG. 52.** (See legend next page)

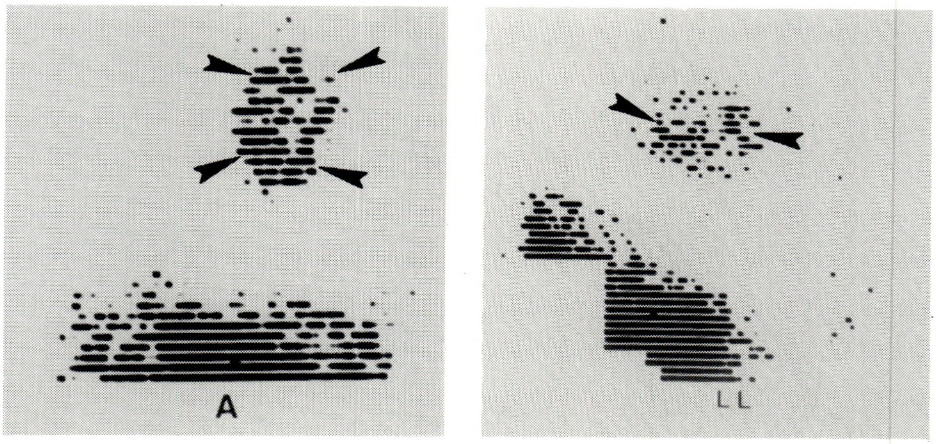


ANT 4 hours L LAT

**FIG. 52. BRAIN ABSCESS.** Initial imaging at 1 hour shows evidence of a rounded space-occupying lesion, just to the left of the midline, in the left frontoparietal region. The central core of absent radioactivity, as seen on the initial study in the anterior position, represents the abscess cavity. The lesion is visualized because of the presence of radioactive material in the pericapsular blood vessels. At 4 hours, when the blood radioactivity has fallen considerably, imaging in the anterior position fails to demonstrate pericapsular activity, and the lesion appears small. This is probably associated with the entrance of the radioactive technetium into the abscess cavity after it leaves the pericapsular blood vessels. This sequence is different from that usually observed with a tumor of the brain parenchyma, in which there is continued accumulation and accretion of radioactive material.

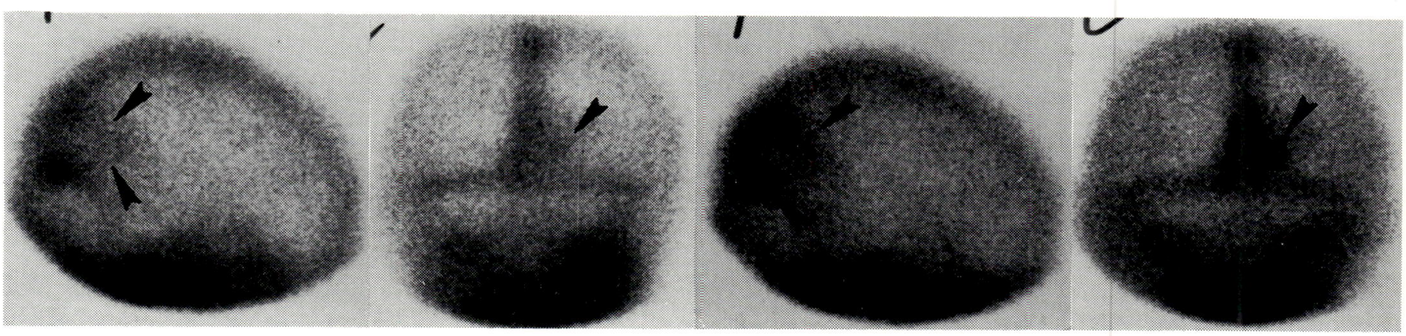

A R LAT POST B R LAT POST

**FIG. 53. BRAIN ABSCESS.** An occipital lobe abscess is seen well in the right lateral and posterior positions. **A.** Imaging at one hour in the right lateral position shows a circular rim of increased radioactivity (arrows) surrounding a zone of reduced radioactivity. The rim of increased activity is probably associated with the presence of radioactive material in the pericapsular vessels. The lesion is seen to lie close to the midline in the posterior position (arrow). **B.** Imaging at 2 hours shows a slight increase in localization, but there is no evidence of markedly increased activity in the abscess cavity (Tc-99m DTPA). (Courtesy of Dr. Emmett M. Cooper, Lancaster General Hospital, Lancaster, PA)

## Suggested Reading

Barnes BD, Finklestein S, Winestock DP: Radionuclide angiography: a sensitive diagnostic test for anterior circulation ischemia. Neurology 28:775–781, 1978

Barnes BD, Winestock DP: Dynamic radionuclide scanning in the diagnosis of thrombosis of the superior sagittal sinus. Neurology 27:656–661, 1977

Brown R, Wever PM, dos Remedios LV: Dynamic/static brain scintigraphy: an effective screening test for subdural hematoma. Radiology 117:355–360, 1975

Buonanno FS, Moody DM, Ball MR: Radionuclide sinography: diagnosis of lateral sinus thrombosis by dynamic and static brain imaging. Radiology 130:207–213, 1979

DeLand FH: *Cerebral Radionuclide Angiography.* Philadelphia, W.B. Saunders, 1976

Front D: Distinctive imaging characteristics of different types of brain tumors. Clin Nucl Med 4:211–218, 1979

Harbert JC, Rocha AFG: The central nervous system. In Rocha AFG, Harbert JC (eds): *Textbook of Nuclear Medicine: Clinical Applications,* Philadelphia, Lea and Febiger, 1979, pp 51–108

Kirchner PT, (ed): *Nuclear Medicine Review Syllabus.* New York, Society of Nuclear Medicine, 1980, pp 161–187

Mishkin FS: Brain imaging. In Schneiden PB, Treves S (eds): *Nuclear Medicine in Clinical Practice.* Amsterdam, Elsevier/North Holland, 1978, pp 21–37

Mishkin FS: Cerebral radionuclide angiography. Angiography 28:261–275, 1977

Potchen EJ, Adelstein SJ, Hoffer PB, James AE, Jr., McNeil BJ, Siegel BA (eds): *Nuclear Radiology Syllabus.* Chicago, American College of Radiology, 1974, pp 2–121

Rockett JF, Moinuddin M: Dynamic cerebral imaging. Clin Nucl Med 1:166–177, 1976

Rockett JF: The radionuclide cerebral angiogram in stroke diagnosis. Clin Neurosurg 23:245–257, 1976

Siegel BA (ed): *Nuclear Radiology* (*Second Series*) *Syllabus.* Chicago, American College of Radiology, 1978, pp 192–254.

Smoak WM, Sheldon J: Intracranial meningiomas: dynamic and static scintigraphic characteristics. Clin Nucl Med 1:41–44, 1976

Steinbach JJ, Mattar AG, Mahin DT: Alteration of the cerebral blood flow study due to reflux in internal jugular veins. J Nucl Med 17:6–8, 1976

# 7/Radionuclide Cisternography

Radionuclide cisternography is a nuclear medicine procedure for studying the dynamics and anatomic distribution of cerebrospinal fluid. Serial images are obtained after the injection of an isobaric radioactive substance into the subarachnoid space. This material then diffuses with the cerebrospinal fluid (CSF) and migrates cephalad to the basal cisterns and subarachnoid space around the brain.

Several different radiopharmiceuticals are available commercially, each consisting of a carrier labeled with a radioactive element. The most desirable of these agents have physical properties that permit adequate imaging at the lowest possible radiation exposure, offer a low incidence of side effects, and migrate in a manner similar to CSF. The cases presented in this section of the *Atlas* were studied with 500 microcuries of In-111 DTPA.

Cisternography displays the dynamics of CSF flow and absorption. The method is useful in evaluating hydrocephalus (communicating and noncommunicating), in the imaging of anatomic lesions involving the subarachnoid space and contiguous structures (e.g., cysts and hygromas), in assessing the patency of CSF shunts, and in identifying leaks of CSF from the subarachnoid space.

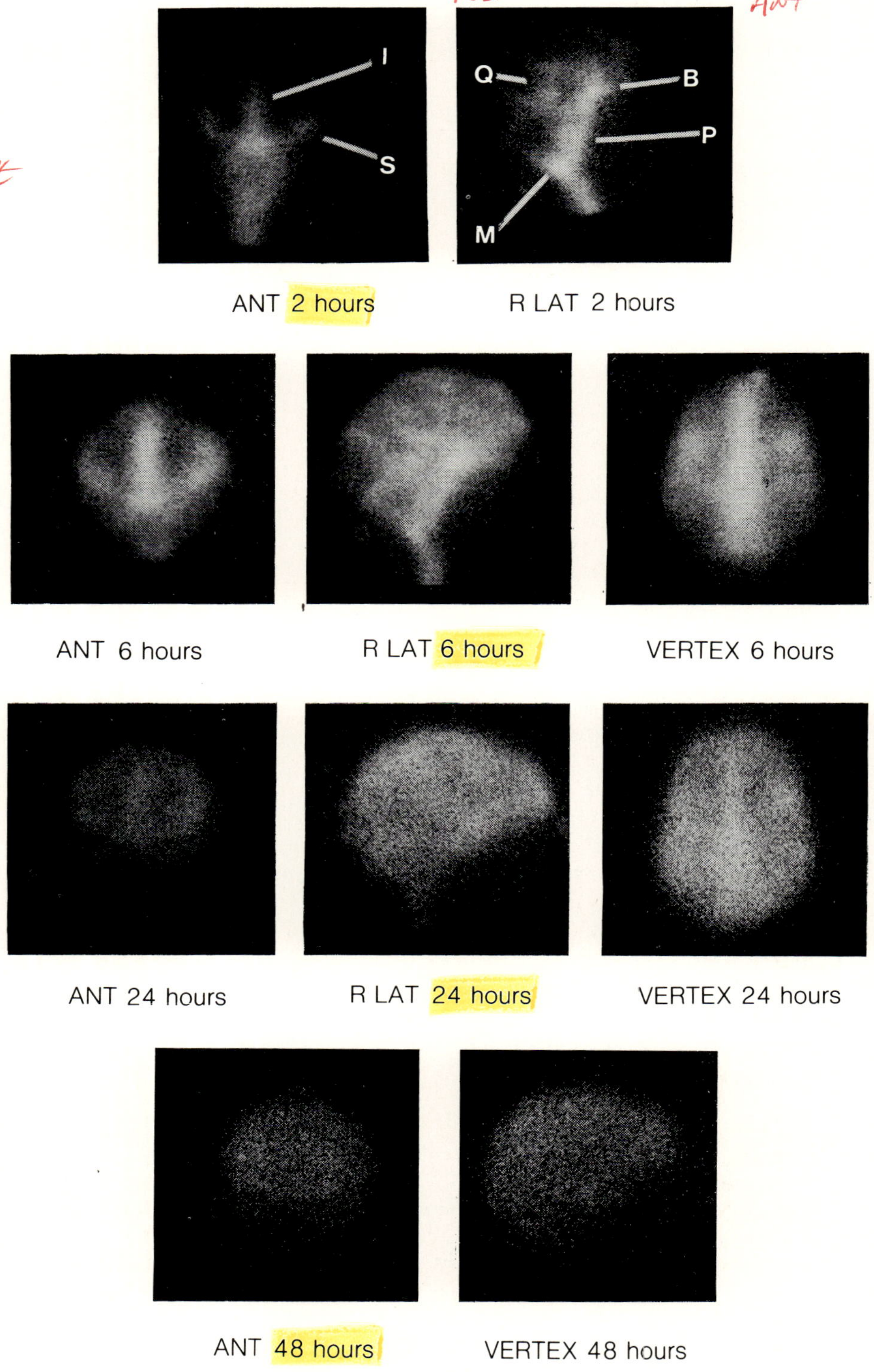


I = INTRAHEMISPHERIC FISSURE; S = SYLVIAN FISSURE; M = CISTERNA MAGNA; B = CISTERNA BASALIS; P = CISTERNA PONTIS; Q = QUADRIGEMINAL CISTERN

**FIG. 1.** (See legend next page)

## CLASSIFICATION OF CISTERNOGRAPHIC PATTERNS

Interpretation of cisternograms is aided by categorizing the studies according to migratory patterns. The following classification is based on the present understanding of the dynamics of CSF pathophysiology. It is directed towards differentiating patients who may be expected to improve with CSF shunt therapy (Type IV) from those who exhibit an abnormal pattern but would not benefit from shunting (Type II, III-A, III-B).

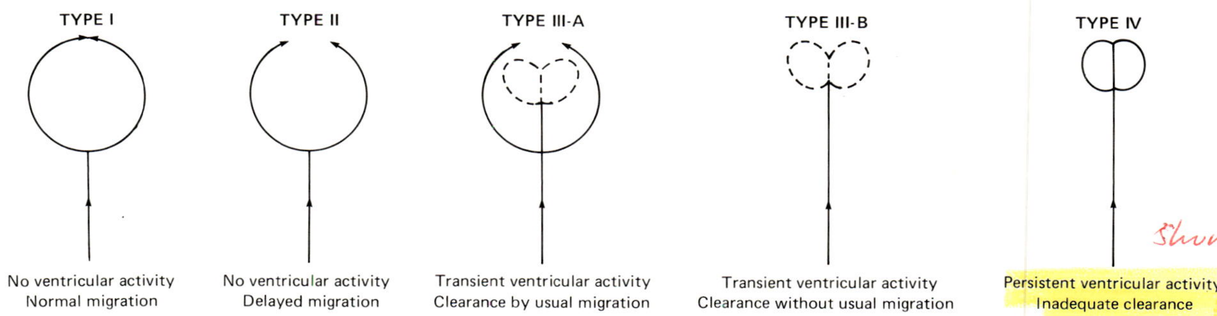


**FIG. 1. CISTERNOGRAM TYPE I. No Ventricular Activity, Normal Migration.** Type I is the pattern seen in normal adults. Following the intrathecal injection of radionuclide, activity is visible in the cisterna magna and other basal cisterns within 2 to 4 hours. Note that the quadrigeminal cistern is clearly visible on the early lateral view. It should not be confused with the lateral ventricle. It is important to obtain multiple views, including vertex, to distinguish basal cisterns from the ventricles. No activity is present in the ventricles in a normal study. At 6 hours the sylvian fissures are clearly visualized. By 24 hours the activity has migrated from the basal cisterns over the convexities and into the parasagittal regions. The radioactivity in the CSF is significantly diminished at 48 hours primarily by absorption through the arachnoid villi. It should be noted that younger patients have more rapid transit of the radionuclide through the subarachnoid space than elderly patients.

**EXAMPLE.** The case is that of a 29-year-old female who sustained head injuries in an automobile accident one month prior to the examination. The patient had persistent confusion, disorientation, and memory loss. On physical examination, there were no localizing findings. The skull x-rays and brain scan were normal. The normal cisternogram excluded the diagnosis of communicating hydrocephalus.

**COMMENT.** Type I is the pattern of normal CSF dynamics. It is seen in normal individuals, patients with noncommunicating hydrocephalus following surgical correction, and patients with spontaneous resolution of communicating hydrocephalus.

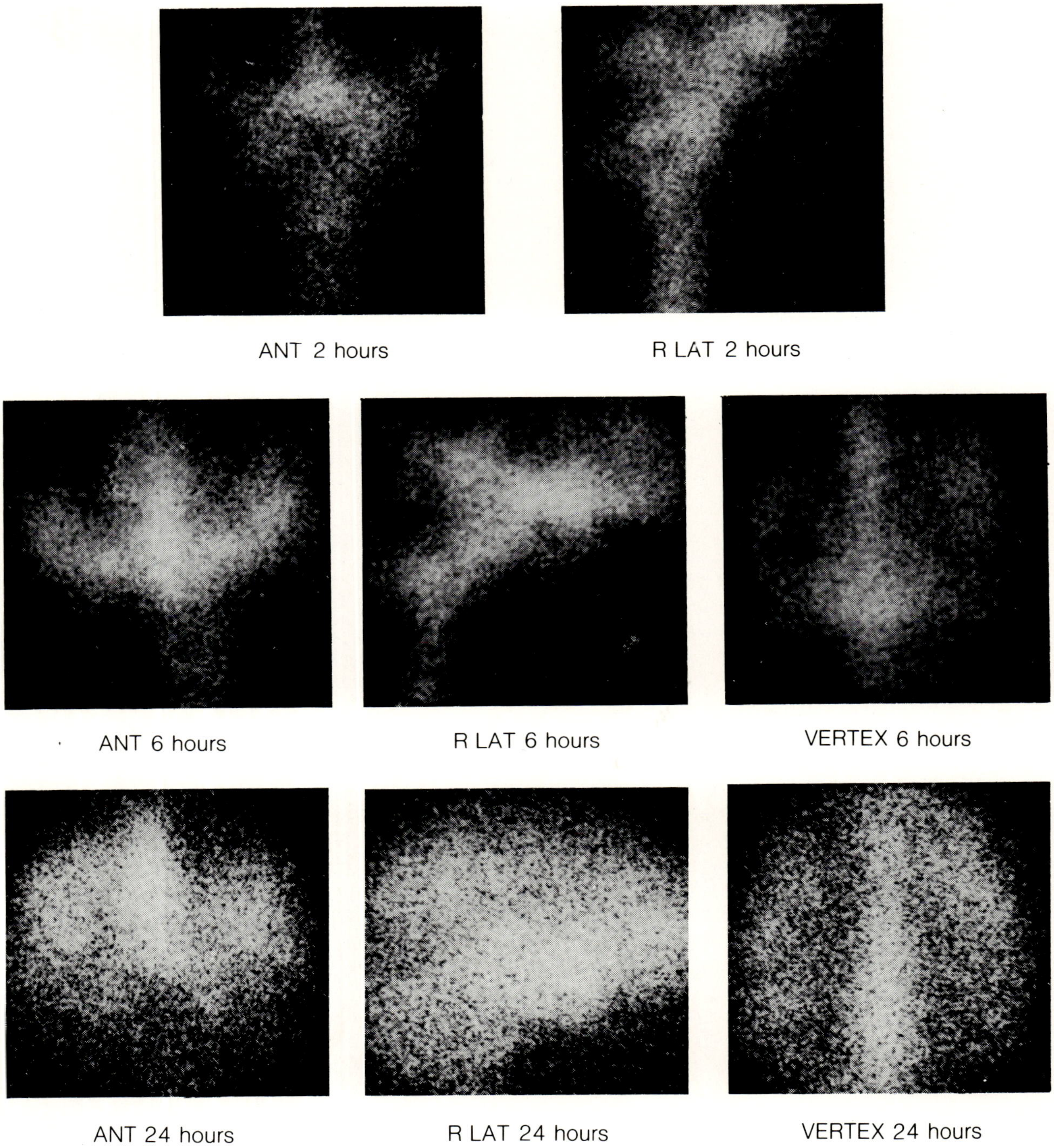


**FIG. 2.** (See legend next page)

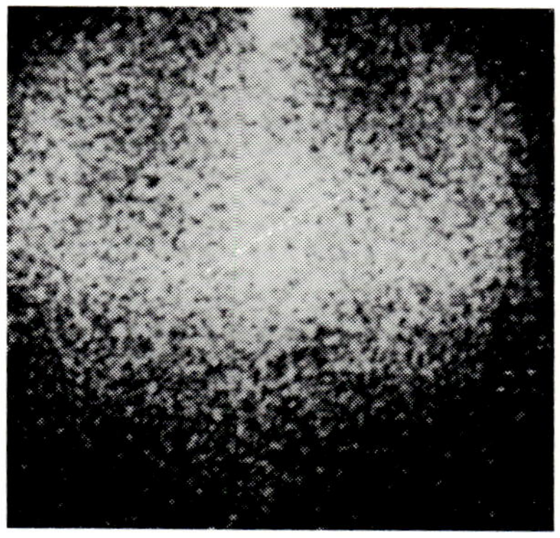

ANT 48 hours

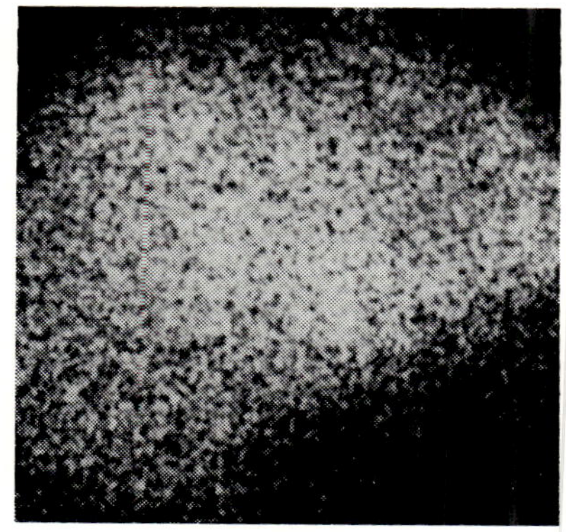

R LAT 48 hours

**FIG. 2. TYPE II. No Ventricular Activity, Delayed Migration.** The Type II pattern differs from the normal in that a longer time is required to complete the migration. Again, there is no ventricular activity at any time during the study.

**EXAMPLE.** The case is that of a 50-year-old male with presenile dementia and no focal neurologic signs.

Activity present in the basal cisterns at two hours persists at six hours, and by 24 hours is just beginning to migrate over the convexities. At 48 hours migration is still incomplete, and the slight decrease in count rate is due primarily to physical decay of the radionuclide. Slight asymmetry is present in the migration over the convexities.

**COMMENT.** The Type II pattern of delayed migration is seen in patients with cerebral atrophy, increased intracranial pressure, noncommunicating hydrocephalus, and advanced age.

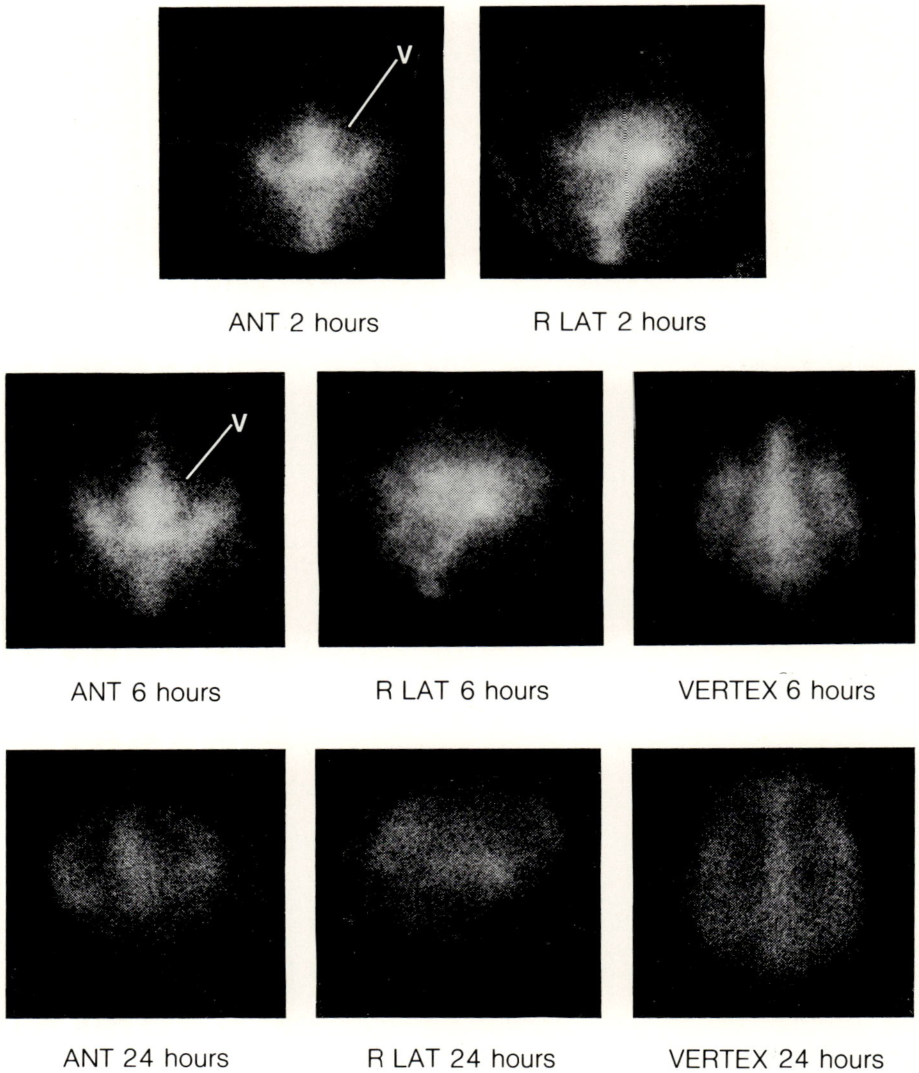


V = LATERAL VENTRICLE

**FIG. 3.** (See legend next page)

**FIG. 3.** **TYPE III-A. Transient Ventricular Activity, Clearance by Usual Migration.** Ventricular activity is present in the Type III-A pattern. This abnormality, however, is transient. The subsequent ventricular clearing is followed by migration over the convexities. The time required for migration and absorption generally is prolonged.

**EXAMPLE.** The case is that of a 53-year-old ex-pugilist with progressive memory loss and dementia. There were no localizing signs, and the gait was normal.

The cisternogram shows ventricular activity at two hours, which becomes more intense at 6 hours. By 24 hours the activity has diminished in the ventricles as it migrates over the convexities. At 48 hours no ventricular activity is present as parasagittal absorption continues.

Subsequent pneumoencephalogram demonstrated cerebral atrophy with slight dilatation of the lateral ventricles.

**COMMENT.** The Type III-A pattern may be seen with evolving or resolving communicating hydrocephalus, as well as with cerebral atrophy.

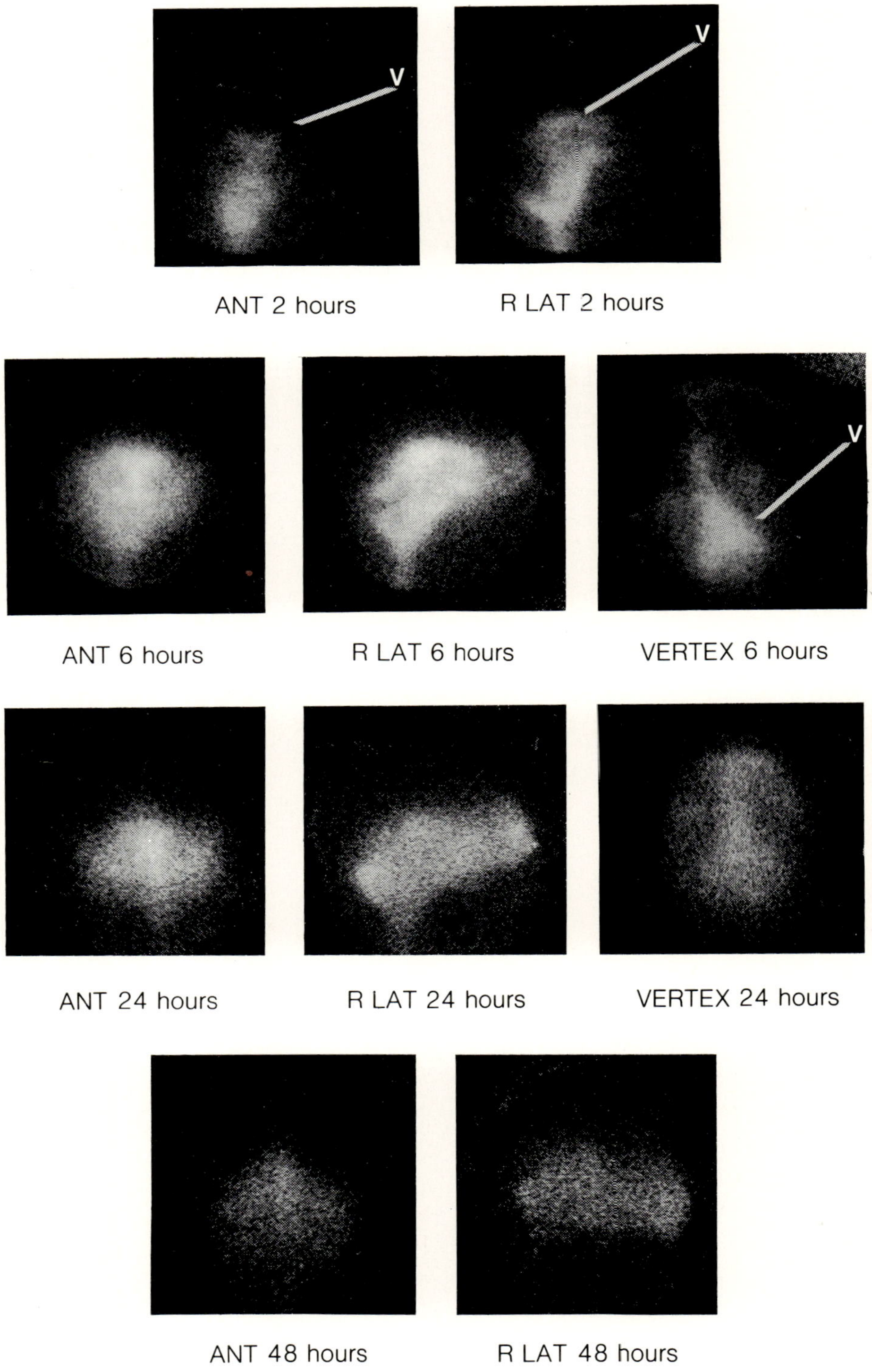


V = LATERAL VENTRICLE

**FIG. 4.** (See legend next page)

**FIG. 4. TYPE III-B. Transient Ventricular Activity, Clearance without Usual Migration.** Ventricular activity is present in the Type III-B pattern but is not persistent. Unlike Type III-A, clearance occurs without the usual migration over the convexities.

**EXAMPLE.** The case is that of a 60-year-old male who was demented and dyskinetic and walked with a broad-based gait.

On his cisternogram, ventricular activity is present at 2 hours, with good delineation on the lateral views. This finding is more intense at 6 hours, and is clearly visible on the vertex view. It substantially decreases by 24 hours, and resorption continues by the same mechanism at 48 hours. The clearance of ventricular activity, however, is not accompanied by the usual migration over the convexities.

**COMMENT.** These findings indicate the presence of an alternative pathway, primarily transependymal resorption. The rapidity with which this occurs suggests that it is an adequate compensatory mechanism. Surgical shunting would therefore not be expected to improve the CSF dynamics.

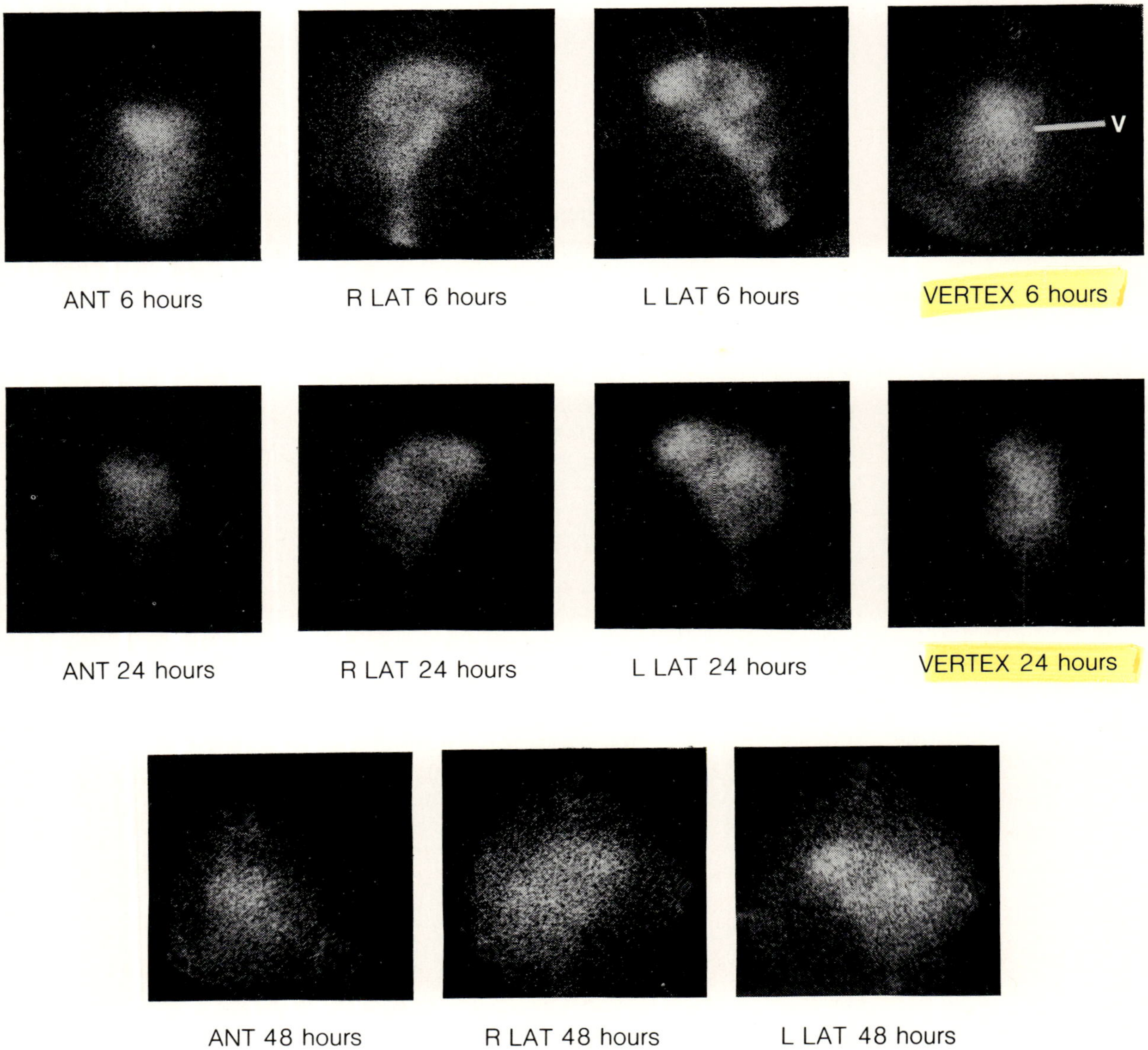


V = LATERAL VENTRICLE

**FIG. 5.** (See legend next page)

**FIG. 5. TYPE IV. Persistent Ventricular Activity, Inadequate Clearance.** The Type IV pattern is characterized by early appearance of ventricular activity, which persists at 48 hours. There is no migration over the convexities. The transependymal pathway of resorption is inadequate, as evidenced by the prolonged activity in the ventricles. Lack of compensatory resorption distinguishes this pattern from Type III-B.

**EXAMPLE.** The case is that of a 40-year-old male who 5 years ago had a hemorrhage from a basal ganglion arteriovenous malformation. He was rehospitalized for recent mental deterioration, with memory loss and confusion. His gait was abnormal. He had no urinary incontinence.

The ventricular activity seen at 6 hours is unchanged at 24 hours, and persists at 48 hours. Throughout the study, the ventricles are clearly visible, signifying inadequate clearance. Note the absence of migration over the convexities.

Pneumoencephalogram supported the cisternographic findings of enlarged, dilated ventricles and communicating hydrocephalus. CSF pressure measured at the time of PEG was normal. Subsequent ventriculo-atrial shunting led to clinical improvement.

**COMMENT.** The classic triad of dementia, gait disturbance, and urinary incontinence characterizes the syndrome of communicating hydrocephalus without elevated CSF pressure. The triad is not always complete in every patient. Furthermore, an imperfect correlation exists between the clinical signs, cisternographic findings, and surgical results. Among the various causes of this discrepancy is an inability to differentiate between reversible and nonreversible changes in the afflicted individual. Cisternography provides a relatively noninvasive, low-morbidity method of evaluating patients suspected of harboring this syndrome. The use of a classification, based on pathophysiology, will aid in the understanding of this complex phenomenon, and will serve to differentiate patients who have achieved their own mechanism of compensation from those who have not.

## FUNCTIONING SHUNT
## LOCALIZED SUBARACHNOID PATHOLOGY
## ANATOMIC LESIONS

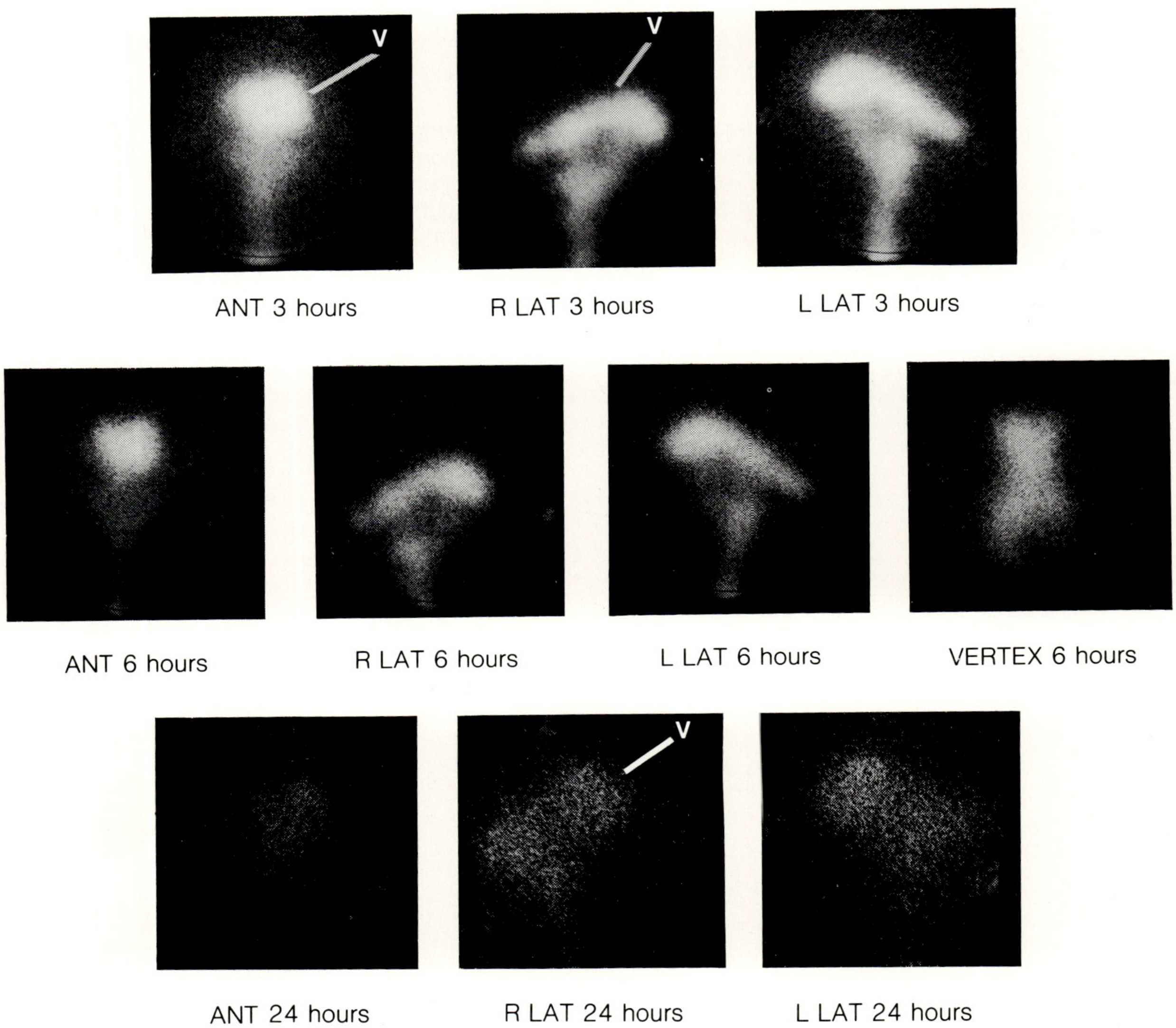


V = LATERAL VENTRICLES

**FIG. 6.** (See legend next page)

**FIG. 6. EVALUATION OF SHUNT FUNCTION.** The function of ventricular shunts can be determined by cisternographic techniques. There are two methods of evaluating shunt patency: (1) recording the migration and disappearance time of radionuclide after injection into the subarachnoid space; (2) recording the rate of disappearance of radionuclide injected directly into the shunt reservoir.

**EXAMPLE.** The first method is used in this case of a 43-year-old male who had a ventriculo-atrial shunt for 15 years. Radionuclide injected into the lumbar subarachnoid space migrates cephalad, moving freely into the ventricles, where a large amount of activity is present at 3 hours. There is no subsequent migration out of the ventricles over the convexities. However, by 6 hours the count rate decreases to 38 percent of the 3-hour level. Only a trace amount of activity remains in the ventricles by 24 hours, with a count rate reduced to 5 percent, indicating patency of the shunt. Note that visualization of activity within the shunt is uncommon, and is not necessary to prove shunt patency.

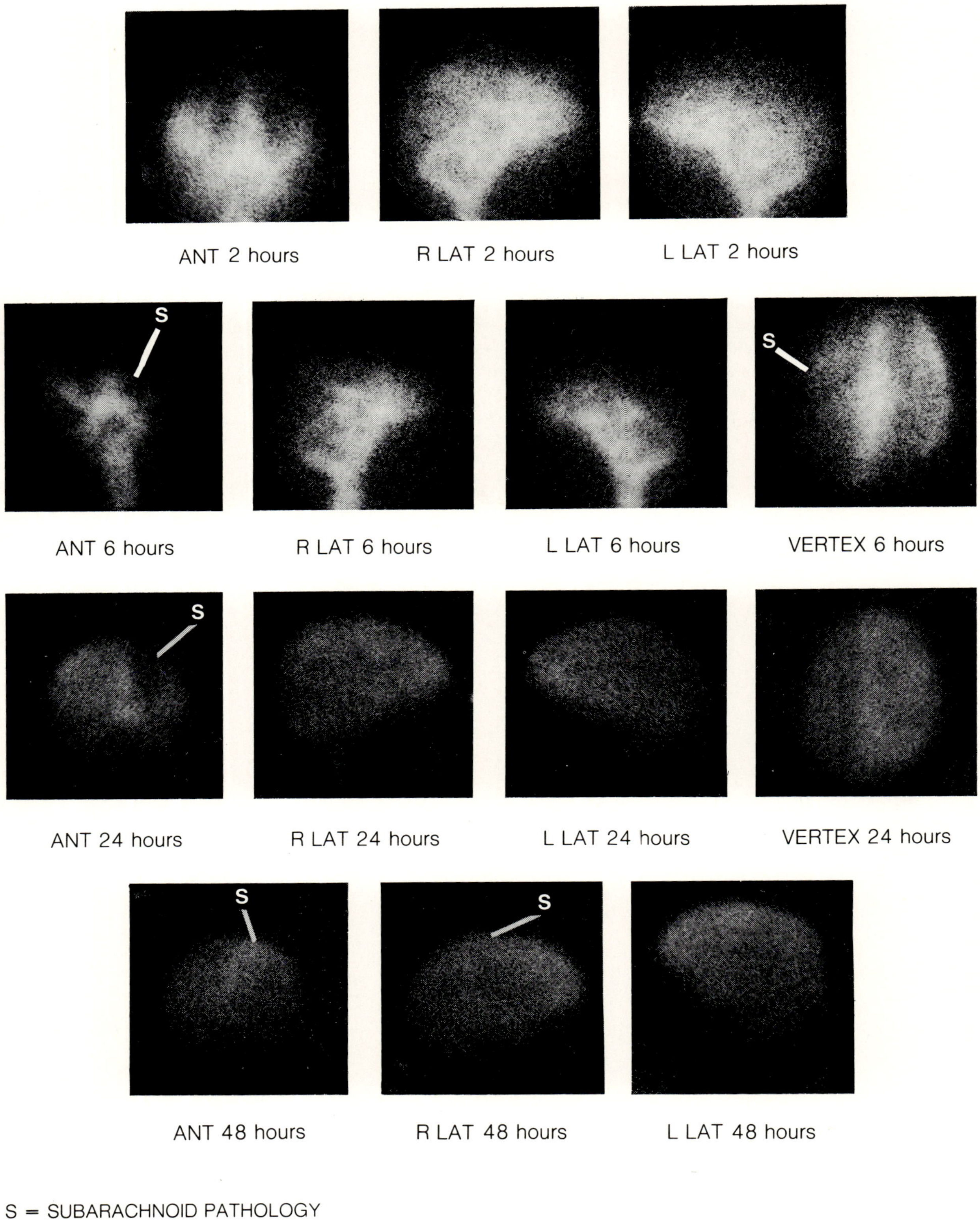


**FIG. 7.** (See legend next page)

**FIG. 7. SUBARACHNOID PATHOLOGY WITH NORMAL CSF DYNAMICS.** Localized obliteration of the subarachnoid space may impede CSF flow to varying degrees. The net effect ranges from negligible to significant obstruction requiring surgical intervention. The effect of a specific lesion can be determined and classified according to its migratory pattern.

Shown as an example is the cisternogram of a 32-year-old female who 7 years ago recovered from a subarachnoid hemorrhage. An aneurysm of the anterior communicating artery was treated by surgical clipping. She was reevaluated because of recent headaches and syncope.

On the 2-hour anterior view, activity is present in the right sylvian fissure. On the left side there is no ascent beyond the basal cisterns. The asymmetry continues at 6 and 24 hours. The radionuclide reaches the parasagittal region on the left side only after 48 hours, implying interference with migration through the left subarachnoid space. It is important to note that there is no ventricular activity, and no delay in migration on the right side. The abnormality of the left subarachnoid space does not adversely affect the overall dynamics.

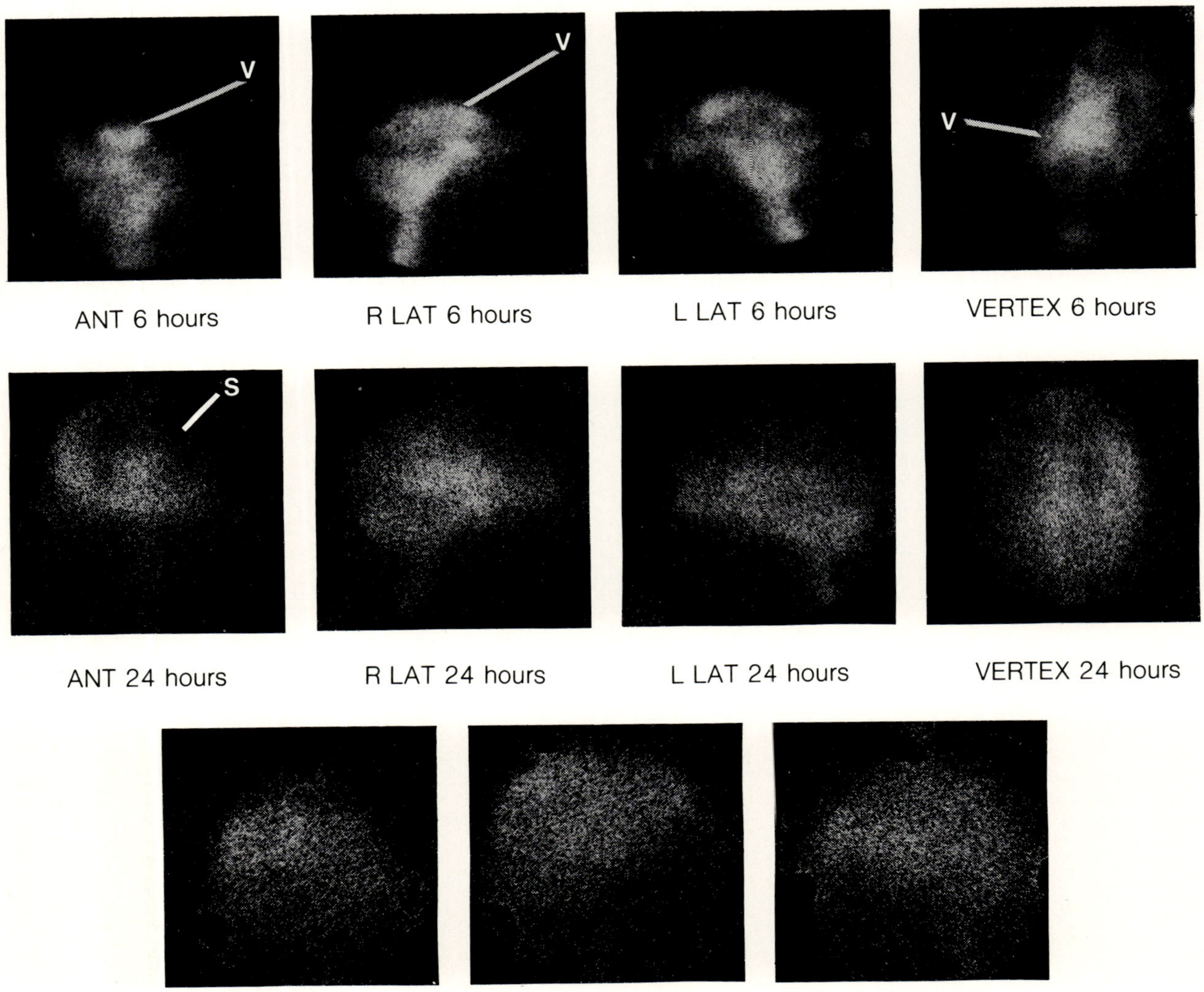


ANT 6 hours — R LAT 6 hours — L LAT 6 hours — VERTEX 6 hours

ANT 24 hours — R LAT 24 hours — L LAT 24 hours — VERTEX 24 hours

ANT 48 hours — R LAT 48 hours — L LAT 48 hours

**FIG. 8. SUBARACHNOID PATHOLOGY WITH ABNORMAL CSF DYNAMICS.** Subarachnoid pathology that interferes locally with CSF migration may adversely affect overall dynamics. This is demonstrated by ventricular activity and general delay in absorption of the radionuclide.

The cisternogram shown is that of a 66-year-old female with documented pulmonary and CNS tuberculosis. She had headaches, dementia, and a wide-based gait.

Ventricular activity is present early in the cisternogram. Migration over the convexities is delayed bilaterally, with a severe obstruction on the left side. On later views there is clearance of the radionuclide from the ventricles. The total activity decreases beyond that due to physical decay, signifying partially compensated CSF dynamics.

Over the next 14 months, antituberculous therapy resulted in slow improvement in the patient's clinical course.

V = LATERAL VENTRICLE S = SUBARACHNOID PATHOLOGY

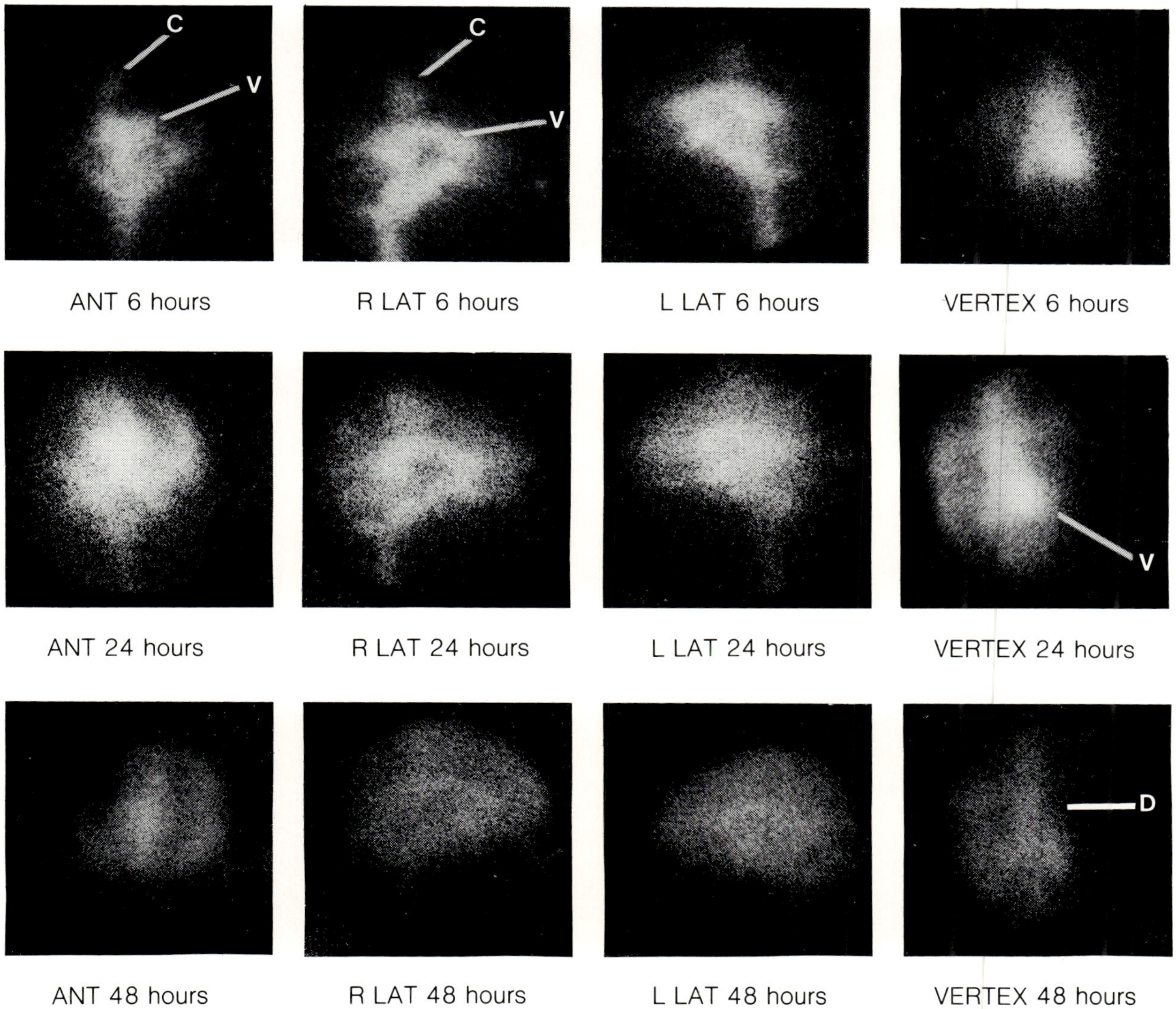


**FIG. 9. PORENCEPHALIC CYST.** Lesions that communicate with the ventricles or subarachnoid space, such as porencephalic cysts, may be visualized with cisternography. Activity can appear in the lesion early or late in the study. This depends on the degree of patency between the cyst and ventricle.

**EXAMPLE.** A 50-year-old female had previous head trauma resulting in intracranial hemorrhage. She remained demented after blood cleared from the CSF.

**COMMENT.** The important feature of this cisternogram is the focal accumulation of activity in the right parietal region above the lateral ventricle. The early appearance of activity in the lesion corresponds to the time of arrival of activity in the ventricles. Furthermore, migration over the right convexity is delayed, and does not contribute to the parietal activity. This porencephalic cyst therefore communicates with the ventricle.

C = PORENCEPHALIC CYST D = DELAY MIGRATION V = LATERAL VENTRICLES

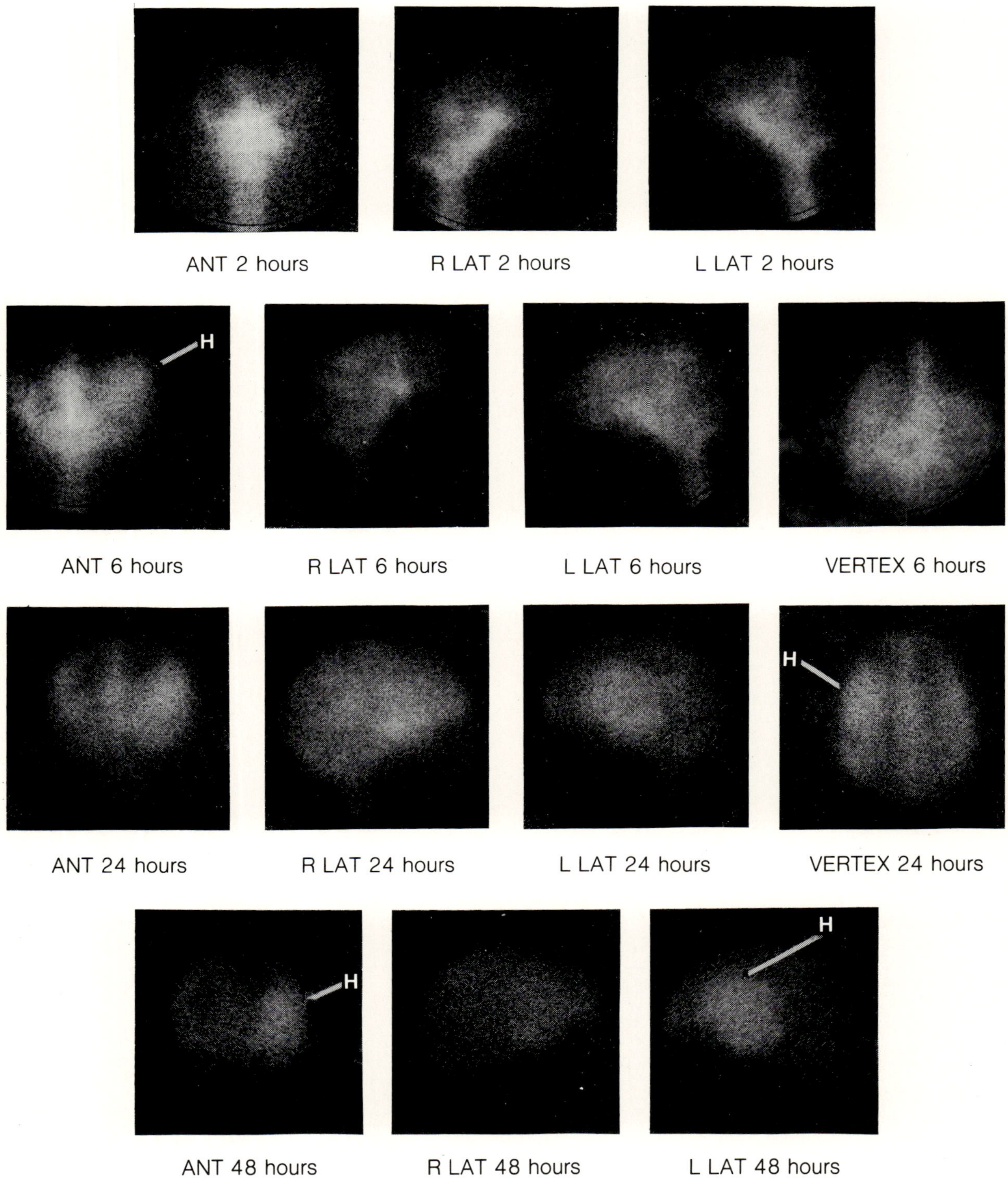


H = SUBDURAL HYGROMA

**FIG. 10.** (See legend next page)

**FIG. 10. SUBDURAL HYGROMA.** A lesion peripheral to the subarachnoid space can contain CSF through communicating channels. Subdural hygromas resulting from tears of the arachnoid membrane may be seen during cisternography.

**EXAMPLE.** A 61-year-old male with head injury had persistent headaches and mental confusion. Evaluation included cerebral angiography, which demonstrated posterior and medial displacement of the left sylvian vessels by an avascular extracerebral mass.

**COMMENT.** The cisternogram demonstrates an abnormal collection of radionuclide in the left frontotemporal region. There is atypical migration in this area at 2 hours, followed by abnormally increased accumulation at 6 hours. The activity is most pronounced at 48 hours because of further accumulation of radionuclide within the hygroma. There is also transient ventricular activity with delayed migration. Pneumoencephalography was performed, and the delayed film at 4 hours showed air in the hygroma.

## Suggested Reading


Enzmann, Norman D, Price DC, et al: Metrizamide and radionuclide cisternography. Radiology 130:681–686, 1979

Harbert JC, McCullough DC, Schellinger D: Computed cranial tomography and radionuclide cisternography in hydrocephalus. Semin Nucl Med 7:197–200, 1977

Harbert JC: Radionuclide cisternography in adult hydrocephalus. Proc R Soc Med 66:827–830, 1973

Hosain F, Som P: Chelated $^{111}$In: an ideal radiopharmaceutical for cisternography. Br J Radiol 45:677–679, 1972

James AE, Jr.: Cerebrospinal Fluid Imaging (Cisternography). In Gottschalk A, Potchen FJ (eds): *Diagnostic Nuclear Medicine.* Baltimore, Williams and Wilkins, 1976, pp 303–340

James AE, Jr., DeLand FH, Hodges FJ, et al: CSF imaging, anatomical considerations. Amer J Roentgen 110:74–87, 1970

Lusins J, Nakagawa H, Sorek M, et al: Cisternography and CT scanning with $^{111}$In-DTPA in evaluation of posterior fossa arachnoid cysts. Clin Nucl Med 4:161–163, 1979

Sty JR, Babbitt DP, D'Souza B: Pediatric radionuclide ventriculography. Clin Nucl Med 4:417–421, 1979

Welch DM, Coleman RE, Siegel BA: Cisternography imaging patterns: effects of partial extra-arachnoid radiopharmaceutical injection and post injection CSF leakage. J Nucl Med 16:267–269, 1975

# 8/ Blood Flow Studies

Blood vessels may be imaged with a remarkable degree of detail with techniques of nuclear medicine. Identification of major arteries and veins is now commonly performed with radionuclide angiography and venography.

Blood flow studies usually involve the sequential imaging of a particular area at intervals of 1 to 3 seconds following the intravenous injection of a radioactive material. Since the radionuclide is administered through the venous route, it is the large venous structures that may be seen in greatest detail (e.g., superior and inferior vena cava, innominate veins). However, dynamic imaging during the arterial phase results in excellent visualization of many arterial structures, such as the abdominal aorta and major cerebral arteries.

A large number of blood flow studies have been presented and discussed in preceding chapters. The extent to which radionuclide angiography and venography may be employed for blood vessel visualization is almost limitless. Commonly encountered situations in which radionuclide blood flow studies may be usefully employed are presented in this chapter. This coverage is by no means exhaustive, and it should be borne in mind that there are myriads of other entities that merit the application of radionuclide angiography and venography.

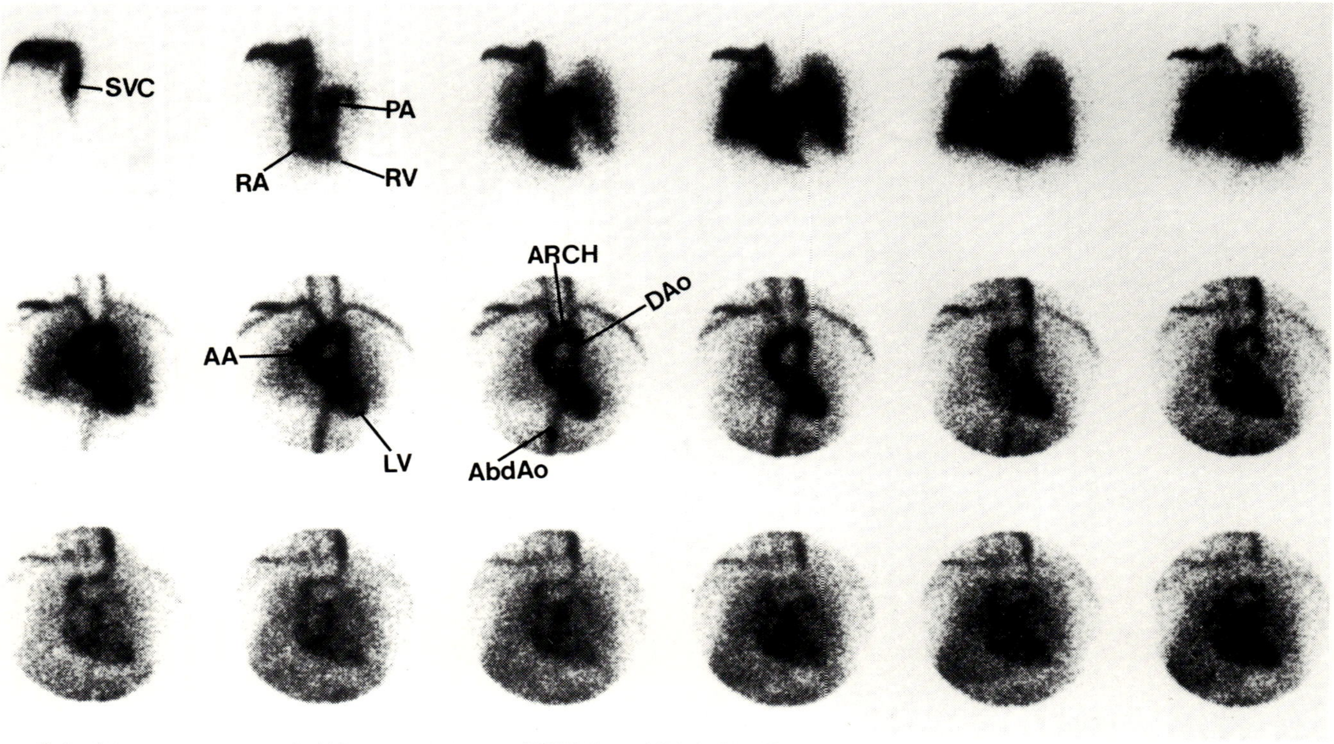


Anterior Blood Flow

**FIG. 1. NORMAL CARDIAC BLOOD FLOW IMAGING.** Following the intravenous injection of Tc-99m in a right upper extremity vein, there is early visualization of the superior vena cava (**SVC**), right atrium (**RA**), right ventricle (**RV**), and main pulmonary artery (**PA**). Following pulmonary arterial perfusion and return of blood via the pulmonary veins to the left heart, there is identification of the left ventricle (**LV**), ascending aorta (**AAo**), arch of the aorta (**ARCH**), descending thoracic aorta (**DAo**), and abdominal aorta (**AbdAo**). Note the continuous visualization and superimposition of arterial and venous structures in the later frames (framing rate: 2 seconds/frame) (Tc-99m-labeled red blood cells).

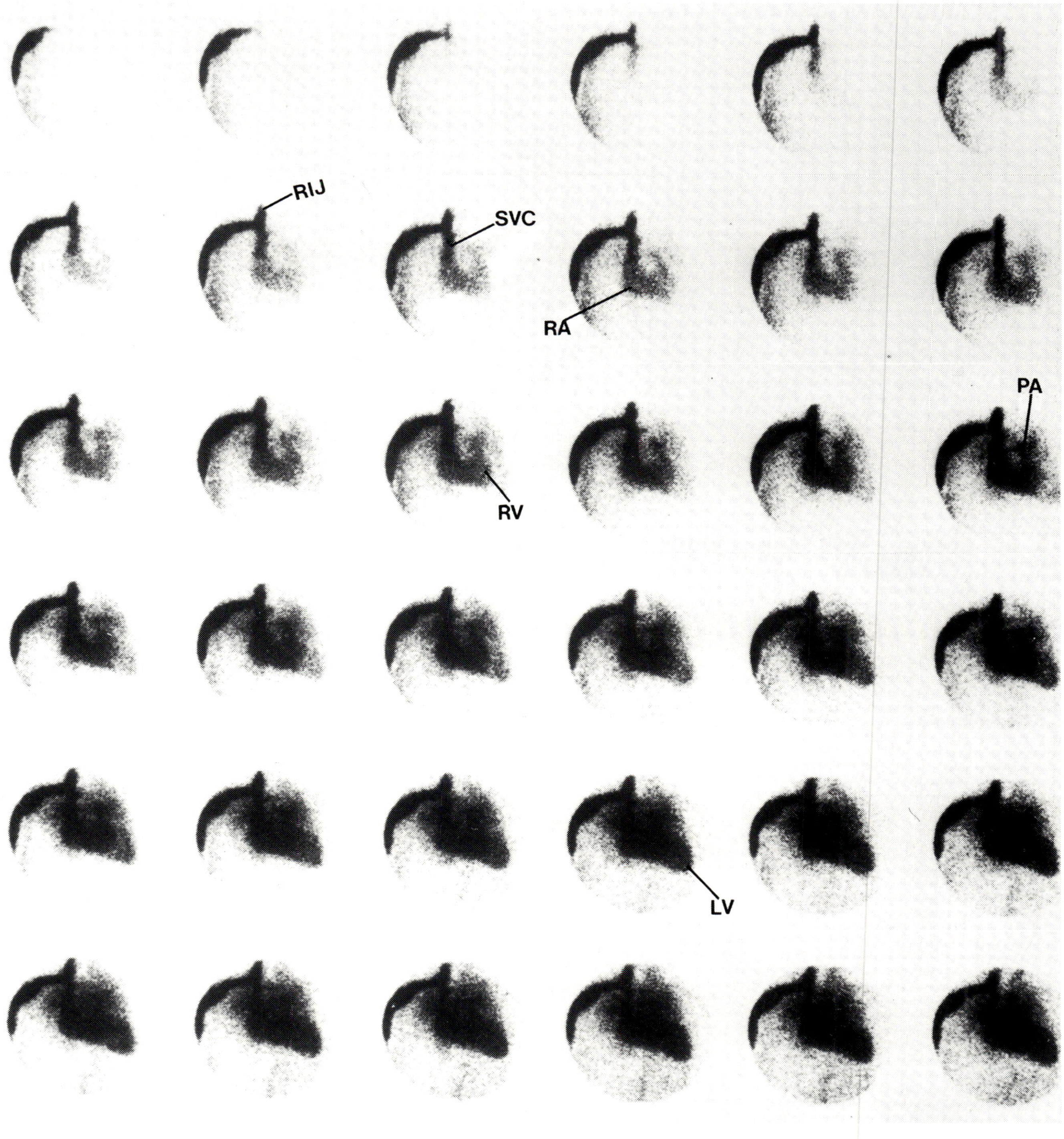


**FIG. 2. ELEVATED SYSTEMIC VENOUS PRESSURE AND CONGESTIVE HEART FAILURE.** There is marked prolongation of the circulation time of the radioactive material. Among the features seen are reflux into the right internal jugular vein (**RIJ**), prolonged visualization of the superior vena cava (**SVC**), slow filling of the right atrium (**RA**) and right ventricle (**RV**), and unusual prolongation in the visualization of the main pulmonary artery (**PA**). There is late identification of the left ventricle (**LV**) (framing rate: 2 seconds/frame) (Tc-99m-labeled red blood cells).

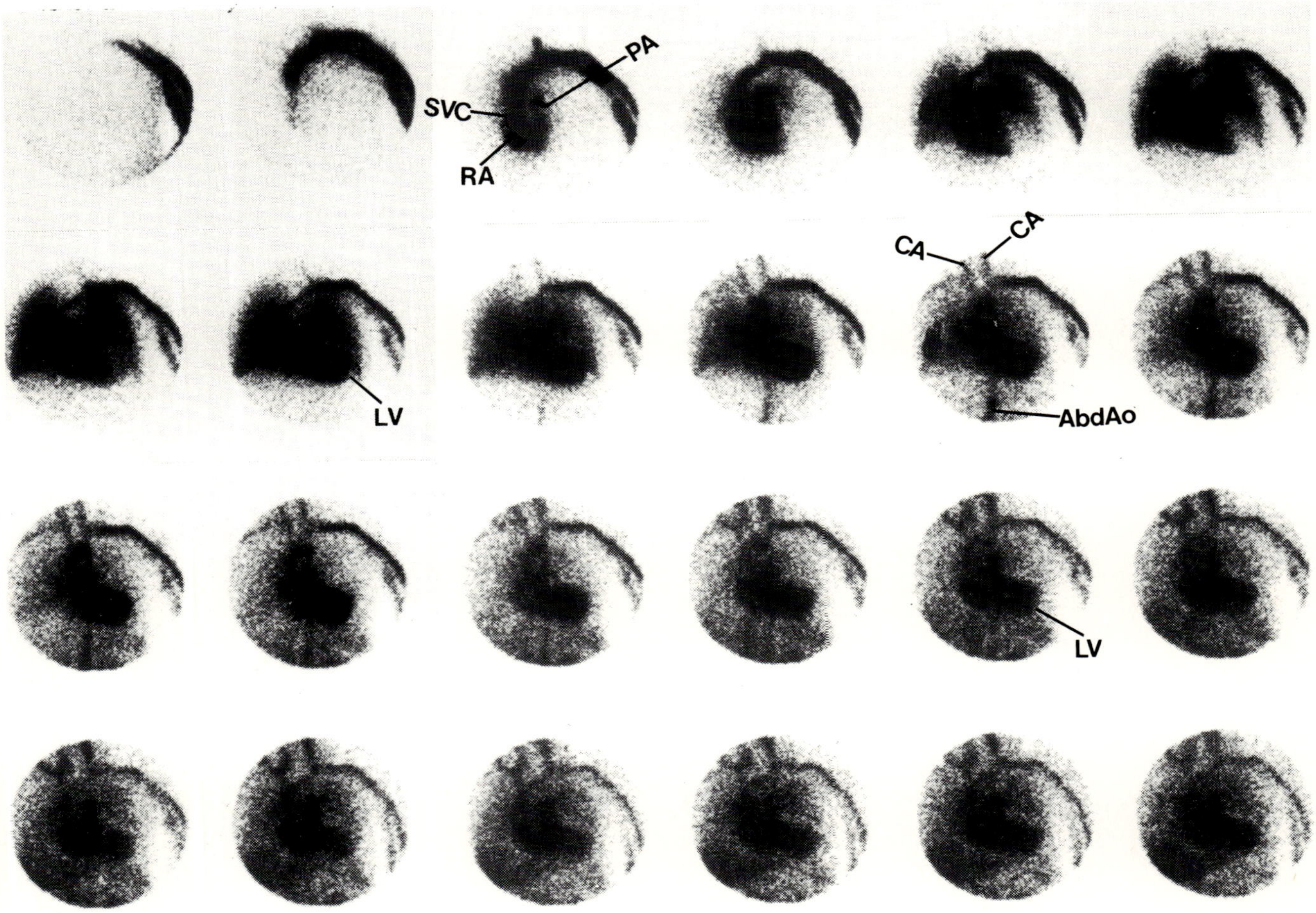


Anterior Blood Flow

**FIG. 3. ANEURYSM OF LEFT VENTRICLE.** Persistence of radioactivity in an enlarged left ventricle usually is seen with a left ventricular aneurysm. During the venous phase, the superior vena cava (**SVC**), right atrium (**RA**), and pulmonary artery (**PA**) are visible. Following the return of blood to the heart through the pulmonary veins, there is prompt visualization of the left ventricle (**LV**), ascending aorta, aortic arch, both common carotid arteries (**CA**), descending thoracic aorta, and abdominal aorta (**AbdAo**). There is persistence in the imaging of the left ventricle throughout, due to aneurysm formation at that site (framing rate: 2 seconds/frame) (Tc-99m sodium pertechnetate).

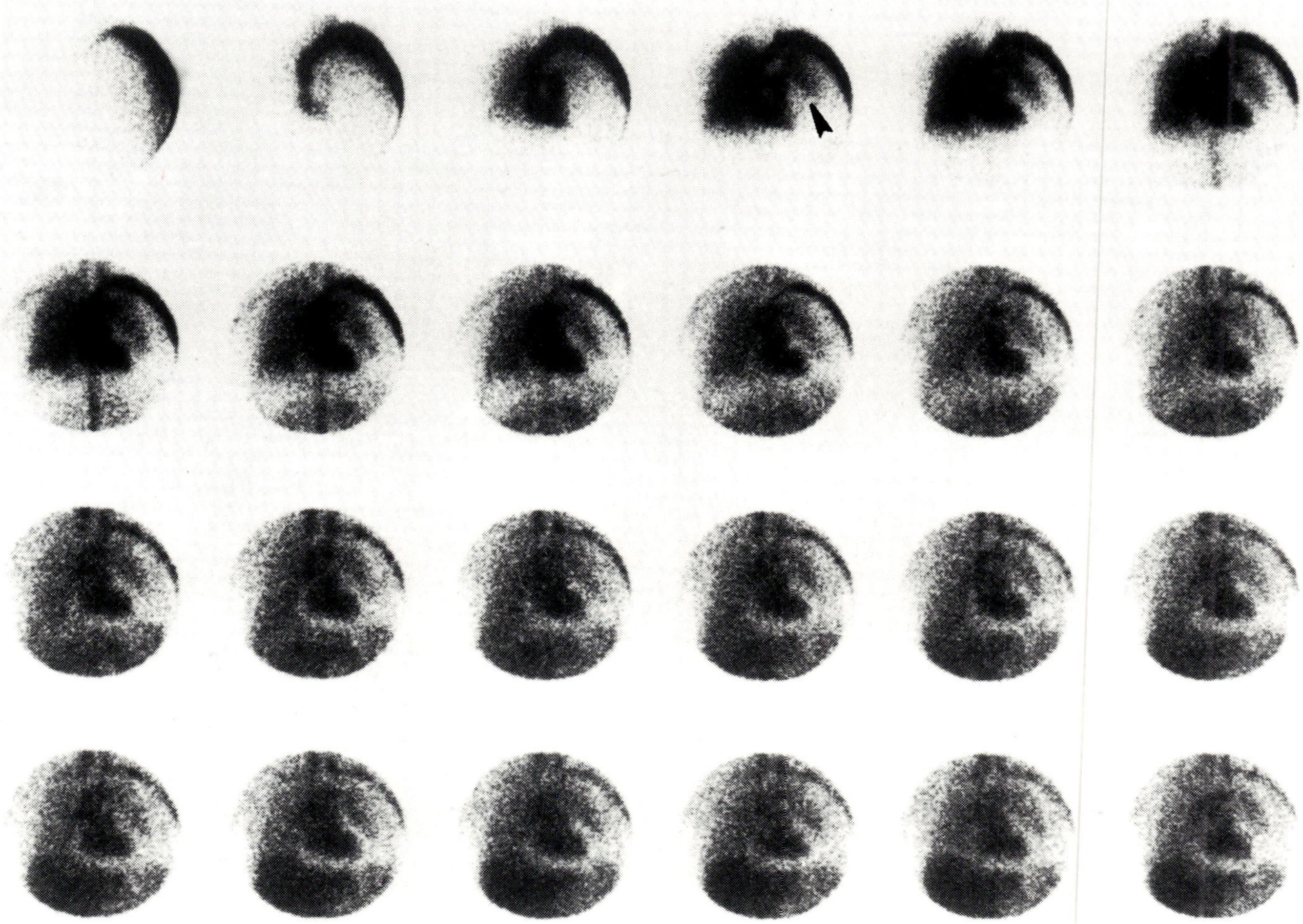

Anterior Blood Flow

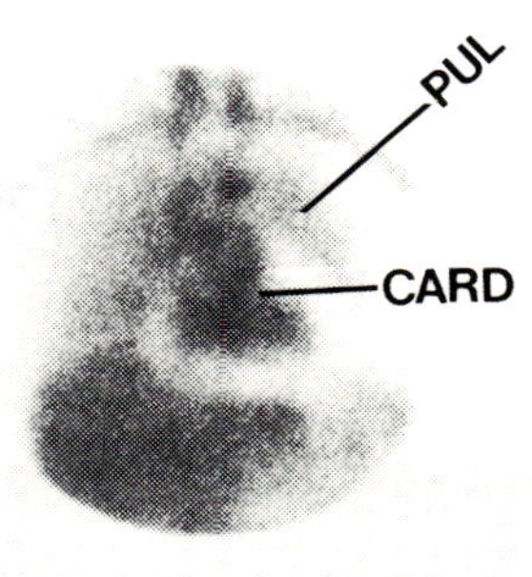


Anterior, Static

**FIG. 4.** (See legend next page)

**FIG. 4. PERICARDIAL EFFUSION.** The "halo" of absent radioactivity due to the presence of the pericardial effusion is visible as early as frame 4 (arrow). Subsequent imaging shows the well-defined area of absent radioactivity surrounding the heart (frame 18). In this case, imaging was performed with Tc-99m-labeled red blood cells. When the study is performed with pertechnetate, there may be diffusion of the tracer into the pericardial space, and on subsequent static imaging, there may be an inability to demonstrate the area of the effusion. This is not so with Tc-99m-labeled red blood cells, since this radionuclide is normally confined to the intravascular space (framing rate: 2 seconds/frame) (Tc-99m-labeled red blood cells).

Static imaging performed in the anterior position immediately following the blood flow study demonstrates the area of the effusion even more clearly. The clear space of absent radioactivity between the cardiac vascular pool (**CARD**) and the pulmonary (**PUL**) and hepatic vascularity defines the pericardial effusion.

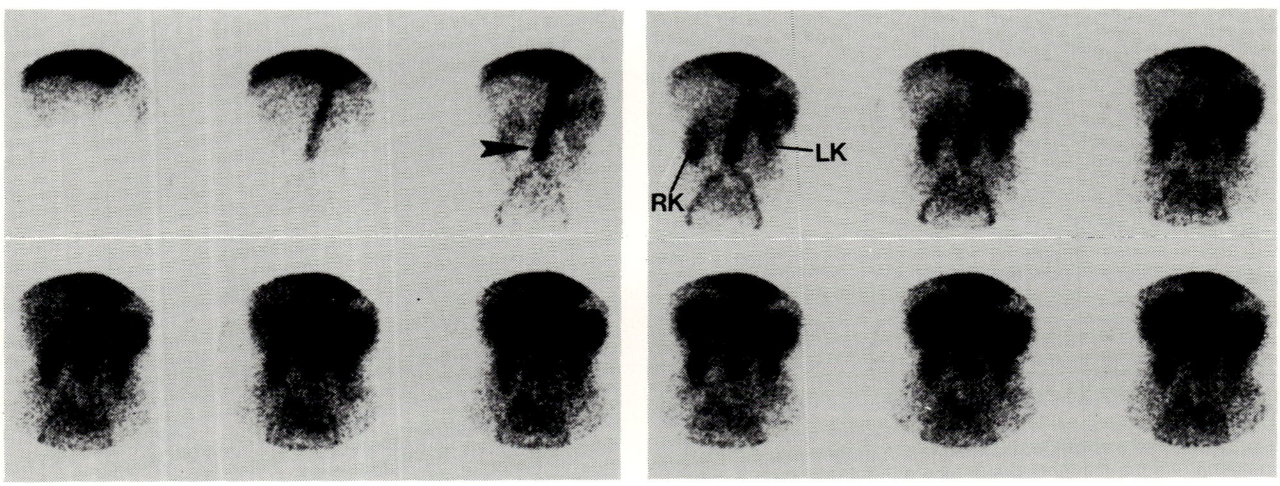


Anterior Blood Flow

**FIG. 5. ANEURYSM OF ABDOMINAL AORTA SEEN ON ANTERIOR BLOOD FLOW STUDY.** Identification of the aneurysm of the distal abdominal aorta (arrow) is made during the arterial phase. Note the persistent visualization in the early venous phase. Despite the aneurysm, there is arterial perfusion of both the right and left kidneys (**RK, LK**) (framing rate: 3 seconds/frame) (Tc-99m diphosphonate).

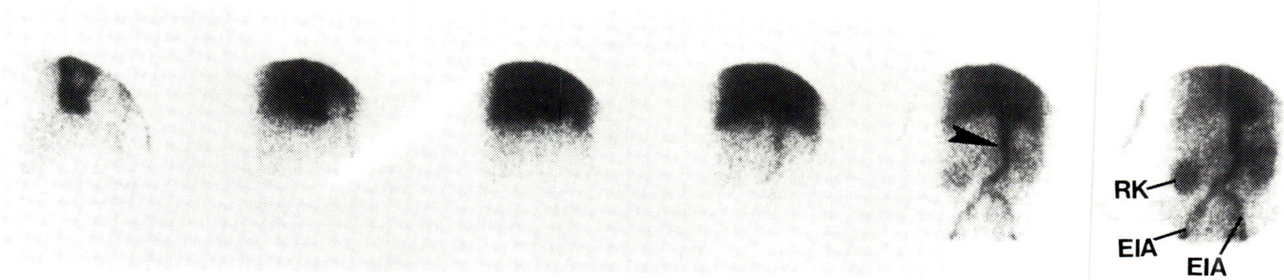


**FIG. 6. MARKED TORTUOSITY OF THE ABDOMINAL AORTA.** Irregularity of the distal abdominal aorta (arrow) can be recognized early in the arterial phase. Note the inferior location of the right kidney (**RK**) and the visualization of the external iliac arteries (**EIA**) (framing rate: 3 seconds/frame) (Tc-99m sodium pertechnetate).

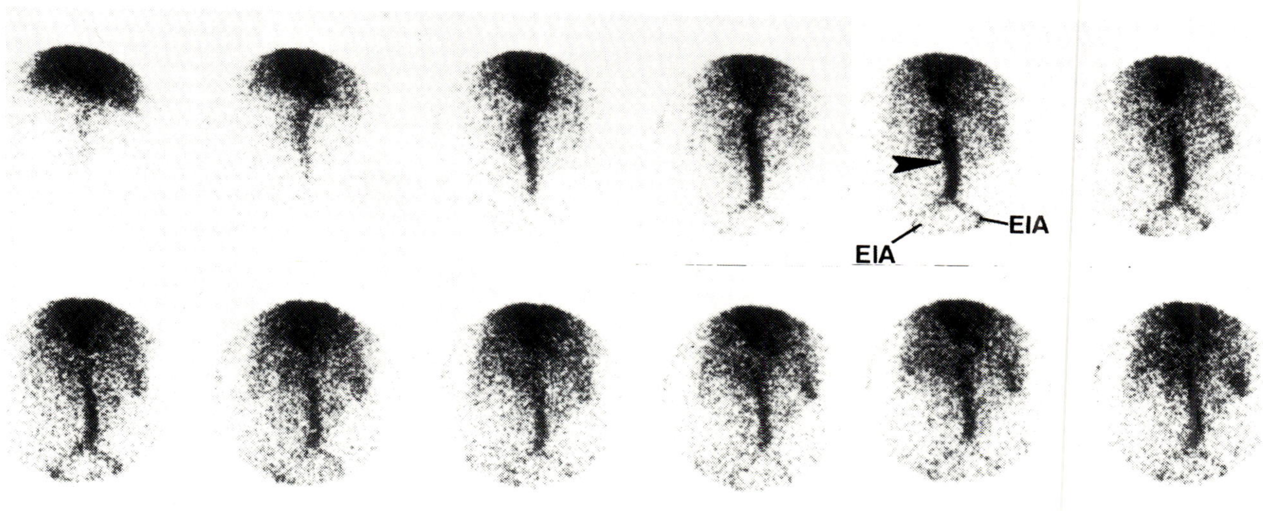


**FIG. 7. VISUALIZATION OF AORTIC GRAFT PROSTHESIS.** An abdominal aortic aneurysm was resected in this patient and a Teflon graft inserted. The site of the inserted graft is identified as the long area of persistently increased radioactivity (arrow). The distal patency of the graft is demonstrated by the visualization of the external iliac arteries (**EIA**). This blood flow study was performed in conjunction with liver–spleen imaging (framing rate: 3 seconds/frame) (Tc-99m sulfur colloid).

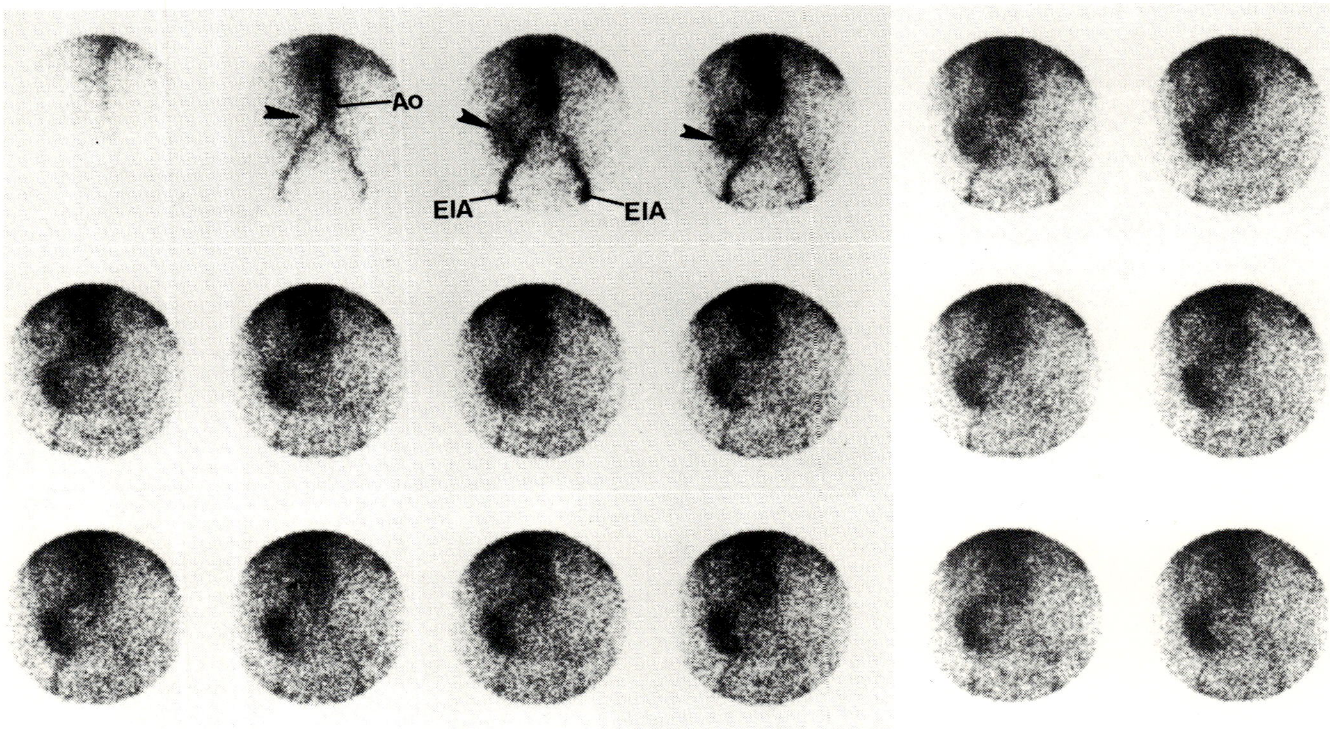


**FIG. 8. DETERMINING PATENCY OF ARTERIAL SUPPLY TO A TRANSPLANTED KIDNEY.** Serial imaging during the arterial phase (frames 2, 3, and 4) shows evidence of arterial perfusion to the transplanted kidney (arrows). The abdominal aorta (**Ao**) and external iliac arteries (**EIA**) are clearly identified at this time (framing rate: 3 seconds/frame) (Tc-99m-DTPA).

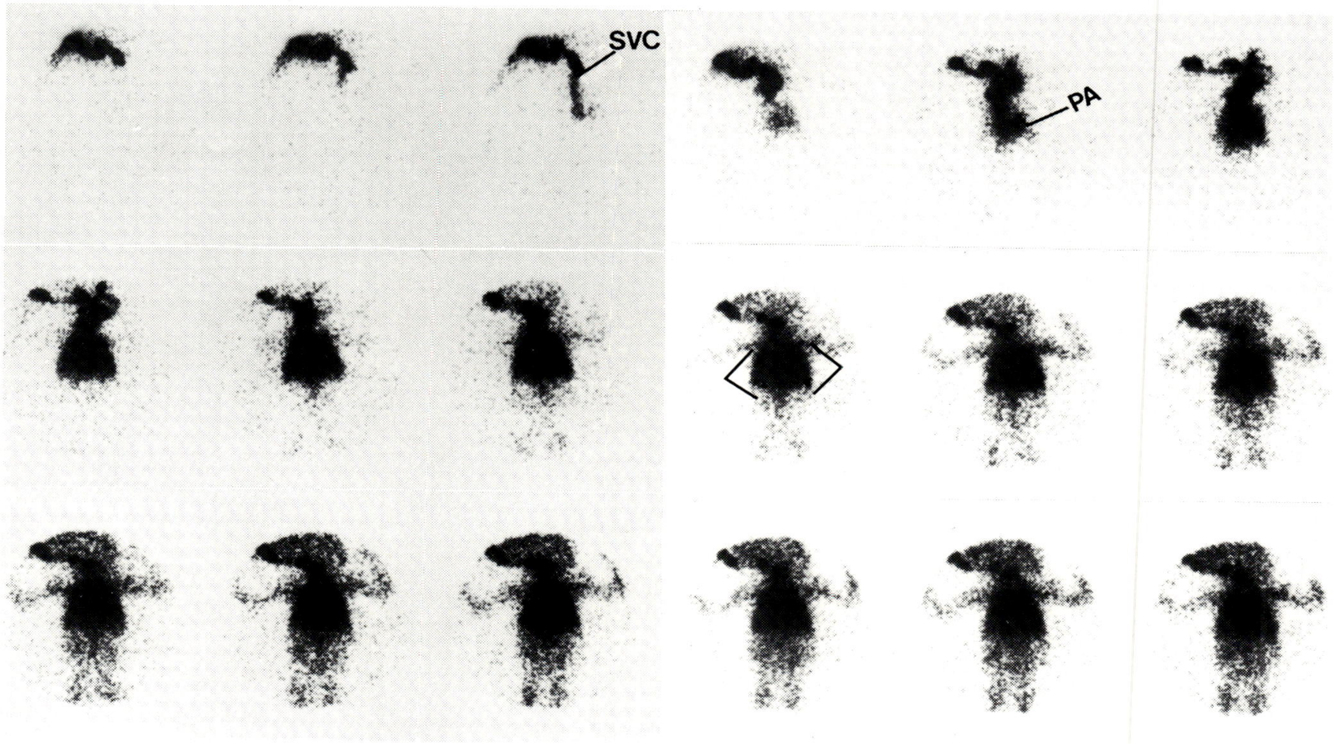


Anterior Blood Flow

**FIG. 9. LEFT-TO-RIGHT SHUNT IN AN INFANT (PATENT DUCTUS ARTERIOSUS).** This blood flow study was performed in conjunction with liver–spleen imaging. The superior vena cava (**SVC**) and main pulmonary artery (**PA**) are visualized on early studies. Following initial pulmonary perfusion, there is continuous pulmonary visualization (brackets) as the radioactive material leaving the left ventricle and ascending aorta is returned to the pulmonary artery through the patent ductus arteriosus. The continued pulmonary imaging makes cardiac identification impossible (framing rate: 2 seconds/frame) (Tc-99m sulfur colloid).

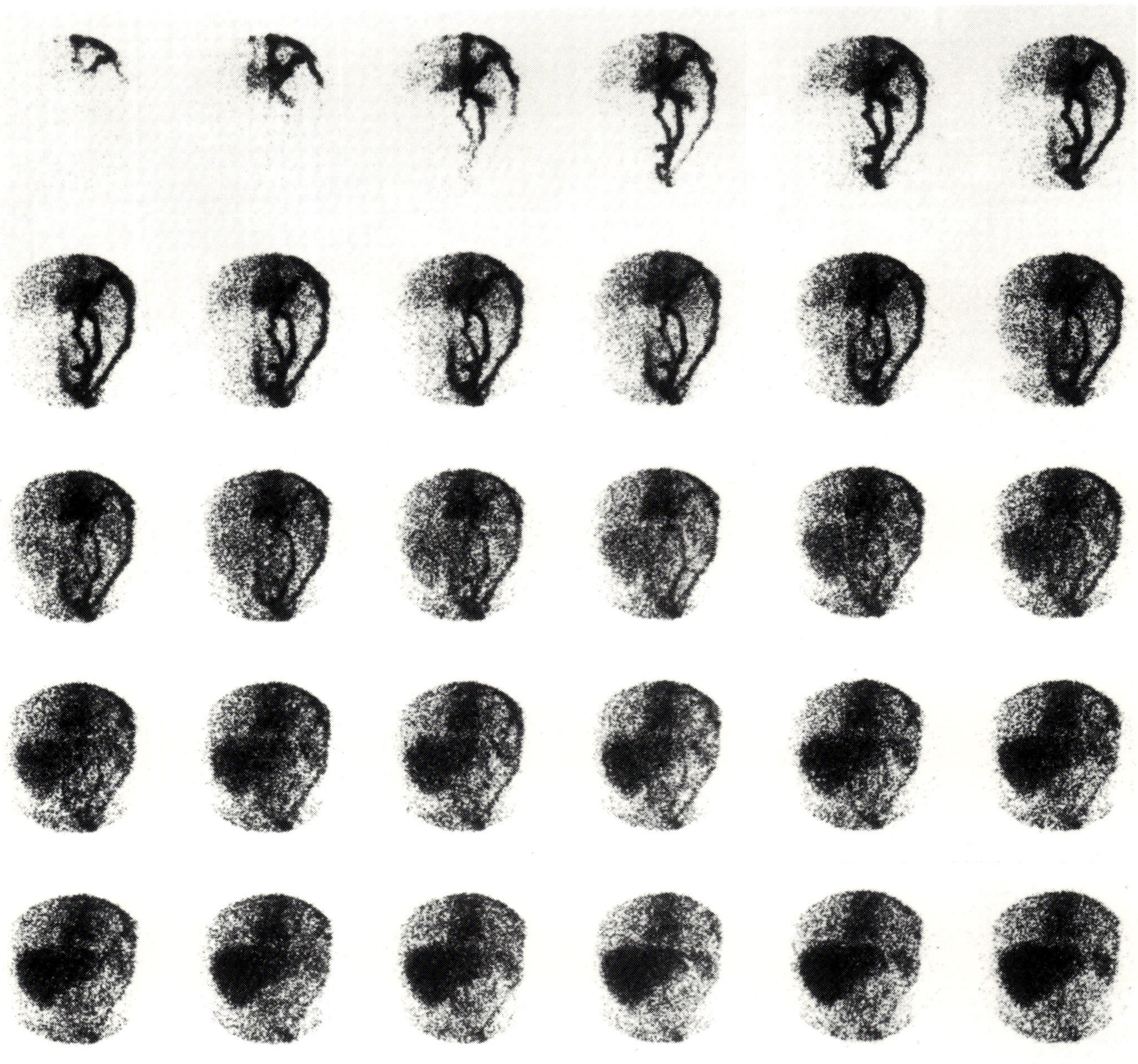


**FIG. 10, A.** (See legend next page)

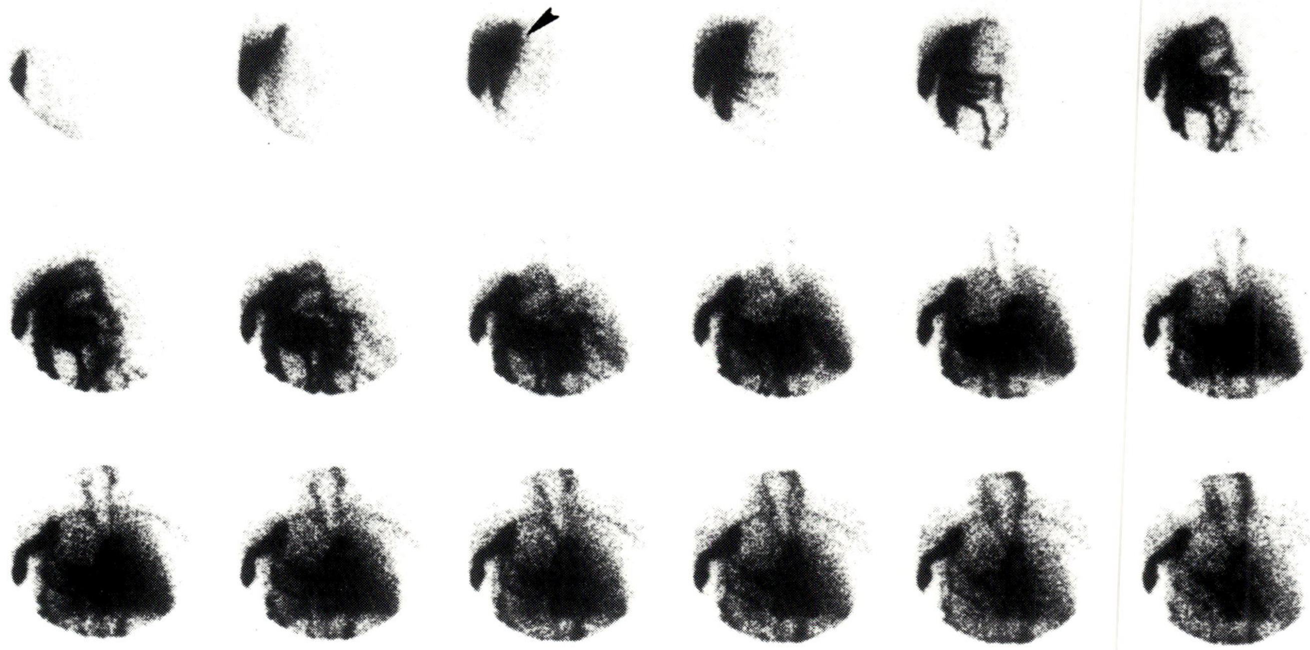

B

Anterior Blood Flow

**FIG. 10. SUPERIOR VENA CAVA SYNDROME WITH RIGHT SUBCLAVIAN VEIN AND SUPERIOR VENA CAVA OBSTRUCTION.** The initial imaging evidence that suggested the presence of a superior vena cava syndrome came at the time of the blood flow study performed in conjunction with Tc-99m sulfur colloid liver imaging (**A**). The network of extensive collaterals visible almost immediately after radionuclide injection in a left upper extremity vein suggested the nature of the abnormality. The patient was found to have a lung carcinoma of the right upper lobe (framing rate: 3 seconds/frame). **B.** Blood flow study following right upper extremity injection shows blockage in the region of the right subclavian vein (arrow) with extensive collateral vessels. **C.** Injection in a left upper extremity vein demonstrates the incomplete obstruction of the superior vena cava (arrow) (framing rate: 2 seconds/frame) (**B** and **C**, Tc-99m sodium pertechnetate).

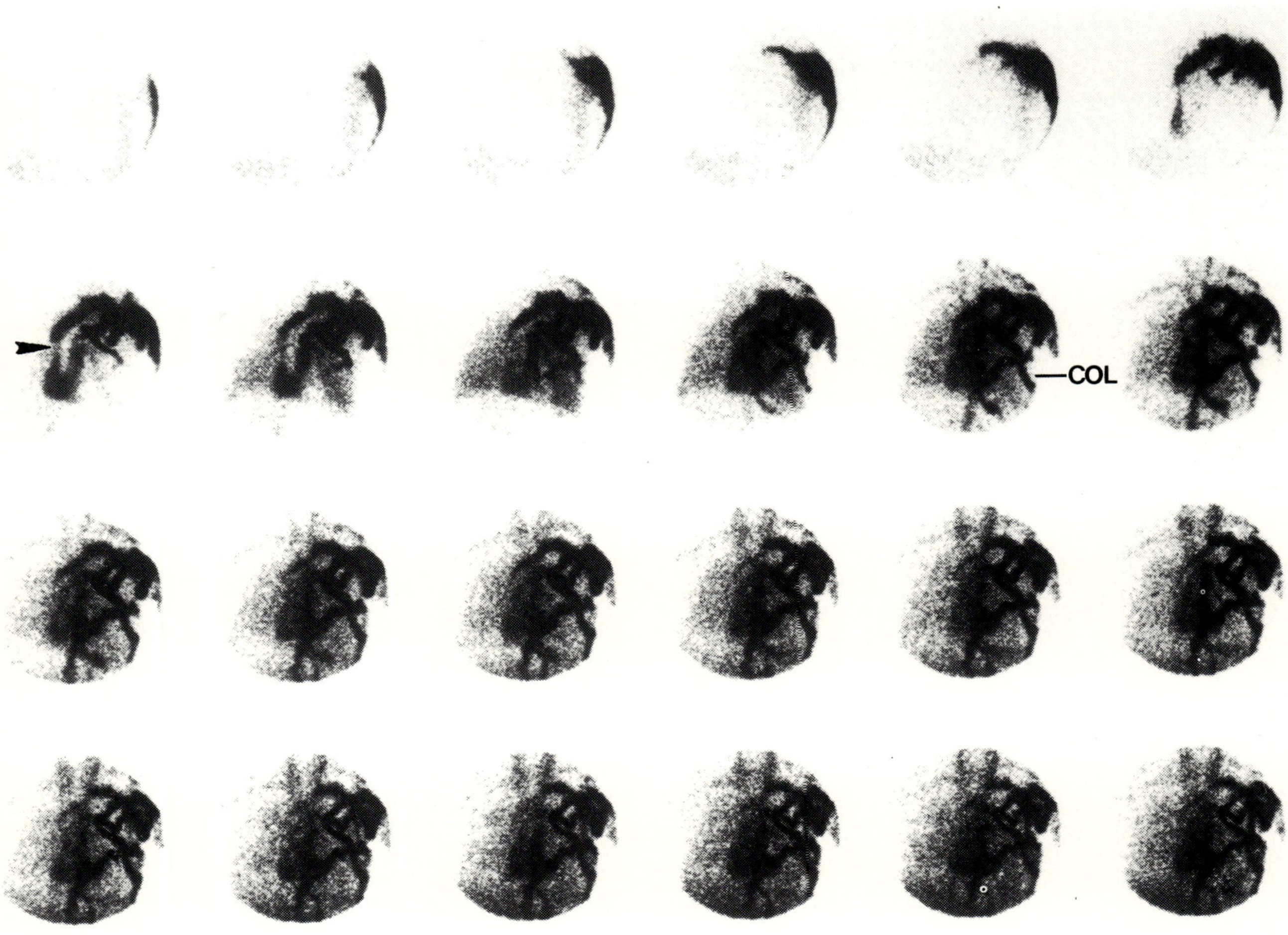


C Anterior Blood Flow

**FIG. 10. C.** (See legend previous page)

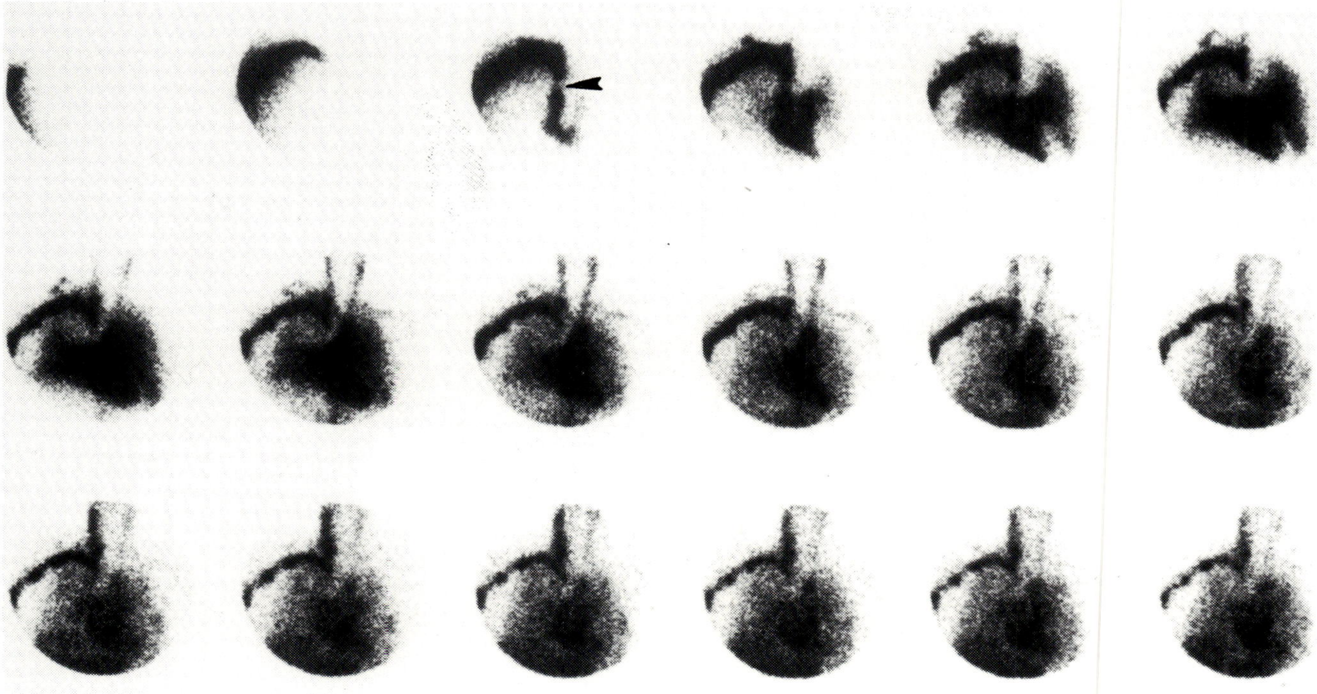

A

Anterior Blood Flow

**FIG. 11. SUPERIOR VENA CAVA CONSTRICTION, LEFT INNOMINATE VEIN OBSTRUCTION.** This patient had lung carcinoma of the right upper lobe with associated venous blockade. **A.** Blood flow study performed after right upper extremity injection shows evidence of superior vena cava constriction (arrow) as early as frame 3, and that constriction continues to be visualized. However, there is continued flow through the constricted superior vena cava without collateral formation. **B.** Blood flow study performed after left upper extremity injection shows evidence of venous blockade (arrow) in the region of the left innominate vein with numerous collateral veins demonstrated (some designated by **COL**). The area of the constricted superior vena cava (arrow) is again identified (framing rate: 2 seconds/frame).

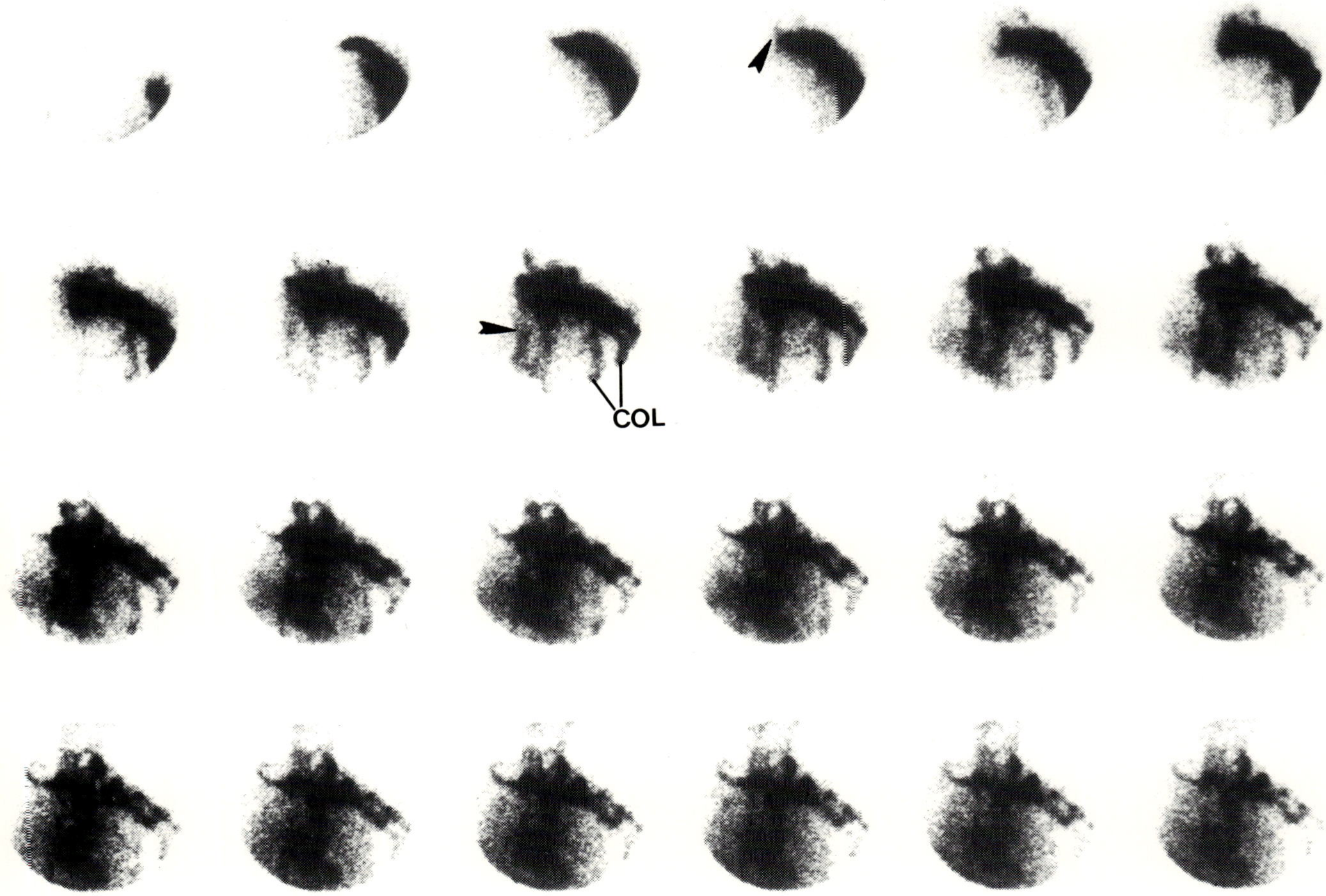


B

Anterior Blood Flow

**FIG. 11. B.** (See legend previous page)

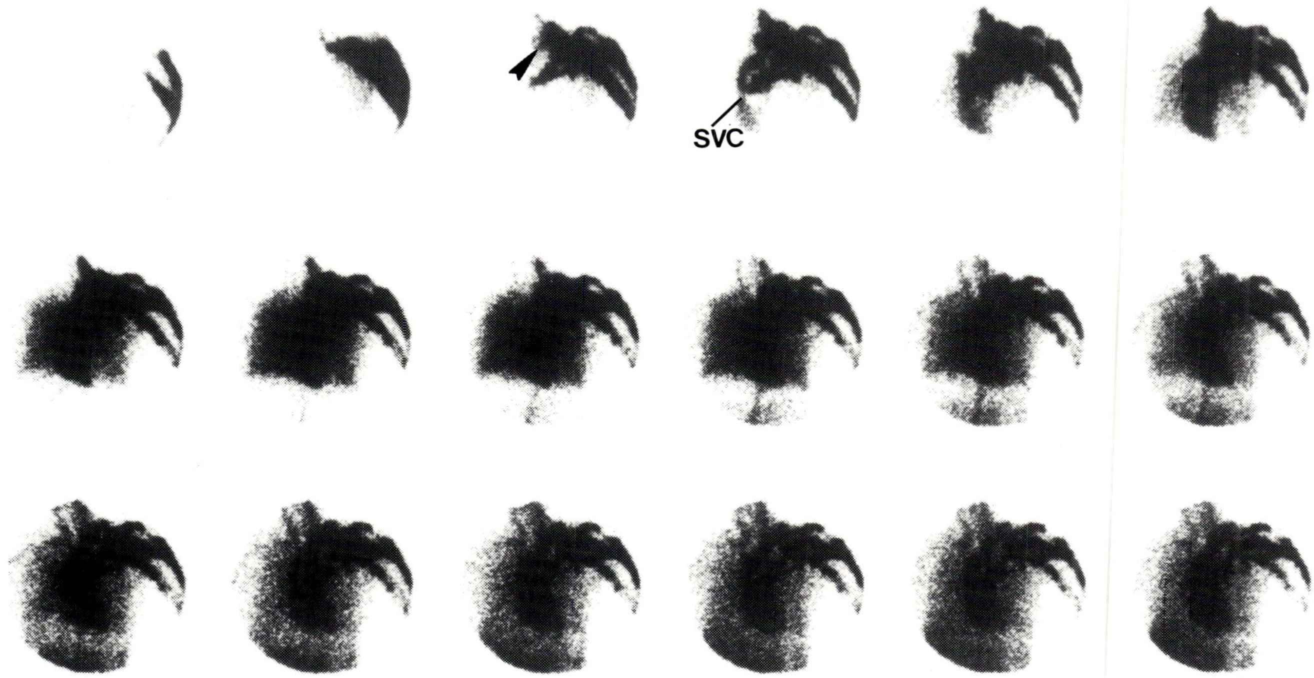


A Anterior Blood Flow

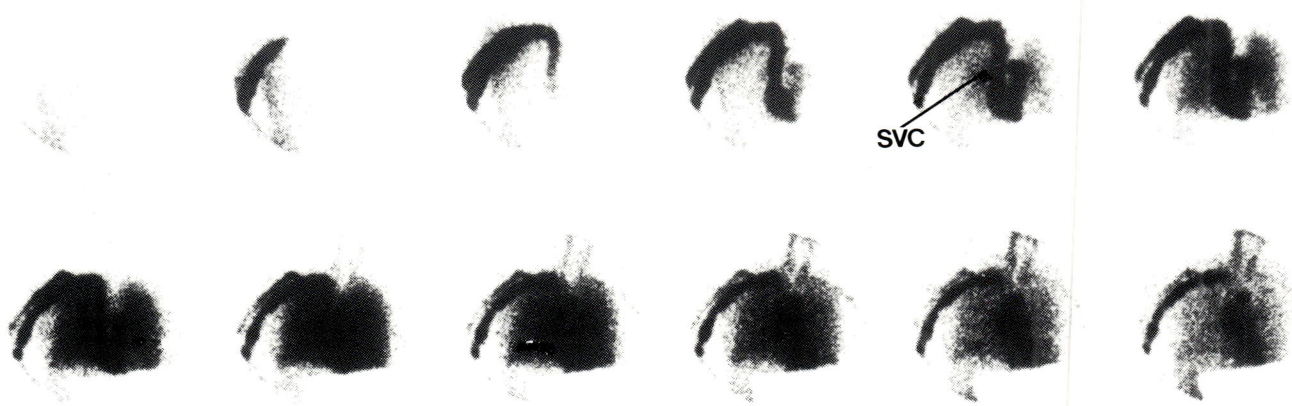


B Anterior Blood Flow

**FIG. 12. IDENTIFYING THE SITE OF VENOUS OBSTRUCTION.** The location of the venous obstruction in this 30-year-old woman with dilated neck veins was uncertain prior to radionuclide blood flow studies. **A.** Imaging performed following a left upper extremity injection shows no flow in the region of the left subclavian vein (arrow) in addition to multiple collateral veins. The superior vena cava (**SVC**) appears to be supplied from collateral vessels. **B.** Blood flow study after radionuclide administration in a right upper extremity vein shows no evidence of venous obstruction. The superior vena cava (**SVC**) shows direct filling (framing rate: 2 seconds/frame) (Tc-99m sodium pertechnetate).

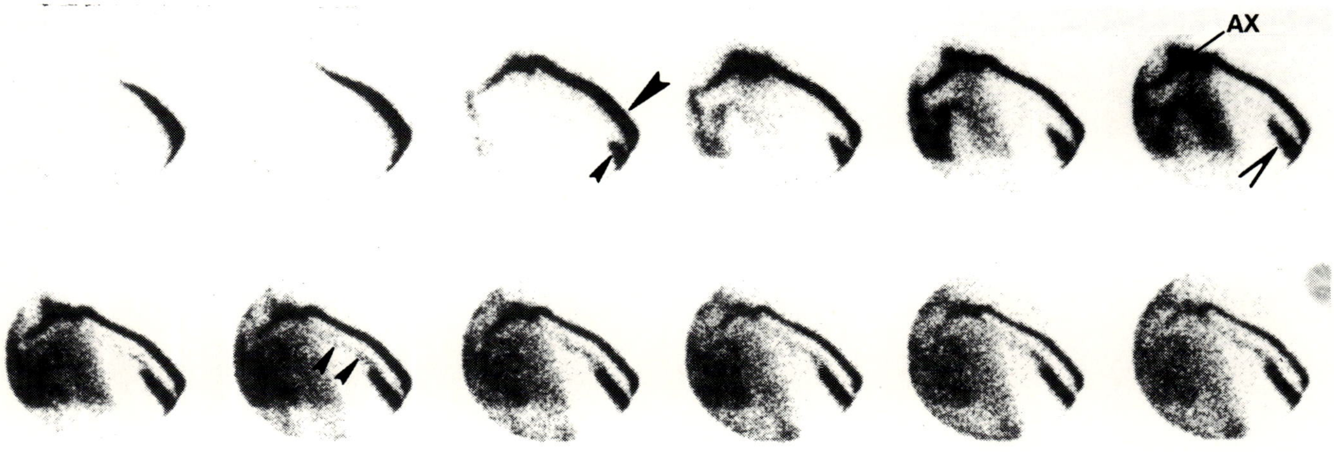


Anterior Blood Flow

**FIG. 13. LEFT BASILIC VEIN OBSTRUCTION.** Following intravenous injection of the radioactive material in an antecubital vein, radioactivity is visible in the basilic (arrow) and cephalic ( larger arrow) veins. Note the point of obstruction in the left basilic vein (open arrow) secondary to thrombus formation. The site of the axillary (**AX**) vein is also identified. The obstruction in the left basilic vein and some visualization of the balance of the left basilic vein and its entry into the axillary vein can be seen (small arrows) (framing rate: 2 seconds/frame) (Tc-99m sodium pertechnetate).

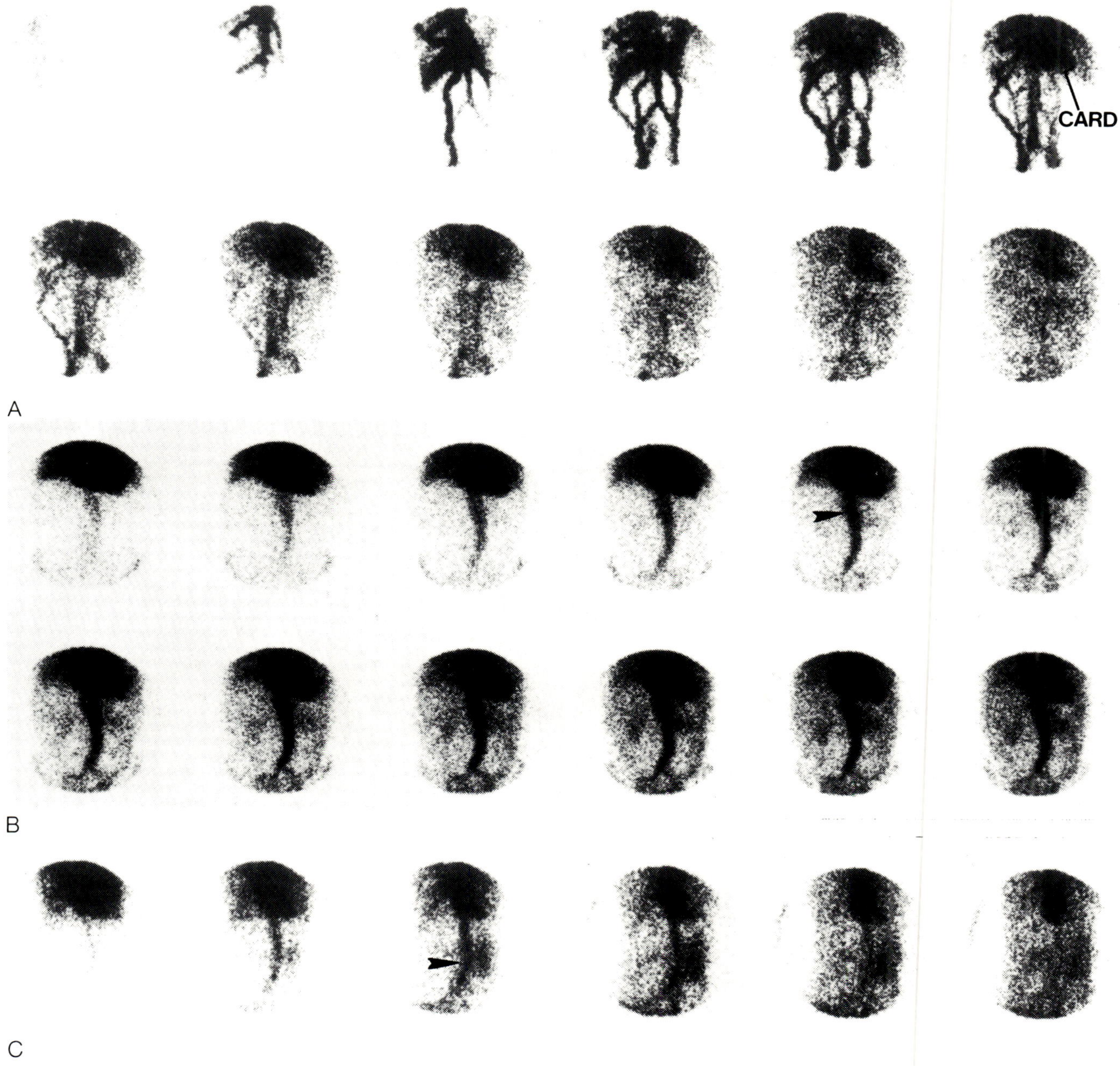


**FIG. 14. VASCULAR ABNORMALITIES SEEN ON BLOOD FLOW STUDIES IN CONJUNCTION WITH LIVER–SPLEEN IMAGING.** Even though a relatively small dose of radioactive material was injected in these cases (3 mCi Tc-99m sulfur colloid), the vascular abnormalities were easily detected. **A.** Extensive superficial collateral vein formation secondary to superior vena cava obstruction. Following the initial appearance of collateral veins, entry of radioactive material into the heart (**CARD**) is visible, and there is ultimately hepatic identification as the radioactive colloid is delivered to the liver via the portal veins. **B.** Visualization of large aortic aneurysm (arrows) during arterial phase. **C.** Marked deviation (arrow) of aorta (framing rate: 3 seconds/frame).

## RADIONUCLIDE PULMONARY ARTERIOGRAPHY

Radionuclide pulmonary arteriography offers a unique method for visualizing the main pulmonary artery and its major branches. Following the intravenous administration of a radiopharmaceutical used for perfusion lung imaging, such as Tc-99m albumin microspheres or macroaggregated serum albumin, dynamic studies are performed and images obtained at frequent intervals (1 to 2 seconds) as the radioactive material travels from a peripheral vein to the right heart and then to the pulmonary artery and its branches. Since the radionuclides administered consist of tagged particles (average diameter 10 to 50$\mu$) that are larger in diameter than the pulmonary capillaries (average diameter 7$\mu$) and precapillary arterioles (average diameter 35$\mu$), the radioactive material becomes lodged in these small vessels. Thus, the radioactive particles do not return to the heart via the pulmonary veins and do not enter the systemic circulation. The radionuclide pulmonary arteriogram is done in conjunction with perfusion lung imaging. (Figures 15-20 are from Baum S, d'Avignon MB, Latshaw RF: Clin Nucl Med 4:461, 1979)

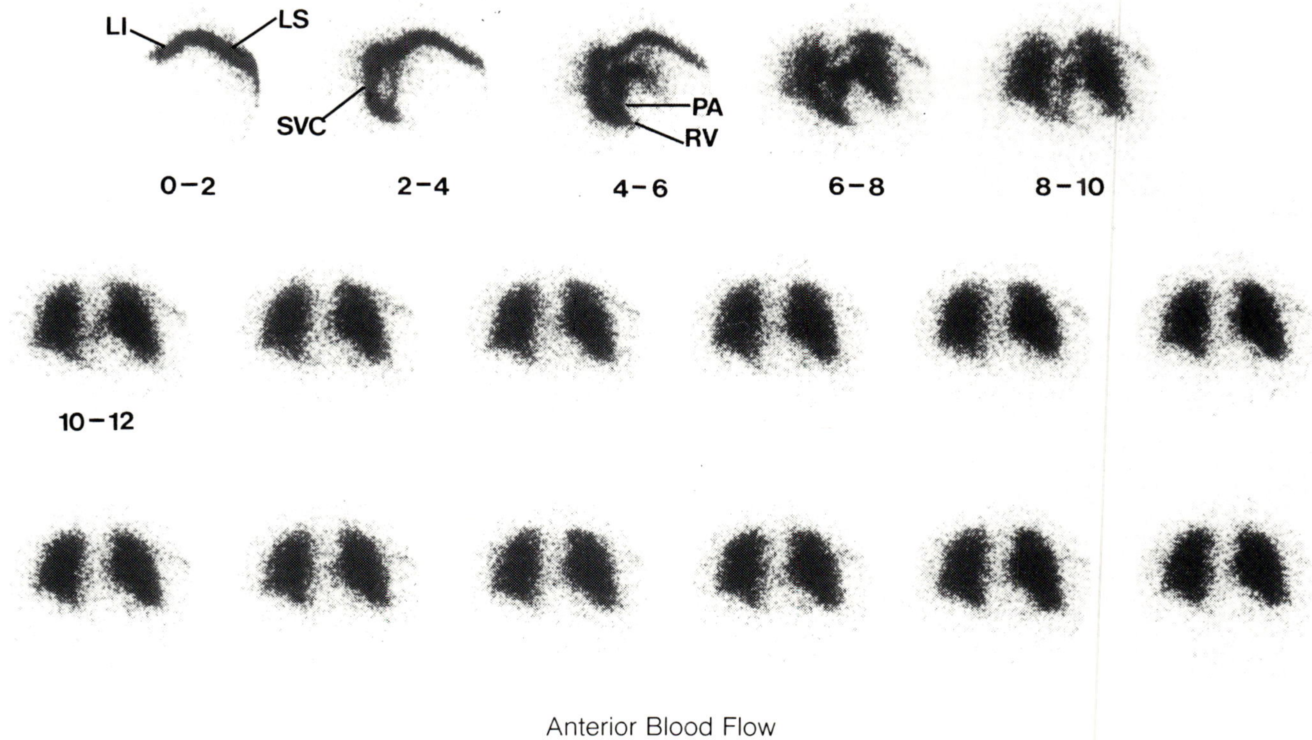


**FIG. 15.** NORMAL RADIONUCLIDE PULMONARY ARTERIOGRAM. A number of vascular structures may be readily and clearly identified. In this normal study, the left innominate vein, superior vena cava, right atrium, and right ventricle are demonstrated as the radionuclide courses through them. The radioactive material has been injected in a left upper extremity vein, and images are obtained at intervals of 2 seconds. In the first frame at 0 to 2 seconds, the left subclavian (**LS**) and left innominate (**LI**) veins can be identified. At 2 to 4 seconds, the superior vena cava (**SVC**) is visible and at 4 to 6 seconds the right ventricle (**RV**) and main pulmonary artery (**PA**) can be identified. The branching into the right and left pulmonary arteries is seen at 6 to 8 seconds. Normally, the maximum duration of clear visualization of the main pulmonary artery is not more than 6 seconds; unusual prolongation of visualization may herald the onset ofor be associated with elevated pulmonary arterial pressure. The radionuclide is rapidly delivered to the peripheral branches of the pulmonary arterial tree. In this normal case, the large radioactive particles have become almost completely trapped in the pulmonary capillaries and precapillary arterioles 12 seconds following the initial appearance of radioactivity in the superior vena cava (framing interval: 2 seconds/frame).

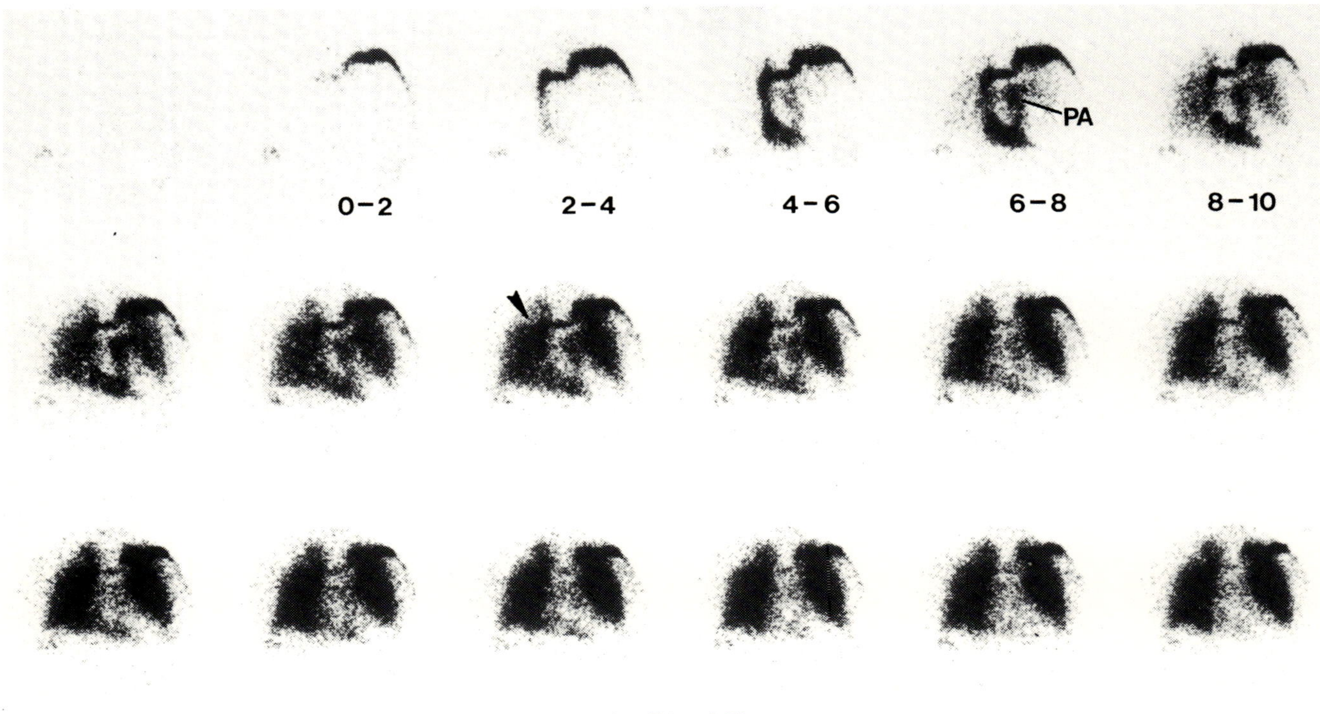


A

Anterior Blood Flow

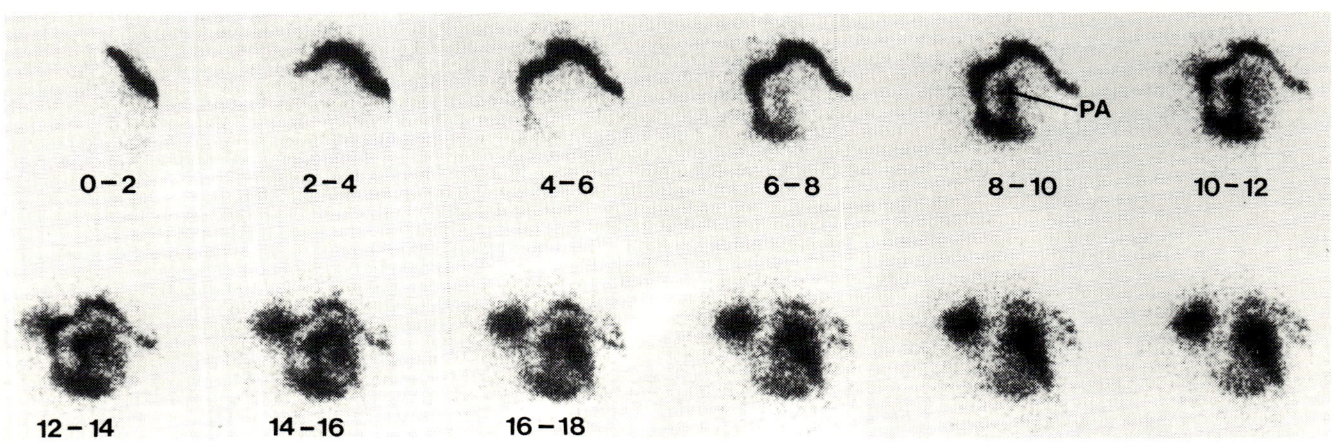


B

Anterior Blood Flow

**FIG. 16.** PULMONARY EMBOLISM. In the patient with pulmonary thromboembolism, there is usually at least a transient increase in pulmonary arterial pressure following the embolic episode. This may be reflected by prolongation in the visualization of the main pulmonary artery and may be the first imaging clue of an alteration in hemodynamics. **A. Pulmonary embolism, right upper lung field.** The main pulmonary artery (**PA**) is clearly visible at 6 to 8 seconds, and this duration of clear visualization of the main pulmonary artery is prolonged to 10 seconds. Reduced perfusion is also visible in the right lung (arrow) at the site of involvement. However, the pulmonary perfusion defect imaged on the blood flow study is not nearly so well defined as that on a static perfusion image. **B. Pulmonary embolism involving right middle and lower lobes.** The duration of visualization of the main pulmonary artery (**PA**) is prolonged to about 12 seconds. The large area of absent perfusion related to the embolic changes can be appreciated early in the blood flow study (framing interval: 2 seconds/frame).

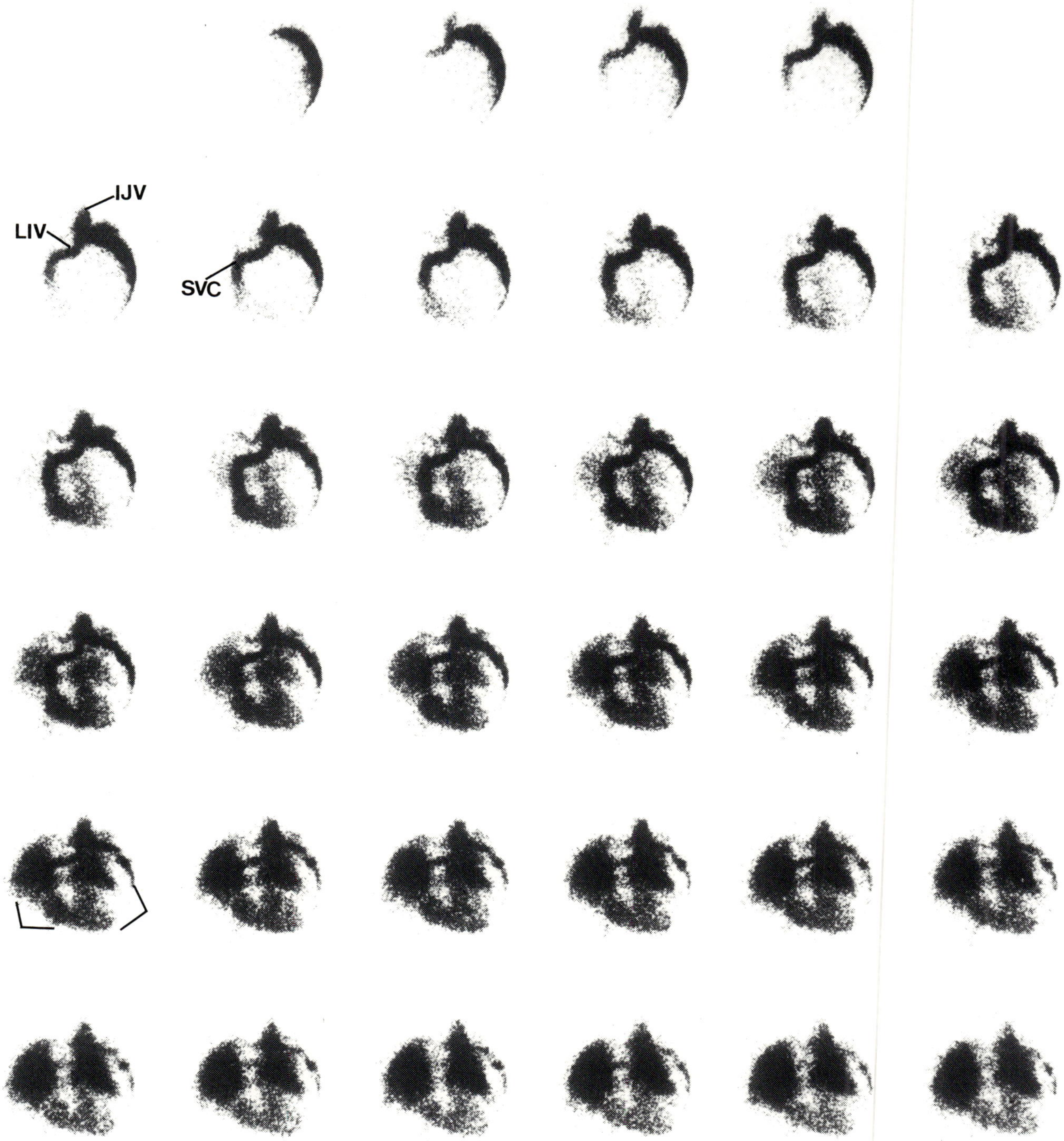


Anterior Blood Flow

**FIG. 17.** (See legend next page)

**FIG. 17. ELEVATED SYSTEMIC VENOUS PRESSURE AND CONGESTIVE HEART FAILURE.** Imaging findings related to elevated systemic venous pressure and shunting of blood to the upper lung fields may be seen in the patient with congestive heart failure. In this case, the transit of radioactive material from the left axillary vein to the right ventricle is greatly prolonged. The elevated systemic venous pressure is manifested by the continued imaging of the large veins [left innominate (**LIV**), superior vena cava (**SVC**)] and the reflux of radioactive material into the left internal jugular vein (**IJV**). Normally, the superior vena cava should not be visible for more than 6 seconds, while in this case visualization persists for almost 40 seconds. A further manifestation of congestive failure is the shunting of pulmonary arterial blood flow to the upper lung fields; there is a relative reduction in pulmonary arterial perfusion to the lower lung fields (brackets). The right atrium is clearly identified at 22 seconds, and there is prolonged visualization of the main pulmonary artery (**PA**).

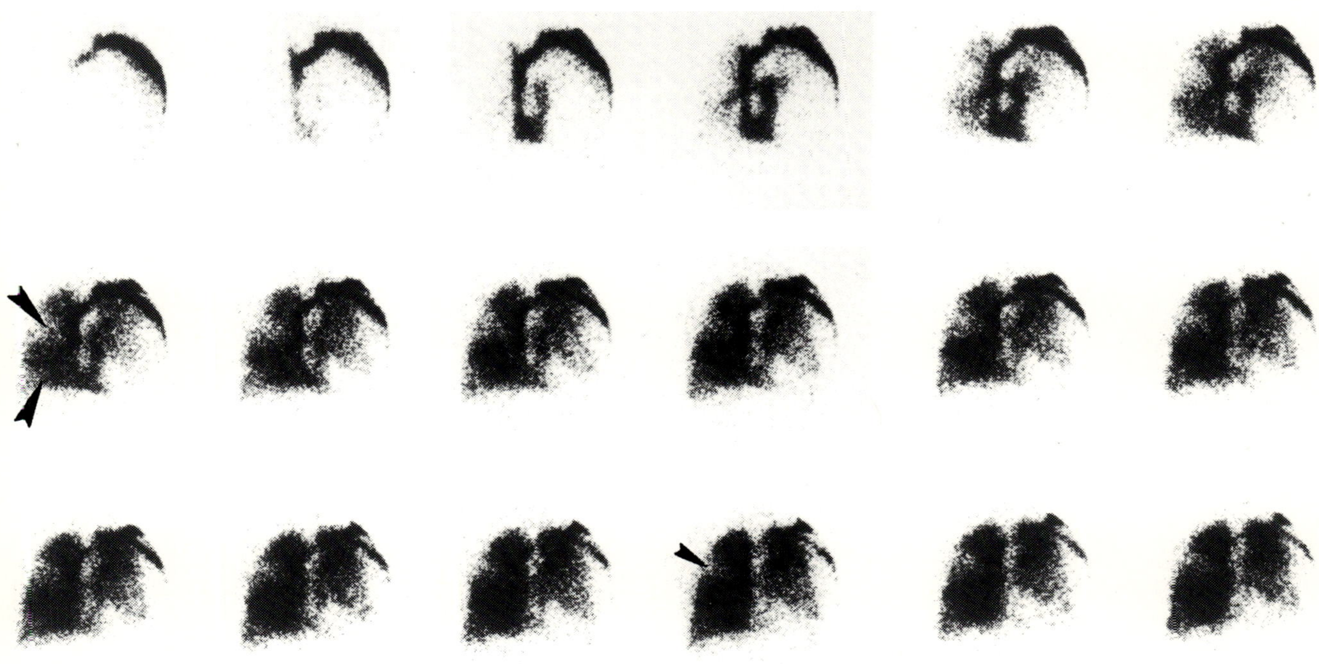

Anterior Blood Flow

**FIG. 18. PULMONARY EMPHYSEMA AND CARCINOMA OF RIGHT UPPER LOBE.** The patient with pulmonary hypertension, regardless of the etiology, will show prolonged visualization of the main pulmonary artery and perhaps one or more of its major branches. In this patient with carcinoma of the right upper lobe and chronic obstructive pulmonary disease, the main pulmonary artery continues to be visualized for at least 14 seconds. In addition, the tumor has resulted in localized pulmonary arterial blockade (small arrow)akin to what might be seen with pulmonary embolism. The magnitude of reduced pulmonary arterial blood flow associated with both the tumor and the regions more severely involved with pulmonary emphysema ( larger arrows) is clearly identified during the initial phases of the blood flow study (12 to 24 seconds).

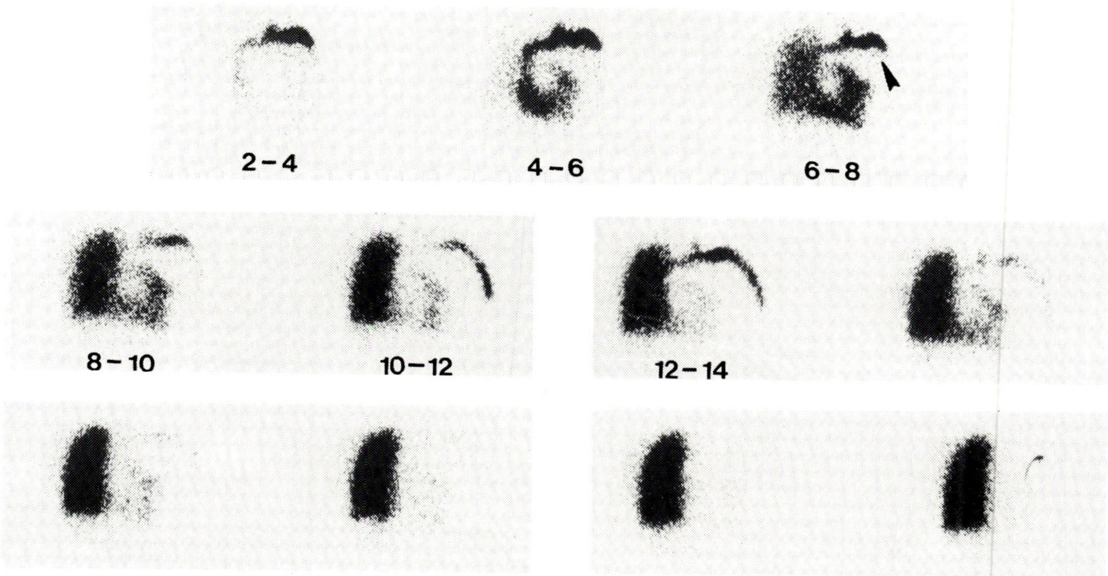


Anterior Blood Flow

**FIG. 19.** STENOSIS OF LEFT PULMONARY ARTERY. The patency may be determined of one of the major branches of the pulmonary artery and this may be delineated without interference from radioactivity in the systemic circulatory tree. The suspicion that there is stenosis of the left pulmonary artery in this patient with tetralogy of Fallot who had undergone corrective surgery is confirmed in this study. The right pulmonary artery is clearly visible, and the site of stenosis of the left pulmonary artery is readily identified (arrow) at 35 minutes.

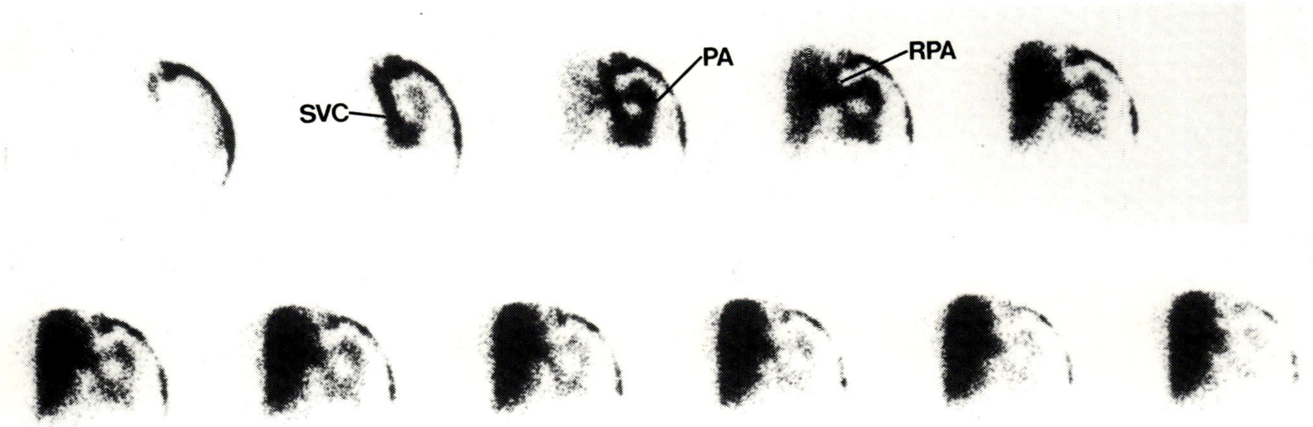


**FIG. 20.** **LEFT PNEUMONECTOMY.** There is no visualization of the left pulmonary artery. The superior vena cava (**SVC**), main pulmonary artery (**PA**), and right pulmonary artery (**RPA**) are clearly visible.

## Suggested Reading

Bentley PG, Hill PL, de Haas HA, et al: Radionuclide venography in the management of proximal venous occlusion. A comparison with x-ray contrast venography. Br J Radiol 52:289–301, 1979

Bentley PG, Kakkar VV: Radionuclide venography for the demonstration of the proximal deep venous system. Br J Surg 66:687–690, 1979

Hurlow RA, Strachan CJ: The clinical scope and potential of isotope angiology. Br J Radiol 51:682–686, 1978

Matin P, Glass EC, Villarica J: Peripheral radionuclide angiography. JAMA 242:1781–1784, 1979

Moss CM, Rudavsky AZ, Veith FJ: Isotope angiography: technique, validation and value in the assessment of arterial reconstruction. Ann Surg 184:116–121, 1976

Moss CM, Rudavsky AZ, Veith FJ: The value of scintiangiography in arterial disease. Arch Surg 111:1235–1242, 1976

Muroff LR, Freedman GS: Radionuclide angiography. Semin Nucl Med 6:217–230, 1976

Nillus AS, Lindvall R, Nylander G: Dynamic radionuclide phlebography. A clinical study in patients after total hip replacement. Eur J Nucl Med 3:161–167, 1978

Sy WM, Lao RS, Bay R, et al: ($^{99m}$Tc) Pertechnetate radionuclide venography—large-volume injection without tourniquet. J Nucl Med 19:1001–1006, 1978

Sy WM, Lao RS, Nissin A: Occlusion of inferior vena cava—features by radionuclide venography. J Nucl Med 19:1013–1019, 1978

# 9/Gallium Imaging

Gallium was first introduced in 1965 as a bone-scanning agent. However, it was soon found to concentrate in soft tissue tumors and later in sites of inflammation. The mechanism of gallium localization in tumors and other tissues is not precisely known. Electron microscopic radioautographic studies have demonstrated that gallium is bound to intracellular particles that are lysosomal in nature. Following the intravenous injection of gallium-67 citrate, in a dose of 50 $\mu$Ci/kg of body weight, about one third of the dose of gallium-67 is bound to transferrin and other plasma proteins.

Ga-67 has a physical half-life of 77.9 hours with four primary gamma emissions, 93 keV (45 percent), 184 keV (24 percent), 300 keV (22 percent), and 388 keV (7 percent). In normal subjects the total body dose is estimated at 0.25 rad/mCi with the target organ, the large bowel, receiving about 0.9 rad/mCi. Gallium-67 is slowly excreted from the body and has a biologic half-life of two to three weeks in normal patients. About 40 percent of the dose is excreted in the first 5 days after injection, 20 to 25 percent by the intestinal tract, and 15 to 20 percent by the kidneys. In the first 24 hours the major mode of excretion is through the kidneys with clearance of 12 percent of the injected dose. After the first day, the bowel excretion predominates and necessitates bowel preparation for imaging at 48 to 72 hours, when the target/background and tumor/nontumor ratios reach a maximum.

Abnormal gallium-67 concentration is not tumor-specific. Inflammatory lesions have been visualized, especially pyogenic infections, as well as active granulomatous lesions. Fresh surgical wounds and salivary glands following radiation therapy may also take up the radiotracer. Among tumor localizations, Hodgkin's disease, malignant lymphoma, primary pulmonary malignancies of various histology, primary hepatoma, and brain tumors concentrate gallium in approximately 70 to 90 percent of the cases.

The energies of gallium-67 are suitable for imaging with either a rectilinear or scintillation camera. On one single pulse height analyzer, a single large window is commonly used to encompass the 184- and 300-keV peaks. In general, the rectilinear scanner has proved to be superior to the scintillation camera for imaging Ga-67. In performing the scan on a rectilinear scanner, one should attempt to obtain an information density of at least 500 counts per square centimeter. Using a dual-probe scanner, with 5:1 or 2:1 minification, the patient is scanned from the top of the head to the mid-thigh region. Further improvement

A

B POST

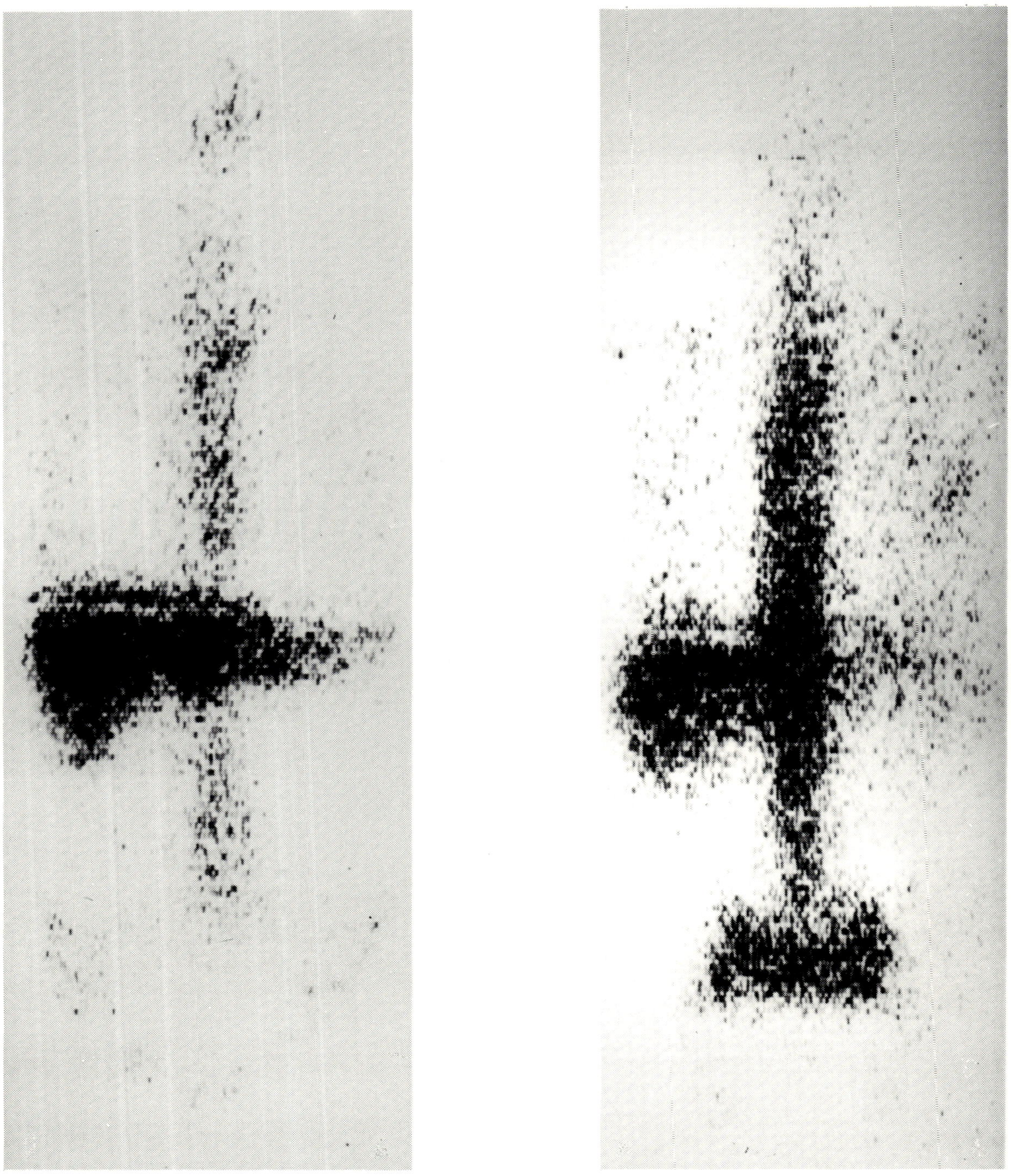

**FIG. 1. A, B.** (See legend next page)

in image quality can be achieved by the use of devices with spatial resolution superior to that of 5-inch rectilinear scanner systems such as the Anger tomographic scanner.

It should be pointed out that the images of this chapter are presented in the more traditional roentgenographic designation. Thus the right side is *always* on the viewer's left for images performed in both the anterior *and* posterior positions.

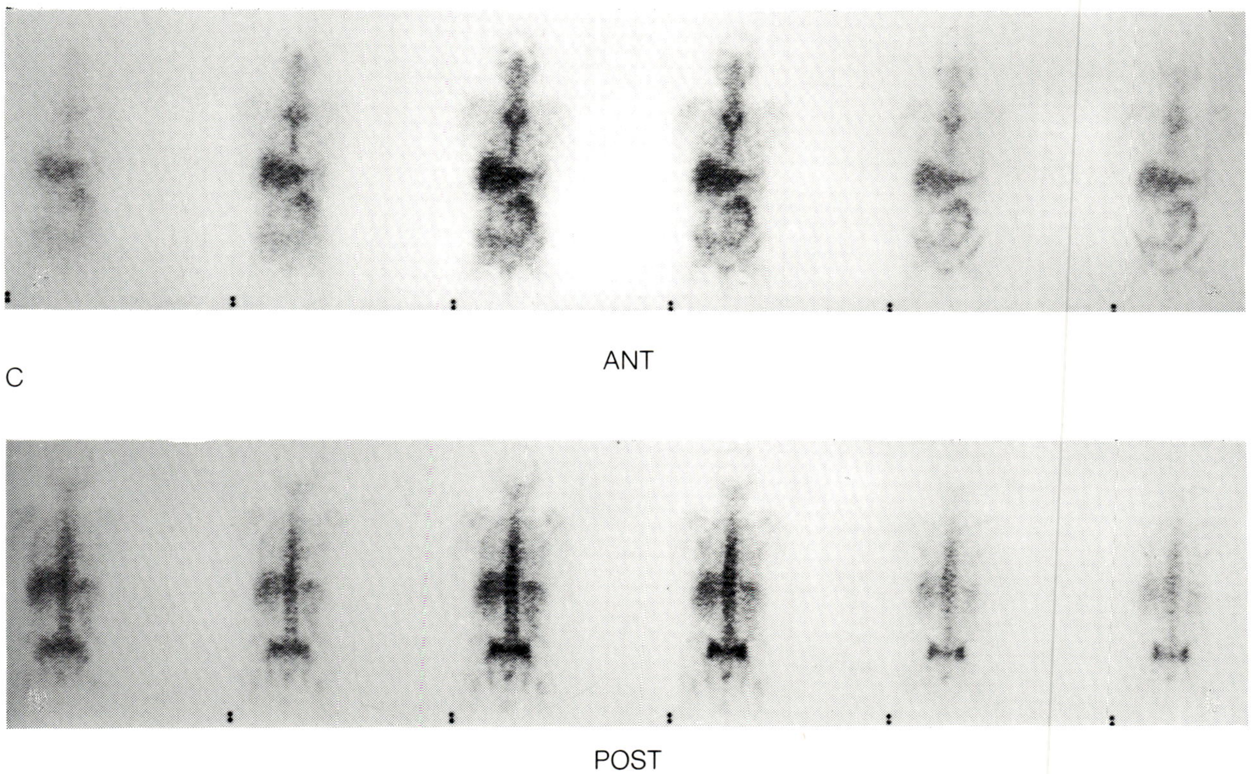


**FIG. 1.** NORMAL Ga-67. **A. Anterior Rectilinear Scan.** On the anterior view, the normal appearance includes uptake in the lacrimal glands, which may be asymmetrical. Nasopharyngeal activity, often the most prominent accumulation in the head and neck regions, can mask lymphomatous involvement of Waldeyer's ring. The liver contains the greatest accumulation of gallium. Other areas normally visualized are the breasts, especially in postpartum women; bone and bone marrow, with faint to moderate activity; and large intestine, especially when the bowel preparation is inadequate. **B. Posterior Rectilinear Scan.** On the posterior view, structures normally visible are the nasopharynx, bone and bone marrow, liver, and, faintly, the spleen. **C. Normal Pho-Con Tomo Scan.** The lacrimal glands, nasopharynx, liver, breasts, bone, and bone marrow are the same as with a regular rectilinear scanner except for the tomographic depth effect. The depth of each "cut" is about 2.75 cm. Tomography is useful in separating activity in the bowel lumen from retroperitoneal accumulation.

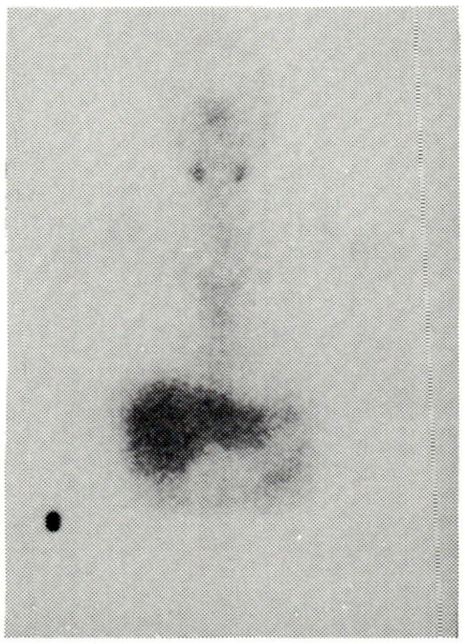

**FIG. 2. INCREASED SALIVARY GLAND UPTAKE FOLLOWING IRRADIATION.** A 28-year-old male with a lymphoma, which presented as a large mediastinal mass that resolved following radiation therapy. Increased salivary gland uptake normally occurs after irradiation and should not be mistaken for recurrent cervical lymph node involvement by lymphoma or Hodgkin's disease.

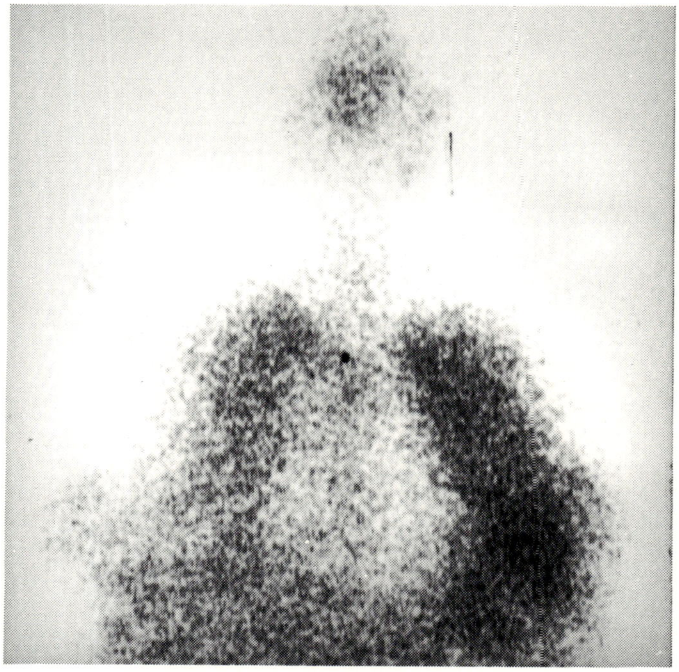

**FIG. 3. DIFFUSELY INCREASED PULMONARY UPTAKE IN PATIENT TREATED BY CYTOTOXIC CHEMOTHERAPY.** A 21-year-old female with chronic myelogenous leukemia who was on Busulfan treatment had intense lung uptake of gallium. A lung biopsy showed drug toxicity. Interstitial pneumonia associated with bleomycin therapy may also result in diffuse gallium localization and may be difficult to differentiate from diffuse pulmonary lymphangitic tumor metastases, infection, or radiation pneumonitis. The diffuse, uniformly increased uptake is also common in those studies performed immediately after lymphangiography.

ANT POST

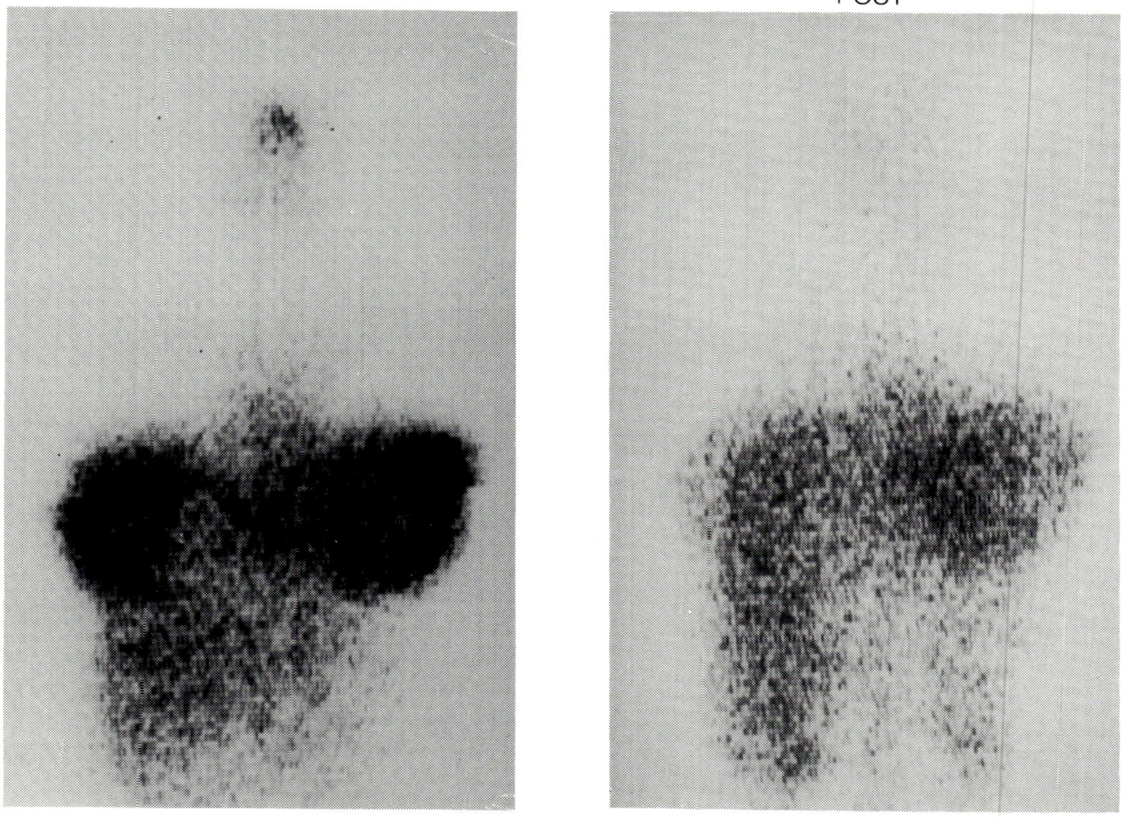

**FIG. 4. BREAST UPTAKE.** A 23-year-old female with a known history of fibrocystic disease of the breast showed markedly increased breast uptake. This has also been noted in the postpartum female. Benign or malignant tumor or inflammatory disorders may cause similarly increased uptake in breast.

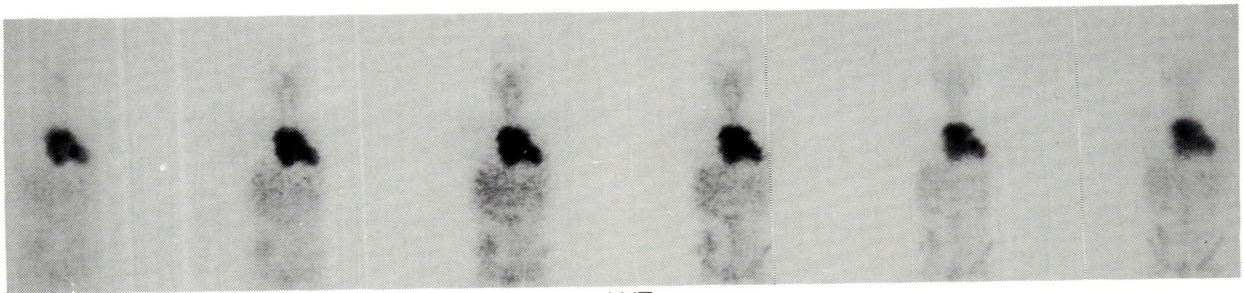

ANT

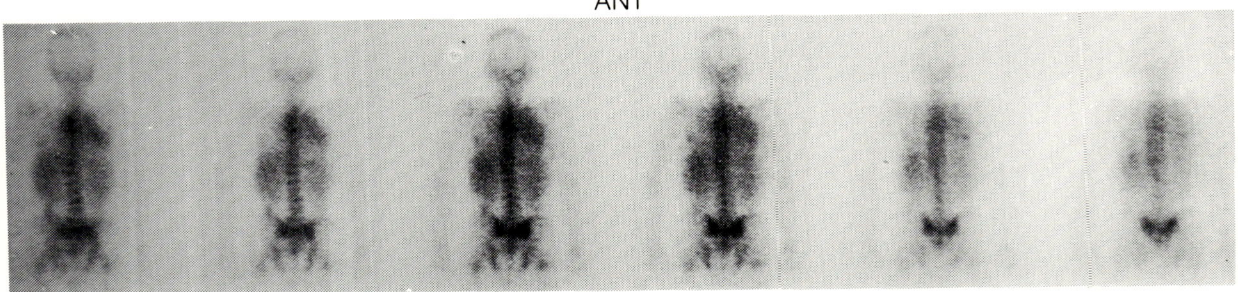

POST

**FIG. 5. HODGKIN'S DISEASE.** A 49-year-old male with recurrent Hodgkin's disease (nodular sclerosing type) six years following initial diagnosis and treatments with radiation and chemotherapy. Tomographic gallium imaging demonstrated anterior mediastinum and left chest wall involvement. In general, the gallium scan manifests about 70 to 75 percent of these lesions and plays an important role in the follow-up of such patients.

ANT

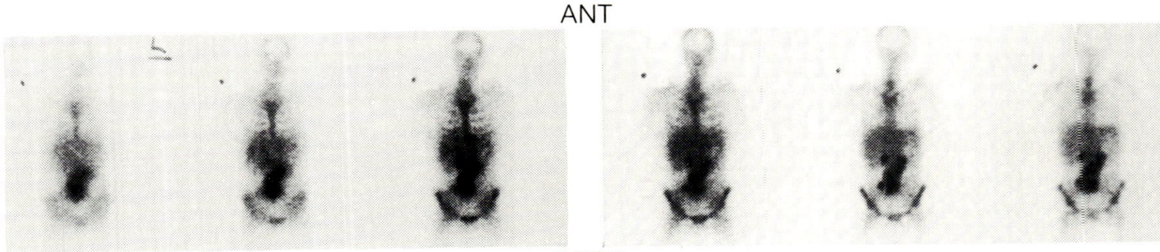

POST

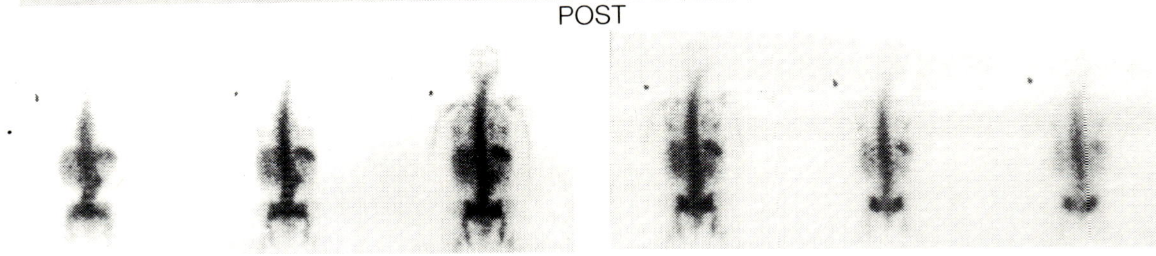

**FIG. 6. LYMPHOMA.** Malignant lymphoma in a woman aged 64. Tomographic gallium imaging showed periaortic lymph node and splenic involvement. Of histologically proven sites of malignant lymphoma, there is only a 50 percent overall sensitivity rate. The yield will vary with the histology. The better results were obtained with well-differentiated lymphocytic lymphoma, 86 percent; and histiocytic lymphoma, 71 percent. Poorly differentiated lymphocytic lymphoma had the lowest yield at 31 percent. As with Hodgkin's disease, in the case of lymphoma, gallium scans have very few false positive findings. Because of the very low false positive rate, gallium scanning contributes significantly to a determination of the extent of lymphomatous disease.

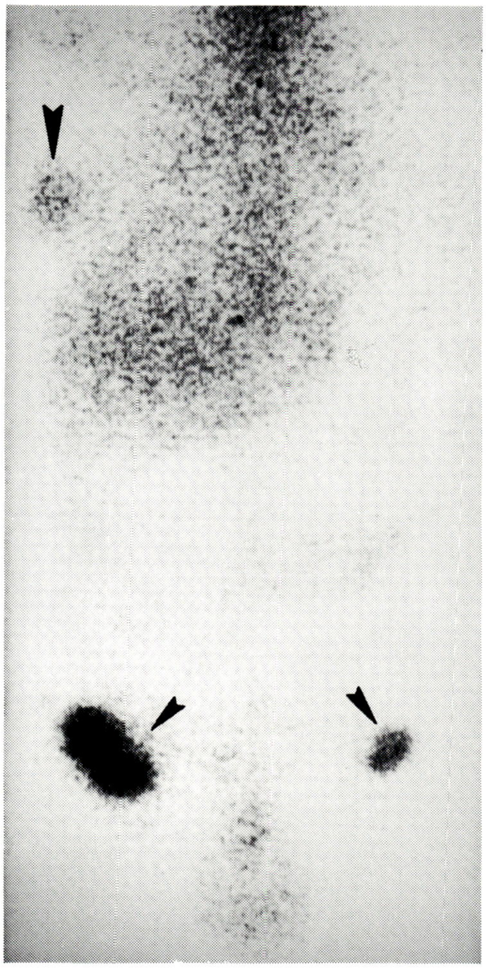

A ANT

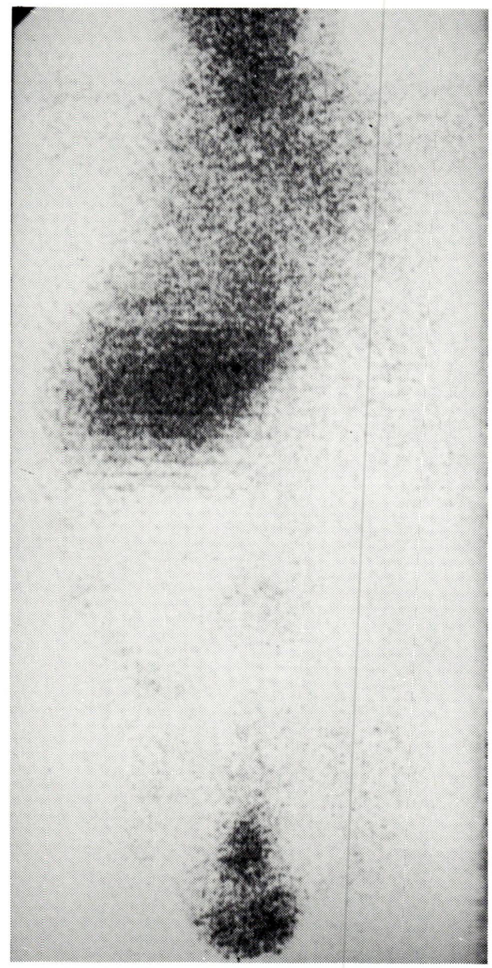

B ANT

**FIG. 7. 1, A, B.** (See legend next page)

ANT

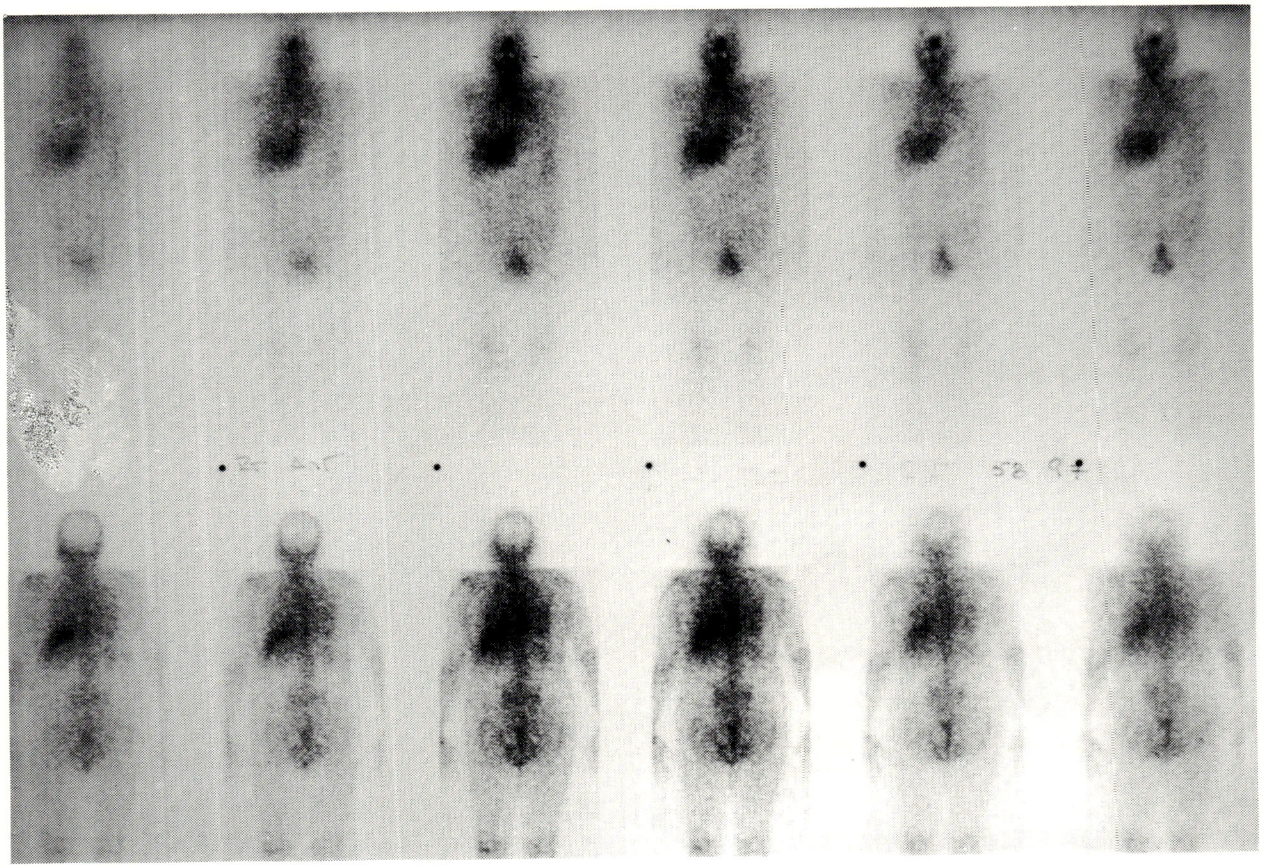

C

POST

**FIG. 7. LYMPHOMA.** An 83-year-old male with malignant lymphoma, poorly differentiated. **A.** Initially there was marked uptake bilaterally in the inguinal region (arrows) and the right axilla ( larger arrow). **B.** Six months later the study showed significant improvement following chemotherapy. **C.** At 15 months, the tomographic scan was essentially normal. The cause of the diffuse uptake in the lungs throughout the studies was not identified but was most probably drug toxicity.

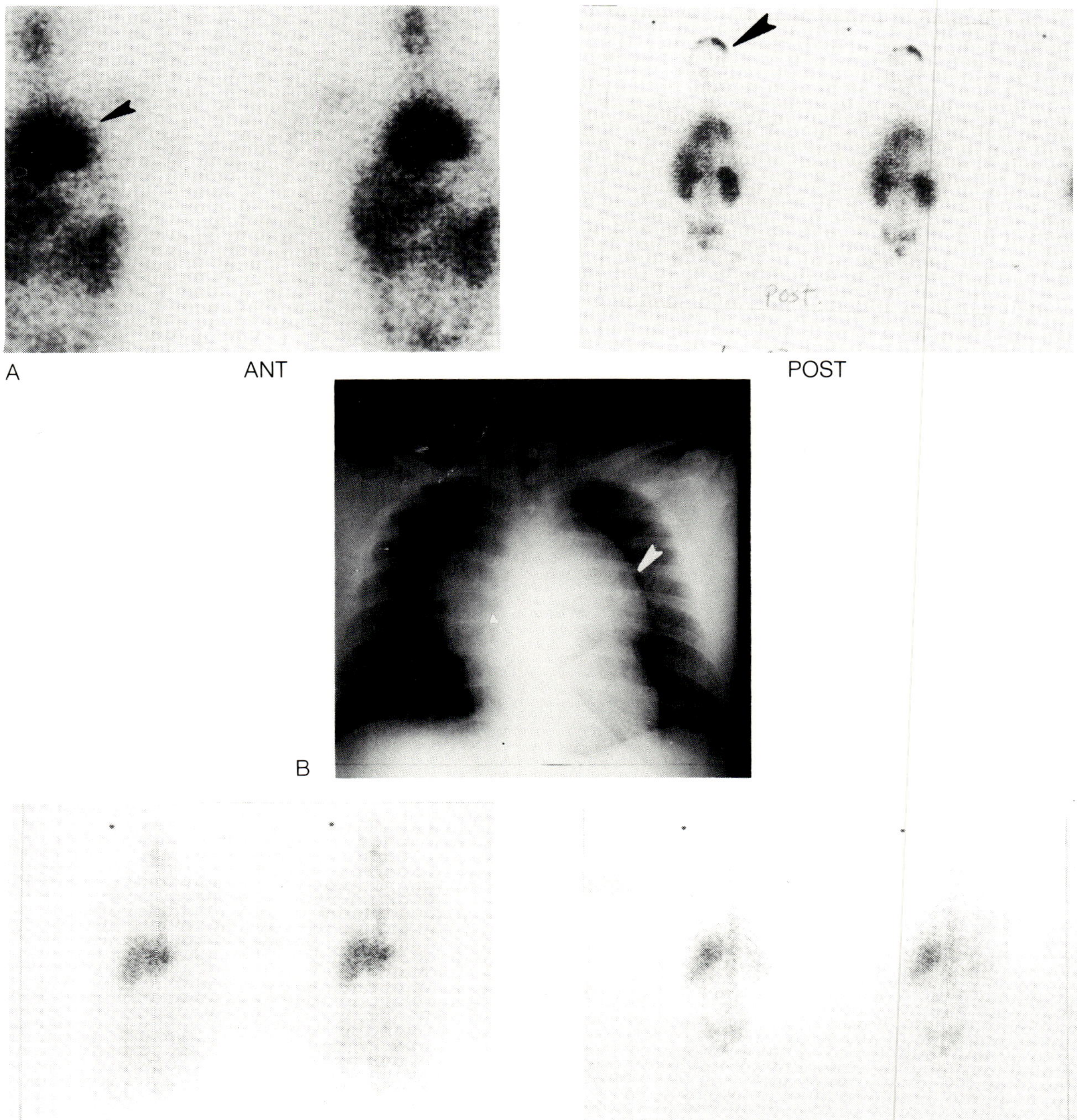


**FIG. 8.** LYMPHOMA. A 30-year-old male with poorly differentiated lymphoma. **A.** At 48 hours gallium tomographic scan demonstrated intense accumulation of gallium in the anterior mediastinum (arrow) and left occipital and parietal regions of the skull ( larger arrow)—areas of known metastasis, as well as increased renal uptake bilaterally. **B.** Chest x-ray showed the mediastinal lymphomatous mass (arrow). **C.** Four months later the gallium study was essentially negative after the patient received chemotherapy. The gallium scan remained normal 10 months later as the patient continued in remission.

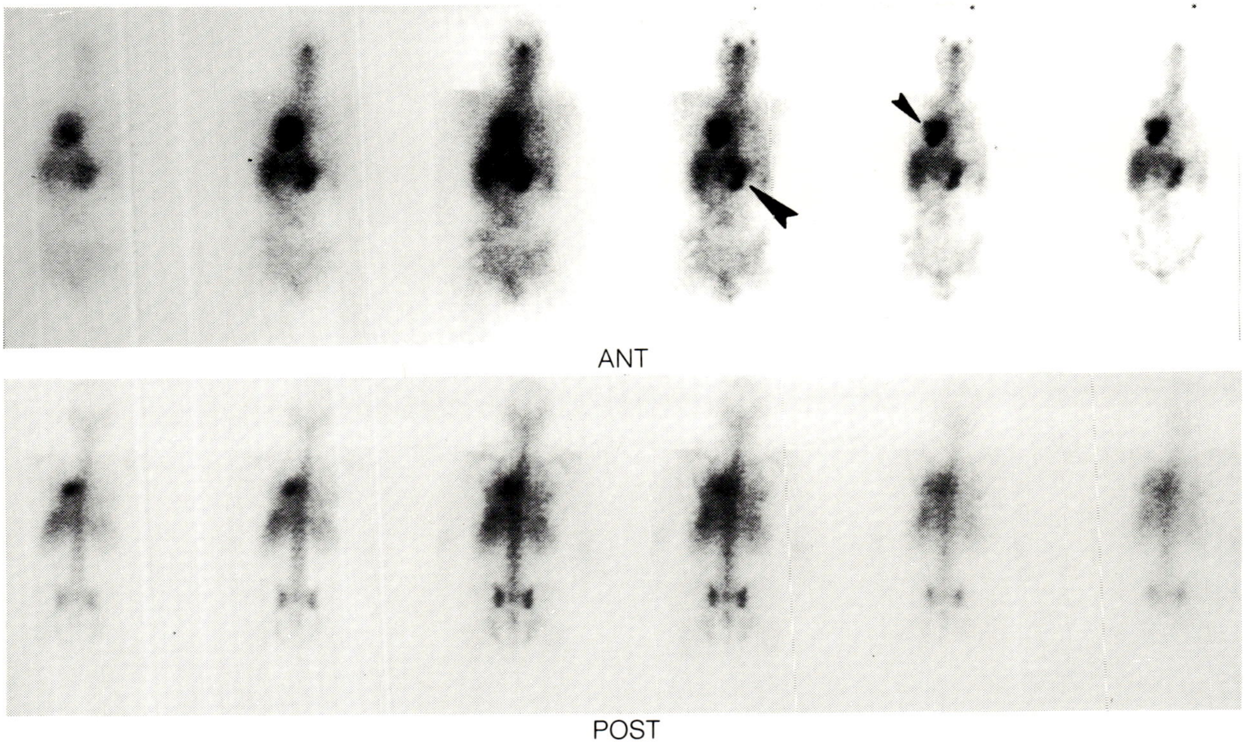


**FIG. 9.** LYMPHOMA. A 31-year-old male with lymphocytic lymphosarcoma. Tomographic gallium imaging demonstrated mainly right hilar node involvement (arrow). The uptake in left upper quadrant identified the primary site of duodenal involvement ( larger arrow).

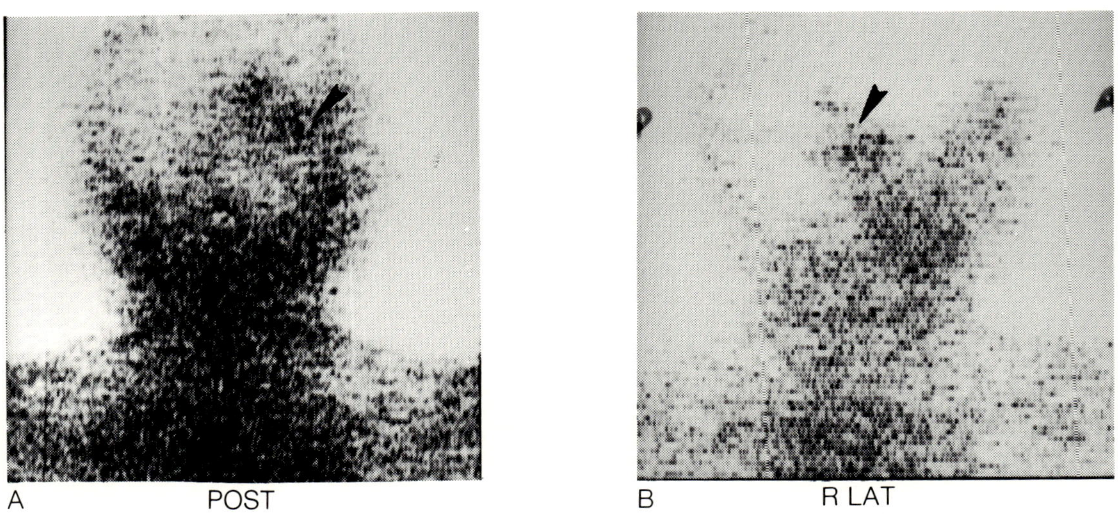


**FIG. 10.** LYMPHOMA. A 67-year-old man with reticular cell sarcoma. The gallium scan demonstrated a metastatic intracranial lesion in the left temporal region (arrows). **A.** Posterior view. **B.** Right lateral view. Steroid therapy may "mask" abnormal gallium accumulation in cases of neoplastic brain lesions.

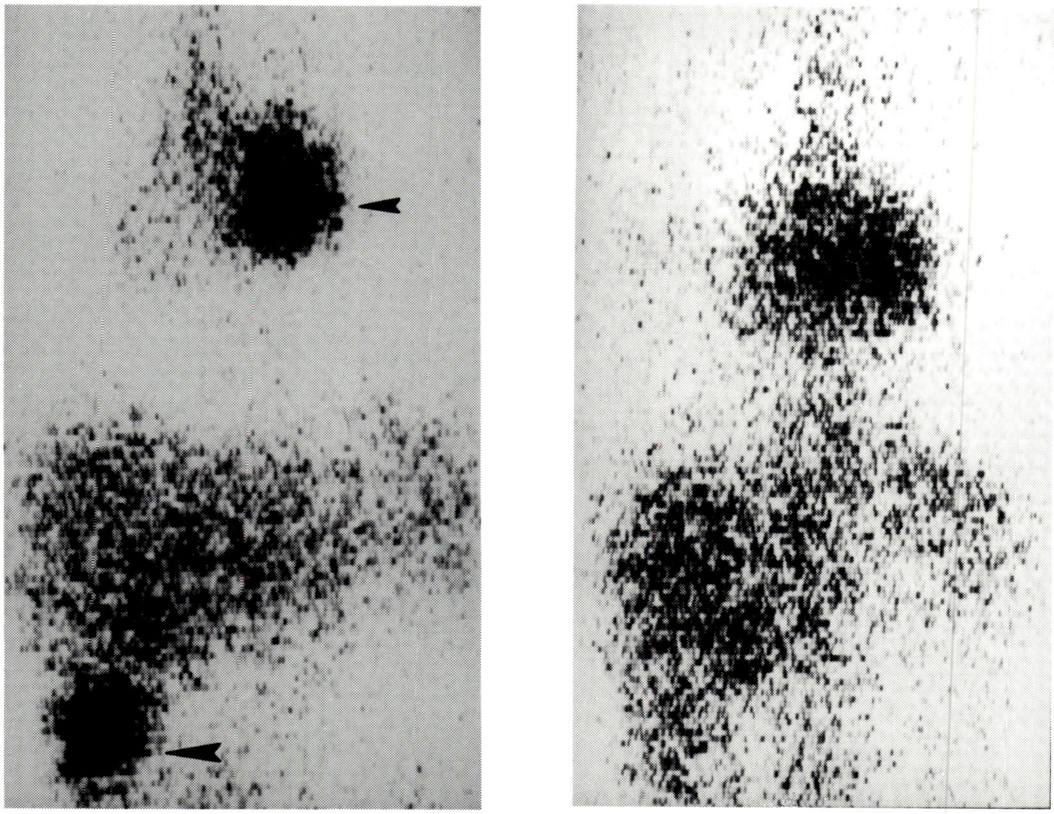

ANT POST

**FIG. 11. PULMONARY NEOPLASM.** Bronchogenic squamous cell carcinoma in a 64-year-old male. The gallium scan showed the primary lesion near left hilum ( small arrow) and a metastatic lesion in the inferior tip of right hepatic lobe ( large arrow). Primary pulmonary malignancies of various histology have been clearly visualized with an 85 to 95 percent success rate. Unfortunately, a variety of benign pulmonary lesions also accumulates gallium. Gallium scans detect about 80 percent of regional lymph node metastases but only about 50 percent of proven metastases to distant organs, i.e., bone and brain. Such imaging is useful in determining the resectability of a tumor.

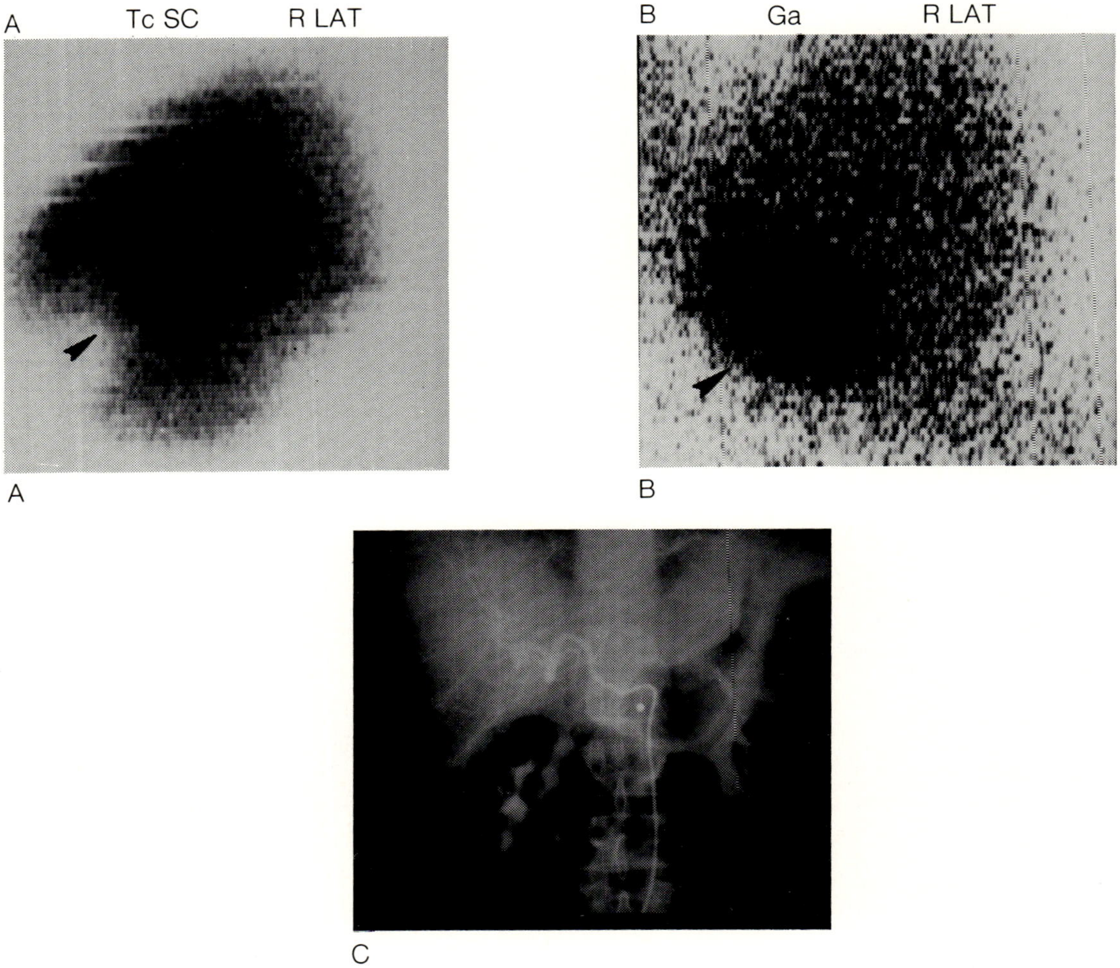


**FIG. 12.** HEPATOMA. A 57-year-old male with primary hepatoma. **A.** A Tc-99m SC liver scan showed a defect posteriorly in the right lobe (arrow). **B.** Gallium scan demonstrated increased accumulation in the region with decreased Tc-99m SC uptake (arrow). Several series have shown increased gallium accumulation in primary hepatomas (70 to 90 percent). In general, nonmalignant disease, such as cirrhotic fibrosis (Fig. 13) and ischemic necrosis (Fig. 19), have shown decreased gallium concentration. Metastatic tumors to the liver accumulate gallium in about one third of the cases. Hepatic abscesses may mimic the findings of a primary hepatoma and must be differentiated clinically and with ultrasonography. **C.** A selective coeliac and hepatic artery angiogram showed a highly vascular lesion in the right lobe of liver. Intravenous radionuclide hepatography may be useful in demonstrating increased perfusion to a primary hepatoma in contradistinction to an abscess.

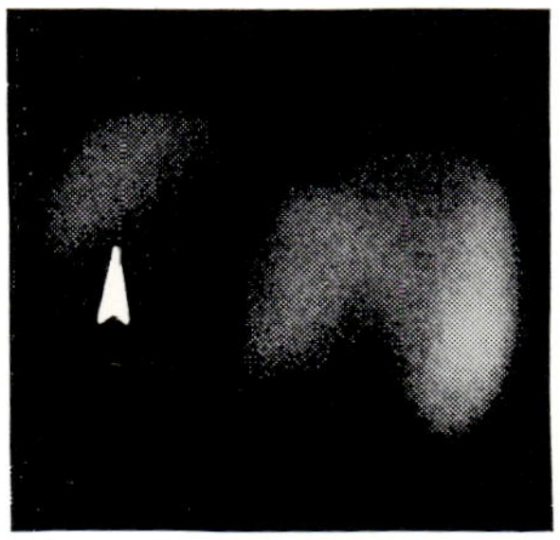

A ANT

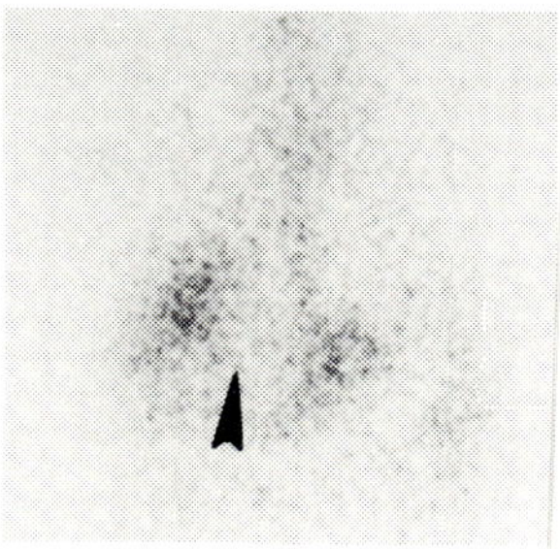

B ANT

**FIG. 13. HEPATIC CIRRHOSIS.** A 53-year-old male with a history of heavy ethanol intake. **A.** The Tc-99m-SC liver scintigram demonstrates a large photon-deficient area in the right hepatic lobe anteriorly (arrow). **B.** Gallium scan with a defect matching Tc-99m colloid scan (arrow) (Gallium scan was obtained by Pho-Con tomo-scanner).

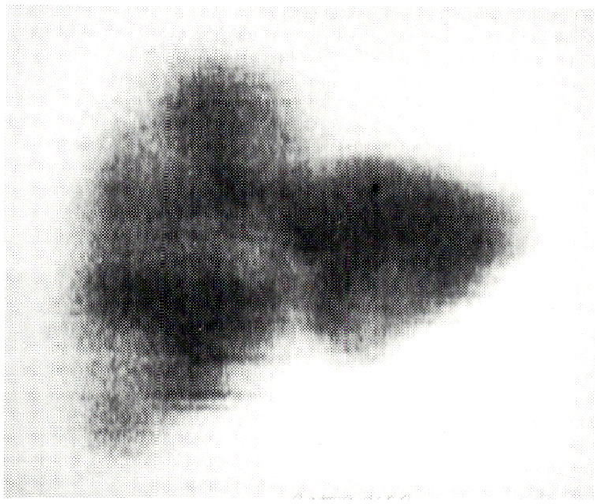

A Tc SC ANT

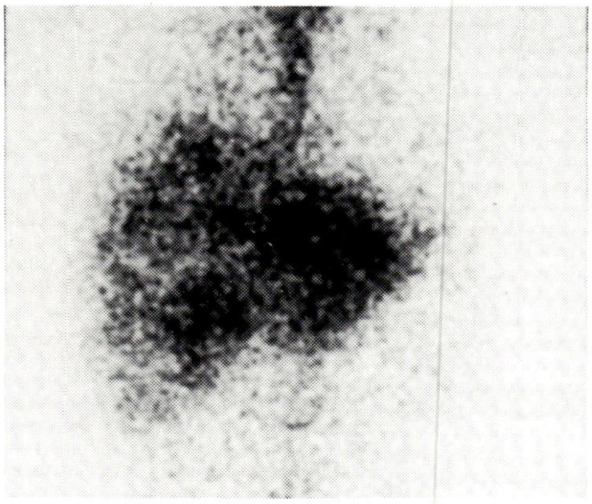

B Ga ANT

**FIG. 14. ANGIOSARCOMA OF LIVER.** Disseminated angiosarcoma in a woman aged 57. **A.** The Tc-99m SC liver scintigram demonstrates multiple lesions. **B.** Gallium scan shows essentially matching defects.

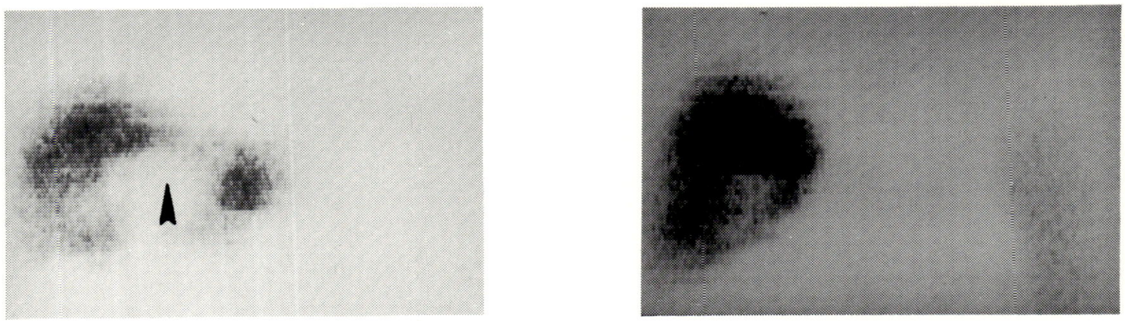

A ANT POST

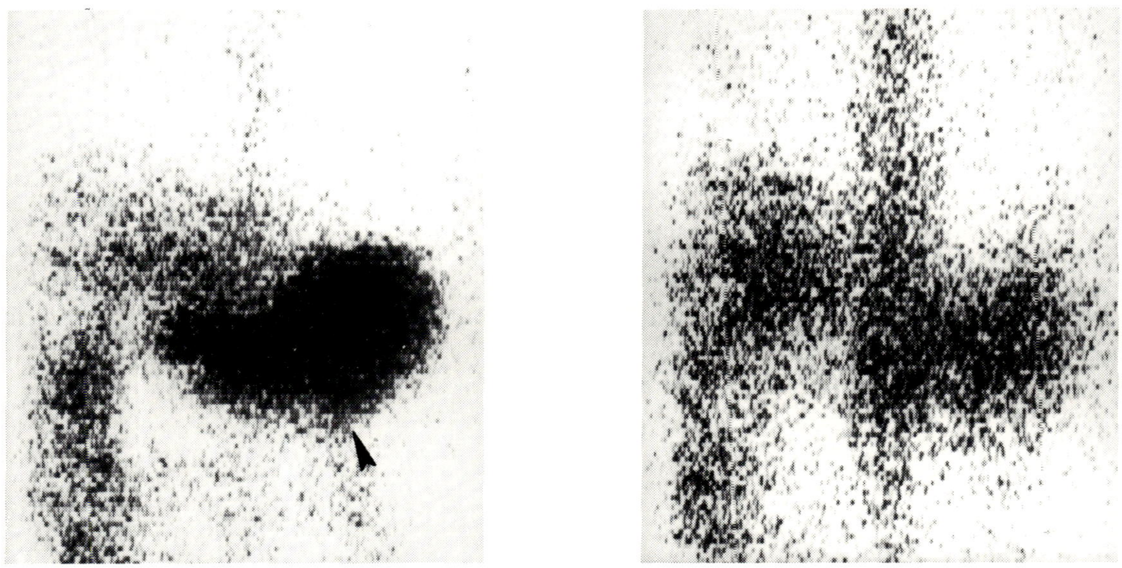

B ANT POST

**FIG. 15.** PANCREATIC CARCINOMA. Large cell carcinoma of the pancreas with liver metastases. Studies of a 57-year-old male with a three-month history of weight loss and an epigastric mass on physical examination are shown. **A.** The Tc-99m SC scintigram shows a large lesion in the region of the porta hepatis (arrow). **B.** Gallium scan shows a large area of intensely increased activity in the epigastrium corresponding to the palpable mass (arrow). In addition there is a mild concentration of gallium in the defect demonstrated on Tc-99 scintigraphy. Bowel activity is present in both the right and left lateral abdomen. Autopsy performed 2 weeks after the study revealed large cell carcinoma of the pancreas with extensive liver metastasis.

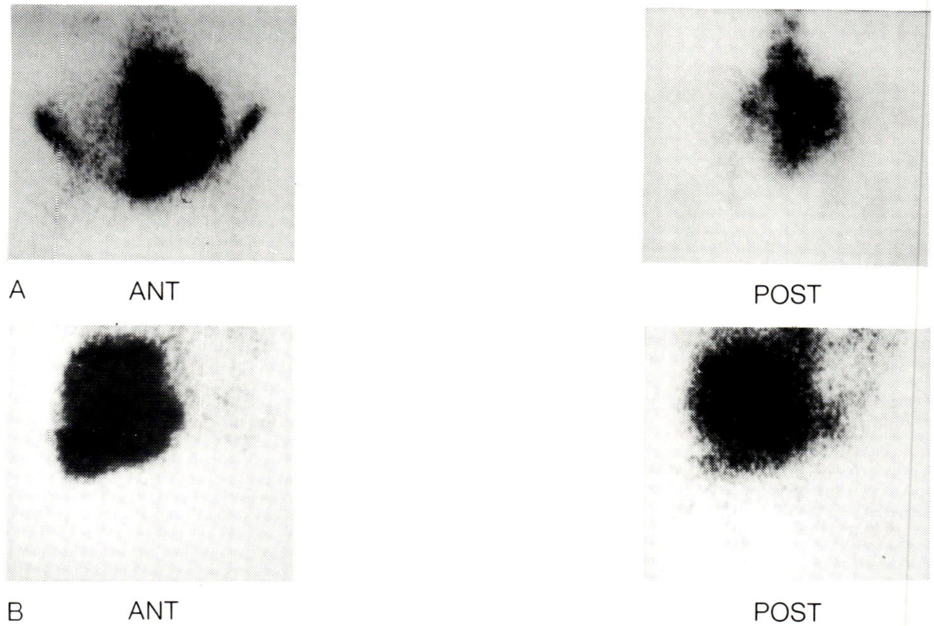


**FIG. 16. BLADDER CARCINOMA.** Papillary transitional cell carcinoma of the urinary bladder with metastasis to right pelvis. **A.** Bone scan with Tc-99m diphosphonate demonstrates a deformed and distended bladder, which occupies mainly the left half of the pelvis. **B.** Gallium scan demonstrates intensive activity in the right side of the pelvis corresponding to the massive, palpable mass.

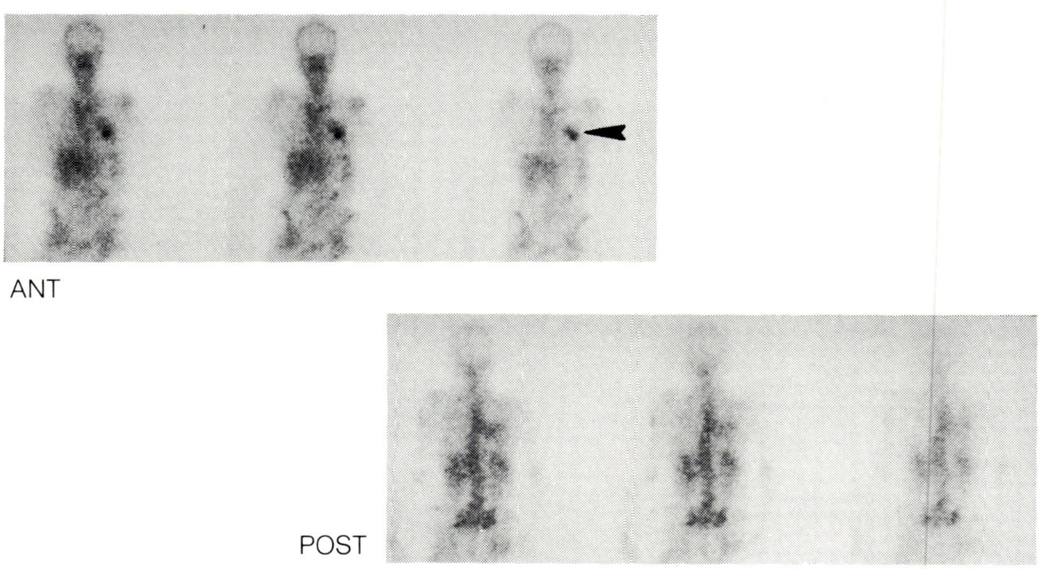


**FIG. 17. LUNG ABSCESS.** Lung abscess in a woman aged 57. Tomographic gallium scan initially showed a focal area of gallium accumulation in left lower lobe (arrow). Three months after treatment, the gallium scan of the lung appeared normal.

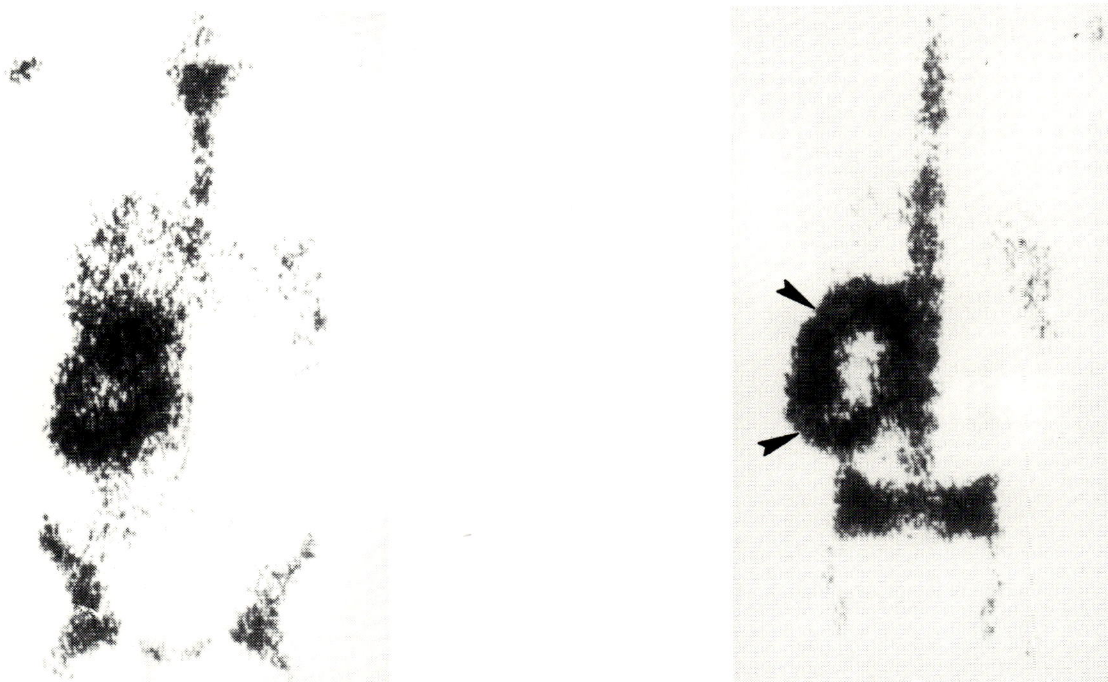

ANT POST

**FIG. 18. PERINEPHRIC ABSCESS.** Rectilinear gallium scan reveals a strikingly intense accumulation around the right kidney(arrows)with a central area of reduced activity. The abscess was surgically drained of over a liter of exudate.

Tc SC Ga-67

A R LAT B

**FIG. 19. HEPATIC ISCHEMIC NECROSIS.** A 42-year-old male with right upper quadrant pain, persistent low grade fever, and abnormal liver function tests. **A.** Tc-99m colloid liver scintigram showed decreased activity in the centro-lateral portion of right hepatic lobe. **B**. Gallium scan shows a similar defect. Open liver biopsy disclosed only ischemic necrotic tissue.

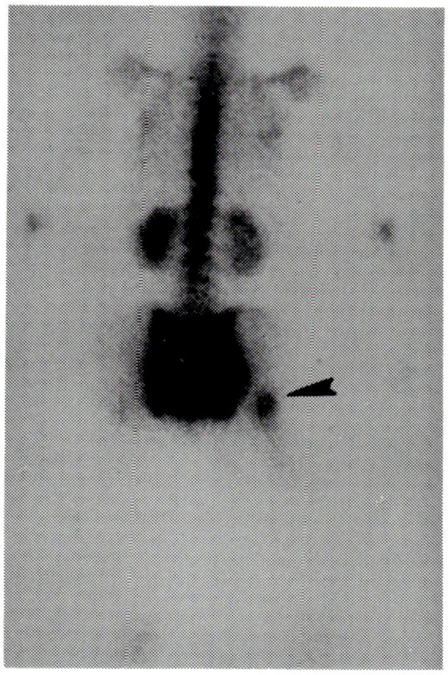

A POST

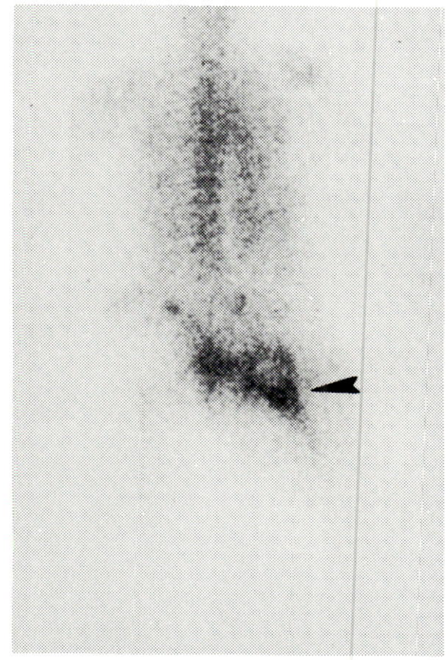

B POST Ga 6 hours

**FIG. 20.** OSTEOMYELITIS. Streptococcal osteomyelitis involving the left femoral head and acetabulum. A 30-year-old female diabetic with a history of uterine mesodermal sarcoma 5 years earlier developed persistent left hip pain and septicemia following bone marrow biopsy. **A.** Markedly increased concentration of Tc-99m pyrophosphate in the left femoral head and acetabulum (arrow). **B.** A 6-hour gallium scan revealed decreased activity in the femoral head but increased activity surrounding the head (arrow).

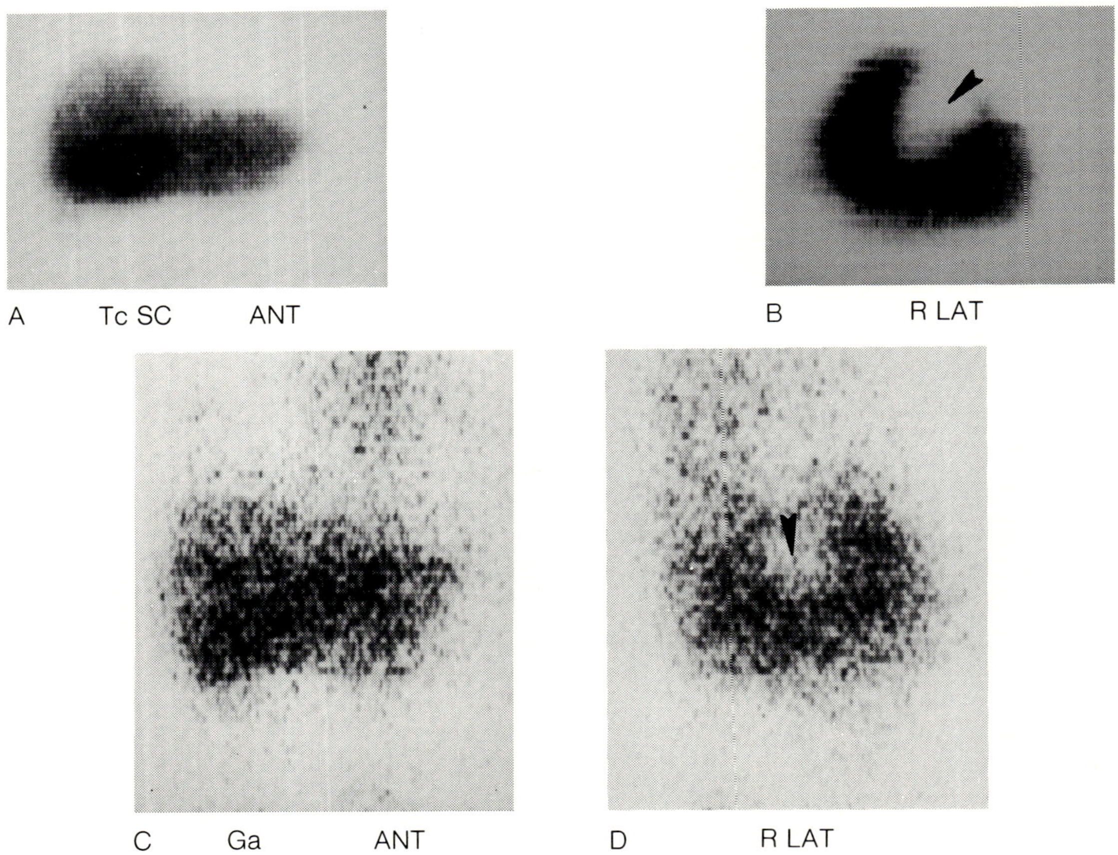


**FIG. 21.** CHRONIC AMOEBIC ABSCESS. A 45-year-old male with a history of vague abdominal pain, mild fever, and weight loss. Hemagglutination test for amoeba histolytica was positive at 1:520 dilution. Anterior (**A**) and lateral (**B**) views of the Tc-99m SC liver scintigram demonstrated an elliptical defect in the antero-superior aspect of the right hepatic lobe (arrow). Anterior (**C**) and lateral (**D**) views of gallium scan showed no significant gallium accumulation in the defect seen on Tc-99m SC liver imaging (arrow).

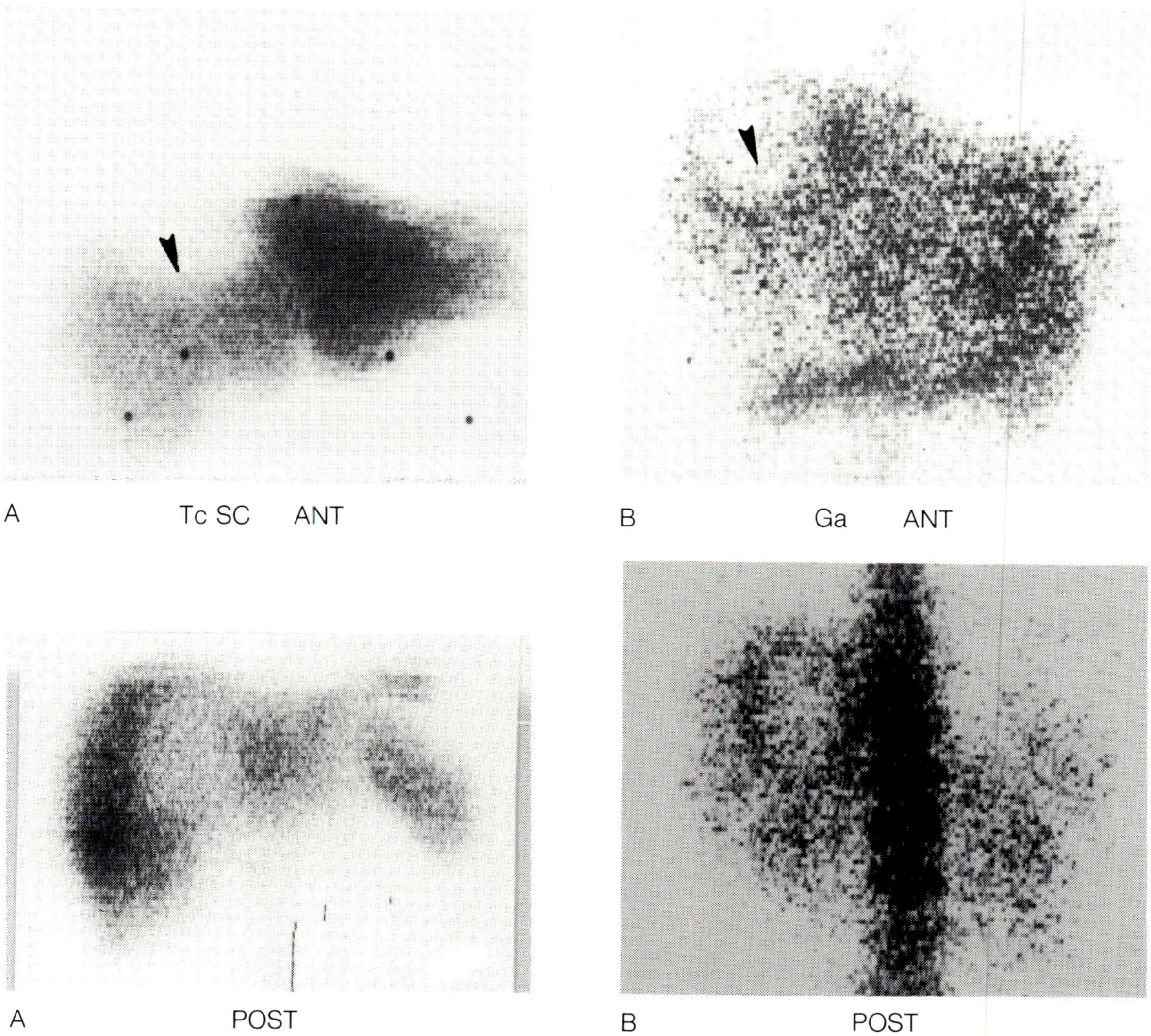


**FIG. 22. ACUTE AMOEBIC ABSCESS. A.** A Tc-99m-SC scintigram demonstrated a round focal defect in the anterosuperior aspect of the right hepatic lobe (arrow). **B.** The Ga-67 liver scan exhibited a smaller defect bordered by a rim of increased activity in the region of the colloid scan defect (arrow). (Courtesy of Dr. Ramesh Verma, UCLA and Oliveview Medical Center)

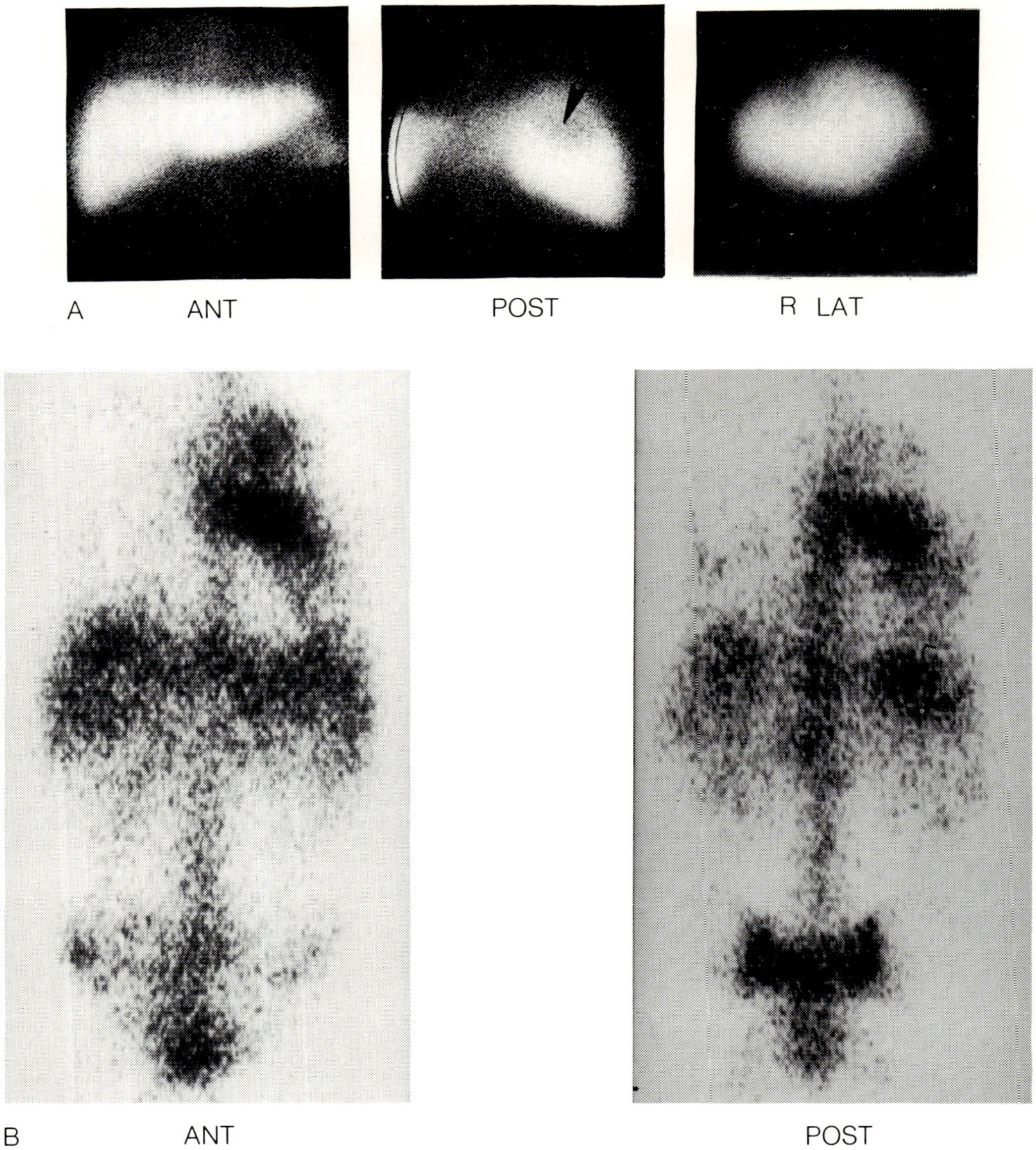


**FIG. 23. A, B.** (See legend next page)

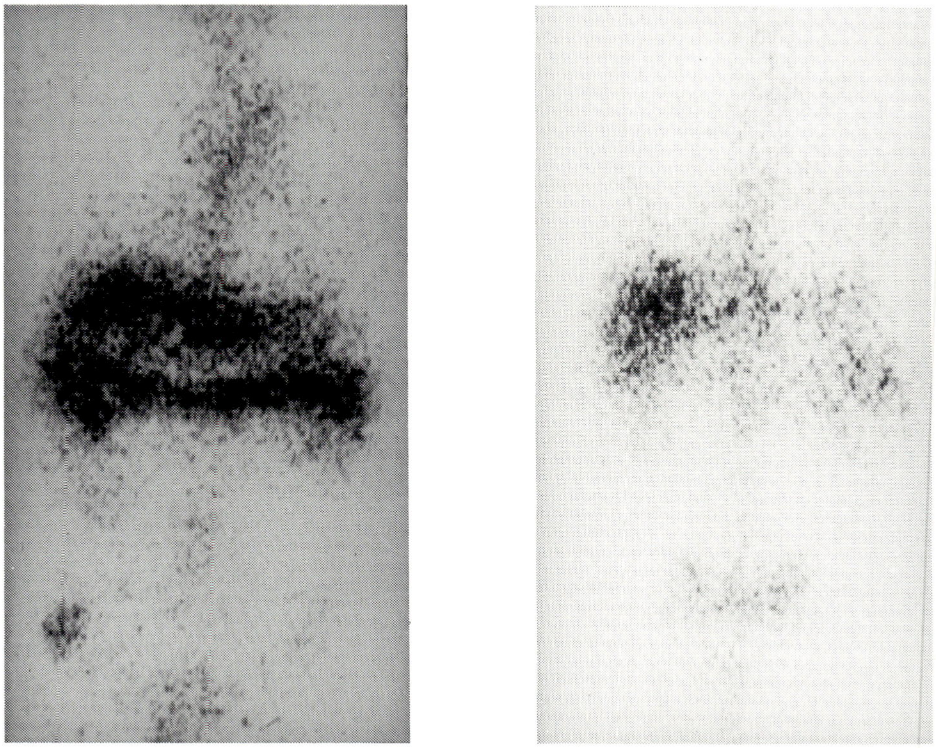

C ANT D POST

**FIG. 23. DISSEMINATED COCCIDIOMYCOSIS IN A PATIENT WITH PRIMARY HEPATOMA.** A 48-year-old male known to have pulmonary coccidiomycosis. **A.** Tc-99m SC liver scintigram demonstrates an abnormality in the superior-posterior portion of right hepatic lobe (arrow). **B.** Gallium scan shows intense activity in the left side of the neck posteriorly, in the spleen, and right lower quadrant (caecum). The posterior view of the liver reveals a slight increase in gallium uptake. **C.** Six months later, following intense antifungal medication, a repeat colloid liver study again contains a defect with no definite interval change. **D.** A repeat gallium scan shows only a minimal increase in activity in the left upper anterior chest and dome of the liver posteriorly. Linear and focal activity in the epigastrium and right lower quadrant are due to bowel activity. The patient died of bronchopneumonia 3 weeks following the gallium study. On autopsy, primary hepatoma was found in the superiorposterior portion of the liver, with chronic disseminated coccidiomycosis involving the lungs, adrenal glands, lymph nodes (including hepatic, gastric, pancreatic, omental, paraesophageal, thoracic, periaortic, and inferior cervical nodes), and spleen.

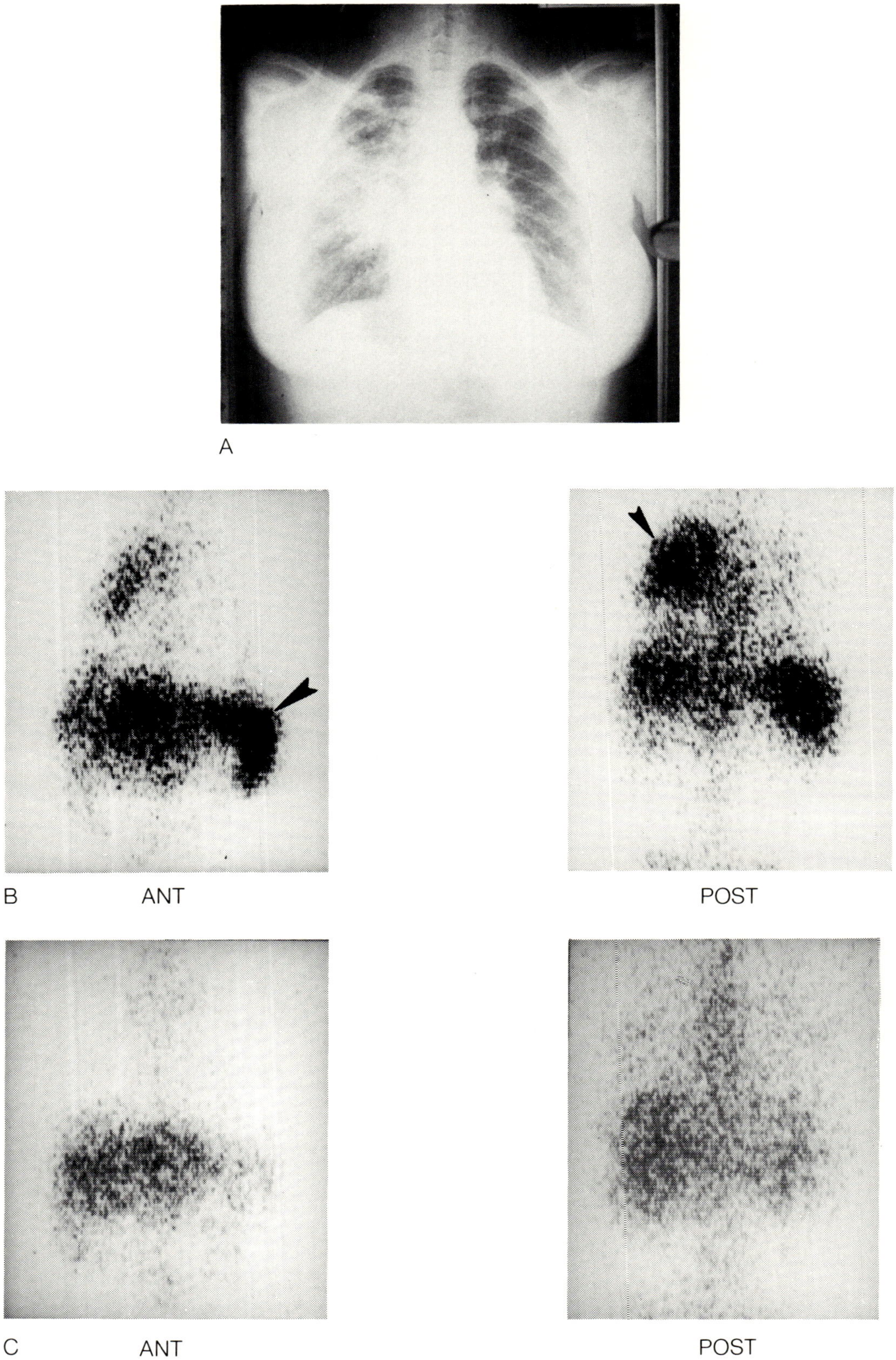


**FIG. 24.** (See legend next page)

**FIG. 24.** SARCOIDOSIS. A 42-year-old woman with known sarcoidosis was evaluated by gallium scan. **A.** Prior to steroid therapy, intense uptake is seen in the right hemithorax (arrow in B) corresponding to chest x-ray changes of hilar adenopathy and pulmonary infiltration. **B.** Increased gallium accumulation in the enlarged spleen ( larger arrow ) may be due to splenic involvement but is nonspecific. **C.** Follow-up gallium scan, 5 months after the onset of steroid therapy, demonstrates the clearing of abnormal activity in the chest and spleen. The gallium scan is useful in the follow-up of patients with sarcoidosis. Increased gallium accumulation in the chest usually suggests an active granulomatous processes even when distinct or persistent signs of scarring can be seen on radiographic investigation. It has been reported recently that the concurrent use of an angiotensin-converting enzyme assay, which is often elevated in active cases, and gallium imaging is of value in the diagnosis of sarcoidosis. The results from one study indicate the combination of these two techniques increases the diagnostic specificity from 83 percent to 99 percent without sacrificing sensitivity.

## Suggested Reading


Donoghue GD, Steinbach JJ, Lee JY: False-positive studies in early $^{67}$Ga citrate scintigraphy. Clin Nucl Med 4:56–58, 1979

Handmaker H, O'Mara RE: Gallium imaging in pediatrics. J Nucl Med 18:1057–1063, 1977

Hoffer P: Gallium: mechanisms. J Nucl Med 21:282–285, 1980

Hoffer P: Gallium and infection. J Nucl Med 21:484–488, 1980

Hoffer PB, Miller-Catchpole R, Turner DA: Demonstration of lactoferrin in tumor tissue from two patients with positive gallium scans. J Nucl Med 20:424–427, 1979

Larson SM: Mechanisms of localization of gallium-67 in tumors. Semin Nucl Med 8:193–203, 1978

Lentle BC, Castor WR, Khaliq A, et al: The effect of contrast lymphangiography on localization of $^{67}$Ga citrate. J Nucl Med 16:374–376, 1975

Levenson SM, Warren RD, Richman SD, et al: Abnormal pulmonary gallium accumulation in P. carinii pneumonia. Radiology 119:395–398, 1976

Levin J, Kew MC: Gallium-67 citrate scanning in primary cancer of the liver: diagnostic value in the presence of cirrhosis and relation to alphafetoprotein. J Nucl Med 16:949–951, 1975

Levitt RG, Biello Dr, Sagel SS, et al: Computed tomography and $^{67}$Ga citrate radionuclide imaging for evaluating suspected abdominal abscess. Am J Roentgen 132:529–534, 1979

Lomas F, Dibos PE, Wagner HN, Jr.: Increased specificity of liver scanning with the use of $^{67}$Ga citrate. N Engl J Med 286:1323–1329, 1972

Mendez G, Morillo G, Alonso M, et al: Gallium-67 radionuclide imaging in acute pyelonephritis. Am J Roentgen 134:17–22, 1980

# 10/ Nuclear Cardiology

There are three general types of nuclear cardiology procedures: myocardial infarction imaging, myocardial perfusion imaging, and dynamic measurement of ejection fraction and myocardial wall motion. Myocardial infarction and myocardial perfusion imaging can be performed with any standard high resolution gamma camera. Although techniques have been described for estimating the left ventricular ejection fraction by ECG-gated static images, more commonly the ejection fraction is computer generated as are the cinematic wall motion studies.

Radiotracer measurement of cardiac dynamics dates back to the early days of nuclear medicine. The first paper presented at the first meeting of the Society of Nuclear Medicine in 1954 was on measurements of cardiac output. In the 1960s several agents were developed and tested for imaging the myocardium. In the 1970s major advancements were achieved in nuclear cardiology with the introduction of Tc-99m pyrophosphate infarct imaging, and thallium 201 (Tl-201) myocardial imaging. Meanwhile, the availability of relatively low-cost microprocessors allowed rapid growth and expansion into the area of dynamic cardiac imaging and physiologic measurement.

## PYROPHOSPHATE MYOCARDIAL SCINTIGRAPHY*

Technetium-labeled phosphates will generally be deposited in tissues and organs in the same manner as calcium and phosphorus. Under the regulatory influences of parathormone and calcitonin, calcium and the phosphates will be deposited in bone and other tissues that contain hydroxyapatite or hydroxyapatitelike radicals. With the usual aerobic state, intracellular calcium content will be held at a fixed level. Under anaerobic conditions, such as those that occur during myocardial ischemia, the cell membrane becomes permeable to calcium, which freely enters the cell and attaches to hydroxyapatitelike structures. Technetium-labeled phosphates are also free to enter the cell and are either laid down along with newly entering calcium or replace other anions, such as lactate, that have been linked to previously laid calcium. This mechanism is the basis for technetium pyrophosphate myocardial scintigraphy. Whether the cell must be irreversibly damaged by oxygen deprivation and calcium influx in order for phosphate labeling to occur or if the process may occur during reversible ischemia remains an unsettled issue. Still others believe that the mechanism of phosphate scintigraphy is unrelated to calcium labeling of hypoxiapatite but due merely to phosphate adherence to cellular proteins extruded from dying myocardial cells. Regardless of which method accounts for the concentration of pyrophosphate in dead or dying cells, the technique has been effectively applied to the diagnosis of acute myocardial infarction.

The overall sensitivity for detecting acute infarction generally runs greater than 90 percent; however, as with all sensitive tests, the specificity is not especially high. Several systems of grading and interpreting the results of pyrophosphate scintigraphy have been proposed. The study may be interpreted according to the intensity of radioactivity seen in the myocardium, the pattern of activity as either diffuse or localized, or a combination of both. In this section, the grading system used is based on intensity. Its four levels range from zero to three-plus based on a comparison to bone activity. Other grading systems go from zero to four-plus and split grade one into two grades, thus yielding five grades. A three-plus on the five-step grading system would therefore be equal to a two-plus on the four-grade system and a four-plus would be equal to the three-plus on the system used in this atlas. Both systems have the same threshold for positivity in that grades three- and four-plus of the five-step grading system are considered positive for acute infarction as are the equivalent levels of two- and three-plus of the four-step grading system presented here.

Pyrophosphate scintigraphy is not specific for acute myocardial infarction as it has been shown that up to one third of positive studies will not normalize following acute myocardial infarction. Other entities including unstable angina, without actual infarction as classically defined, may cause a positive scintigram. A refinement of the grading system according to a pattern of activity, either diffuse or localized, lessens the sensitivity of the test but significantly increases the specificity for acute myocardial infarction. The study may therefore be interpreted according to the intensity of myocardial activity for optimal sensitivity, or according to intensity plus pattern for increased specificity.

Although pyrophosphate scintigraphy has become a useful test for the diagnosis of acute myocardial infarction, it has not replaced, nor was it in-

* The section on pyrophosphate imaging was done in collaboration with Dr. Harold Olson.

tended to replace, the standard ECG and serum enzymes. It is a valuable adjunct to the standard tests when additional information is needed to establish or strengthen the diagnosis. Furthermore, in the absence of acute myocardial infarction, pyrophosphate scintigraphy has prognostic significance for patients with unstable angina or previous myocardial infarction. Patients with a positive study during episodes of unstable angina have a worse prognosis than similar patients whose pyrophosphate scintigram is negative. The predictive value of the scintigram is independent and additive to the information from other known prognostic indicators. The incidence of cardiac death, acute myocardial infarction, and congestive failure are increased when the scintigram is positive in patients with unstable angina. If the pyrophosphate scintigram remains positive following acute myocardial infarction, the chances of cardiac complications will be greater than if the scintigram resolves in the usual fashion. It seems likely, therefore, that a positive scintigram in the absence of acute myocardial infarction is the result of significant cardiac disease. The phosphate may concentrate in cells during reversible hypoxia or in scattered foci of necrotic cells. In either case abnormal cardiac activity signifies significant cardiac disease and should not be considered a "false positive" even in the absence of acute myocardial infarction.

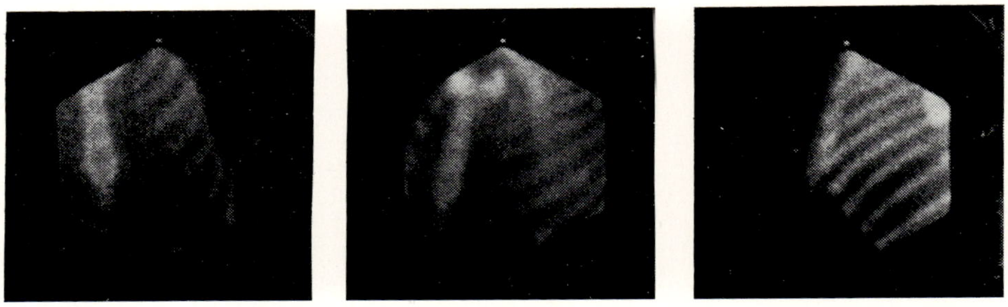

A O L

**FIG. 1.** **NORMAL.** Pyrophosphate is the agent of choice for "hot spot" infarct imaging. It is the phosphate derivative from which most of the data concerning phosphate myocardial scintigraphy has been developed. The method involves the injection of 20 mCi of radiotracer containing the minimal amount of tin that will yield effective binding and result in a radiotracer that passes the usual radio and chemical purity analyses. Images are obtained 2.5 to 3 hours after injection using a high resolution camera and collimator. The standard views of the thorax are the left anterior (**A**), 45 degree left anterior oblique (**O**), and left lateral (**L**) projections. Normally, no radiotracer is present in the region of the heart. An image of good quality consists of a high concentration of radiotracer in the sternum and ribs with low soft tissue background.

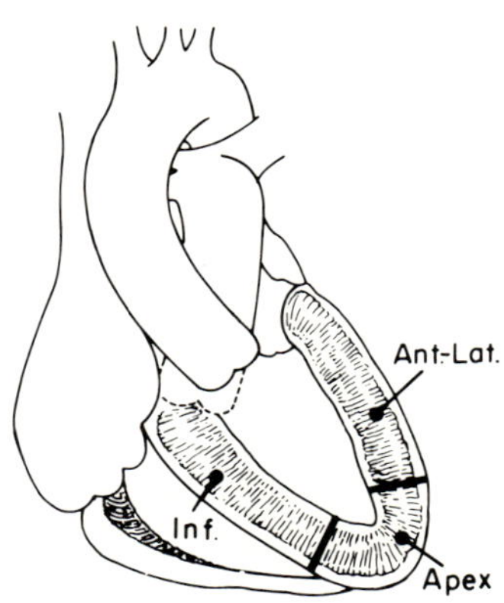


**FIG. 2.** **ANTERIOR SCHEMATIC.** This image is a schematic of the heart in the anterior view. The left ventricular walls seen in this view are the anterolateral wall, apex, and the inferior wall. The right ventricle even when infarcted would rarely be visible on the anterior view. Involvement of the septum or posterior wall on this view would appear to be diffuse and nonlocalized.

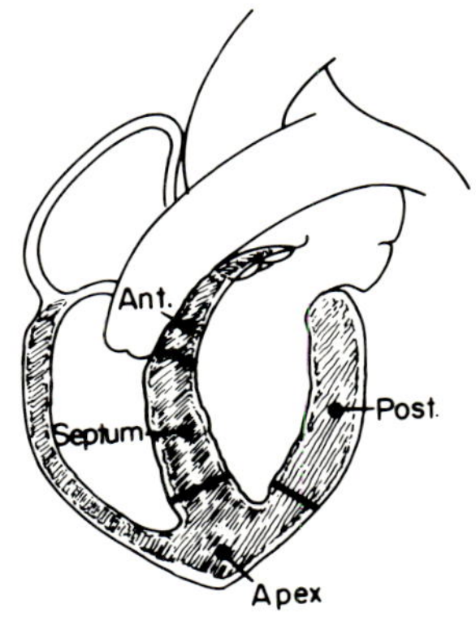


**FIG. 3. LAO SCHEMATIC.** In the left anterior oblique view the posterior wall, apex, septum, and a small portion of the anterior wall can be seen. This is the best view for evaluating right ventricular infarction. Involvement of the posterior wall or septum will be visible on this view. Depending on the axis of the heart, the inferior wall and the apex may be superimposed. Evaluation of these areas is more accurate on the two other views.

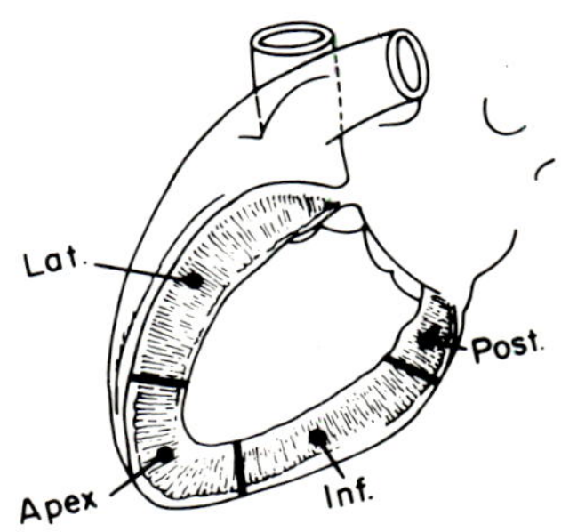


**FIG. 4. LEFT LATERAL SCHEMATIC.** Shown is the heart in the left lateral projection. This view is similar to the anterior view in that the inferior wall and apex are clearly visualized. The lateral wall makes up the roof of the left ventricle with some contribution from the anterior wall depending on the rotation of the heart. A small portion of the posterior wall is sometimes visible on this projection. This nomenclature may differ somewhat from that used in angiography. Contrast coronary angiography gives a better three-dimensional display as secondary and tertiary branches of the arteries outline walls in an *en face* position. Myocardial scintigraphy results in a more tomographic effect with visualization of the walls perpendicular to the face of the detector. As with a subdural hematoma when the lesion is rotated parallel to the surface of the collimator, it becomes less perceptible. Myocardial walls parallel to the face of the camera are not clearly visible

whereas those walls that are positioned on-end are most easily detectable. Unlike angiography, this makes the anterior wall difficult to see on the anterior view and the lateral wall relatively invisible on the LAO view.

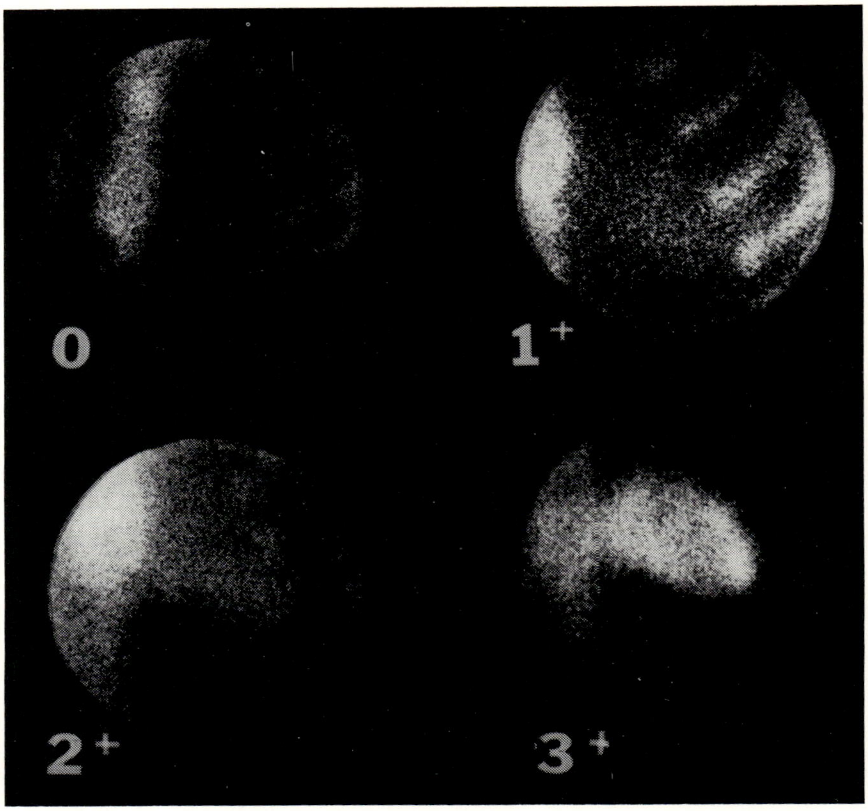


**FIG. 5.** **GRADING SYSTEM.** Images are graded on a scale of zero to three-plus according to the amount of radiotracer in the heart relative to the adjacent bone. The radiotracer present in the infarcted myocardium results in a hot lesion in a cold background. This situation potentially yields a high sensitivity. When there is no concentration of radioactivity in the region of the heart, the study is normal and receives a grade of zero (0). A grade of one-plus is assigned for faint activity in the heart that is less than that of the adjacent ribs. One-plus activity is not considered positive for acute myocardial infarction. This pattern has been seen in patients with known heart disease such as ischemia or congestive heart failure. It has been postulated that pyrophosphate concentration in the heart other than during acute myocardial infarction may be due to a low-grade focal necrosis. A grade of two-plus is given when the cardiac activity is equal to or greater than that in the adjacent ribs. Acute myocardial infarction, especially subendocardial infarction, may result in two-plus activity. The activity may be either diffuse or localized. Discrete localization is more specific for acute transmural myocardial infarction than for the other causes of two-plus activity, such as

ischemia, unstable angina, previous myocardial infarction, aneurysm, electrocardioversion, or pericarditis. A grade of three-plus is for cardiac activity equal to or greater than that of the sternum. This intensity is usually associated with acute myocardial infarction especially if the pattern is localized. The anterior, LAO, and left lateral views should be used in grading the intensity of myocardial activity. The study is graded according to the highest intensity present on any one of the views. Abnormalities may appear as one-plus in intensity on one view and two-plus in intensity on another projection as the lesion is rotated into a plane perpendicular to the face of the detector. As an example, an anteroseptal myocardial infarction may be diffuse and one-plus in intensity on the anterior view and appear as two-plus and localized on the LAO view. The proper grading in that instance would be two-plus localized. (From J Nucl Med 19:1117, 1978)

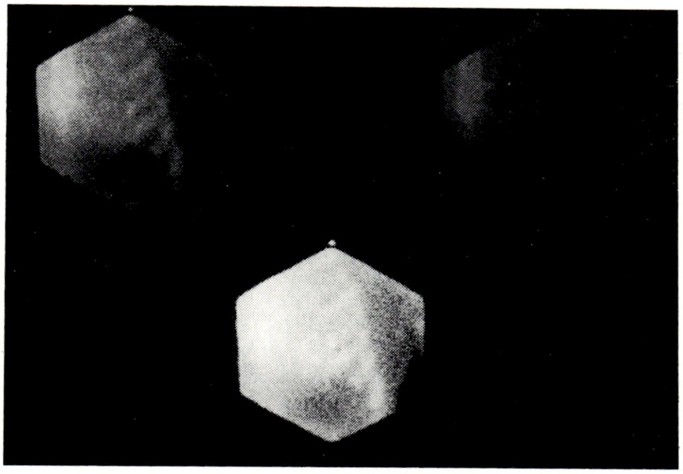

**FIG. 6. TRIPLE-LENS POLAROID READOUT.** A triple-lens Polaroid camera readout is useful when assigning a grade to the myocardial activity. The three levels of exposure should be adjusted to produce suppression of the rib intensity on the darker image in order to determine if myocardial activity fades earlier or later than rib activity and is therefore of higher or lower intensity. In this figure, radiotracer is present in the heart, and in the heavily exposed lower image the myocardial activity is striking. Even in the middle intensity exposure seen on the upper left, the diffuse pattern of myocardial activity is graded at one- to two-plus intensity. It is only in the lowest exposure on the upper right with myocardial activity sufficiently suppressed that the grading is shown to be one-plus. As noted in that view, the sternum and ribs are still visible as the myocardial activity is lost. According to the grading system defined in Fig. 5, the myocardial activity that is present is less than that of the adjacent ribs and, therefore, is given a grade of one-plus. This figure should be compared with Fig. 9, which shows a two-plus diffuse pattern.

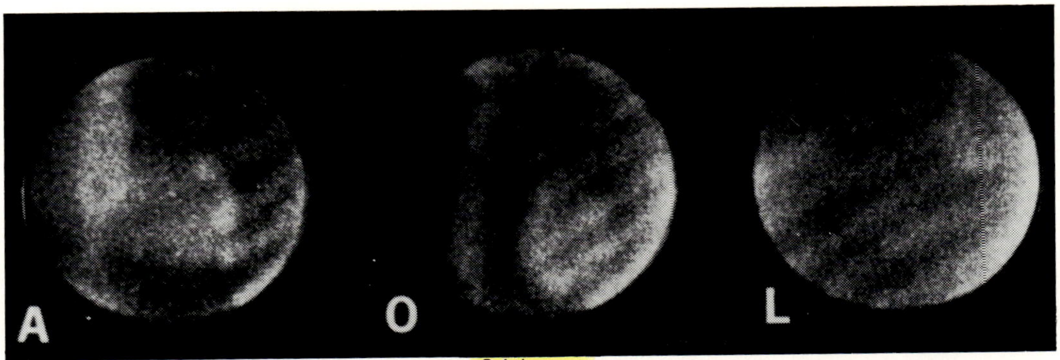


24 hours

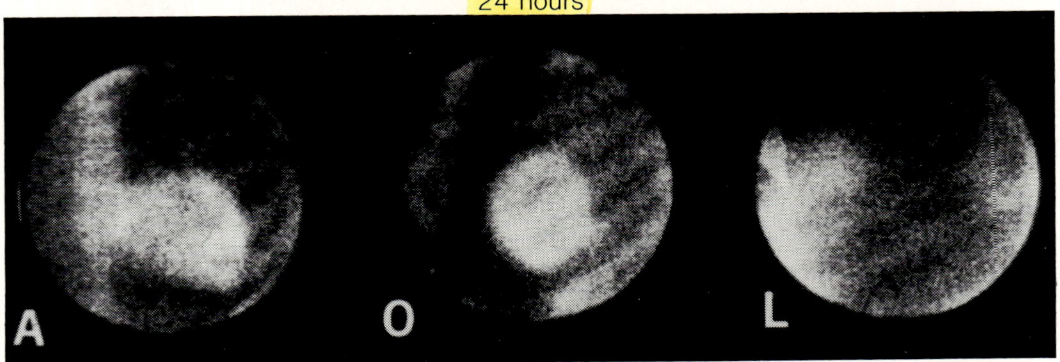


3 days

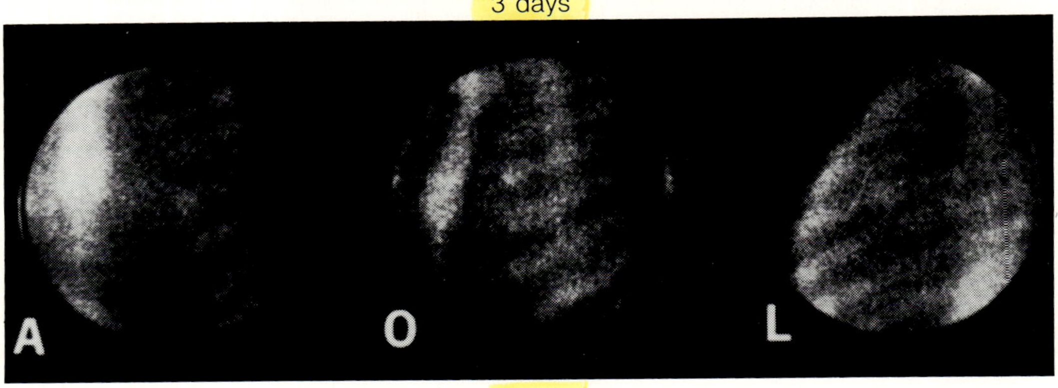


14 days

**FIG. 7.** **TIME COURSE.** This is representative of the usual time course for myocardial pyrophosphate scintigraphy during acute myocardial infarction. Scintigraphy may become positive during the first 24 hours following acute myocardial infarction. The peak sensitivity, however, will occur between one and three days after infarction. Therefore, studies that are negative soon after the infarction should be repeated in one to two days before one concludes that the examination is negative. Usually, the abnormal myocardial activity will fade over the next two weeks. In the top panel of this figure, the study is clearly positive at 24 hours; however, the activity has reached an intensity of only two-plus, and the pattern is just beginning to become localized. Two days later, when the infarct is three days old, the abnormality is more pronounced, with a three-plus intensity and discrete localization in the anterolateral and anteroseptal walls as seen in the middle panel. In the bottom panel, no abnormal myocardial activity is present at 14 days after acute myocardial infarction. This pattern is followed in approximately two thirds of the cases. In the remaining third, abnormal myocardial activity may persist after acute myocardial infarction for weeks to months. The persistence of abnormal myocardial activity correlates with the level of cardiac symptoms and generally portends a worse prognosis.

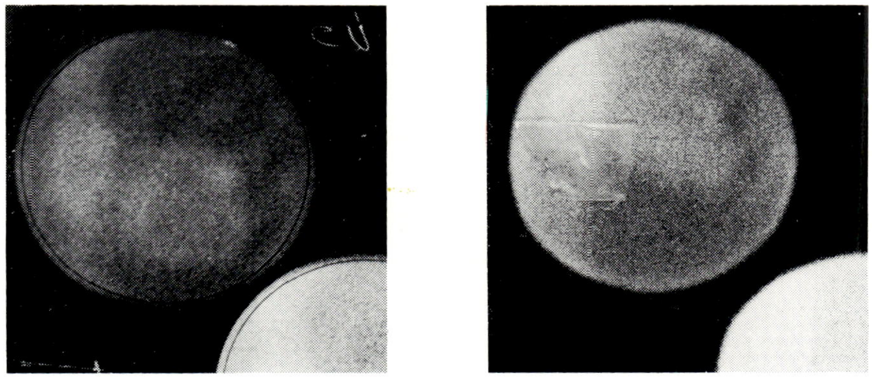

A B

**FIG. 8.** PERSISTENT ABNORMALITY. In one third of the cases, the pyrophosphate study will remain positive weeks to months following an acute myocardial infarction although the intensity will usually diminish. The persistent abnormality is usually of a two-plus intensity and the pattern diffuse. In this figure, **A** is the acute study three days following infarction and **B** is taken eight months later. The grade of the remote study is two-plus diffuse. A persistent abnormality is generally associated with the presence of angina or congestive heart failure. The persistence of an abnormality has prognostic significance in that those patients will generally fare worse than their counterparts whose scintigrams become normal when repeated two to three weeks following infarction. The incidence of subsequent cardiac death, recurrent myocardial infarction, and congestive heart failure is two times higher if the myocardial scintigram remains positive than if it turns negative in the remote period after acute myocardial infarction. (From J Clin Nucl Med, 1:256, 1976)

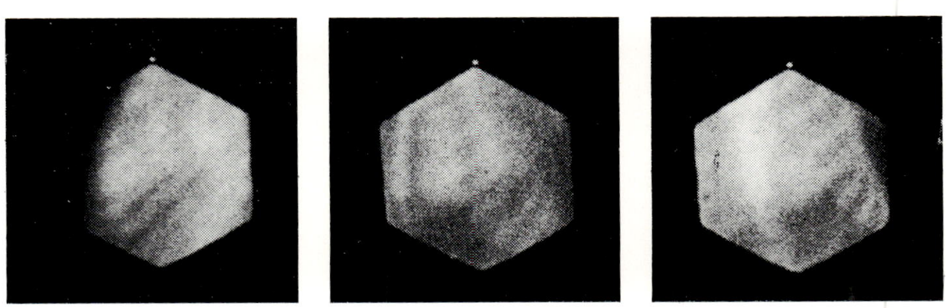

A O L

**FIG. 9.** (See legend next page)

**FIG. 9. SUBENDOCARDIAL INFARCTION.** Shown is a patient with an acute subendocardial myocardial infarction. The intensity of myocardial activity is two-plus and the pattern is diffuse. The two-plus diffuse pattern is less specific than a pattern with an intensity of three-plus or localized for acute myocardial infarction. The majority of acute subendocardial myocardial infarctions will show a two-plus diffuse pattern as will one third of the transmural myocardial infarctions. Other causes of this finding in the absence of acute myocardial infarction are unstable angina, pericarditis, uncompensated congestive heart failure, previous myocardial infarction, and myocardial injury from radiation or chemotherapy. When the abnormality is two-plus diffuse during an acute infarction, the study should be repeated in 3 to 4 weeks. A decrease in intensity of myocardial activity on the convalescent study from the two-plus diffuse pattern of the acute phase strengthens the diagnosis of acute myocardial infarction. The repeat examination will also serve as a nonacute baseline for future use.

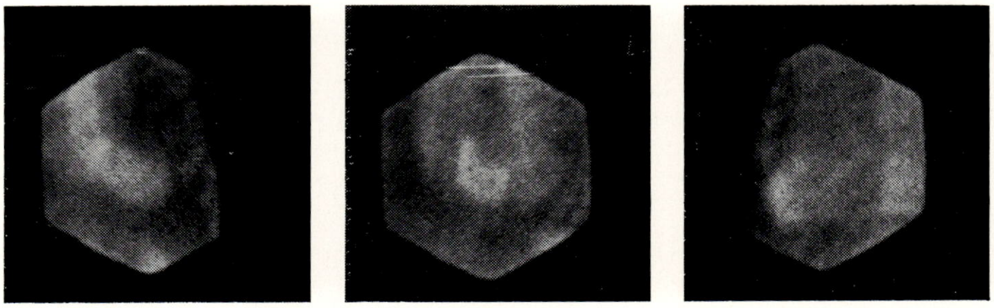

A O L

**FIG. 10. THREE-PLUS LOCALIZED PATTERN.** This is an example of a three-plus intensity abnormality with a localized pattern. The concentration of myocardial activity is equal to that of the sternum. On the three views it can be seen that the abnormality is localized to the anteroseptal and apicoinferior walls. A three-plus localized pattern has a high specificity for an acute transmural myocardial infarction. Occasionally, a subendocardial infarction will also show this pattern as may ventricular wall aneurysms, calcified valves, and myocardial trauma. Unstable angina and persistent abnormalities from previous myocardial infarctions will rarely cause a three-plus localized pattern. Although the sensitivity of a three-plus localized pattern is lower than the sensitivity of the test based on a grading by intensity only, the specificity of this finding, especially in the clinical setting of acute myocardial infarction, is greater than 95 percent.

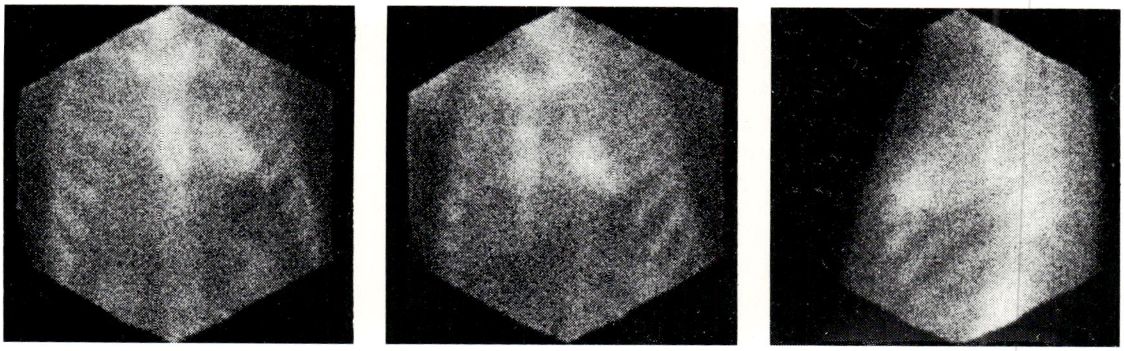

A O L

**FIG. 11.** **ANTEROLATERAL MYOCARDIAL INFARCTION.** On the anterior view, myocardial activity is localized in the lateral wall extending from the anterior basal segment to the apex. Activity can also be seen below the lateral wall in the anterior wall and septum. This extension is best appreciated on the LAO view. The intensity of the activity is equal to that of the sternum and is, therefore, graded at three-plus. The localized pattern makes the overall grading a three-plus localized lesion, which carries a high specificity for acute myocardial infarction. (Courtesy of Dr. Hilliard W. Green, Ridgecrest, CA)

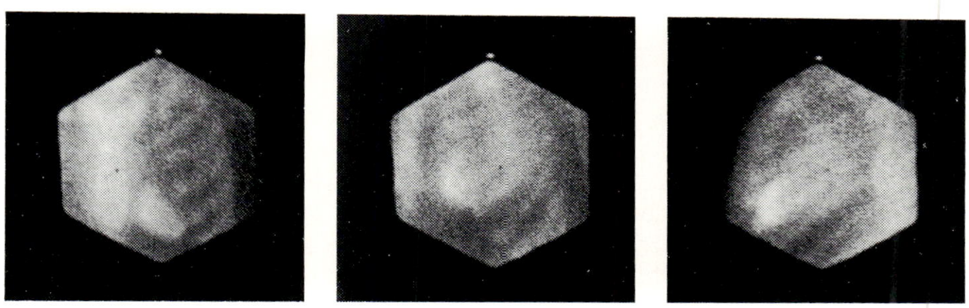

A O L

**FIG. 12.** **ANTEROSEPTAL INFARCTION.** On the anterior view, there is a diffuse pattern of increased activity as the anteroseptal wall is visible *en face*. The intensity is equal to the sternum's and therefore graded at three-plus. On the LAO view, the abnormality becomes localized and the infarction can be seen to involve the anterior wall and septum. On the left lateral view, involvement of the apex can be appreciated, as well as some extension to the anterolateral and anterobasal segments. The three-plus intensity and localized pattern in this patient clinically suspected of having an acute myocardial infarction is highly specific.

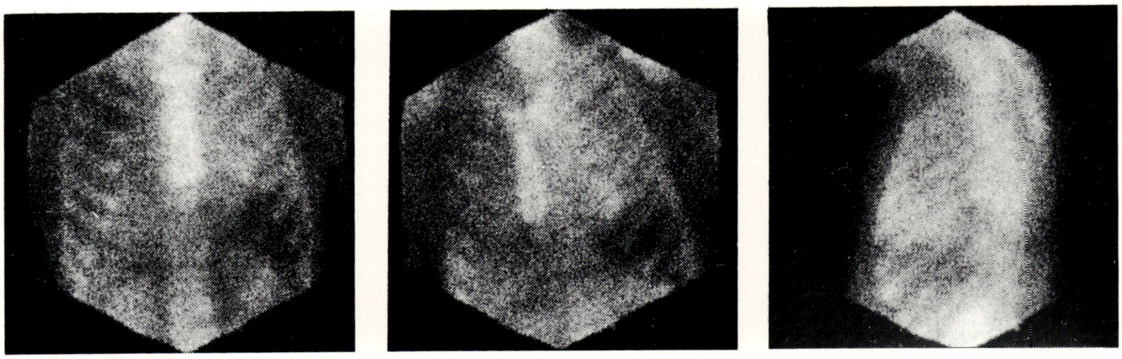

A O L

**FIG. 13. POSTERIOR WALL INFARCTION.** A posterior wall lesion results in a diffuse abnormality on the anterior view. In this example, the anterior view shows an ill-defined area of diffuse activity that is equal in intensity to that of the adjacent ribs but is not a very prominent finding. On the LAO view the posterior wall is imaged end-on and is now visible as a definite abnormality of two-plus intensity and localized to the posterior wall. On the left lateral projection abnormal activity can still be seen in the region of the heart but the finding becomes diffuse and less striking than on the oblique image. In this regard, anterior and posterior wall infarctions are similar in that they are less optimally seen on the anterior and lateral views and projected best on the oblique image. This image should be compared to Fig. 11 of an anterior wall lesion. On the oblique view the anterior and posterior walls are oriented in an axis perpendicular to the collimator face and, therefore, show their localized nature. The anterior wall is situated just behind the sternum, whereas the posterior wall lies deeper within the thorax and is projected as a more posterior structure on the oblique image. (Courtesy of Dr. Hilliard W. Green)

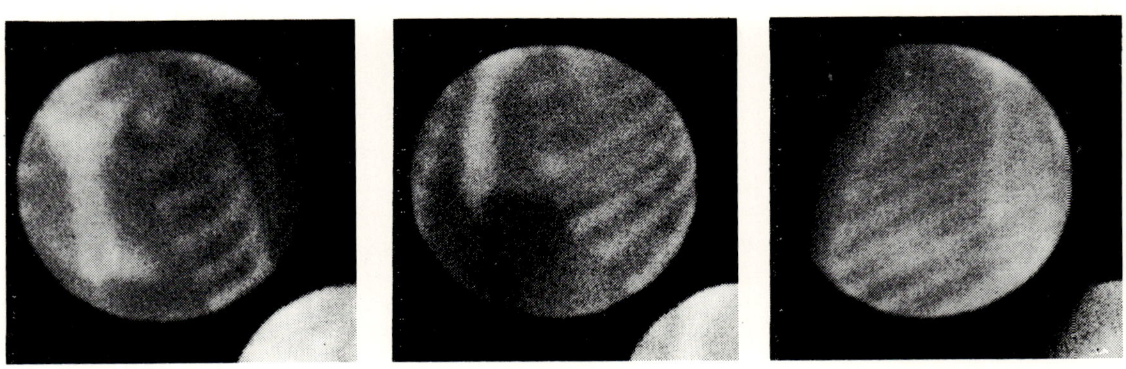

A O L

**FIG. 14. INFERIOR WALL INFARCTION.** This abnormality will be most clearly visible on the anterior view as a linear band of activity extending laterally from the tip of the sternum. It may be confused with, or simulated by, increased concentration of radiotracer in the costal cartilage. Although the abnormal myocardial activity may be less intense on the LAO and left lateral views, it is important to see the lesion on these projections. As the relationship of the thorax and the detector head is changed from the anterior to the LAO view, chest wall activity will rotate as a peripheral structure and maintain a fixed relationship with the sternum. On the LAO view the heart, lying within the chest, will change its relationship with the sternum and be visible as a separate structure. Inferior wall abnormalities are difficult to detect and careful methodologies are necessary to achieve good sensitivity. On the LAO view, especially when the heart assumes a vertical axis, the inferior wall may be poorly visualized. Angling the detector head 10 to 15 degrees cephalad may bring the inferior wall into a more perpendicular axis to the collimator face, thereby enhancing the finding.

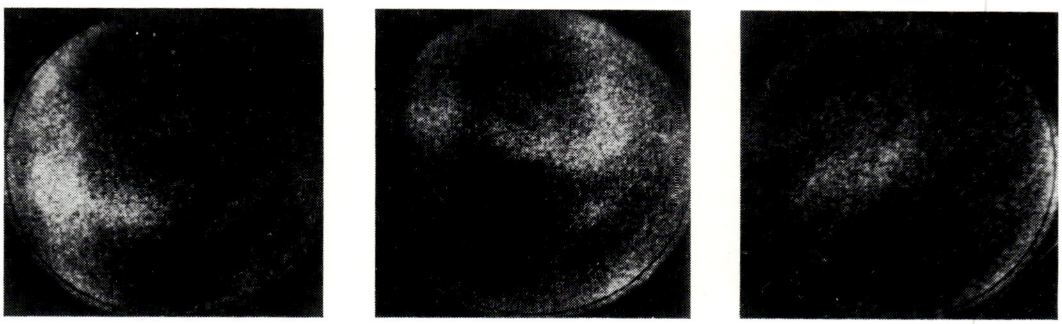

A O L

**FIG. 15.** RIGHT VENTRICULAR INFARCTION. The diagnosis of right ventricular infarction is difficult to establish by the usual criteria of elevated serum enzymes or changes on ECG. Infarction of the right ventricle is invariably accompanied by injury to the thicker and more massive left ventricle, which will dominate the changes occurring in the ECG. The elevation of serum enzymes can also be attributed to the left ventricular infarction, and therefore right ventricular infarction can be suspected only on clinical grounds. As seen in this example, the pyrophosphate scintigram can be helpful in substantiating the diagnosis. On the anterior projection the right ventricle overlies the left ventricle and cannot be distinguished as a separate structure. On the LAO view, however, the two ventricles are positioned side by side, and the abnormality involving the right ventricle can be seen behind the sternum as an extension of the infarction involving the inferior wall and septum. The overall abnormality is W-shaped with the right ventricle forming the left arm of the W.

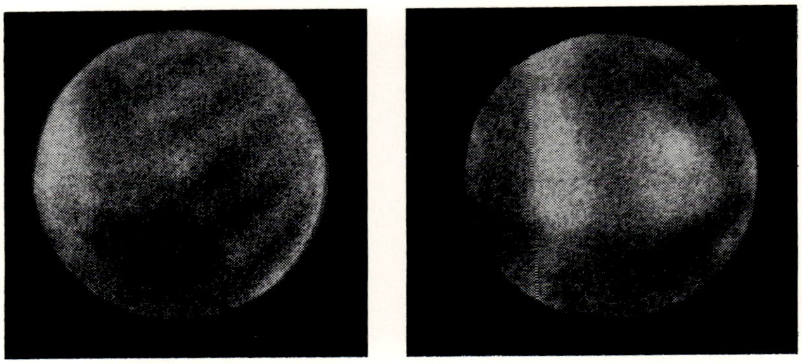

A B

**FIG. 16. PERIOPERATIVE INFARCTION.** Acute myocardial infarction may complicate coronary artery bypass surgery. The incidence commonly quoted in the literature ranges between five and twenty percent. The actual incidence may be much higher. Based on scintigraphic criteria, perioperative infarction may be as common as 30 to 40 percent. A preoperative study is necessary for forming a baseline against which the postoperative scintigram can be compared. The preoperative study should be performed as close to the date of surgery as possible, and the postoperative study on the second or third day following surgery. In this figure the preoperative study (**A**) shows two linear bands of activity which are in the chest wall. The postoperative study (**B**) taken 3 days after surgery contains a new large abnormality of three-plus intensity. (From, J Nucl Med 19:1119, 1978)

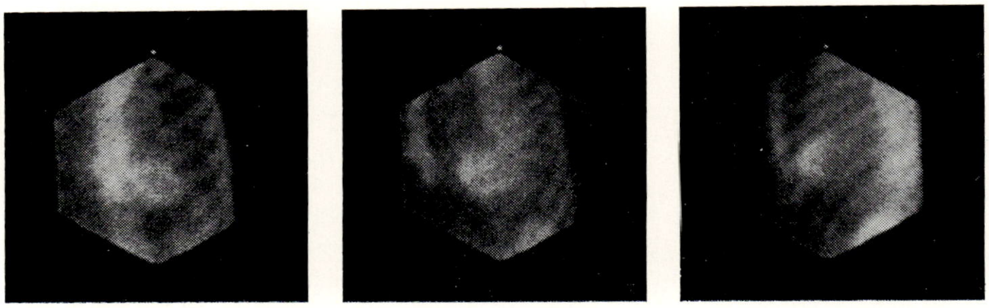

A O L

**FIG. 17. DOUGHNUT PATTERN.** In all three views of this figure, the heart contains an intense concentration of radiotracer, which is localized primarily to the anteroseptal wall. On the anterior view, the activity is greatest around the periphery of the lesion with a central area of decreased activity. This has been labeled the "doughnut" pattern and has been shown to carry a worse prognosis than a diffuse or more regionalized pattern. The development of the doughnut pattern is presumably due to areas of decreased perfusion in the center of a large infarction. The doughnut pattern may be equated with an extensive infarct; the increased morbidity is due to the magnitude of the lesion. In this particular instance there is extensive involvement of the anterior wall with extension to the adjacent anteroseptal and anterolateral segments.

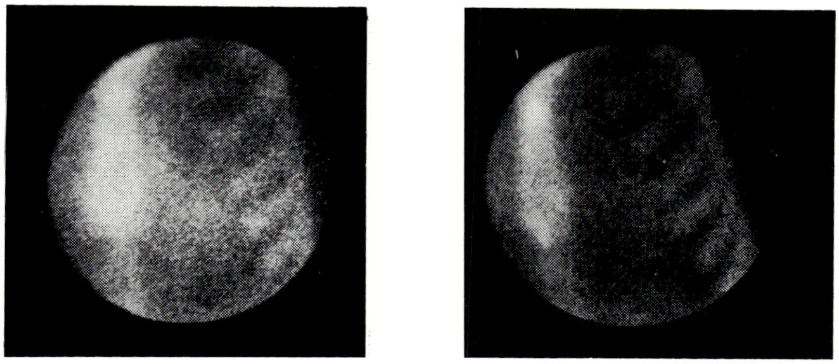

A B

**FIG. 18.** CHANGES WITH CORONARY ARTERY BYPASS SURGERY. In the absence of acute myocardial infarction, when the myocardial scintigram is positive prior to coronary artery bypass surgery (**A**), the study may become normal (**B**) when repeated during the early postoperative period. The causes of normalization following surgery are unknown. Preoperative abnormalities are generally of the two-plus diffuse type (**A**), and the incidence of positivity correlates with the severity of the patient's symptoms. Following surgery the symptoms usually abate; however, the improvement in symptoms does not necessarily correlate with improvement or lack of improvement of the myocardial scintigram. There is a positive correlation with the presence of an abnormal scintigram prior to coronary artery bypass surgery and the surgical mortality. Patients with a positive preoperative scintigram have a higher surgical mortality than do similar patients whose preoperative scintigram shows an intensity less than two-plus. (From J Nucl Med 19:1118, 1978)

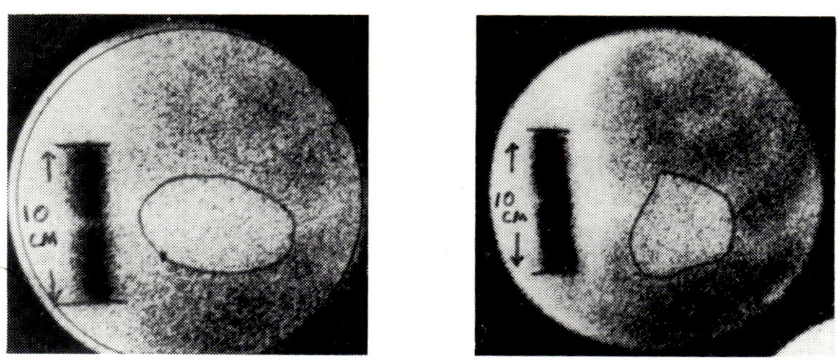


A B

**FIG. 19.** SIZING INFARCTIONS. Acute infarctions may be sized with pyrophosphate scintigraphy by mapping out the area of increased activity and then estimating the size by planimetry. Good correlation has been shown with other standard methods of sizing infarction such as enzyme elevation. The limitations of this procedure are that only those infarcts visible in full relief can be sized by this procedure. For the most part, this limits the technique to the sizing of anteroseptal wall lesions. The technique may underestimate the size of infarctions of other walls when the entire wall is not imaged in a plane parallel to the detector. Overestimations of infarct size may occur when significant radiotracer concentration occurs in the peri-infarction zone surrounding the region of actual infarction. In this example the edge of the abnormality is estimated and a line drawn around the area of abnormal activity. By use of a standard size reference, the area within the perimeter can be computed and the volume of the infarct estimated. Pyrophosphate scintigraphy is better suited to estimating the extent of infarction simply by determining the regions involved. Wall segments and even entire walls adjacent to a major infarction may be involved without producing additional changes on the ECG to indicate their involvement.

A O L

**FIG. 20. DIFFERENTIAL DIAGNOSIS.** At times pyrophosphate scintigraphy may be the most reliable examination for the establishing of a diagnosis of acute myocardial infarction. This is especially true in patients in whom other diseases coexist with acute infarction and mask or falsely alter the serum enzymes and ECG changes. In this example of a 59-year-old male who had a documented pulmonary embolism, his serum enzymes were already elevated when he had a recurrence of chest pain. The ECG showed a loss of the anterior forces, which could be due to a recurrent pulmonary embolus or a new myocardial infarction. The pyrophosphate scintigram showed a three-plus regional abnormality involving the anteroseptal wall, which carried a high specificity for acute myocardial infarction. The patient, who was being treated with parenteral heparin for his previous pulmonary embolus, thus had his condition accurately diagnosed as a complicating acute myocardial infarction rather than as a recurrent embolus. Obviously a mistaken diagnosis at that point would have resulted in surgery on the inferior vena cava, which would have been ill advised in the face of acute myocardial infarction.

## THALLIUM IMAGING

Thallium 201, as thallous chloride, behaves in a manner similar to potassium and enters viable cells. If, for example, a coronary occlusion with resultant myocardial infarction has occurred, the Tl-201 will not be able to gain entry to the involved myocardial cells and radionuclide imaging will show a localized area of absent radioactivity (''cold spot'' imaging). The delivery of Tl-201 to the myocardium is dependent on its arterial perfusion to specific regions; any alteration associated with reduced or absent blood flow, as in myocardial ischemia or injury, will be reflected on imaging as an area of absent perfusion (or radioactivity).

This is in contrast to Tc-99m pyrophosphate imaging, in which the area of myocardial infarction is visible as an area of increased radioactivity (''hot spot'' imaging).

Theoretically, once an infarction has occurred and scarred tissue remains, the area of involvement should continue to be represented as an area of absent radioactivity on all future thallium studies. However, such visualization becomes less prominent over time with the restoration of blood flow through collateral vessels to the infarcted area.

There continues to be some controversy in regard to the use of Tl-201 for the documentation of a myocardial infarction. This is, in part, related to the location in which a gamma camera is situated in the hospital. If, for example, a scintillation camera is present at the patient's bedside, thallium imaging may be usefully employed to assist in the diagnosis of myocardial infarction and to follow the patient's progress serially. On the other hand, if imaging facilities are not available in the patient's unit, Tl-201 imaging should be reserved for those cases in which the diagnosis may be difficult to make (e.g., nonspecific electrocardiogram and enzyme changes) or if the more traditional diagnostic methods prove unrewarding (e.g., a left bundle branch block on electrocardiogram).

One of the most useful applications of Thallium-201 is in stress imaging. By exercising a patient to maximum tolerance, then administering Tl-201 and having him undergo immediate myocardial imaging, areas of ischemia resulting from such stress can be identified as areas of absent activity. If a resting thallium study has shown no abnormalities, the stress imaging may thereby geographically identify sites of myocardial ischemia. The introduction of Tl-201 for stress imaging has made an enormous impact on modern medicine. The results of such studies have been most informative and have aided in the monitoring of patients with known or suspected coronary artery disease.

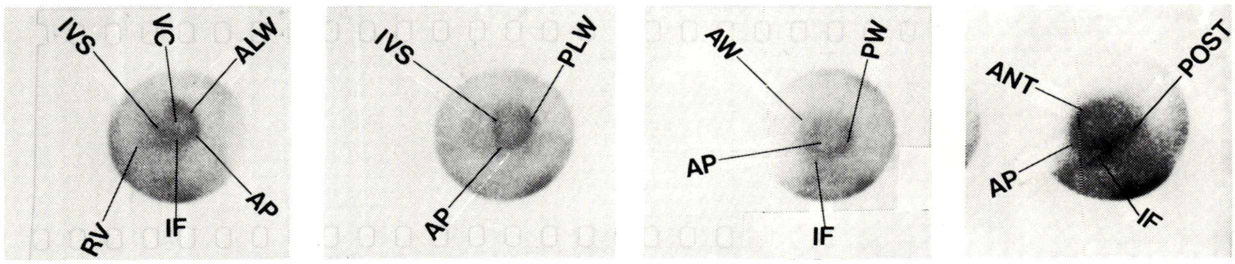


A ANT B LAO 45 degrees C LAO 70 degrees D L LAT

**FIG. 21.** NORMAL, RESTING THALLIUM IMAGING. Imaging is usually performed in the anterior, 45 degree left anterior oblique, 70 degree left anterior oblique, and left lateral positions. Since imaging in the two latter positions gives much the same information, *either* a 70 degree LAO or left lateral study is usually sufficient. For completeness, some groups prefer that imaging be performed in all four positions. In the patient's resting state, the background radioactivity in both the blood and extracardiac structures is relatively high. This results in relatively poor definition of the resting myocardial image. Radioactivity in the liver, spleen, kidneys, stomach, and small intestine is visible. Although each of the studies illustrated is normal, there are marked differences among them. **A. Anterior position.** The anterolateral (**ALW**) or anterior wall, inferior wall *and* the interventricular septum (**IVS**) are demonstrated. Radioactivity from the stomach and liver interfere with the clarity of the image of the interventricular septum. The central area of reduced radioactivity is the ventricular cavity (**VC**). There are no obvious areas of absent radioactivity in the somewhat horseshoe-shaped image. **B. 45 degree LAO position.** It is in this view that the definition of the myocardial image is best, probably because of the closeness of the myocardium to the collimator. The interventricular spectum and posterolateral (**PLW**) (or lateral) wall are clearly visualized. **C. 70 degree LAO position.** Both the anterior (**ANT**) and posterior (**POST**) walls are clearly visible. The apical (**AP**) region is sharply demonstrated. **D. Left lateral position.** As in the 70 degree LAO position, the image is dominated by the anterior and posterior walls of the left ventricle. The inferior wall (**IF**) and apical area are clearly visible.

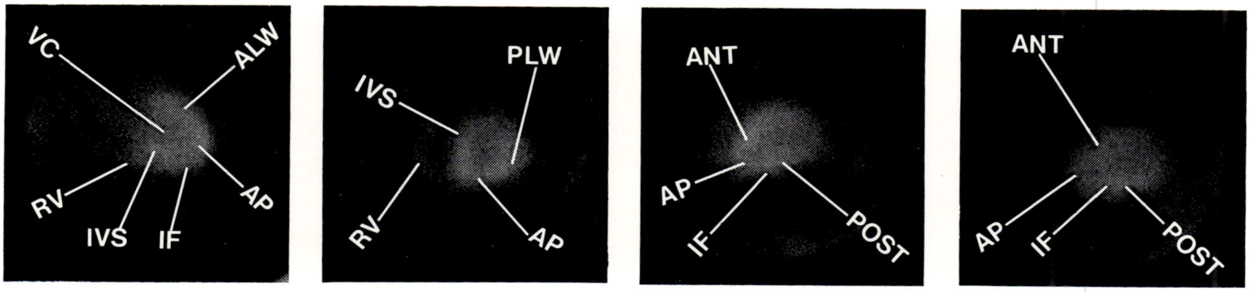


ANT

LAO
45 degrees

LAO
70 degrees

L LAT

**FIG. 22. NORMAL THALLIUM IMAGING FOLLOWING EXERCISE.** If thallium-201 is administered 60 seconds before the cessation of exercise-induced stress (as on a treadmill or bicycle ergometer) and imaging started *immediately* following the completion of the exercise, the thallium image will reflect the increased coronary arterial flow to the myocardium. As a result of increased Tl-201 delivery to the myocardium, the images so produced will be of elegant definition compared to those obtained with the patient at rest. Note the clarity of the cardiac structures (see Fig. 1 for label definitions). It is common to observe the free wall of the right ventricle (RV) on exercise imaging while it is rarely demonstrated in those studies performed with the patient at rest (see Fig. 23 for some exceptions). In the patient with coronary artery disease, reduced perfusion may be induced through exercise, and this will appear on imaging as an area of absent radioactivity.

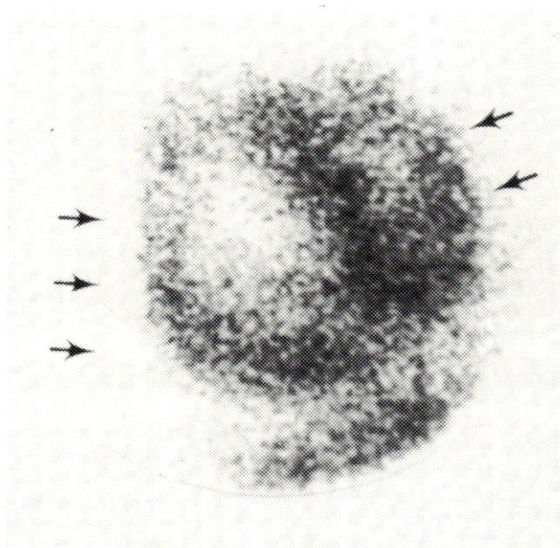

A Pulmonary Hypertension

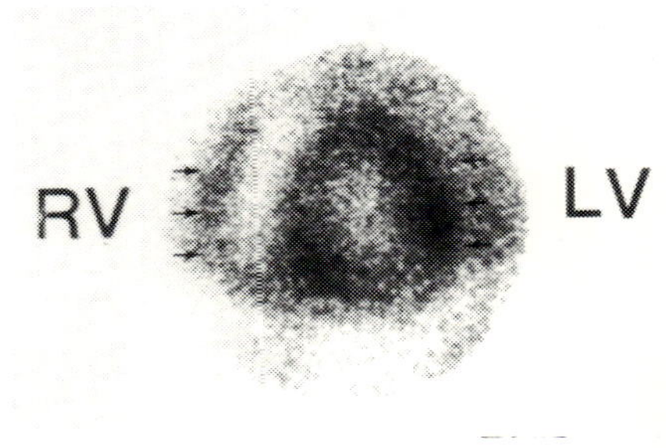


B

Congestive Cardiomyopathy

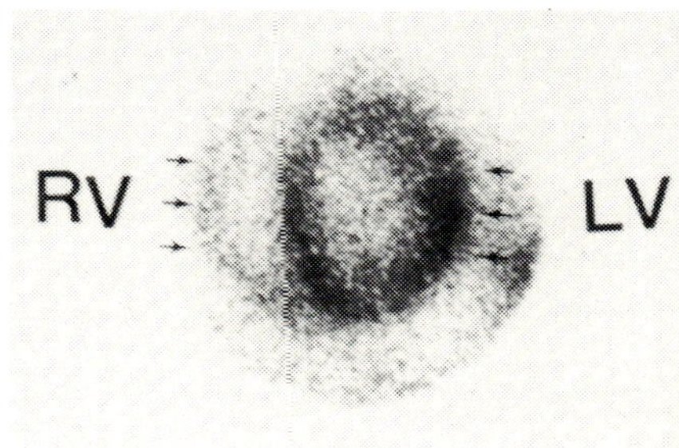


C

Aortic Regurgitation

**FIG. 23. RIGHT VENTRICULAR IMAGING IN THE 45 DEGREE LAO POSITION, IN PATIENTS WITH PULMONARY HYPERTENSION.** Visualization of the right ventricle in the resting state with thallium imaging is uncommon. **A.** Primary pulmonary hypertension. The enlarged right ventricular cavity (large arrow) is readily visible. Compare this to the smaller left ventricle. The right ventricular wall is clearly identified (small arrows). **B.** Pulmonary hypertension secondary to congestive cardiomyopathy. There is unusual clarity in the demonstration of the wall of the enlarged right ventricle. Right ventricular visualization in patients with (**C**) aortic regurgitation is also commonly seen. (From Khaja F, Mohsin A, Goldstein S, et al: Circulation 59:182, 1979)

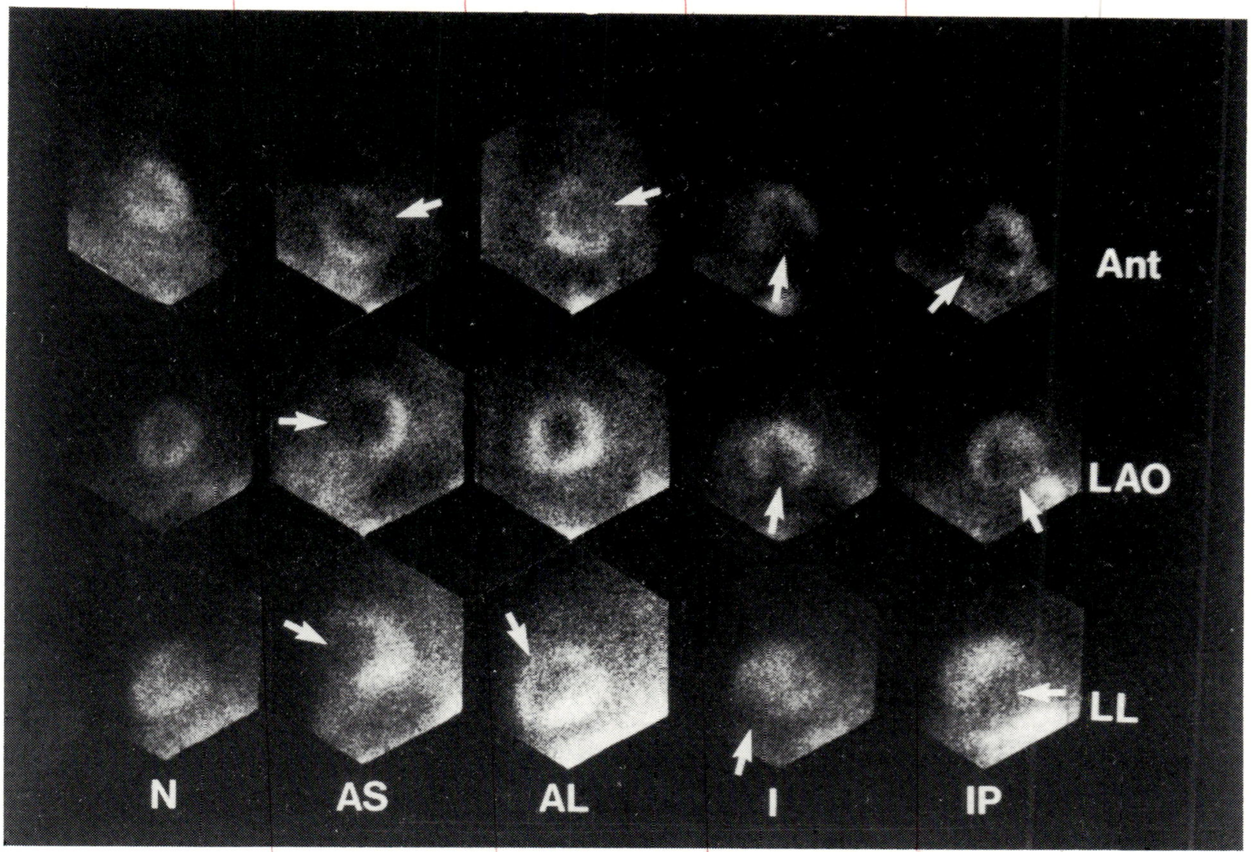


**FIG. 24.** **THALLIUM IMAGING OF MYOCARDIAL INFARCTIONS THAT HAVE OCCURRED AT VARIOUS SITES.** The distinctive feature of a myocardial infarction on thallium imaging is a localized area of absent radioactivity, which is equivalent to an area of absent or reduced arterial perfusion. In this illustration, thallium images in five different patients are shown that were obtained in the anterior, 45 degree LAO and left lateral positions. **A. Normal Images.** The images in the first column are normal. In the subsequent four columns, arrows identify regions of myocardial infarction at various sites. **B. Anteroseptal Infarction.** The area of involvement in the anterior wall is seen in the anterior and left lateral positions, and involvement of the septum is visible in the 45 degree LAO position. **C. Anterolateral Infarction.** The area of absent radioactivity in the anterolateral wall is best seen in the anterior position. The reduction in perfusion in the anterior wall is less marked in the left lateral position. **D. Inferior Wall Infarction.** The area of involvement, including the apex, is sharply demonstrated in all three positions. **E. Inferoposterior Wall Infarction.** Note how clearly this is demonstrated in the left lateral position. (From Wackers FJT, Sokole EB, Samson G et al: Clin Nucl Med 2: 64, 1977)

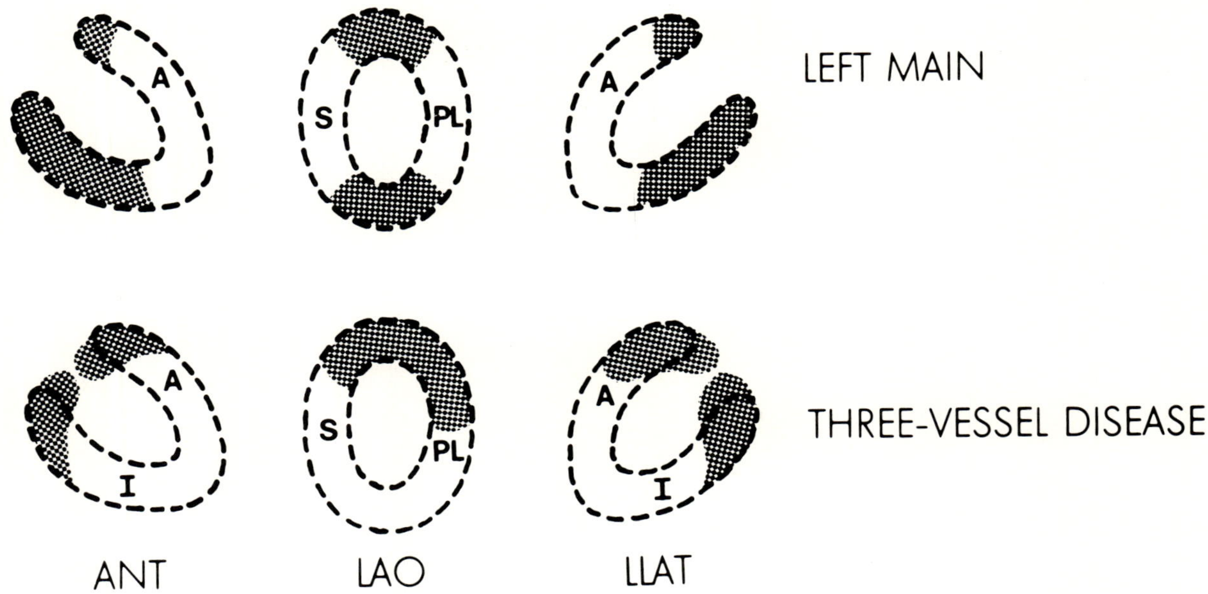


**FIG. 25. ARTERIAL INVOLVEMENT AND THALLIUM IMAGING.** Attempts have been made to *precisely* define the major coronary arteries that might be involved when visualizing areas of absent perfusion on the thallium image. In this schematic representation, imaging findings in cases of left main coronary artery and three-vessel disease are illustrated. The shaded areas represent regions of relatively normal perfusion, while the clear or white areas are indicative of an absence or reduction of perfusion. **Upper panel:** Isolated left main coronary artery disease associated with an absence of radioactivity in the regions of the anterior (A) wall in the anterior and left lateral positions and the interventricular septum (S) and posterolateral wall (PL) in the 45 degree LAO position. **Lower panel:** Three-vessel disease (involvement of the right coronary artery, circumflex artery, and left anterior descending artery). As a result of three-vessel disease, reduced perfusion and absent perfusion are visible in all three views including the anterior, posterolateral, and inferior (I) walls as well as the interventricular septum. (From Dash H, Massie BM, Botvinick et al: Circulation 60: 276, 1979)

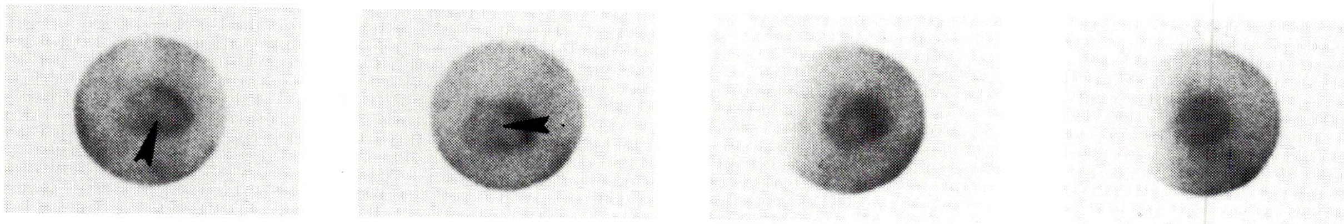

A ANT LAO 45 degrees LAO 70 degrees L LAT

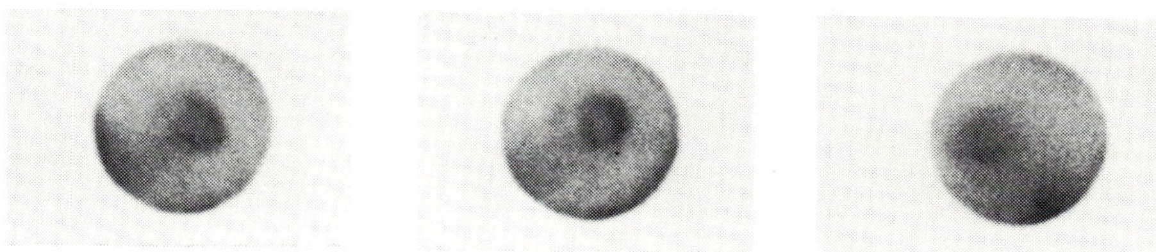

B ANT LAO 45 degrees L LAT

**FIG. 26.** STRESS THALLIUM IMAGING AND SEPTAL ISCHEMIA. Following exercise on a treadmill until anterior chest pain was elicited, 2 mCi of T1-201 was administered intravenously and imaging was started immediately thereafter. **A.** Reduced activity (arrow) in the interventricular septum is consistent with myocardial ischemia at that site, but this interpretation can be made with confidence only if certain other conditions are met. These conditions include normal thallium imaging in the patient's resting state *or* knowledge that a myocardial infarction has not occurred. Although the findings are consistent with ischemia, the single study could also be consistent with a septal infarction. **B.** The term *redistribution study* is commonly used to designate thallium imaging 3 or 4 hours following its injection at the time of exercise. The purpose of redistribution imaging is to demonstrate the altered perfusion to the myocardium in the patient's resting state as compared to that seen during exercise. In many situations, this is an accurate reflection. However, in some cases the findings on redistribution imaging are at variance with those of separate resting studies.

If there is persistence in absent radioactivity on the redistribution image when compared to the exercise study, this *may* be interpreted as being consistent with infarction. However, there may be insufficient circulating Tl -201 available to enter the involved myocardium in the presence only of ischemia; therefore, the study would be incorrectly interpreted as showing infarction. On the other hand, if there has been a prior myocardial infarction with the development of collateral vessels, the stress study may show no evidence of absent radioactivity because of the increased perfusion associated with the collaterals at the time of exercise. The redistribution study in such cases may or may not demonstrate the infarcted area. Thus the insistence on separate thallium imaging with the patient at rest a day or two before or after the stress study.

In the redistribution study shown here, there is reperfusion to the involved area of the septum. This was interpreted as being consistent with ischemia.

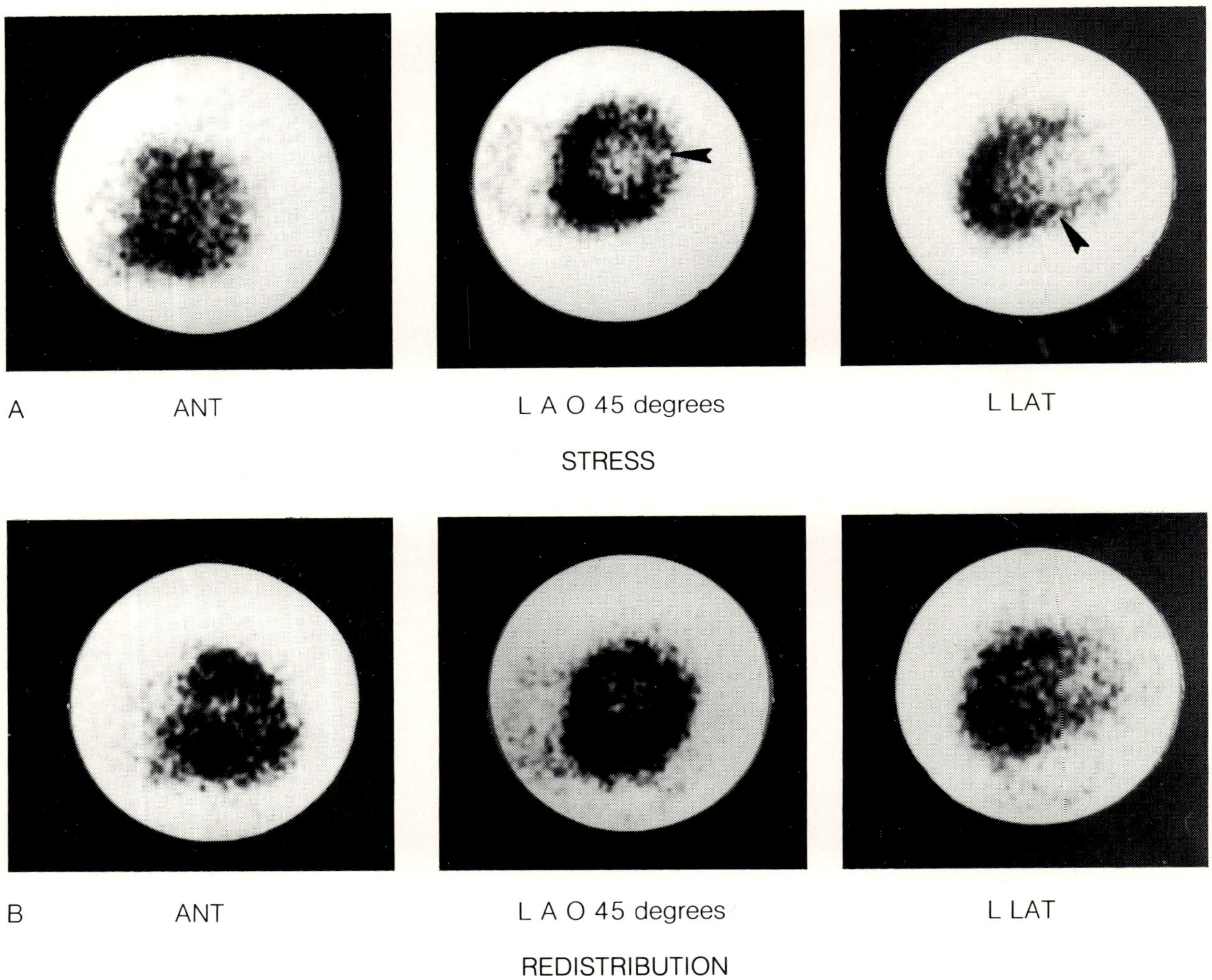


**FIG. 27. MYOCARDIAL ISCHEMIA INVOLVING THE POSTEROLATERAL WALL. A.** Stress imaging shows evidence of reduced activity in the area of the posterior and posterolateral wall (arrows). **B.** Redistribution study shows evidence of reperfusion at these sites, findings that are consistent with myocardial ischemia. (Courtesy of Dr. John F. Rockett, Baptist Memorial Hospital, Memphis, TN)

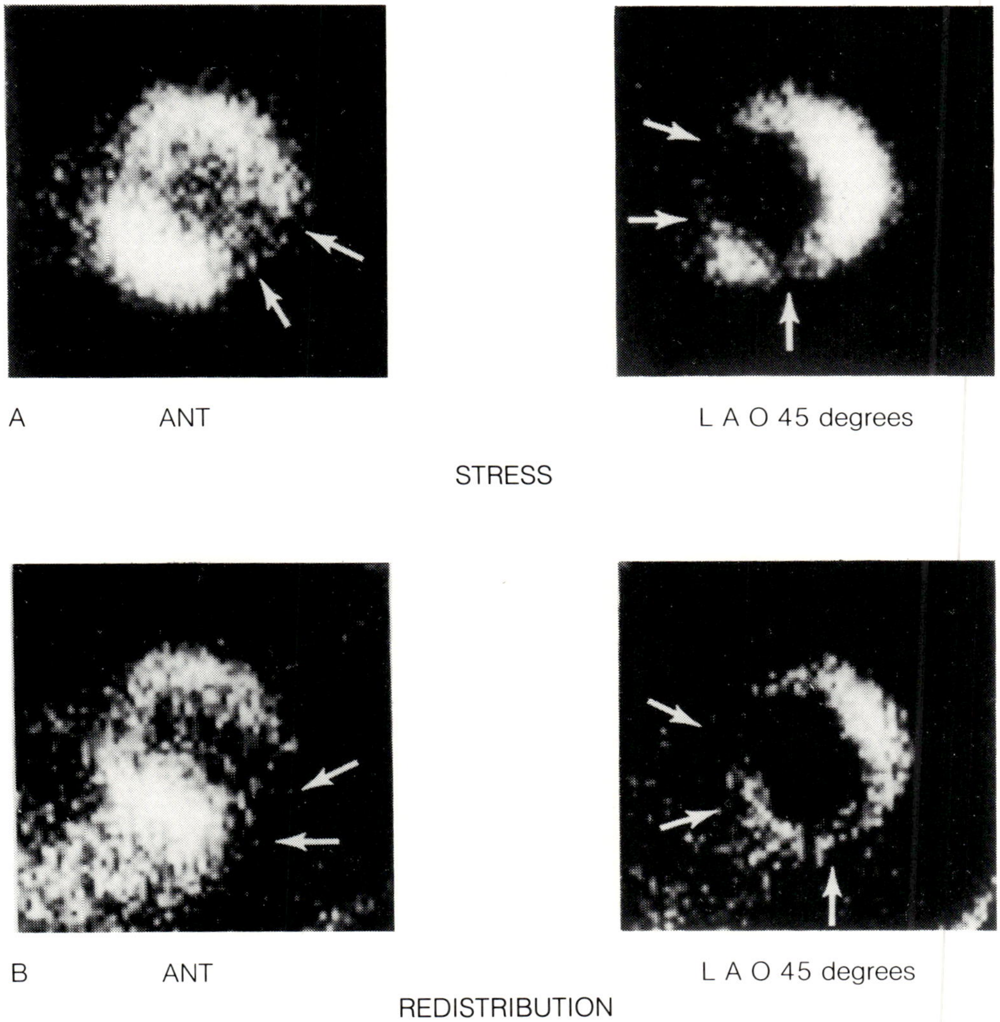


**FIG. 28. STRESS THALLIUM IMAGING AND DELAYED RESTING STUDIES IN A PATIENT *WITH* PRIOR KNOWN MYOCARDIAL INFARCTION: NO REDISTRIBUTION.** There is persistence in the areas of absent radioactivity in this patient with a known history of anterolateral infarction. **A.** Stress imaging shows areas of absent perfusion in the anterior apical wall in the anterior position and in the septum and apex in the LAO position (arrows). **B.** Delayed redistribution imaging performed 4 hours following the stress study shows no evidence of redistribution, with persistent absence of perfusion at the sites of the previously infarcted areas. These findings suggest no evidence of collateral supply to the previously infarcted myocardium and is the imaging picture commonly seen in the patient with prior myocardial infarction. (From Verani MS, Jhingran S, Attar M: Am J Cardiol 43:1114, 1979)

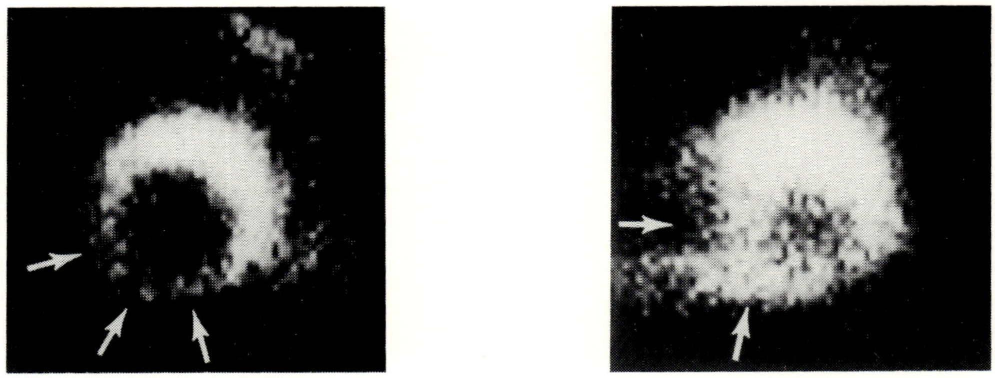

A ANT L A O 45 degrees

STRESS

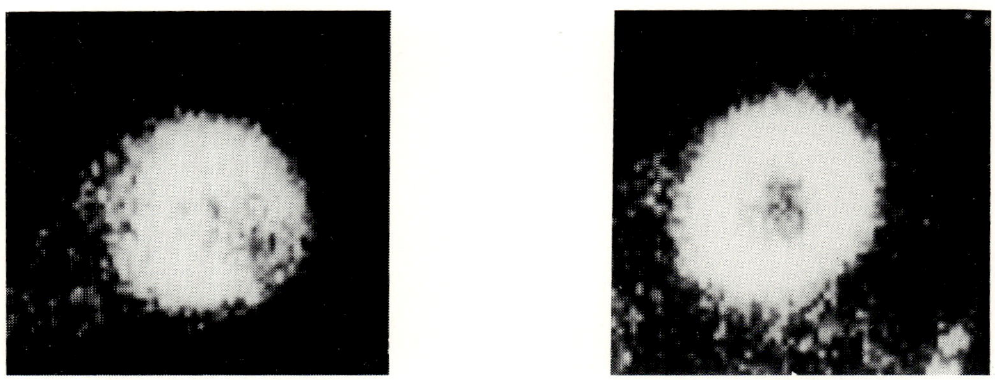

B ANT L A O 45 degrees

REDISTRIBUTION

**FIG. 29.** STRESS THALLIUM IMAGING AND DELAYED RESTING STUDIES IN A PATIENT *WITH* PRIOR KNOWN MYOCARDIAL INFARCTION: REDISTRIBUTION. Although the patient with a known myocardial infarction in the past should exhibit a corresponding area of absent radioactivity on imaging in the absence of stress, this is not always the case. **A.** Stress imaging in a patient with a history of inferior and anteroseptal infarctions shows areas of absent perfusion in the inferior and apical regions in the anterior position and in the septum and inferior wall in the LAO position (arrows). **B.** Delayed redistribution studies performed 4 hours after the start of the stress study show a minimal perfusion defect (arrow) in the apex (arrow) in the anterior position and none in the LAO position. There has been almost complete redistribution in the involved regions in association with perfusion through collateral vessels to the previously infarcted myocardium. In the absence of a prior history of myocardial infarction, this might have been interpreted as showing evidence simply of myocardial ischemia and thus further emphasizes the necessity of separate injection *resting* studies to help document whether or not evidence of a prior myocardial infarction is present. (From Verani MS, Jhingran S, Attar M: Am J Cardiol 43:1114, 1979)

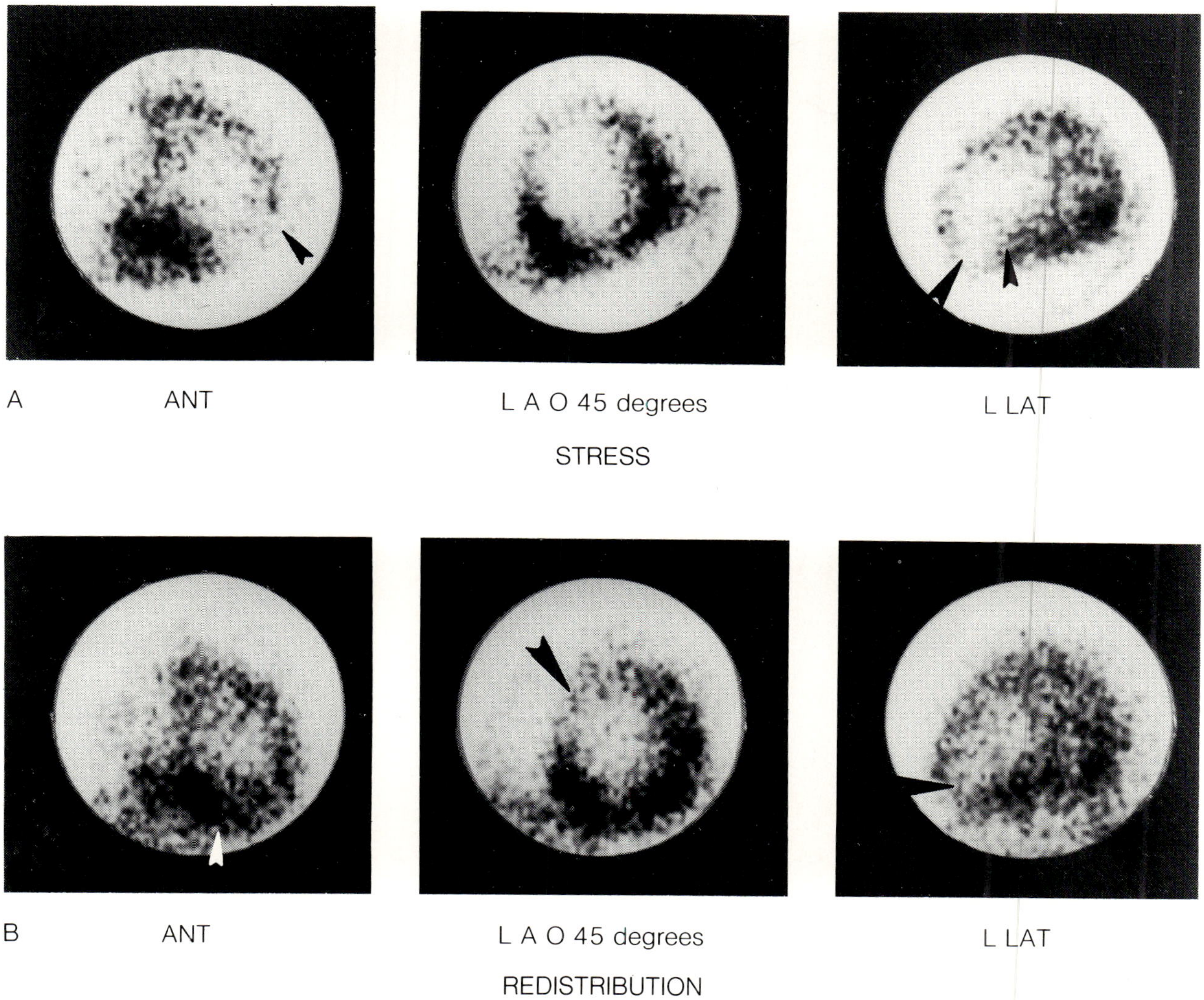


**FIG. 30. INFERIOR WALL ISCHEMIA IN A PATIENT WITH ANTEROSEPTAL AND APICAL INFARCTIONS. A.** Stress study shows absent perfusion (small arrow) in the region of the inferior wall. This finding is clearly demonstrated in the anterior and left lateral positions. Note the manifestations of the anteroseptal and apical infarctions ( larger arrow) in the LAO and left lateral positions. **B.** Redistribution studies at 4 hours show evidence of reperfusion in the region of the inferior wall (small arrow), findings that are consistent with ischemia. However, the persistence of absent radioactivity in the anteroseptal and apical regions suggests that infarction is responsible for this abnormality (larger arrows). (Courtesy of Dr. John F. Rockett, Baptist Memorial Hospital, Memphis, TN)

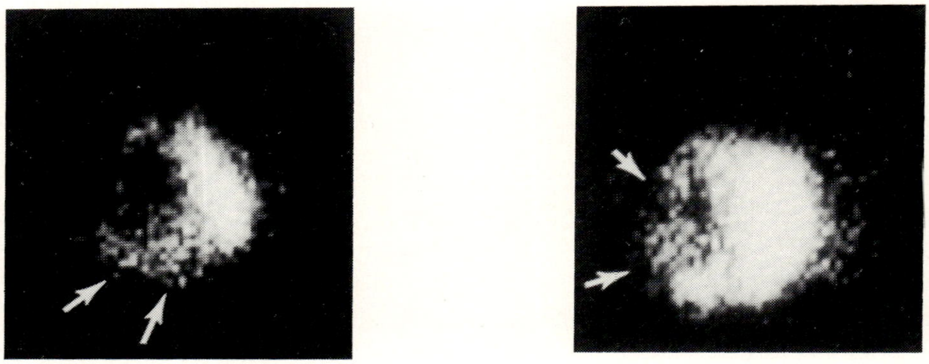

A ANT L A O 45 degrees

STRESS

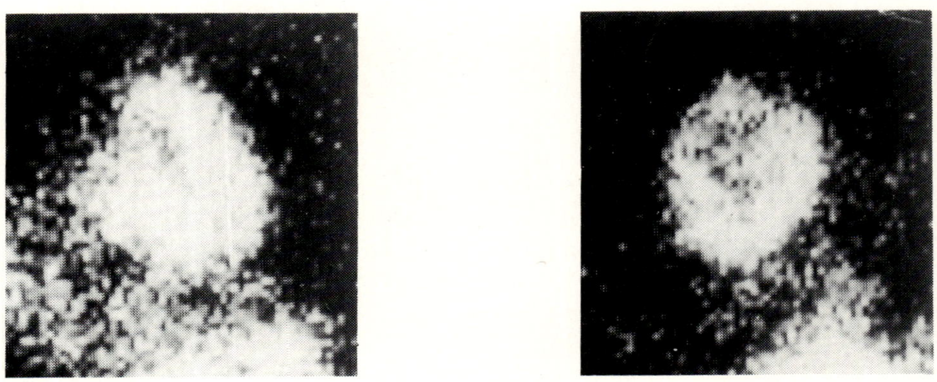

B ANT L A O 45 degrees

REDISTRIBUTION

**FIG. 31.** STRESS THALLIUM IMAGING AND DELAYED RESTING STUDIES IN A PATIENT WITH CORONARY ARTERY DISEASE *WITHOUT* PRIOR MYOCARDIAL INFARCTION: REDISTRIBUTION. If there has been no previous myocardial infarction, it is expected that there should be no areas of absent perfusion on the delayed resting study. **A.** Stress thallium imaging shows evidence of absent perfusion in the inferior wall in the anterior position and in the septum in the LAO position (arrows). **B.** Delayed resting imaging performed 4 hours following the start of the stress study shows no abnormalities and further confirms the interpretation of myocardial ischemia on stress imaging. (From Verani MS, Jhingran S, Attar M: Am J Cardiol 43:1114, 1979)

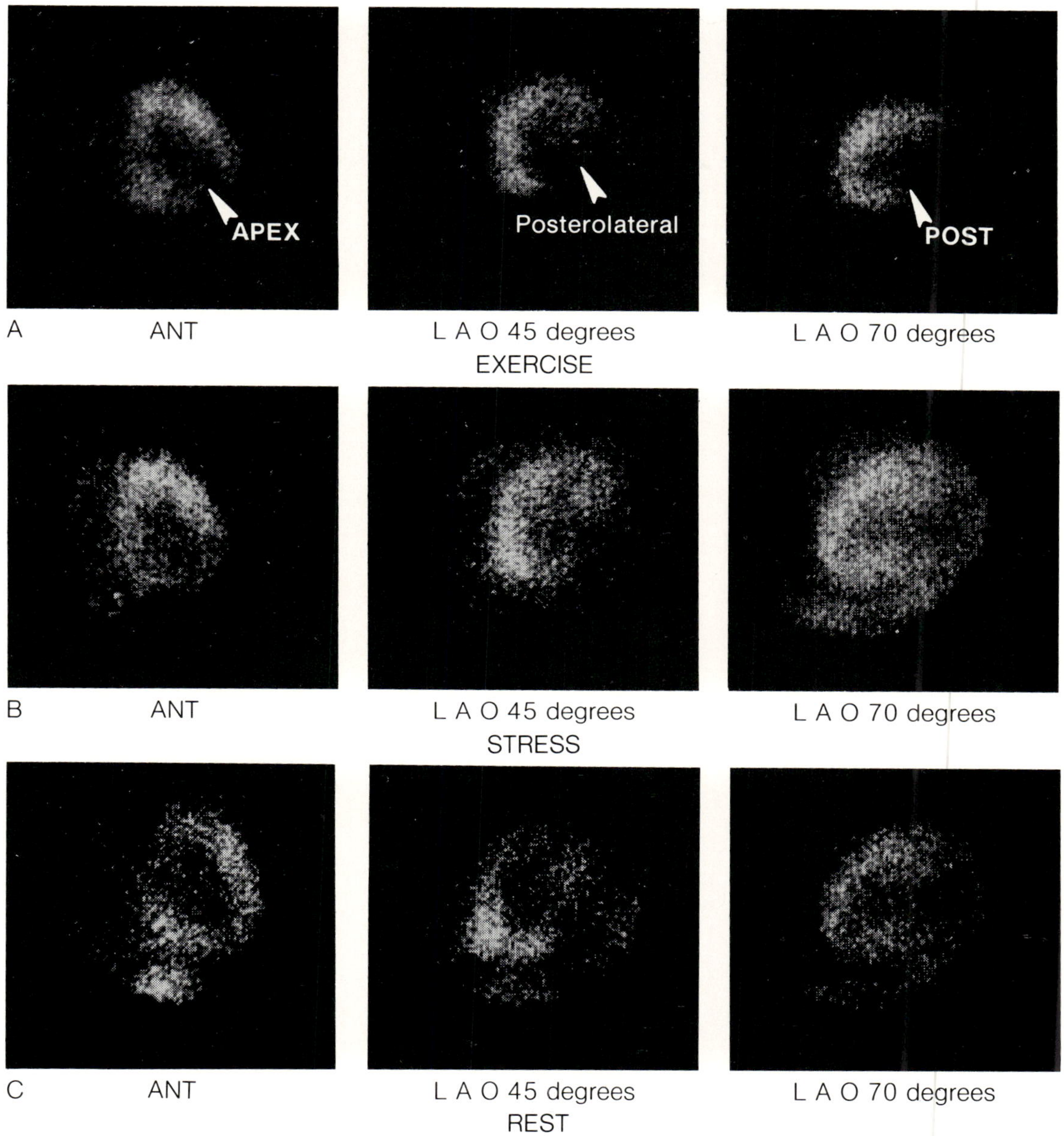


**FIG. 32. MYOCARDIAL ISCHEMIA: EXERCISE AND REDISTRIBUTION STUDIES AT VARIANCE WITH SEPARATE RESTING STUDIES.** **A.** Stress thallium imaging shows large areas of absent perfusion (arrows) in the regions of the apex, inferior, and posterolateral walls. **B.** Similar extensive areas of absent radioactivity are seen on the 4 hour redistribution study. In the absence of further evaluation, the persistence of the stress findings on the redistribution studies could have been interpreted as showing areas of myocardial infarction. **C.** Resting imaging performed one week later shows a relatively normal perfusion pattern and *now* the findings are indicative of myocardial ischemia rather than infarction.

Redistribution imaging may not accurately reflect myocardial perfusion in the patient at rest, as in this case. If possible, it is best to perform resting myocardial imaging as a separate procedure to help determine whether myocardial ischemia or infarction is present. Although logistically more cumbersome, it provides a more meaningful comparison between those images obtained with the patient at rest and those taken during exercise. (Courtesy of Dr. John F. Rockett, Baptist Memorial Hospital, Memphis, TN)

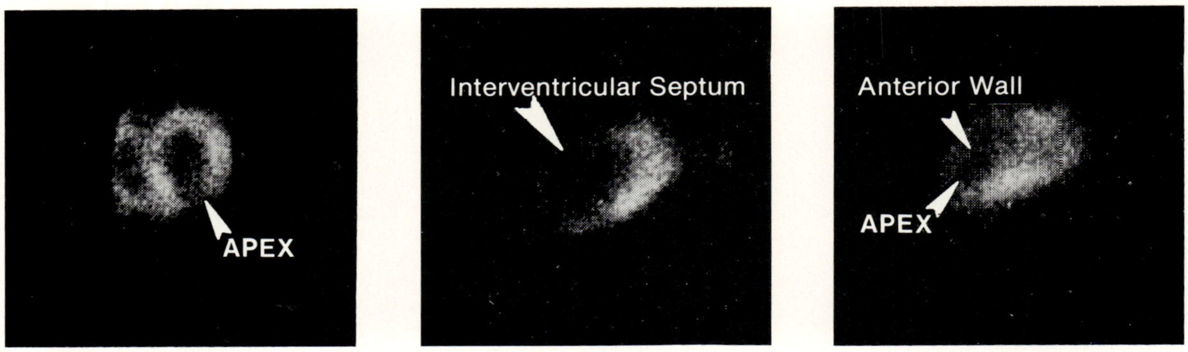


A ANT L A O 45 degrees L LAT

PREOPERATIVE STRESS

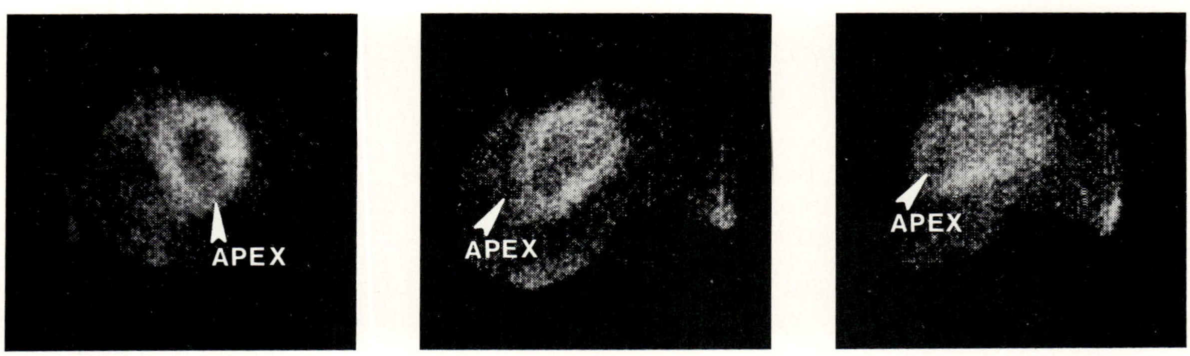


B ANT L A O 45 degrees L LAT

PREOPERATIVE, REDISTRIBUTION

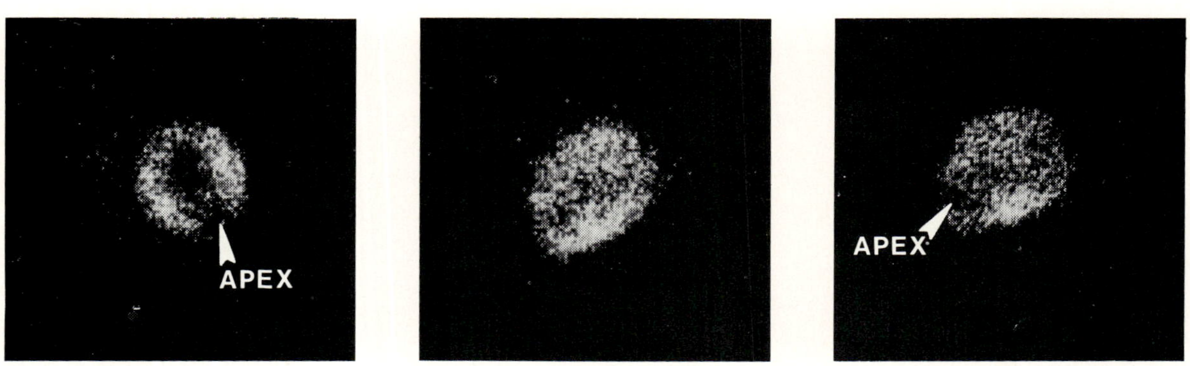


C ANT L A O 45 degrees L LAT

POSTOPERATIVE STRESS

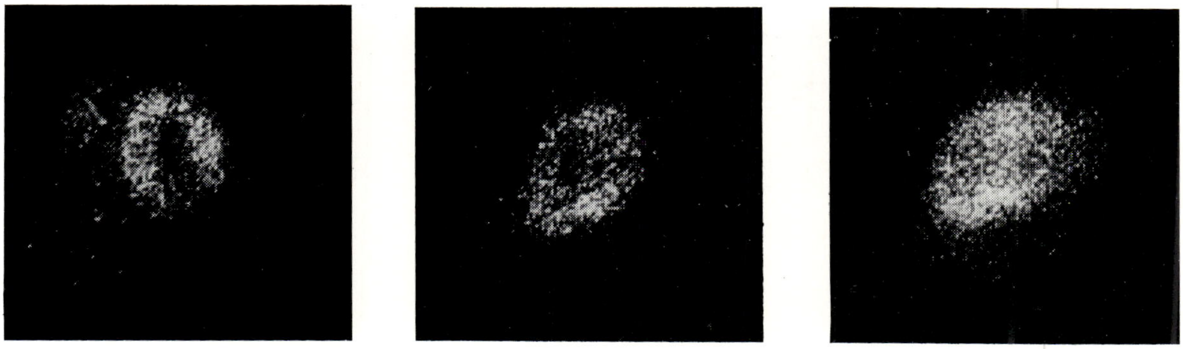

D ANT L A O 45 degrees L LAT

POSTOPERATIVE RESTING

**FIG. 33.** MYOCARDIAL IMAGING AND BENEFICIAL EFFECTS OF CORONARY ARTERY BYPASS SURGERY. **A. Preoperative Stress Imaging.** The absent radioactivity at the apex (arrow) is consistent with a known, prior apical infarction. However, perfusion defects are seen in the 45 degree LAO position in the interventricular septum ( larger arrow) and, in the left lateral position, in the anterior wall. That this is probably due to ischemia is indicated in the redistribution study. **B. Preoperative Redistribution Study.** There has been reperfusion in the comparable septal and anterior wall regions. The apical reduction persists.

A coronary arteriogram showed marked narrowing of the right coronary artery and the circumflex artery and occlusion of the proximal portion of the left anterior descending coronary artery. Coronary artery bypass surgery was performed with resultant symptomatic improvement.

C. **Postoperative Stress Imaging** performed 1 month following surgery shows an absence of apical activity (arrow) at the site of the old infarction. Otherwise, no areas of absent perfusion are noted. Compare this to the preoperative stress study. **D. Postoperative Redistribution Study** shows no changes when compared to the rest imaging. **Comparison of preoperative and postoperative stress imaging in the LAO position** shows the marked change in the perfusion in the regions of the septum and posterolateral wall seen as a result of bypass surgery. (Courtesy of Dr. John F. Rockett, Baptist Memorial Hospital, Memphis, TN)

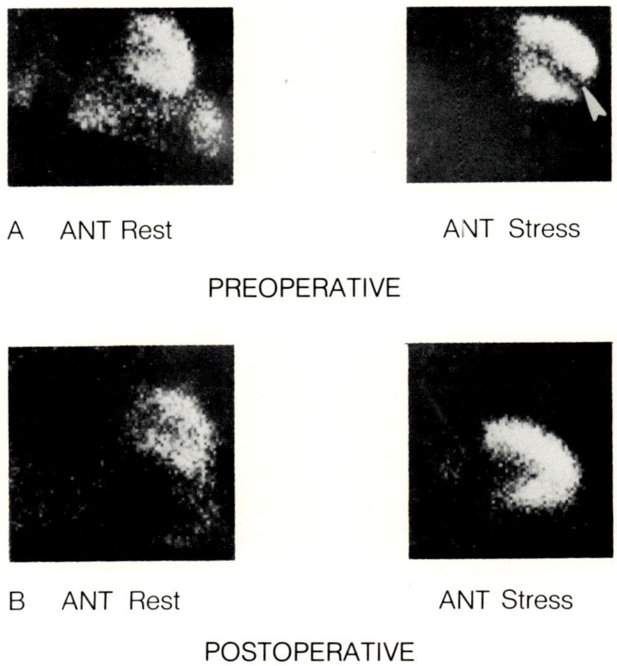


**FIG. 34. REPERFUSION ASSOCIATED WITH CORONARY ARTERY BYPASS GRAFT SURGERY. A.** Preoperative resting imaging performed in the anterior position shows no abnormalities. However, the preoperative stress thallium image shows a localized area of absent radioactivity (arrow) in the apical region. Preoperative coronary arteriography showed a 95 percent stenosis of the left anterior descending coronary artery. **B.** Postoperative resting image shows no abnormalities. In the postoperative stress study, the area of absent perfusion visible on preoperative stress imaging is no longer seen. A coronary arteriogram performed 3 months postoperatively showed a patent graft to the left anterior descending coronary artery. (From Corne RA, Gotsman MS, Atlan H: Am Heart J 97:112, 1979)

## MYOCARDIAL IMAGING WITH THALLIUM AND USING A MULTIPLE PINHOLE COLLIMATOR

Improved identification of areas of absent or reduced arterial perfusion on thallium imaging has been attempted in several ways such as with computerized image enhancement, a multiple pinhole collimator, and emission computerized tomography. With a multiple pinhole collimator, images are obtained in a number of planes and sectional views of the heart are seen. Rather than being limited to a single composite image in any one position in which an area of absent radioactivity may be masked or not sharply demonstrated, the sectional image can bring into focus a discrete area of absent perfusion that may not otherwise be recognized. When compared to the more commonly performed radionuclide imaging procedures, tomographic imaging of the myocardium is infrequently performed. However, illustrating the tomographic studies makes conventional myocardial imaging a bit easier to conceptualize.

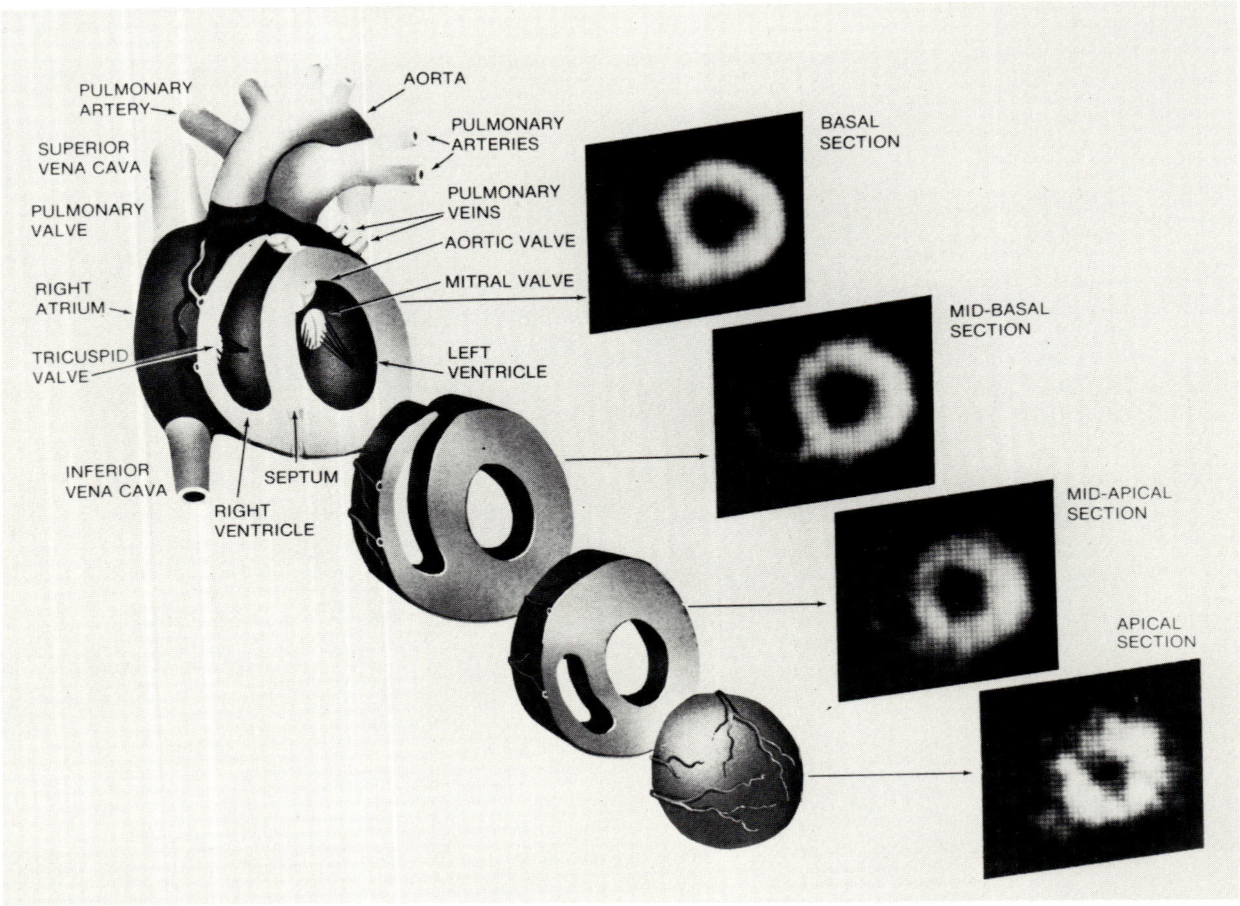


**FIG. 35. THALLIUM TOMOGRAPHIC IMAGING USING A SEVEN PINHOLE COLLIMATOR.** Sectional anterior images as they are related to comparable myocardial sections are shown. Although only four planes are illustrated here, a total of 12 planes had been obtained. In addition to improving the accuracy of the method, such sectional imaging makes the relationship of the myocardial image to the cross-sectional anatomy of the heart more meaningful. (From Vogel RA, Kirch DL, LeFree MT et al: Am J Cardiol 43:787, 1979)

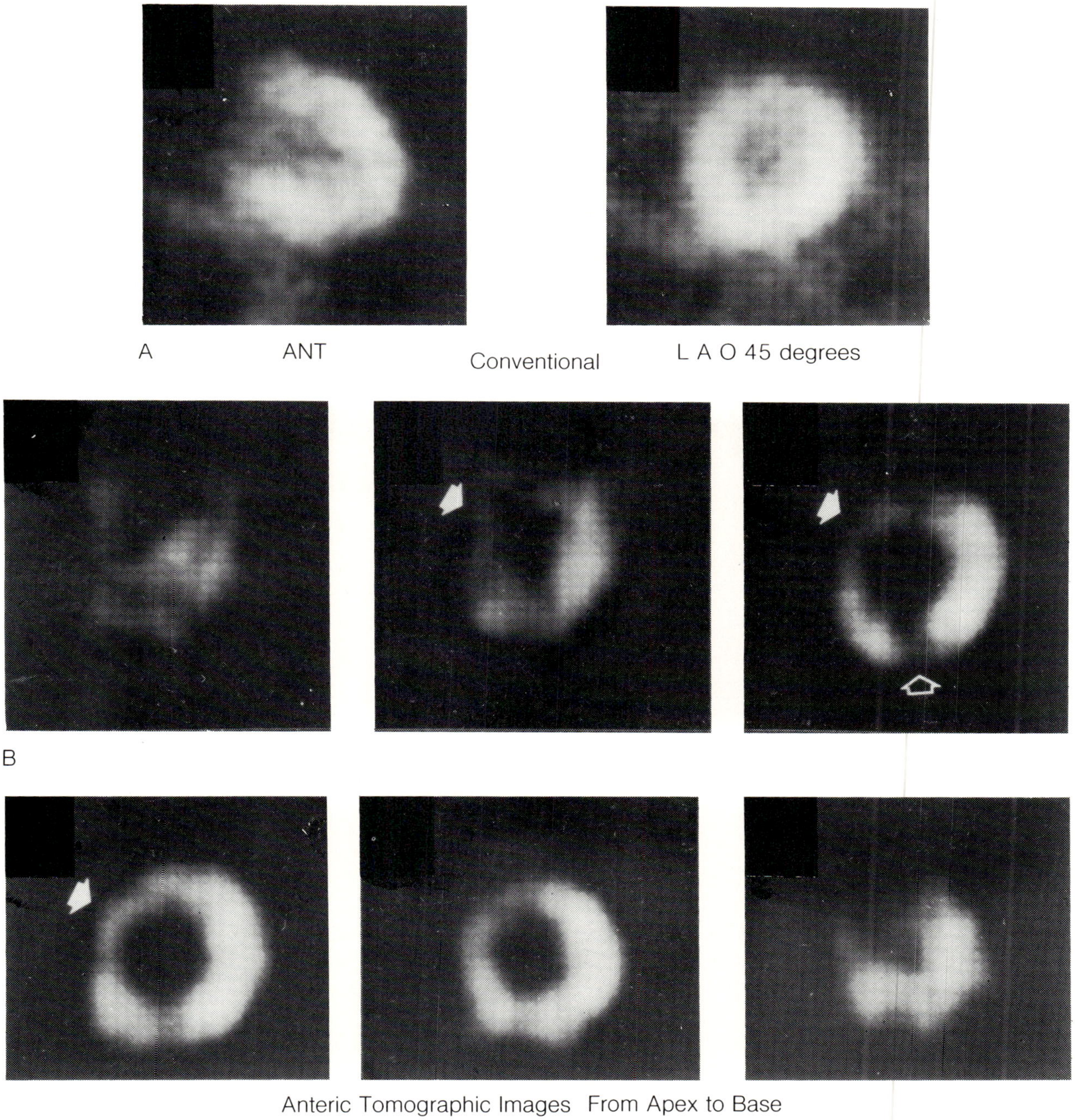


**FIG. 36. ABSENT PERFUSION SEEN ON TOMOGRAPHIC IMAGING ONLY. A.** Conventional thallium imaging in the anterior and 45 degree LAO positions discloses no abnormalities. **B.** Representative anterior tomographic images, from apex to base (left to right) show evidence of absent radioactivity (closed arrows) in the interventricular septum. This patient had 90 percent stenosis of the left anterior descending coronary artery. Unless the tomographic imaging had been performed, the site of absent perfusion could not have been identified. The open arrow indicates the commonly observed apical reduction in radioactivity, which is not abnormal. (From Vogel RA, Kirch DL, LeFree MT et al: Am J Cardiol 43:787, 1979)

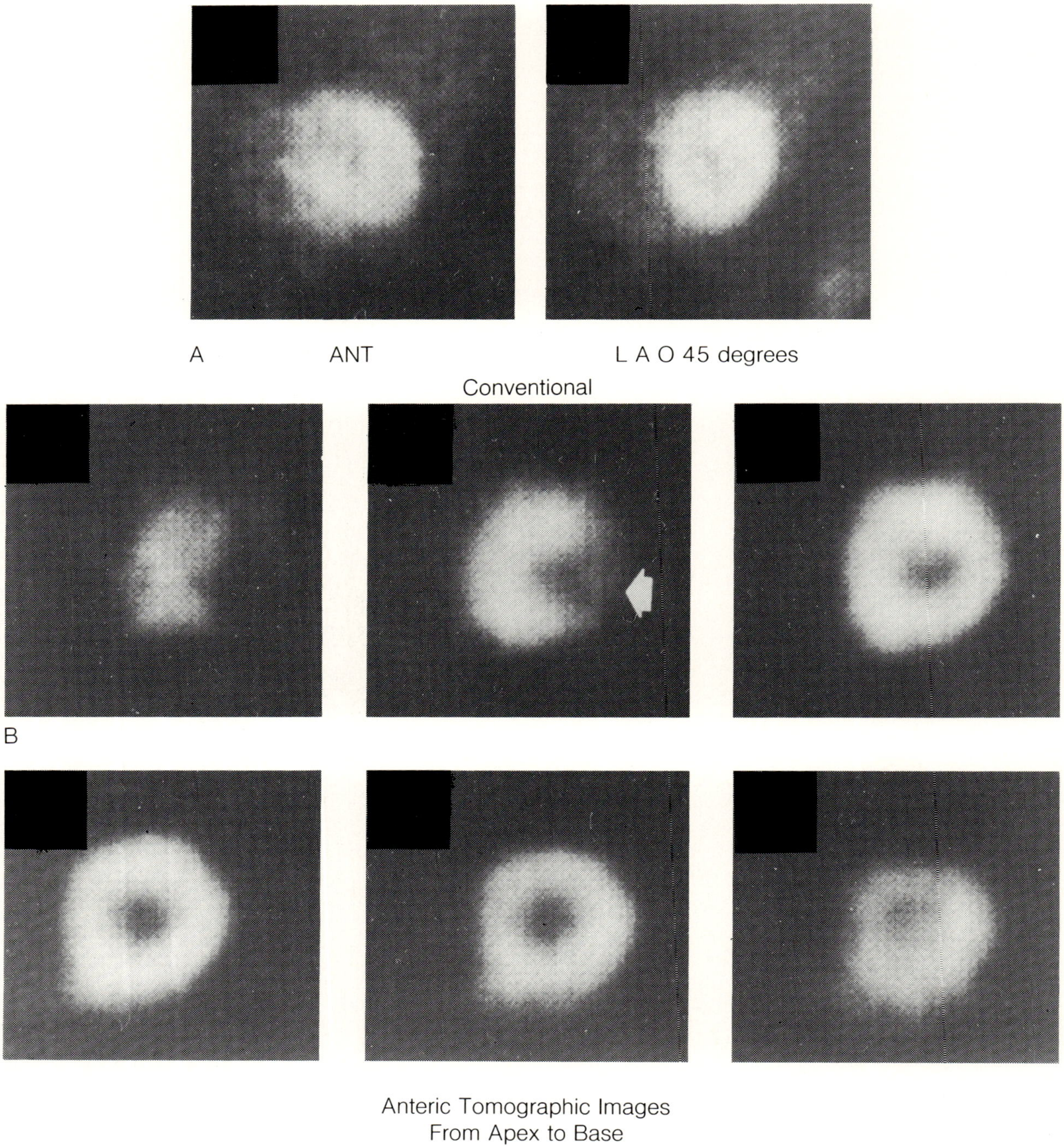


**FIG. 37. AREA OF ABSENT PERFUSION IDENTIFIED ON TOMOGRAPHIC IMAGING ONLY. A.** Conventional imaging in the anterior and 45 degree LAO positions in this patient with three-vessel coronary artery disease shows no abnormalities. **B.** Tomographic pinhole imaging from the apex (left) to base (right) shows a posteroapical area of absent activity (arrow) in a single sectional image. (From Vogel RA, Kirch DL, LeFree MT et al: Am J Cardiol 43:787, 1979)

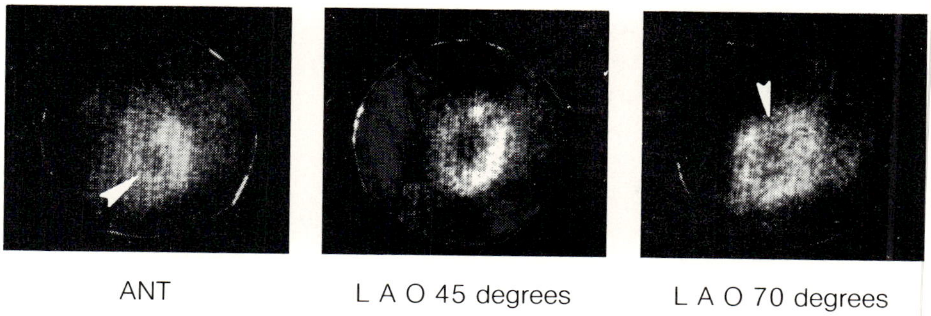


**FIG. 38. CARDIAC AMYLOIDOSIS.** Thallium imaging in this patient with pulmonary and cardiac amyloidosis showed areas of absent radioactivity (arrow) in the interventricular septum and the anterior wall (arrow). The areas of absent activity coincided with sites of amyloid involvement as seen at autopsy. (Courtesy of Dr. John F. Rockett, Baptist Memorial Hospital, Memphis, TN)

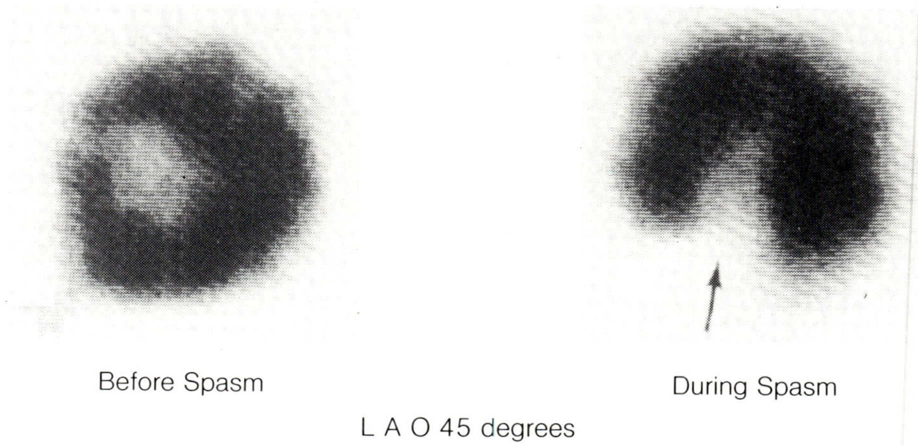


**FIG. 39. MYOCARDIAL ISCHEMIA WITH VARIANT OR PRINZMETAL'S ANGINA.** At the time of chest pain after 4 minutes of exercise, stress thallium imaging showed findings consistent with temporary myocardial ischemia (arrow). This was best demonstrated in the anterior and 45 degree LAO positions. Reduced blood flow to an area supplied by the right coronary artery occurred as a result of spasm in this vessel. (From McLaughlin PR, Doherty PW, Martin RP et al: Am J Cardiol 39:126, 1977)

## CARDIAC IMAGING AND EJECTION FRACTION AND VENTRICULAR WALL MOTION STUDIES

Cardiac imaging is now commonly performed in association with ventricular wall motion studies and ejection fraction determinations. The radionuclides employed in cardiac imaging are confined principally to the intravascular space.

Probably the most commonly used radioactive material for cardiac imaging is Tc-99m labeled red blood cells. The red blood cells may be tagged with the tracer in the following manner. A dose of nonradioactive pyrophosphate, containing at least 2 mg of tin, is injected intravenously, the stannous ion serving as a reducing agent. Thirty minutes later, a dose of 20 mCi of Tc-99m sodium pertechnetate is given intravenously. The stannous ion, from the pyrophosphate injection, reduces the Tc-99m in the sodium pertechnetate from a valence of +7 to a valence of +4. In this reduced state, the Tc-99m red blood cell tag is fairly strong with very little separation during the first 24 hours.

The most common alternative is the use of Tc-99m human serum albumin (HSA), in a dose of 15 or 20 mCi. Since there is usually *at least* a slight albumin leak from the circulatory system, maintenance of steady and high blood radioactivity is more difficult to achieve than with the labeled red blood cell method. However, the use of Tc-99m HSA requires only one intravenous injection rather than two.

Although there are numerous approaches to cardiac imaging and the studies related to this procedure, the most commonly employed methods are related to the employment of gated blood pool imaging with the scintillation camera interfaced to a computer. The camera is connected to a synchronizer (or a gating electrocardiographic control). With ECG leads attached to the patient and an R-wave trigger, images may be obtained, for example, at end diastole and end systole, and by subtracting the difference in radioactivity in each of these two images and dividing by the total radioactivity at end diastole, the ejection fraction may be determined.

When the scintillation camera with ECG synchronizer is interfaced to a computer, information is obtained and stored from comparable sections of the cardiac cycle for up to 1000 or more heart beats. Through this, images of the heart in motion may be reconstructed. Thus, the ejection fraction can be determined by collecting data and observing multiple cardiac images from end diastole to end systole back up to end diastole. Such calculations are determined automatically from specific computer programs.

In addition, by observation of the heart in motion, findings such as those of contrast cineangiography can be made. Thus, the presence or absence of disturbances in left ventricular contraction and motion, such as those seen in akinesia, dyskinesia, and aneurysmal formation, can be determined.

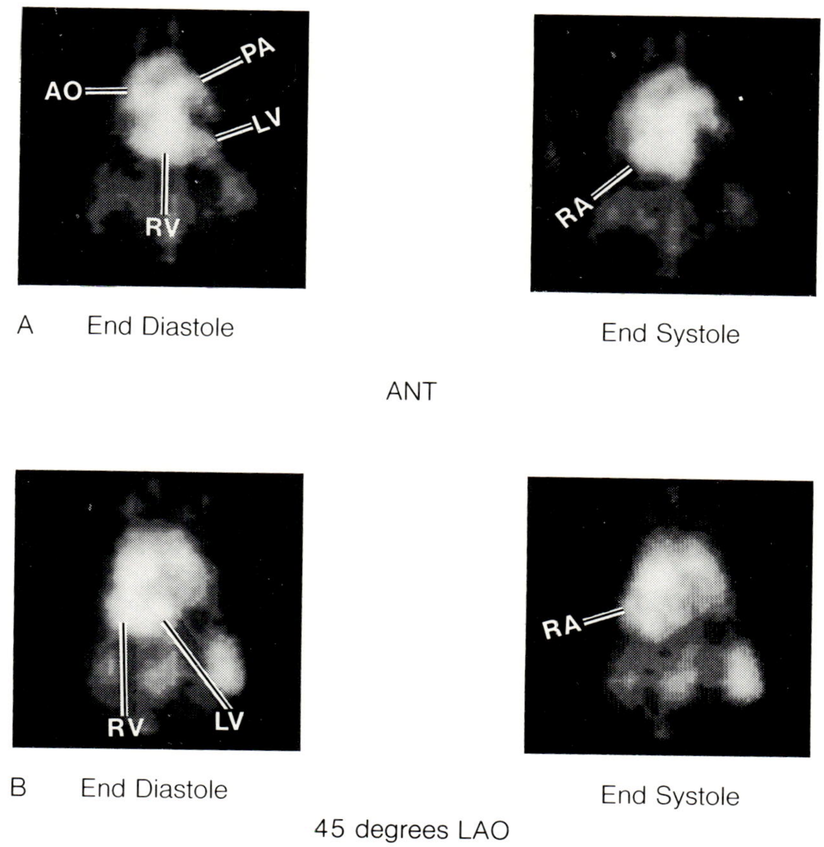


**FIG. 40.** **NORMAL GATED IMAGING. A.** In the normal subject, there is usually scant identification of the contracting left ventricle in the anterior position. During ventricular diastole, the left ventricle is seen but the image is dominated by the right ventricle. Note the pulmonary artery and the ascending aorta. During ventricular systole, the contracted left ventricle is no longer visible in this patient. However, the right atrium is now clearly defined during atrial diastole. **B.** Imaging in the 45° LAO position is usually ideal for the separate demonstration of the right and left ventricles. If the images are not sharply separated, modest accentuation of rotation (to 50 or 60°) may be useful. The ejection fraction is difficult to estimate by observation of the images alone. The differences in the images of the left ventricle during systole and diastole are those that are usually observed in the normal person.

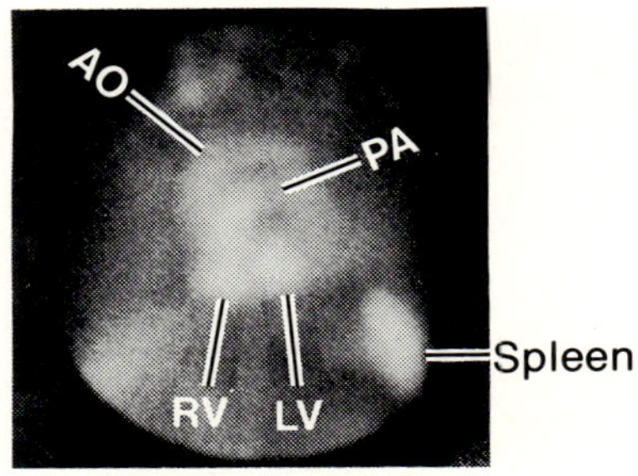


45 degrees LAO

**FIG. 41. ANATOMICAL STRUCTURES DEFINED IN THE 45° LAO POSITION IN A NORMAL SUBJECT.** The right and left ventricles are easily recognized. Note the appearance of the pulmonary artery and its relation to the right ventricle. Superior to the pulmonary artery is the ascending aorta and arch of the aorta. Blood pool imaging of the liver and spleen is visible.

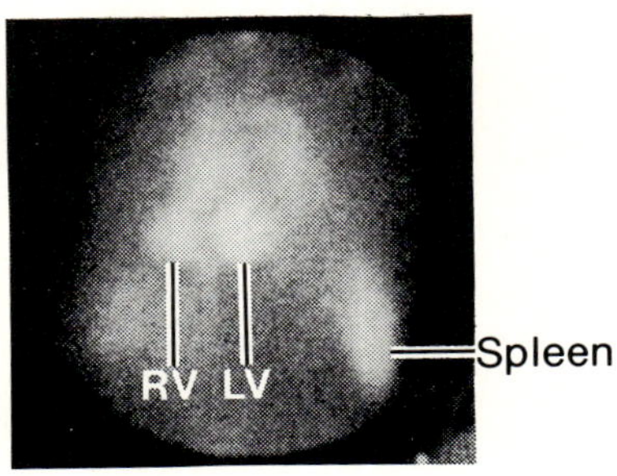


End Diastole

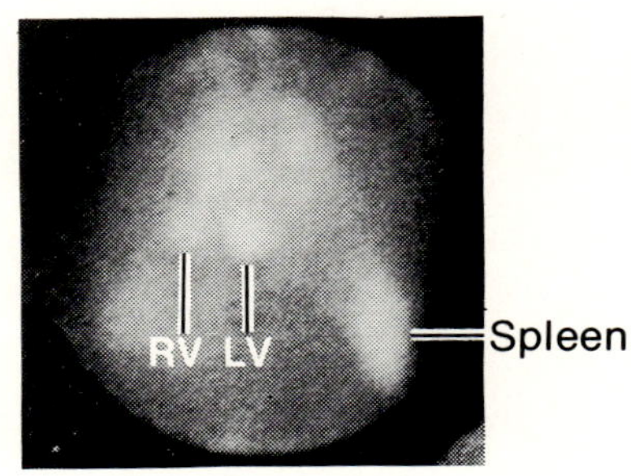


End Systole

Gated Images
45 degrees LAO

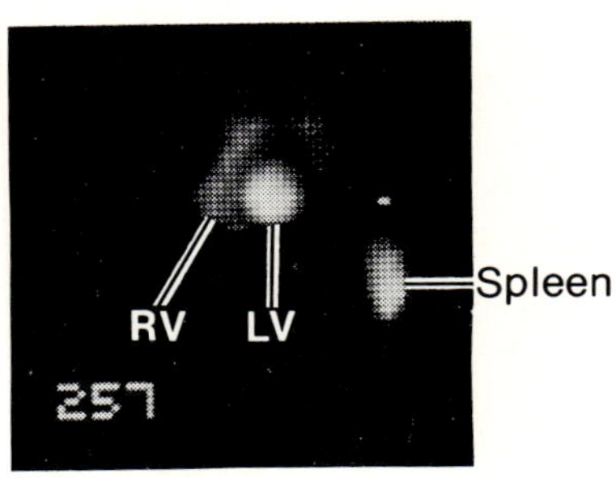


Diastole

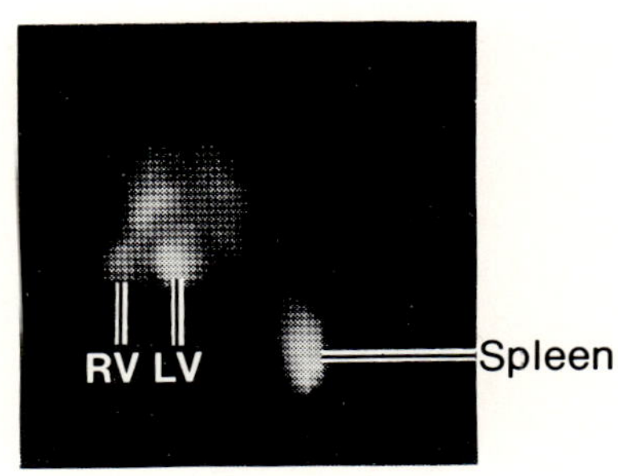


Systole

Selected Frames
from Gated Studies
45 degrees LAO

**FIG. 42. CONGESTIVE HEART FAILURE WITH SLIGHTLY REDUCED EMPTYING OF THE LEFT VENTRICLE.** Imaging in this patient with angina pectoris and congestive heart failure was associated with a left ventricular ejection fraction of 52 percent. Although only slightly reduced from normal, the differences in the images of the left and right ventricles at end diastole and end systole are easily recognized. The changes between systole and diastole are even more sharply illustrated on the selected frames acquired during the gated studies.

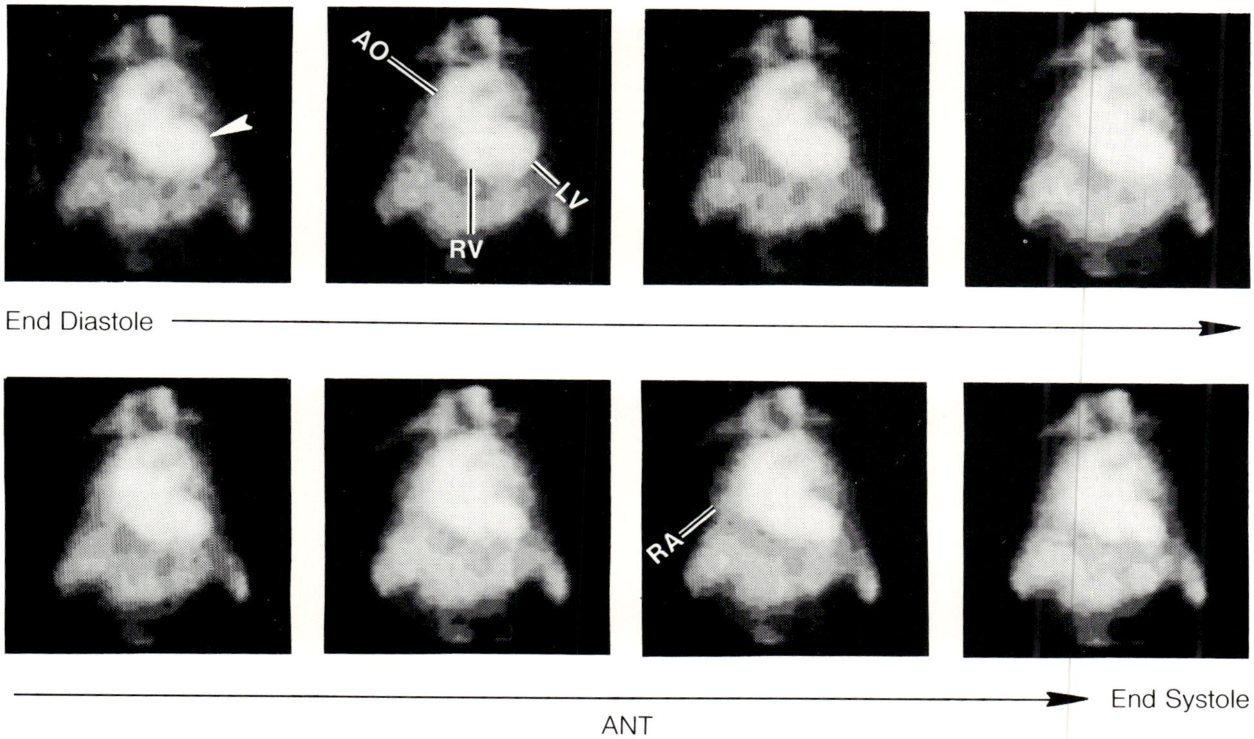


**FIG. 43.** **HYPOKINESIA IN A PATIENT WITH A PREVIOUS MYOCARDIAL INFARCTION.** In this patient with a prioı anterolateral myocardial infarction, gating studies demonstrated evidence of hypokinesia along the anterolateral wall (arrow). During ventricular systole, the involved wall shows barely any contraction as compared to that seen during diastole. Selected sequential frames from end ventricular diastole to end systole are illustrated. The reduced ejection fraction is related to the prior infarction. As a result, there is unusual prominence of the left ventricle in the anterior position. Note the appearance of the right atrium during atrial diastole and the relatively absent radioactivity in this region during atrial systole (in the first frame).

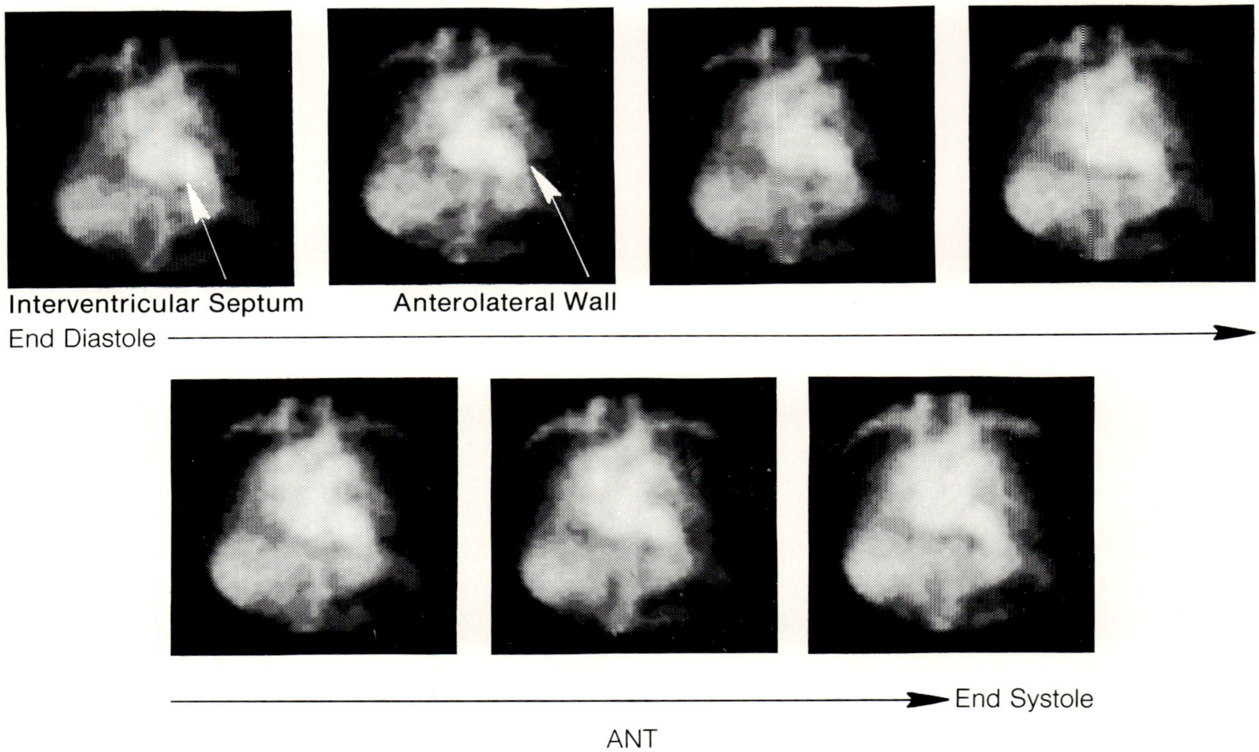


**FIG. 44. HYPOKINESIA FOLLOWING AN ANTEROLATERAL MYOCARDIAL INFARCTION.** Ventricular wall motion studies demonstrated hypokinesia in the region of the anterolateral wall of the left ventricle. The study was performed several weeks after the patient had suffered an anterolateral myocardial infarction. Selected frames from gated imaging are illustrated. Although the figures do not even closely compare to the lack of anterolateral wall contraction visualized on motion studies, the findings are, nevertheless, observed. While the anterolateral wall region remains fairly constant in appearance, sequential changes in the interventricular septum, in association with contraction, are seen. Although the size of the left ventricle continues to decrease in going from from diastcle to systole, the contracting changes are seen in the area of the interventricular septum.

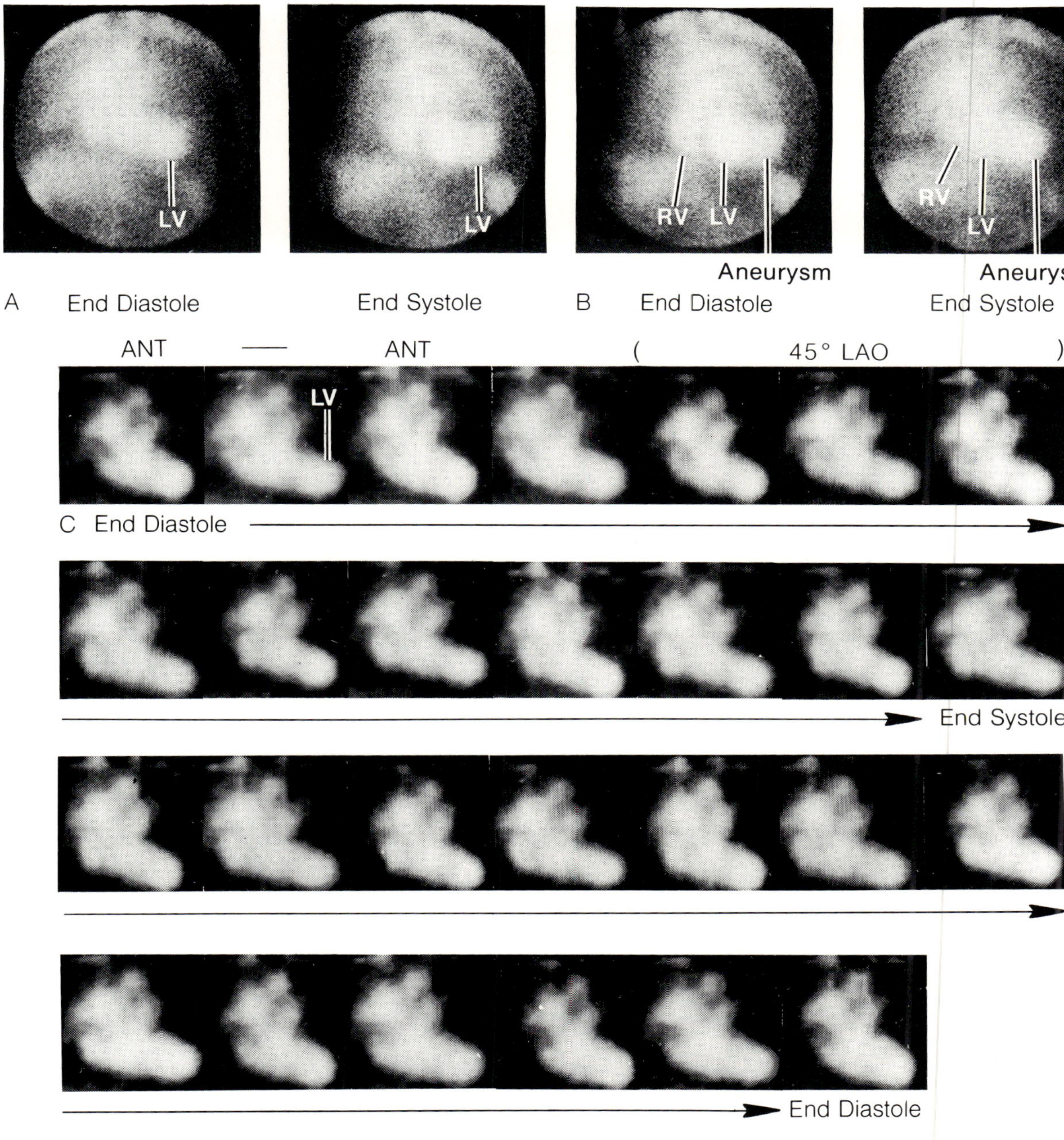


**FIG. 45.** POSTERIOR ANEURYSM OF THE LEFT VENTRICLE. False aneurysms (pseudo aneurysms) of the left ventricle are usually a consequence of rupture of the myocardium, with extension to the pericardium. The communication to the pericardial space becomes walled off by fibrous tissue and an aneurysmal dilatation, or false anerurysm, is created. Most false aneurysms arise from the posterior wall of the left ventricle, which is an unlikely location for a true aneurysm. On blood flow studies in false aneurysms, there is sequential filling, with the left ventricle visualized first and the false aneurysms afterwards. In this patient with a false aneurysm arising from the posterior wall of the left ventricle, imaging in the anterior position does not define the abnormality but shows the left ventricle and pseudoan-

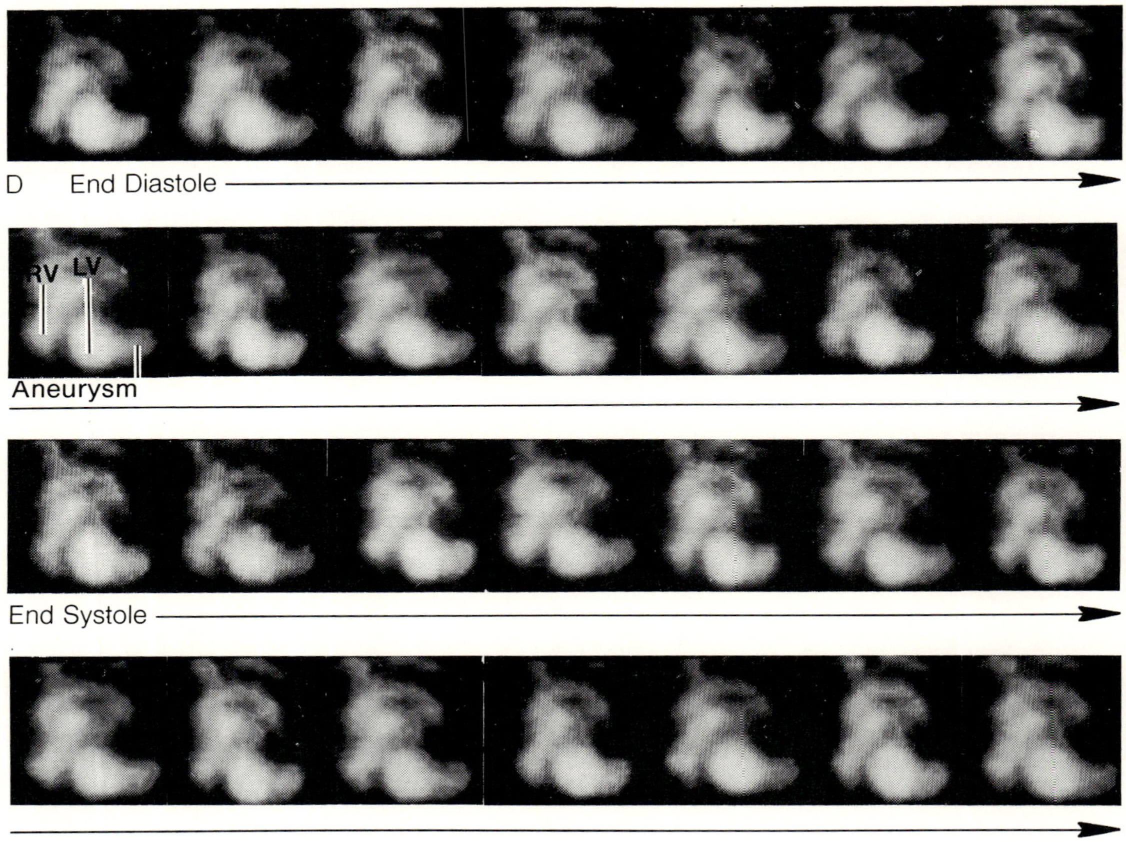


eurysm superimposed. However, in the 45° LAO position, the false aneurysm is sharply demonstrated. **A.** Gated images in the anterior position at end diastole and at end systole. The area of the left ventricle changes very little in appearance from diastole to systole, in part due to the persistence of radioactivity associated with the false aneurysm. Attempts to obtain a left ventricular ejection fraction of functioning left ventricle in the anterior position will not be rewarding in such cases. **B.** Gated images in the 45° LAO position indicate the zone of delineation between the posterior pseudoaneurysm and the remaining portion of the left ventricle, especially when viewed at end systole. **C.** Shown are selected frames from the multiple-gated acquisition study in the anterior position. Note the persistent prominence of the left ventricular area during both diastole and systole. Again, there is no identification of the posterior false aneurysm. **D.** Selected frames from the multiple gated acquisition study in the 45° LAO position are shown. The posteriorly located pseudoaneurysm is now more easily identified. Although it is common for a true aneurysm to increase in size during ventricular systole, the false aneurysm in this patient changes very little during systole and diastole.

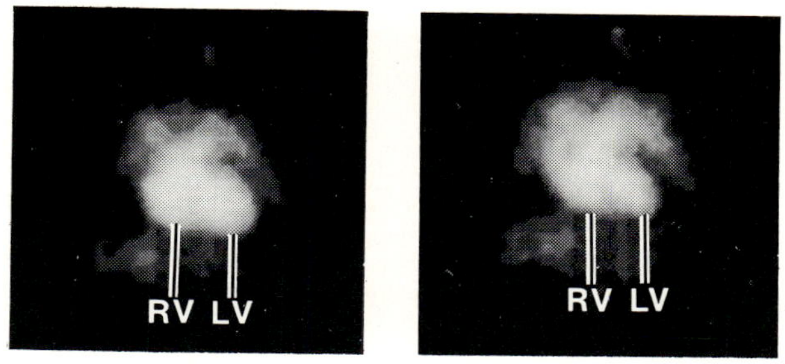


A End Diastole End Systole

ANT

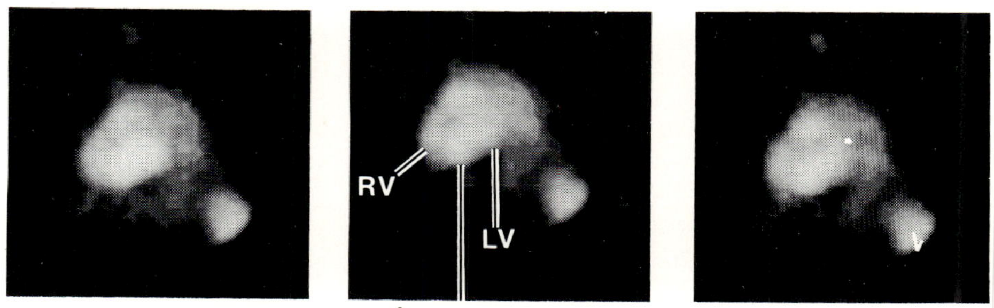


Aneurysm

B End Diastole End Systole

45 degrees LAO

**FIG. 46. ANEURYSM ARISING FROM THE ANTERIOR WALL OF LEFT VENTRICLE. A.** Gated imaging in the anterior position demonstrates the enormous left ventricle at end diastole and the incomplete emptying at end systole. The retained radioactivity is due largely to the anteriorly located aneurysm. **B.** Gated imaging in the 45° LAO position identifies both the aneurysm and the contracting portion of the left ventricle, the latter visible just posteriorly to the aneurysm. The demarcation is more sharply defined *toward* and *at* end systole. Reduced radioactivity is seen in the region of the contracting portion of the left ventricle while the aneurysm itself shows increased radioactivity as it enlarges during ventricular systole.

## Suggested Reading

Ahmad M, Dubiel JP, Logan KW, et al: Limited clinical diagnostic specificity of technetium-99m stannous pyrophosphate myocardial imaging in acute myocardial infarction. Am J Cardiol 39:50–54, 1977

Ahmad M, Dubiel JP, Verdon TA, et al: Technetium 99m stannous pyrophosphate myocardial imaging in patients with and without left ventricular aneurysm. Circulation 53:833–838, 1976

Ahmad M, Logan KW, Martin RH: Doughnut pattern of technetium-99m pyrophosphate myocardial uptake in patients with acute myocardial infarction: a sign of poor long-term prognosis. Am J Cardiol 44:13–17, 1979

Berman DS, Amsterdam EA, Hines HH, et al: New approach to interpretation of technetium-99m pyrophosphate scintigraphy in detection of acute myocardial infarction. Am J Cardiol 39:341–346, 1977

Bonte FJ, Parkey RW, Graham KD, et al: A new method for radionuclide imaging of myocardial infarcts. Radiology 10: 473–474, 1974

Dash H, Massie BM, Botvinick EH, et al: The noninvasive identification of left main and three-vessel coronary artery disease by myocardial stress perfusion scintigraphy and treadmill exercise electrocardiography. Circulation 60:276–284, 1979

Hamilton GW: Myocardial imaging with thallium-201: the controversy over its clinical usefulness in ischemic heart disease. J Nucl Med 20:1201–1204, 1979

Hellman CK, Kamath ML, Schmidt DH, et al: Improvement in left ventricular function after myocardial revascularization. Thorac Cardiovasc Surg 79:645–655, 1980

HolmanBL. Chisholm RJ, Braunwald E; The prognostic implications of acute myocardial infarct scintigraphy with $^{99m}$Tc-pyrophosphate. Circulation 57:320–326, 1978

Isner J, Roberts WC; Right ventricular infarction complicating left ventricular infarction secondary to coronary heart disease. Am J Cardiol 42:885–894, 1978

Khaja F, Alam M, Goldstein S, et al: Diagnostic value of visualization of the right ventricle using thallium-210 myocardial imaging. Circulation 59:182–188, 1979

Klausner SC, Botvinick EH, Shames D, et al: The application of radionuclide infarct scintigraphy to diagnose perioperative myocardial infarct following revascularization. Circulation 56:173–181, 1977

Lyons KP, Olson H, Aronow W, et al: Sensitivity and improved specificity of a localized pattern of Tc-99m pyrophosphate myocardial scintigraphy for the diagnosis of acute myocardial infarction. J Nucl Med 20:660, 1979

Lyons KP, Olson HG, Brown WT, et al: Persistence of an abnormal pattern on $^{99m}$Tc pyrophosphate myocardial scintigraphy following acute myocardial infarction. Clin Nucl Med 1:253–257, 1976

Lyons KP, Olson HG, Kuperus J, et al: Correlations of Tc-99m pyrophosphate myocardial scintigraphy and the results of coronary artery bypass surgery. J Nucl Med 19:1116–1120, 1978

Makler PT, Lederman S, Charkes ND, et al: Myocardial infarct imaging with $^{99m}$Tc-pyrophosphate and $^{99m}$ Tc-methylene disphosphonate: lack of correlation. Clin Nucl Med 4:89–91, 1979

Massie BM, Botvinick EH, Werner JA, et al: Myocardial scintigraphy with technetium 99m stannous pyrophosphate: an insensitive test for nontransmural myocardial infarction. Am J Cardiol 43:186–192, 1979

Olson H, Lyons K, Arnow W, et al: Technetium-99m pyrophosphate and pericardial disease. Circulation 56 (suppl III). 62, 1977

Olson HG, Lyons KP, Aronow WS, et al Follow-up technetium-99m stannous pyrophosphate myocardial scintigrams after acute myocardial infarction. Circulation 56:181–187, 1977

Olson HG, Lyons KP, Aronow WS, et al: Prognositc value of a persistently positive technetium-99m stannous pyrophosphate myocardial scintigram after myocardial infarction. Am J Cardiol 43:889–898, 1979

Onik G, Recht L, Edwards JE: False left-ventricular aneurysm: diagnosis by noninvasive means. J Nucl Med 21:177–180, 1980

Parkey RW, Bonte FJ, Meyer SL, et al: A new method for radionuclide imaging of acute myocardial infarction in humans. Circulation 50:540–546, 1974

Pitt B, Strauss HW; Evaluation of ventricular function by radioisotopic techniques. N Engl J Med 296:1097–1100, 1977

Poliner LR, Buja LM, Parkey RW, et al: Clinicopathologic findings in 52 patients studied by technetium-99m stannous pyrophosphate myocardial scintigraphy. Circulation 59:257–267,1979

Ritchie JL, Albro PC, Caldwell JH, et al: Thallium-201 myocardial imaging: a comparison of the redistribution and rest images. J Nucl Med 20:477–483, 1979

Rossman DJ, Strauss HW, Siegel ME, et al: Accumulation of $^{99m}$Tc-glucoheptonate in acutely infarcted myocardium. J Nucl Med 16:875–878,1975

Rude R, Parkey RW, Bonte FJ, et al: Clinical implications of the "Doughnut" pattern of uptake in myocardial imaging with technetium-99m stannous pyrophosphate. Circulation 55, 56:Suppl III:111–146, 1977

Sabom MB, Curry RC, Curry SL, et al: Technetium pyrophosphate myocardial scintigraphy in patients with stable angina. Circulation 55 and 56:111–162, 1977

Sharpe DN, Botvinick EH, Shames DM et al: The noninvasive diagnosis of right ventricular infarction. Circulation 57:483–490,1978

Verani MS, Jhingran S, Attar M, et al: Poststress redistribution of thallium 201 in patients with coronary artery disease, with and without prior myocardial infarction. Am J Cardiol 43:1114–1122, 1979

Vogel RA, Kirch DL, LeFree MT, et al: Thallium-201 myocardial perfusion scintigraphy: results of standard and multipinhole tomographic techniques. Am J Cardiol 43:787–793, 1979

Wackers FJTh, Sokole EB, Samson G, et al: Value and limitations of thallium-201 scintigraphy in the acute phase of myocardial infarction. N Engl J Med 295:1–5, 1976

Wackers F, Sokole EB, Samson G, et al: Atlas of $^{201}$ Tl myocardial scintigraphy. Clin Nucl Med 2:64–74, 1977

Willerson JT, Parkey RW, Buja LM, et al: Are $^{99m}$Tc-stannous pyrophosphate myocardial scintigrams clinically useful? Clin Nucl Med 2:137–145, 1977

# 11/ Renal Imaging

Renal imaging is commonly performed in association with the functional evaluation of the urinary system. Although a great deal of anatomic information may be obtained from such imaging, it does not approach the detail usually forthcoming from the intravenous urogram and contrast angiography.

A number of radiopharmaceuticals are available for renal imaging, and with them various types of functional and anatomic information may be obtained.

Most renal imaging is performed with Tc-99m diethylenetriaminepentaacetic acid (DTPA). This radionuclide is a true chelate and hence is excreted purely by glomerular filtration. Since the excretion of radioactive material is so rapid, sequential renal imaging is usually performed at intervals during the 30 minutes following tracer injection.

In those instances in which information concerning the renal cortex is desired, an agent such as Tc-99m dimercaptosuccinic acid (DMSA) may be employed. This radiopharmaceutical becomes localized in the proximal tubules, and with it cortical imaging can be obtained without fear of rapid loss of the radioactive material through excretion. It has been especially useful, for example, in the clarification of suspected lesions visible on the contrast intravenous urogram and in determining whether or not there has indeed been destruction or replacement of cortical tissue.

I-131 Hippuran has been employed for renal imaging in those cases in which an agent that is actively secreted by the renal tubules is useful. Such a study may be the procedure of choice if renal identification is necessary in a patient with a markedly elevated blood urea nitrogen. A radionuclide renogram is commonly obtained in association with I-131 Hippuran imaging.

Radionuclide angiography is usually performed in conjunction with Tc-99m renal imaging. Information related to, for example, aortic and renal arterial perfusion may be so obtained.

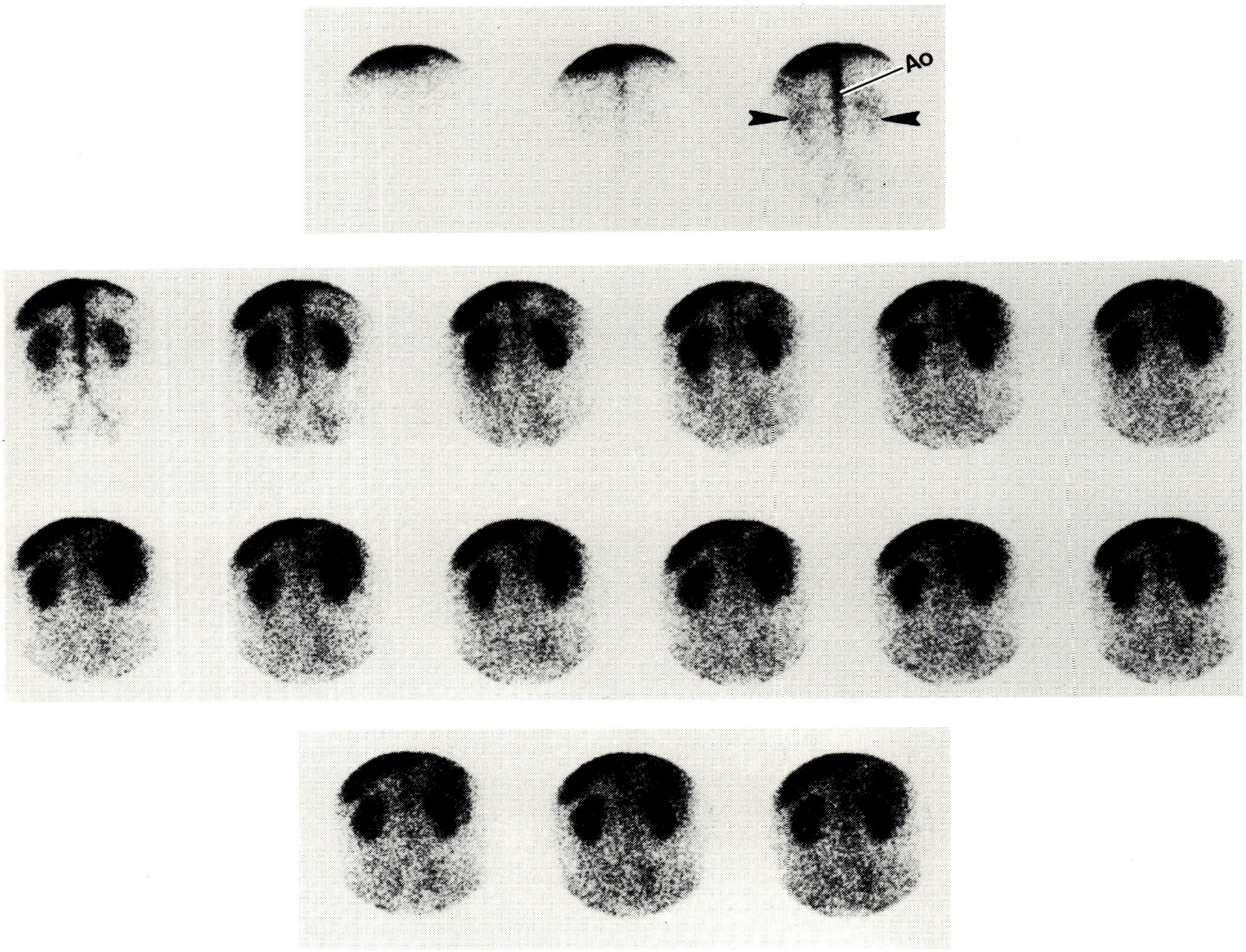


Posterior Blood Flow

**FIG. 1. NORMAL BLOOD FLOW STUDY.** Following the intravenous administration of 20 mCi of Tc-99m DTPA, images are obtained in the posterior position at intervals of 3 seconds. The aorta (Ao) and both kidneys (arrows) are identified in the beginning frames. The visualization of the kidneys during the arterial phase is, of course, indicative of renal arterial perfusion. The kidneys continue to be visualized throughout the study as the radionuclide is taken up to undergo glomerular filtration.

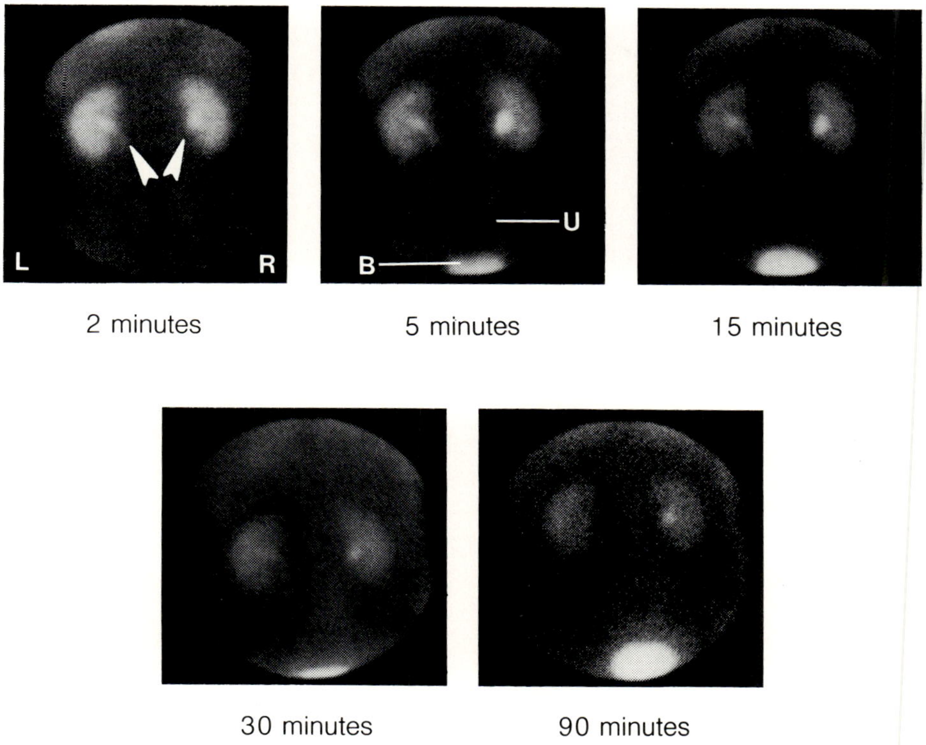


**FIG. 2. NORMAL STATIC IMAGING WITH Tc-99m DTPA.** Imaging performed in the posterior position at 2 minutes demonstrates both kidneys. That excretion is prompt is indicated by the early identification of the renal pelvis (arrows) in each kidney. At 5 minutes, with the rapid excretion through glomerular filtration of the radioactive material, there is diminished cortical activity (as compared to the immediate study). At this time radioactive material is seen coursing through each ureter (U), and the bladder (B) becomes visible. The cortical activity continues to diminish on sequential imaging, and at 90 minutes barely any radionuclide remains in the kidneys.

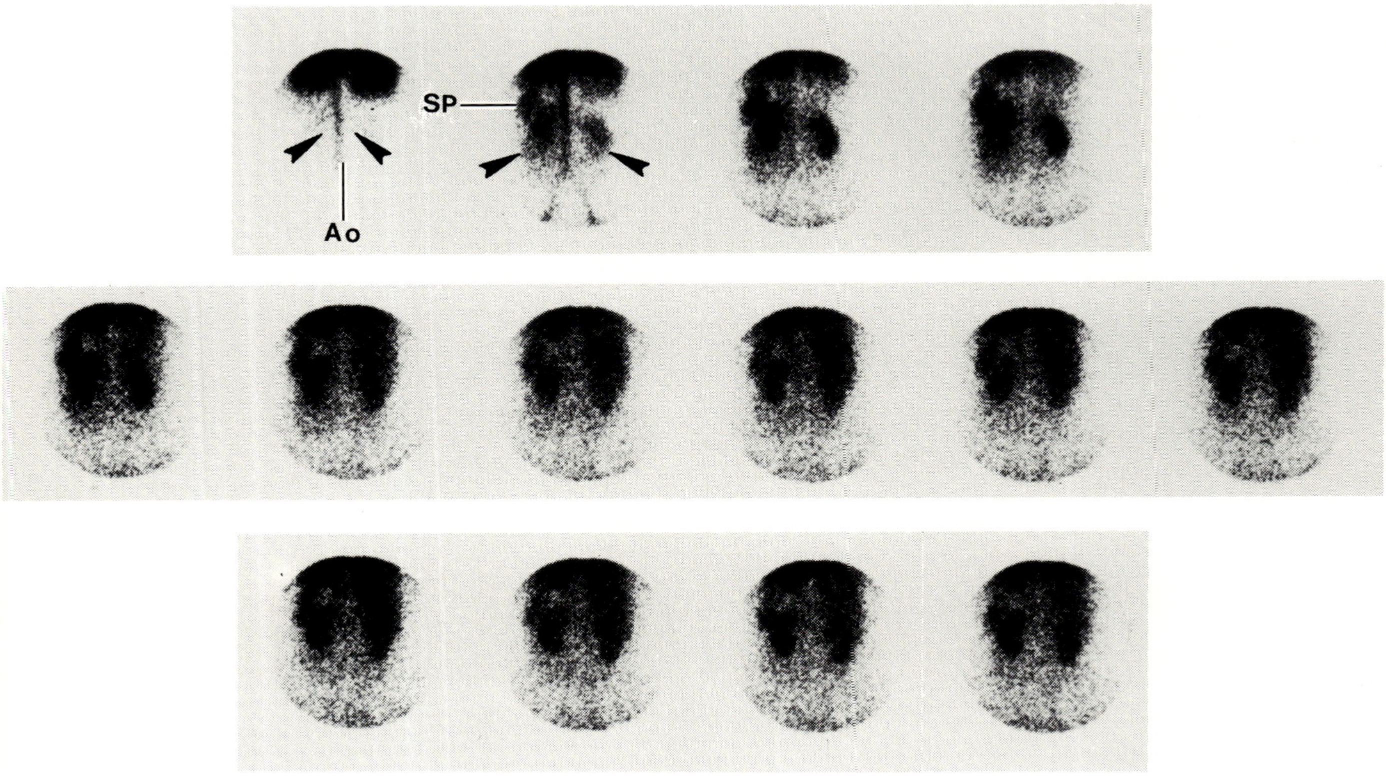


Posterior Blood Flow

**FIG. 3. NORMAL BLOOD FLOW STUDY.** Imaging was performed in the posterior position and frames were obtained at intervals of 3 seconds. The aorta (Ao) and beginning arterial perfusion to each kidney (arrows) are seen in the first frame. Note the visualization of the spleen (Sp) in the second frame and its relation to the left kidney. Splenic and renal visualization are sometimes confused when there is failure to visualize a left kidney. Note the gradual reduction in splenic activity as the radionuclide is taken up in both kidneys.

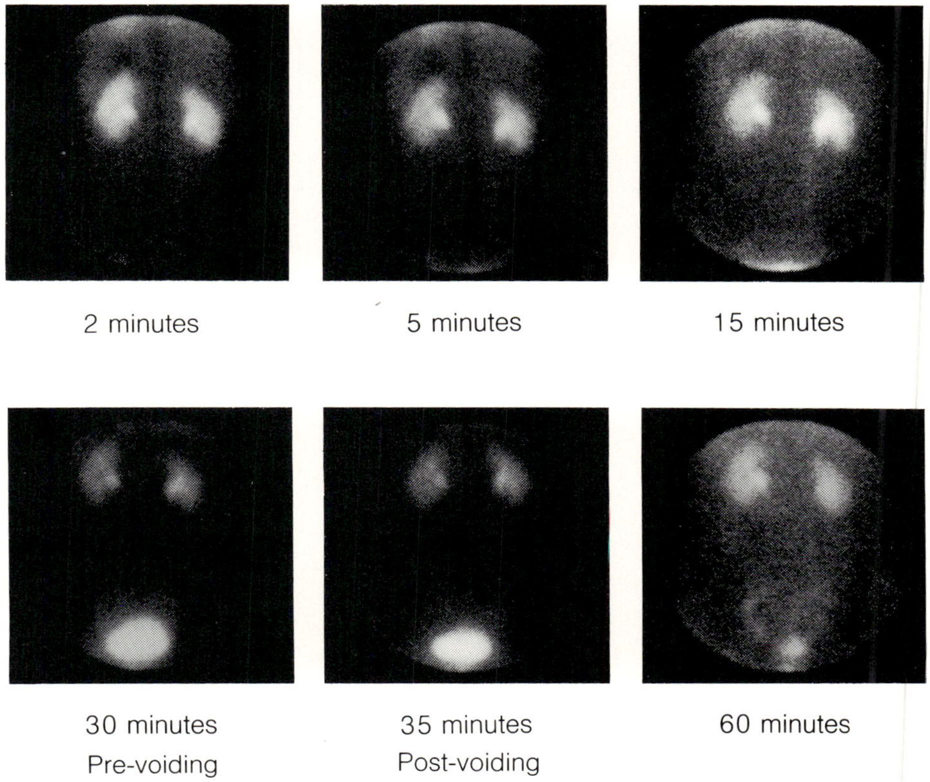


**FIG. 4. NORMAL STATIC IMAGING WITH Tc-99m DTPA.** It is only on the image obtained at 2 minutes that there is satisfactory renal visualization. Thereafter, cortical activity rapidly diminishes as the radioactive material is excreted through glomerular filtration. Gross estimation of residual bladder radioactivity may be made by a comparison of the study done after voiding at 35 minutes with that done at 30 minutes; in this case there has probably been complete emptying.

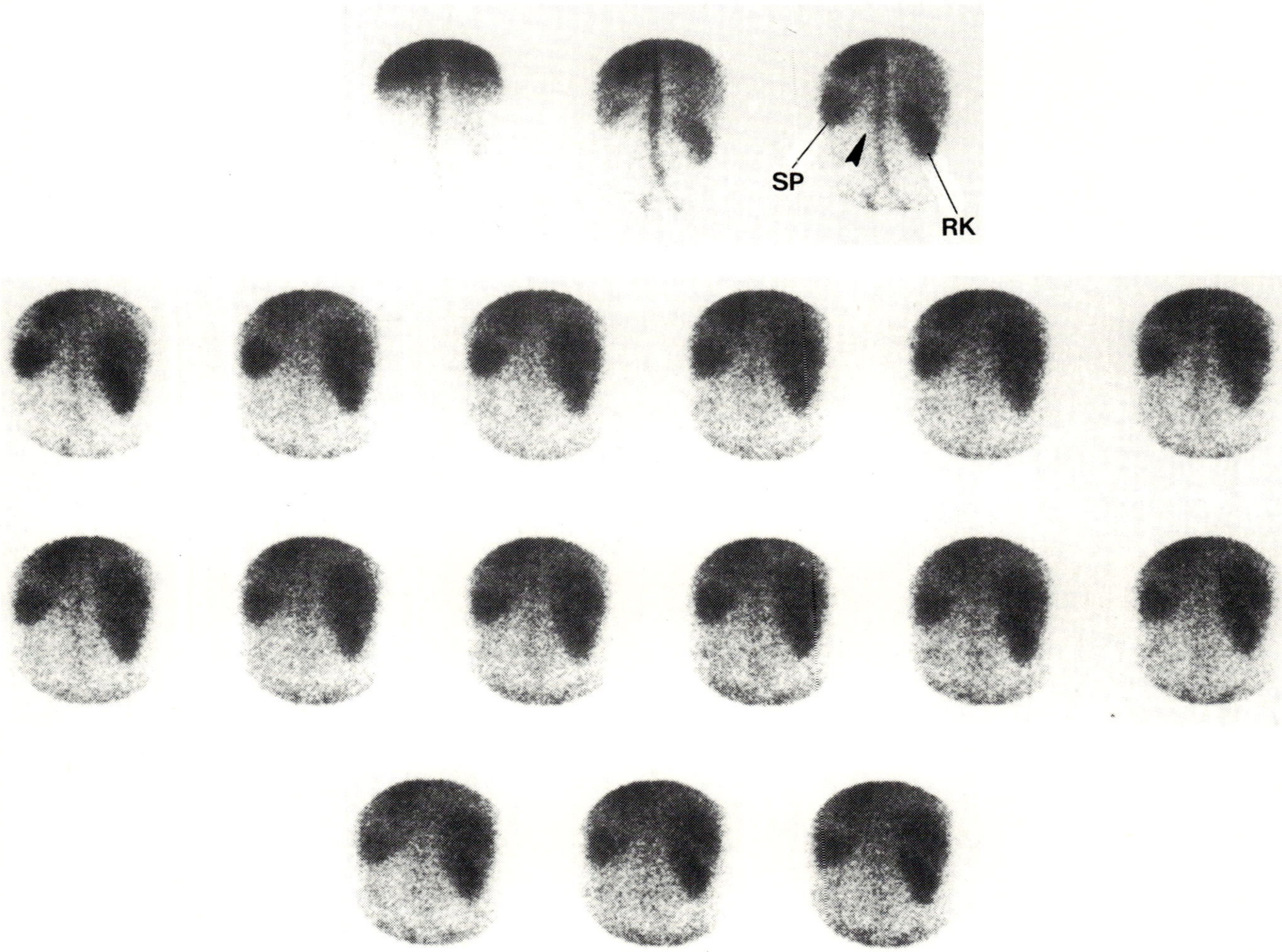


Posterior Blood Flow

**FIG. 5. BLOOD FLOW STUDY IN A PATIENT WITH ABSENT LEFT KIDNEY.** The blood flow study performed in the posterior position identifies the right kidney (RK) and the spleen (Sp); no uptake is noted in the left renal bed (arrow). Continued serial imaging shows reduction in splenic activity due to a fall in vascular radioactivity. Renal radioactivity continues to increase as more Tc-99m DTPA continues to be taken up in the kidney.

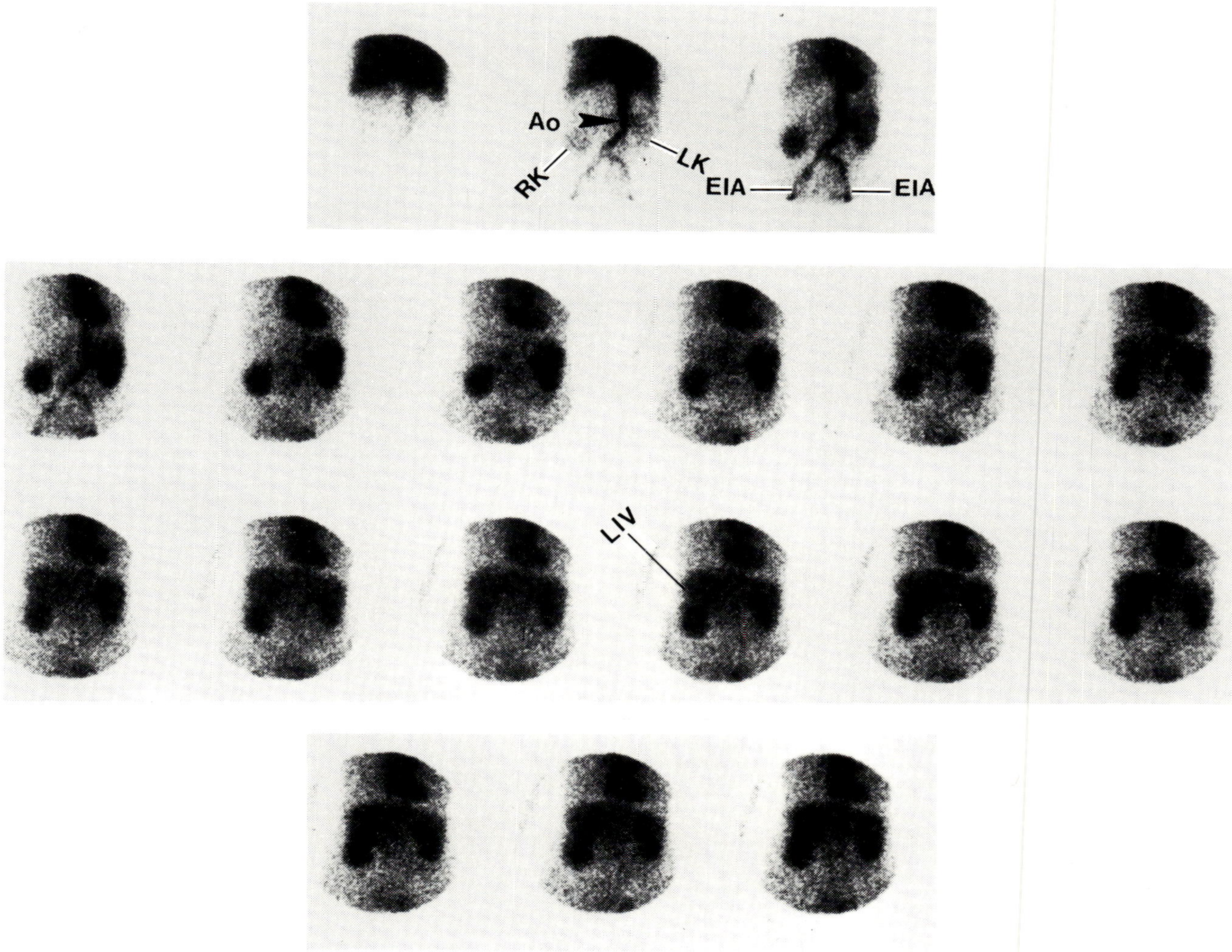


Anterior Blood Flow

**FIG. 6. PTOSIS VISIBLE ON Tc-99m SODIUM PERTECHNETATE BLOOD FLOW STUDY.** Marked ptosis of the right kidney (RK) is seen during the early frames of the radionuclide blood flow study. Note the relation of the ptosed kidney to the tortuous aorta (Ao) and the external iliac arteries (EIA). The left kidney (LK) may also be seen. Although pertechnetate is excreted in part through the kidneys, there is no preferential uptake as with Tc-99m DTPA. Note the hepatic (LIV) radioactivity.

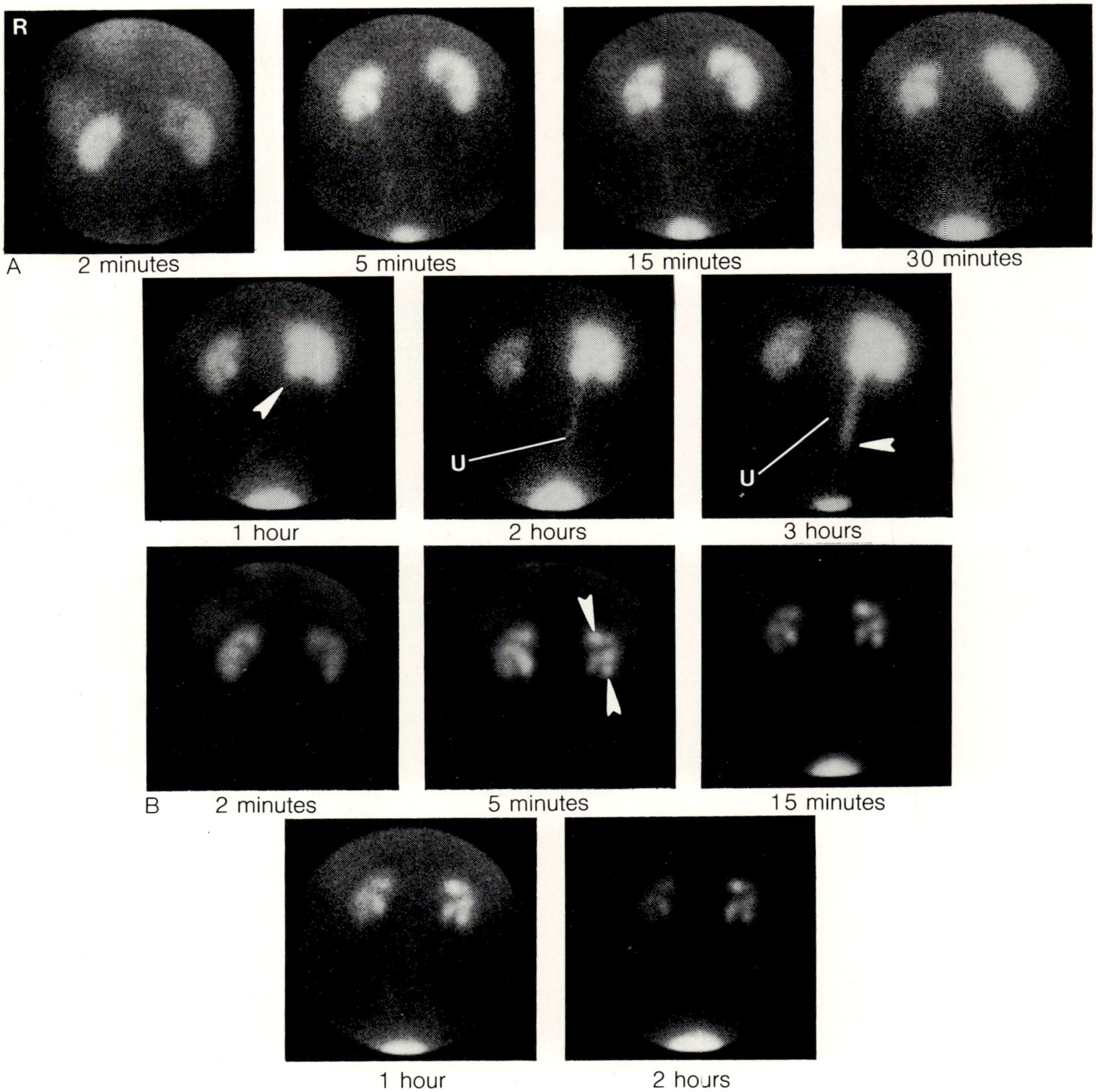


**FIG. 7. URETERAL OBSTRUCTION ASSOCIATED WITH A URETERAL CALCULUS. A.** Static imaging of this patient with a history of calculi and bilateral renal disease was performed at intervals up to 3 hours. Failure of excretion in the right kidney is suggested because of the lack in diminution in cortical activity as late as 30 minutes. At 1 hour, the dilated right renal pelvis (arrow) is identified and at 2 and 3 hours, the right ureter (U) is visualized. The site of the obstructing right ureteral calculus (broken arrow) is demonstrated at 3 hours. It was only with prolonged serial imaging that the site of the obstructing stone could be seen. **B.** Static imaging following the passage of the ureteral calculus no longer demonstrates obstructive uropathy. Although there is evidence of caliectasis (arrows) bilaterally, there is no longer any demonstration of right-sided hydronephrosis or of ureteral obstruction such as was visible on the initial study.

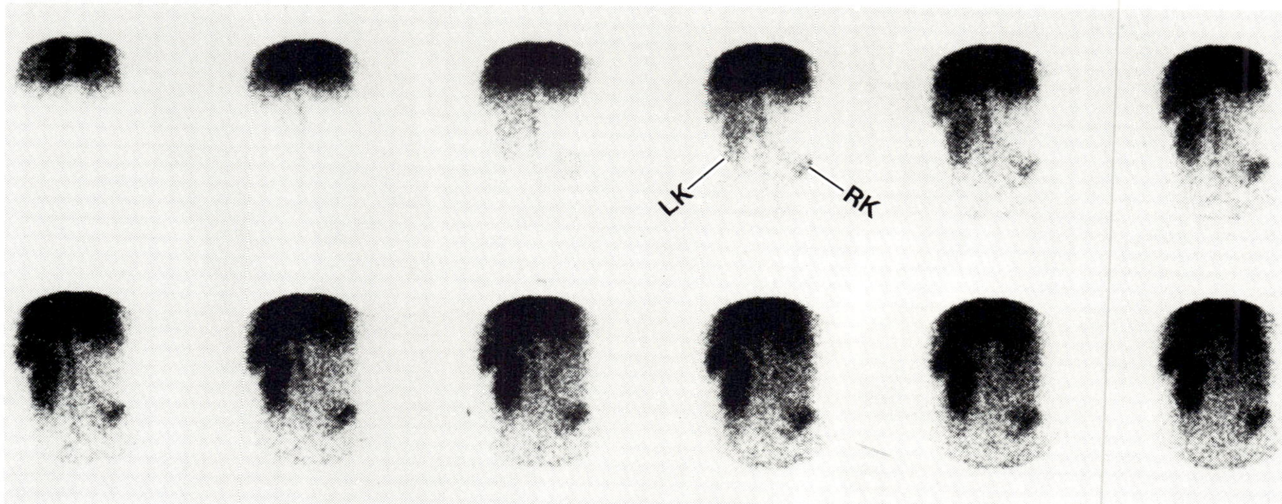


A Posterior Blood Flow

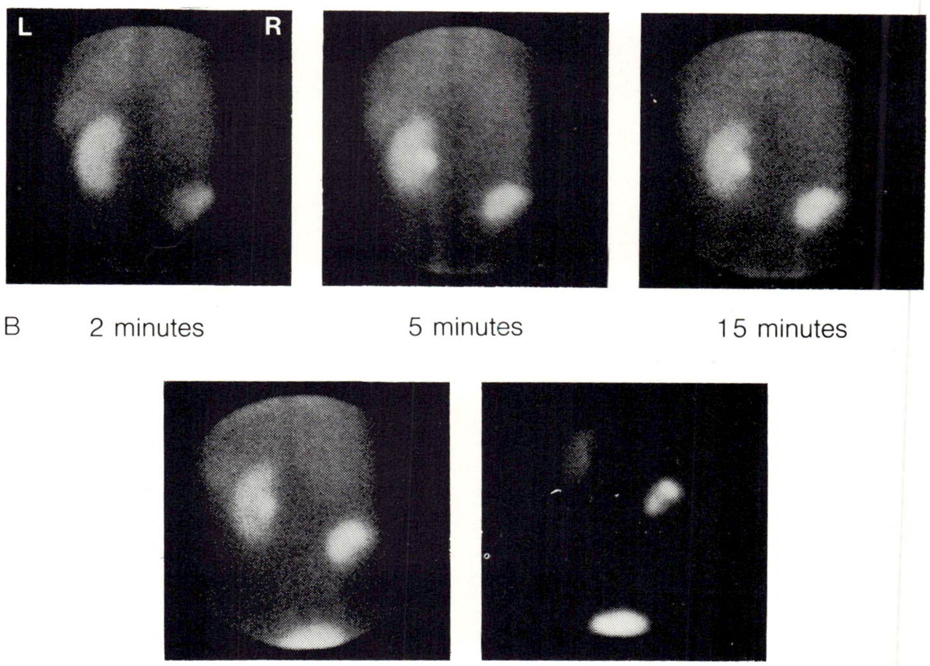


B 2 minutes 5 minutes 15 minutes

30 minutes 2 hours

**FIG. 8 HYDRONEPHROSIS IN A HYPOPLASTIC KIDNEY. A.** Initial frames of blood flow study demonstrate arterial perfusion to both the normal left kidney (LK) and the inferiorly located, hypoplastic right kidney (RK). **B.** Static imaging shows prompt excretion of radioactive material from the left kidney. However, there is a continued increase in radioactivity in the renal pelvis of the hypoplastic right kidney, a finding that suggests hydronephrosis.

In order to distinguish between mechanical obstruction and functional hydronephrosis, a Lasix excretion test may be performed, with a time–activity curve generated on the computer. The Lasix is administered shortly after Tc-99m DTPA injection and if there is a subsequent fall in activity associated with excretion, the hydronephrosis is functional; a plateau or upward sloping curve suggests mechanical obstruction.

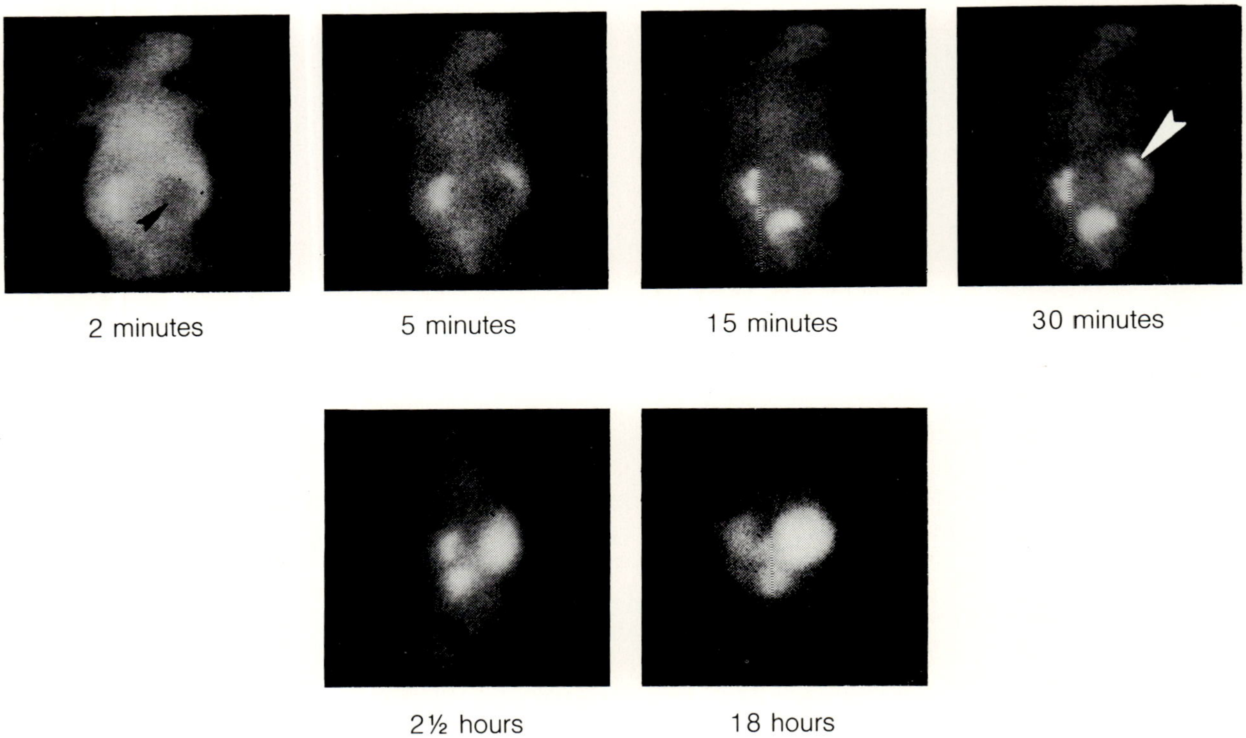


**FIG. 9. DEMONSTRATION OF RENAL FUNCTION IN A NEWBORN WITH OBSTRUCTIVE UROPATHY.** This 4-day-old infant had a large ureteral cyst at the ureterovesicle junction. Imaging at two minutes shows a large, somewhat rounded area of absent activity (arrow) in the right kidney associated with the marked hydronephrosis on that side. However, compressed, functioning renal cortex (larger arrow) can also be seen. Serial imaging continues to show evidence of cortical function, and some excretion into the dilated right renal pelvis begins to be seen at 30 minutes; this is more evident at 2.5 hours. The 18-hour study shows further excretion of radionuclide into the dilated right renal pelvis. There is no evidence of left-sided obstruction. From radionuclide imaging it appeared that there was a functioning right kidney; hence it was decided to reimplant the right ureter into the bladder at surgery following resection of the ureteral cyst.

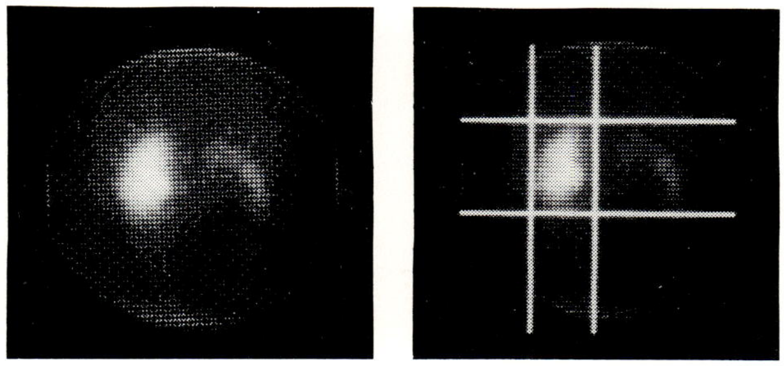

A B

**FIG. 10.** RENOGRAM GENERATION WITH I-131 HIPPURAN IMAGING. This is most easily accomplished with a scintillation camera interfaced to a computer. In the example illustrated here, following the intravenous administration of 300 $\mu$Ci of I-131 Hippuran, 128 images were obtained in the posterior position at intervals of 10 seconds, over a duration of 1280 seconds. In this case, the analysis has been made of the left kidney.

The composite renal image (**A**), which is the image obtained for the entire duration of the study, is identical to the composite image obtained by summing the 128 individual 10-second images. **B.** Region of interest cursors are placed around the entire left kidney on the composite image. **C.** The nuclear medicine images obtained during each 10-second interval indicate the relative location of the tracer at these specific times (cortex, medulla, renal pelvis). The radioactivity at the time of each of these images may be further represented on the renogram (**D**), or time-activity curve. A number of the 10-second images that correspond to specific points on the renogram curve are so indicated.

**E.** The renogram has been outlined to help separate its individual segments. The initial upward rise is the *tracer appearance* and represents the initial blood radioactivity following injection. The more gradually rising second segment is the *accumulation phase* and coincides with the entry of the I-131 Hippuran into the renal tubules. The point of maximum accumulation is the *peak*. The *transit time* includes both the tracer appearance and accumulation phase and normally does not exceed 4 or 5 minutes. The downward sloping segment is the *excretory curve* and indicates the loss of radioactivity as the I-131 leaves the kidney to be excreted into the bladder. Normally, there should be a 50 percent fall from the peak 10 minutes following the start of the tracer appearance. In the case illustrated here, excretion is reduced (24 percent fall from peak at 10 minutes). This impairment in renal function is associated with chronic parenchymal disease.

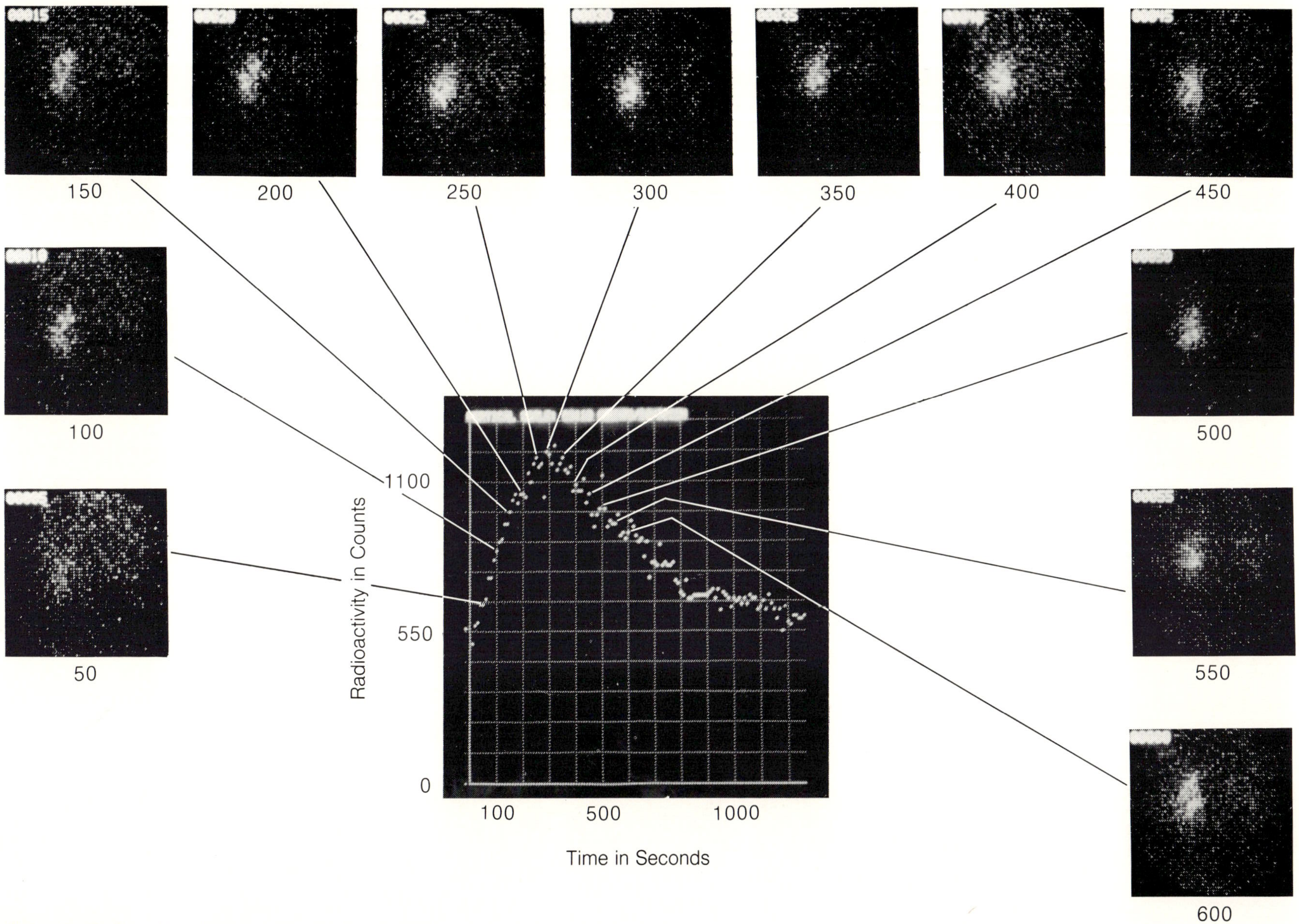


**FIG. 10. C, D.** (See legend on previous page)

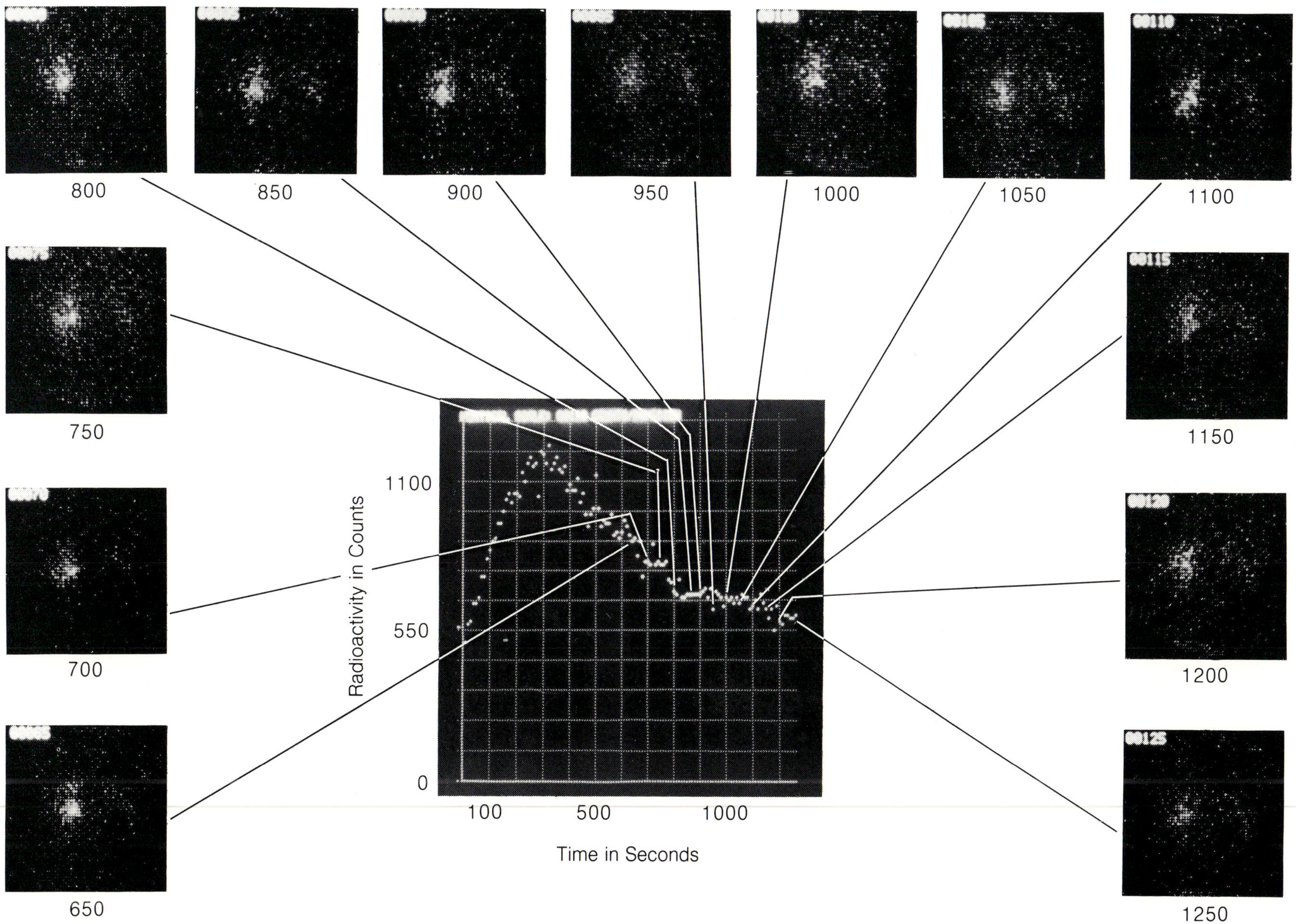


**FIG. 10. C, D.** (See legend on page 395)

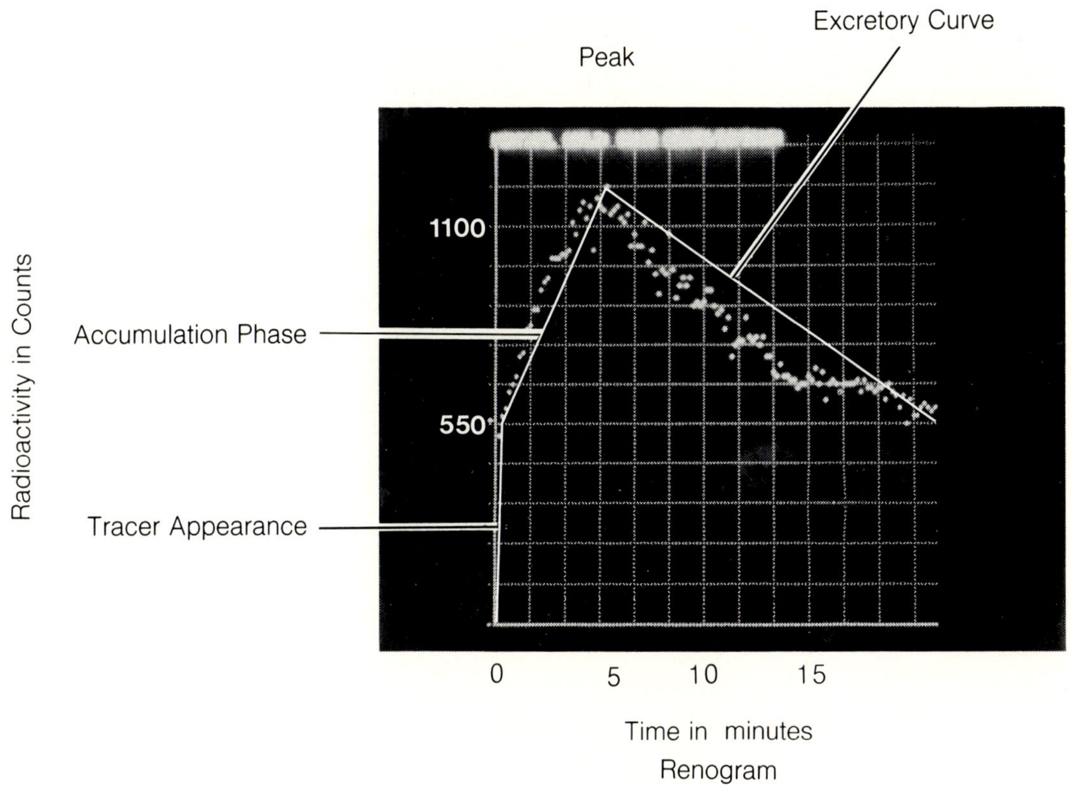


**FIG. 10. E.** (See legend page 395)

A

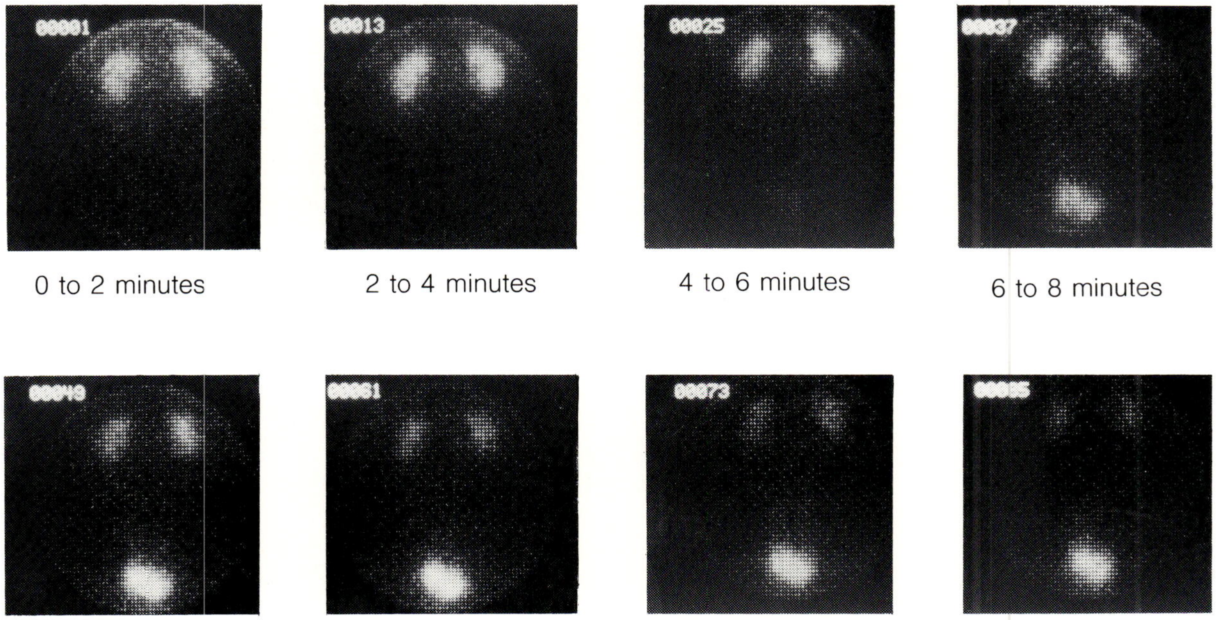


0 to 2 minutes | 2 to 4 minutes | 4 to 6 minutes | 6 to 8 minutes

8 to 10 minutes | 10 to 12 minutes | 12 to 14 minutes | 14 to 16 minutes

B

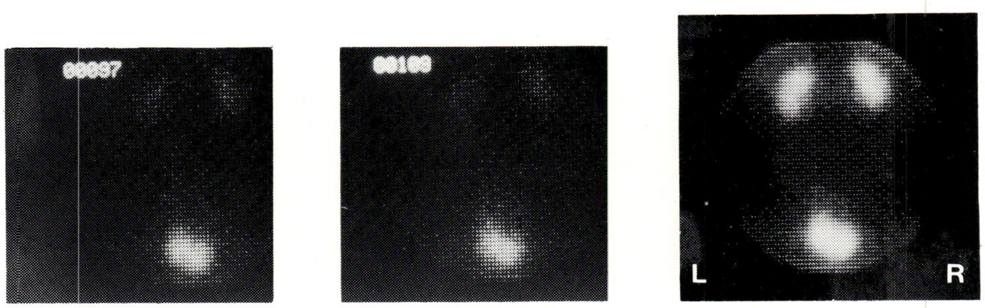


16 to 18 minutes | 18 to 20 minutes | Composite Image

C

Left and Right Renograms Combined

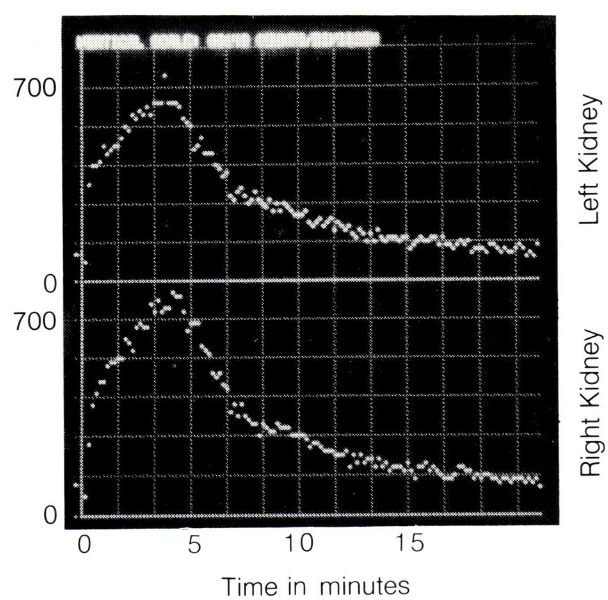


**FIG. 11. A, B, C.**
(See legend next page)

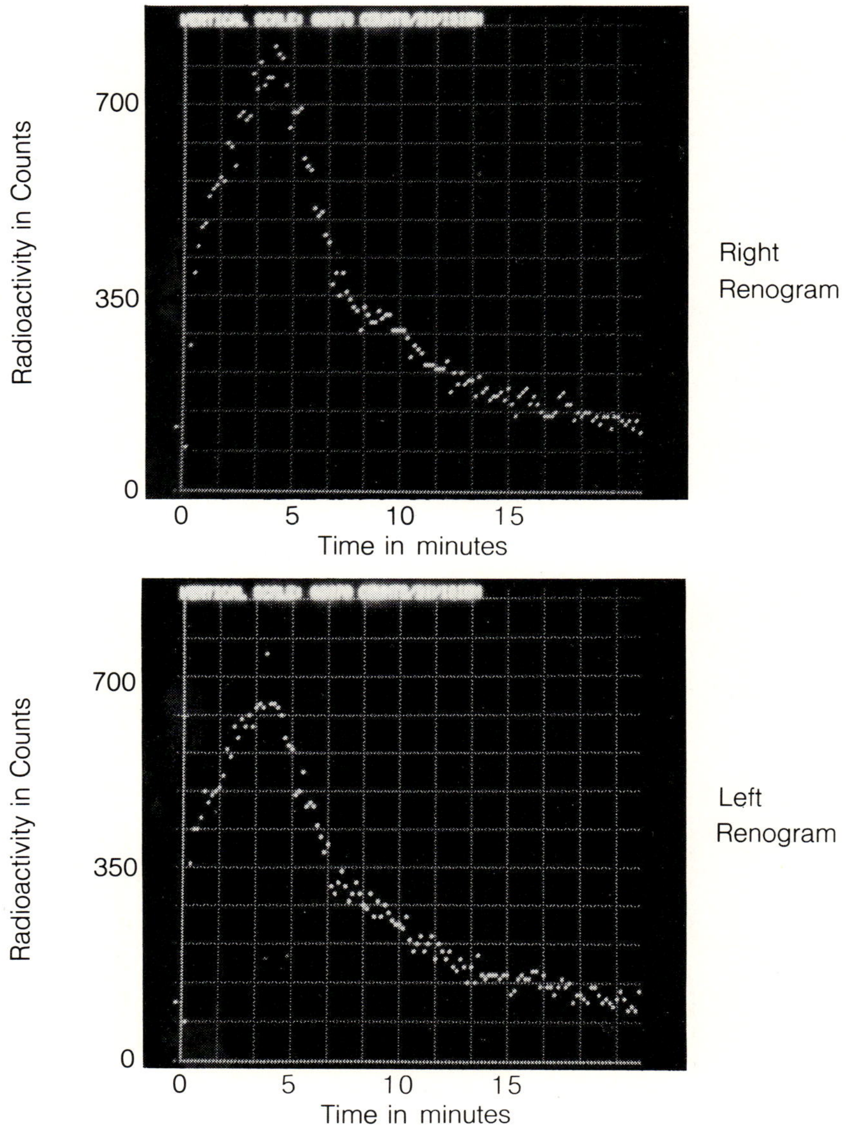


C

**FIG. 11. NORMAL HIPPURAN IMAGING AND RENOGRAM GENERATION.** Following the intravenous administration of 300 $\mu$Ci of I-131 Hippuran, 128 frames were obtained at intervals of 10 seconds, for a total duration of 1280 seconds (a little over 21 minutes). The study was performed in the posterior position. **A. Hippuran imaging.** Images from the computer readout were obtained at intervals of 2 minutes. There is maximum visualization during the 2 to 4 minute interval, and this coincides with the peak or time of maximum radionuclide accumulation as seen on the renogram. During the interval 6 to 8 minutes, there has been perceptible and appreciable excretion of radionuclide. This is evidenced by the relative reduction in renal radioactivity, the faint suggestion of increased radioactivity in the renal pelvis, and the accumulation of radioactivity in the bladder. As imaging continues, the kidneys show progressive loss of radioactivity as the bladder shows continually increased activity with further excretion. **B.** The composite image shows both kidneys to be of similar size. **C. Renogram.** The transit time is approximately 4 minutes for each kidney. On the right side there has been a fall of approximately 60 percent from the peak at 10 minutes while the excretory fall on the left side is about 55 percent. Both values are in the normal range.

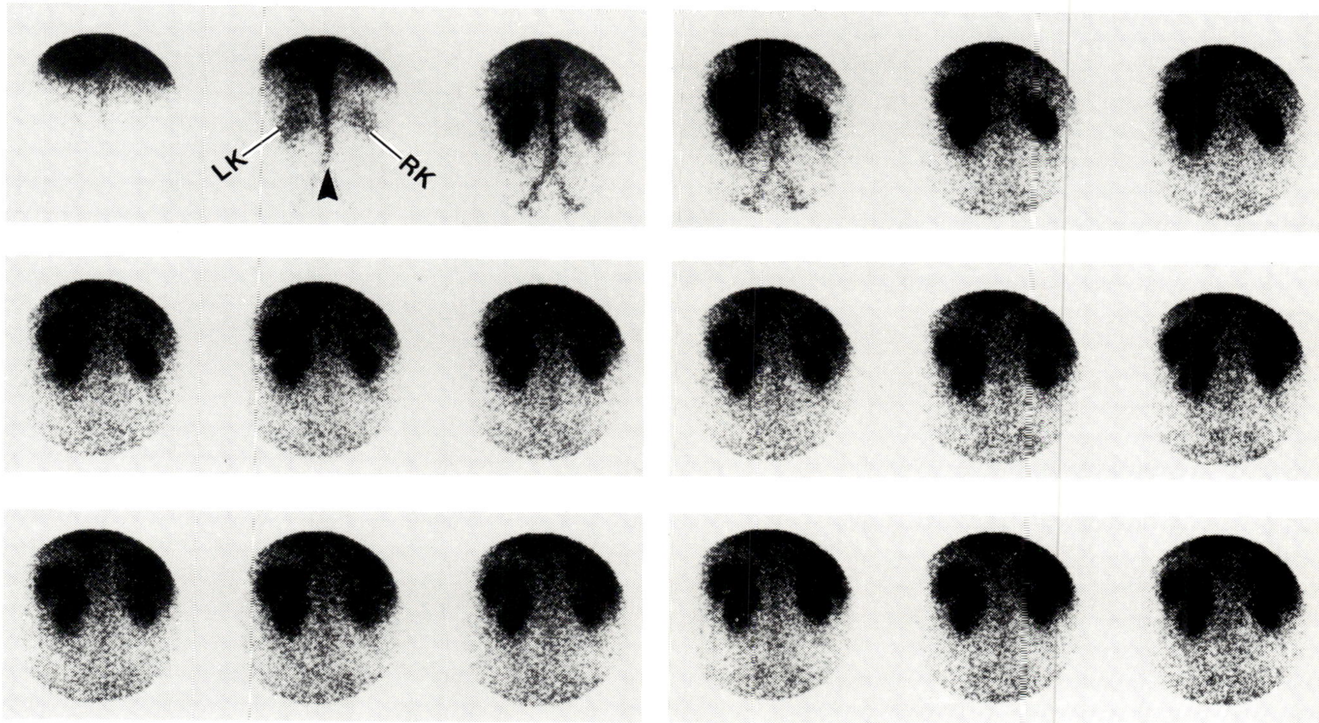


A

Posterior Blood Flow

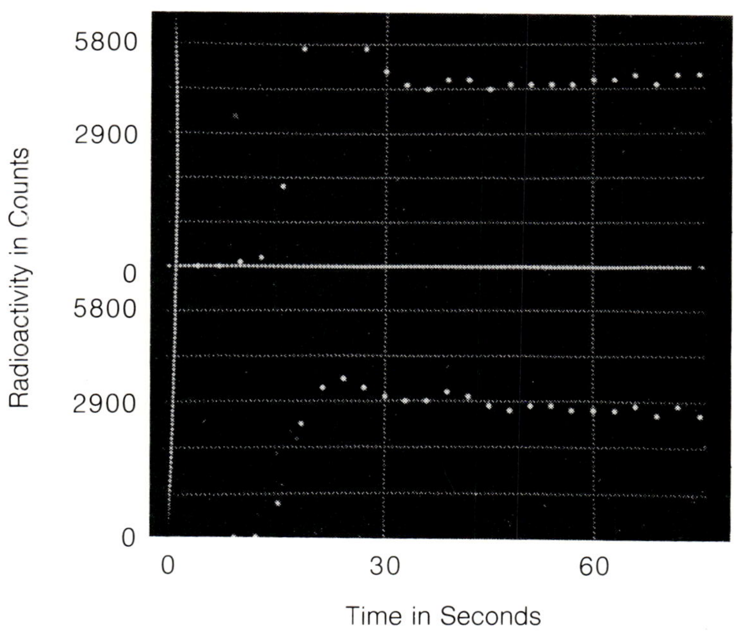


Computerized Analysis
Blood Flow Curve

**FIG. 12. A.** (See legend page 404)

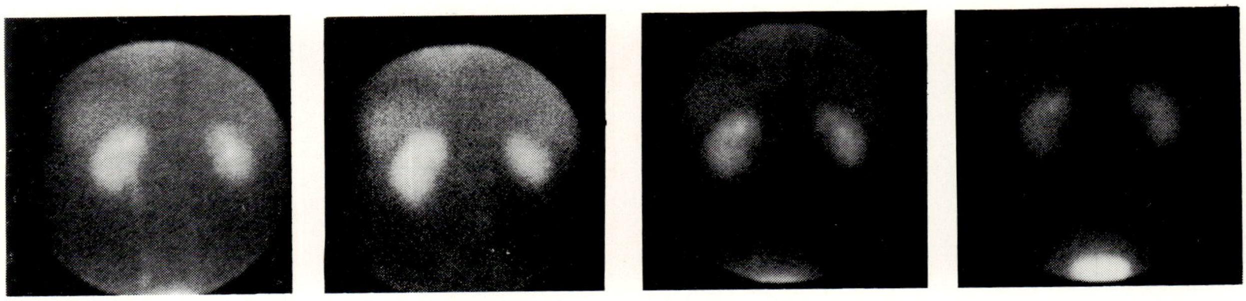

B 2 minutes 5 minutes 15 minutes 30 minutes

Tc-99m DTPA Imaging

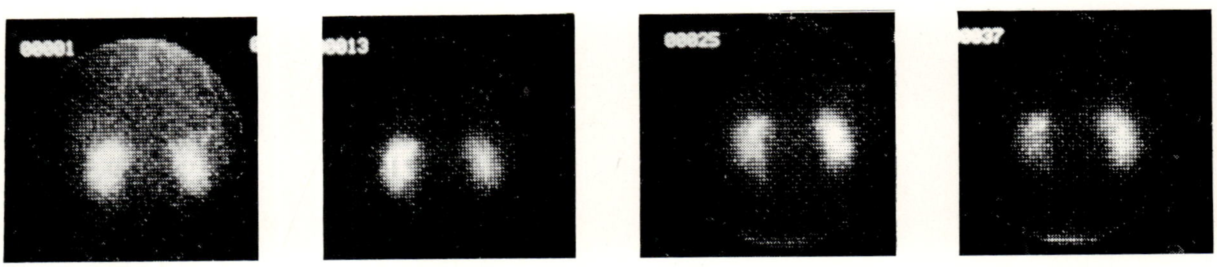

C 0 to 2 minutes 2 to 4 minutes 4 to 6 minutes 6 to 8 minutes

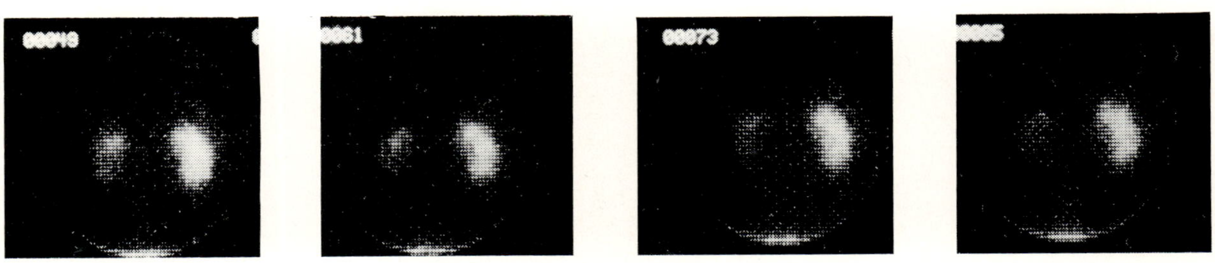

8 to 10 minutes 10 to 12 minutes 12 to 14 minutes 14 to 16 minutes

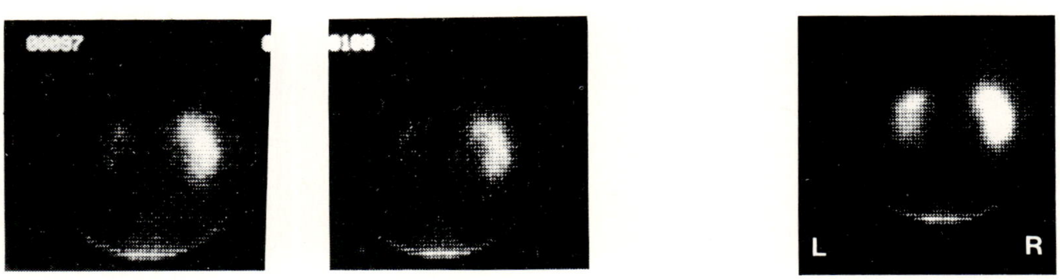


16 to 20 minutes 20 to 22 minutes Composite Image

I-131 Hippuran Imaging

**FIG. 12. B, C.** (See legend page 404)

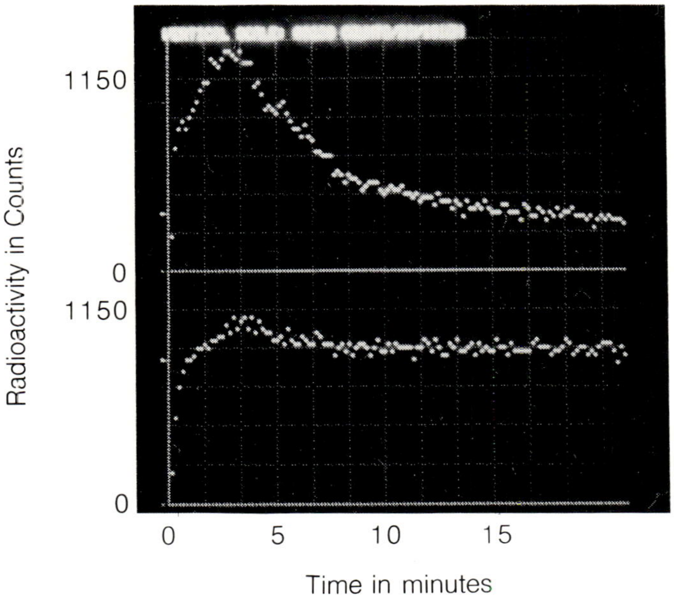


D Renogram

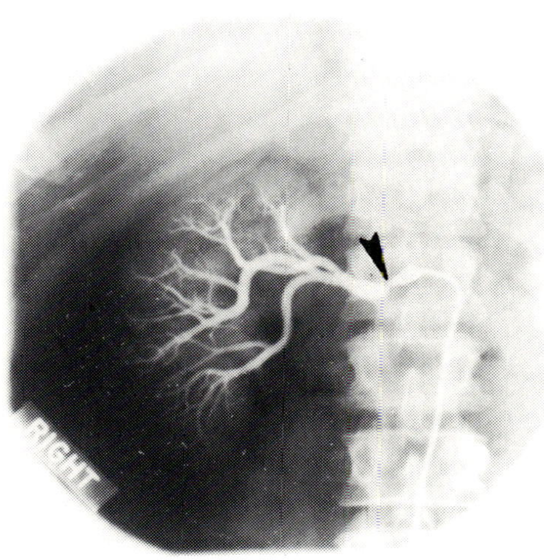


E Renal Arteriogram

**FIG. 12. D, E** (See legend next page)

**FIG. 12.** HYPERTENSION AND UNILATERAL STENOSIS OF AN ACCESSORY RENAL ARTERY. **A. Blood Flow Studies Performed in the Posterior Position with Frames Obtained at Intervals of 3 Seconds.** The abdominal aorta is clearly identified (arrow) and, visually, there appears to be similar perfusion to both the right (RK) and left (LK) kidneys. The perfused right kidney appears slightly smaller than the left. However, the blood flow curve generated from the computer analysis covering frames 1 to 25 shows a difference between the two sides. The arterial perfusion curve of the right kidney (lower curve) shows lower amplitude than that of the left, and the relative flattening of the right curve as compared to the left is related to slower or reduced arterial flow (Tc-99m DTPA). **B. Static Imaging Performed in the Posterior Position Immediately Following Radionuclide Administration and at Intervals Up to 30 Minutes.** The initial image shows that the right kidney is smaller than the left. The initial increase in radioactivity in the left kidney is associated with greater glomerular filtration on that side. Subsequent serial imaging shows slightly less radioactivity on the left side than on the right, a finding related to greater excretion on the left side (Tc-99m DTPA). **C. I-131 Hippuran Imaging.** During the first two frames at 0 to 2 minutes and 2 to 4 minutes, there is increased activity in the left kidney which is associated with more rapid tubular uptake on that side. Afterward, the activity in the left kidney continues to decrease because of excretion on that side. On the other hand, the radioactivity continues to increase in the right kidney due to prolonged uptake and reduced excretion of the radionuclide. **D.** The renogram reflects the Hippuran imaging findings, showing a normal left-sided curve and the described abnormalities on the right (prolonged transit time, reduced excretion). The disparity is consistent with unilateral renal ischemia. **E.** The selective renal arteriogram shows stenosis (arrow) of a right upper renal artery.

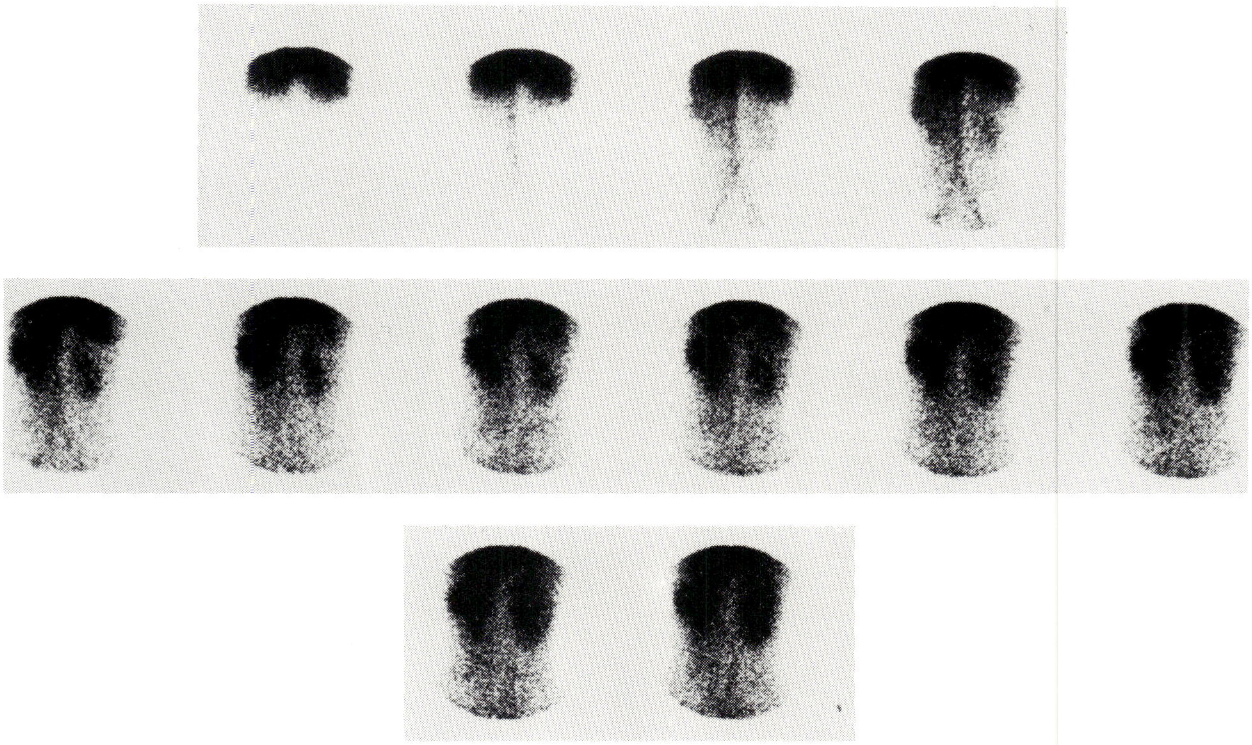

A Posterior Blood Flow

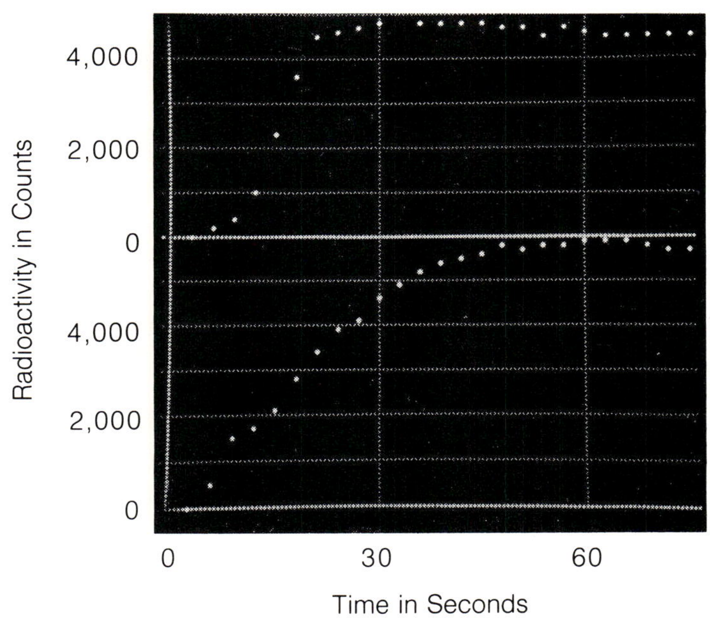


B Computerized Analysis Blood Flow Curve

**FIG. 13. A, B.** (See legend page 407)

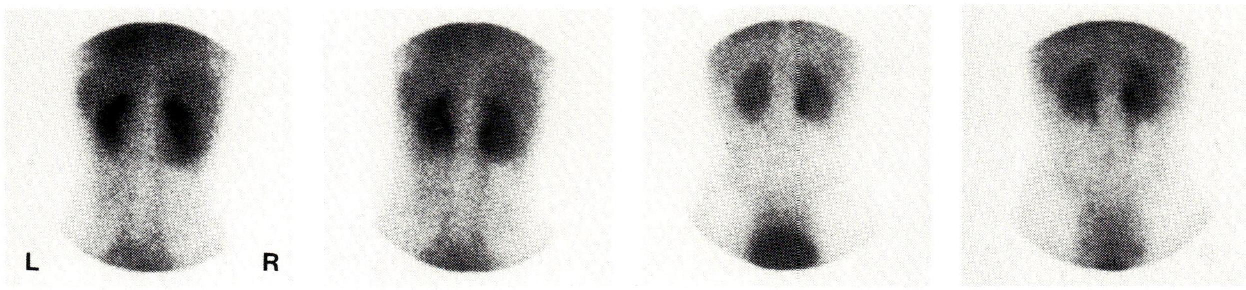


C 2 minutes 5 minutes 20 minutes 30 minutes

Tc-99m DTPA Imaging

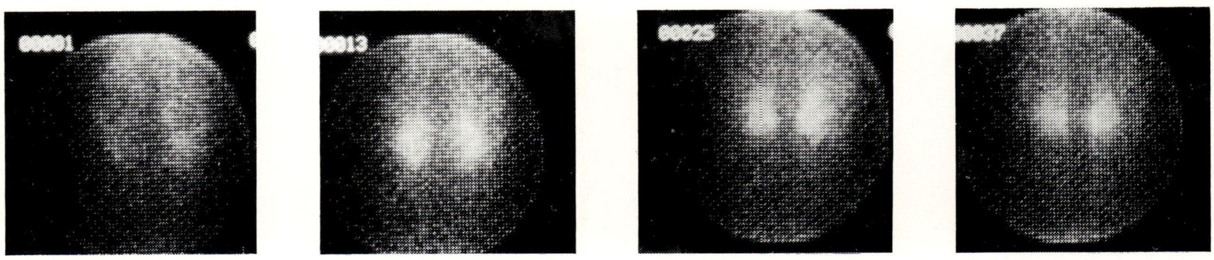

D 0 to 2 minutes 2 to 4 minutes 4 to 6 minutes 6 to 8 minutes

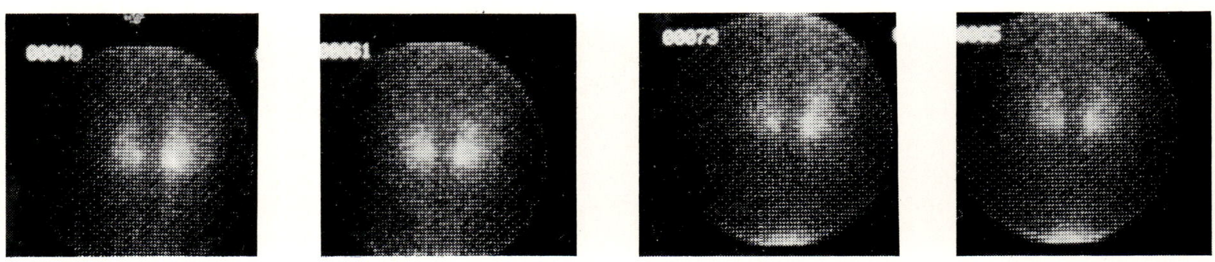

8 to 10 minutes 10 to 12 minutes 12 to 14 minutes 14 to 16 minutes

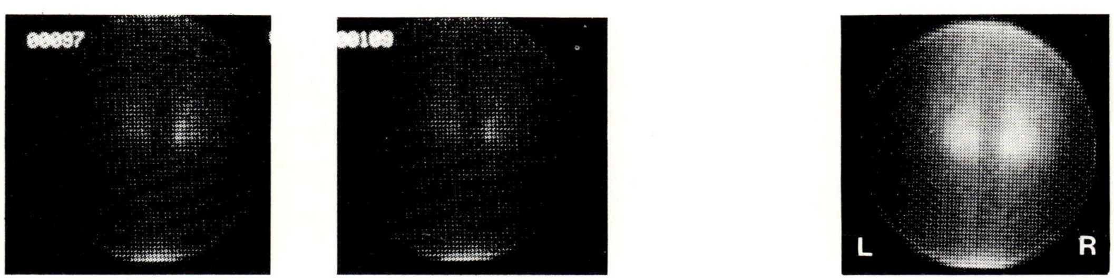


16 to 18 minutes 18 to 20 minutes Composite Image

I-131 Hippuran Imaging

**FIG. 13.** (See legend next page)

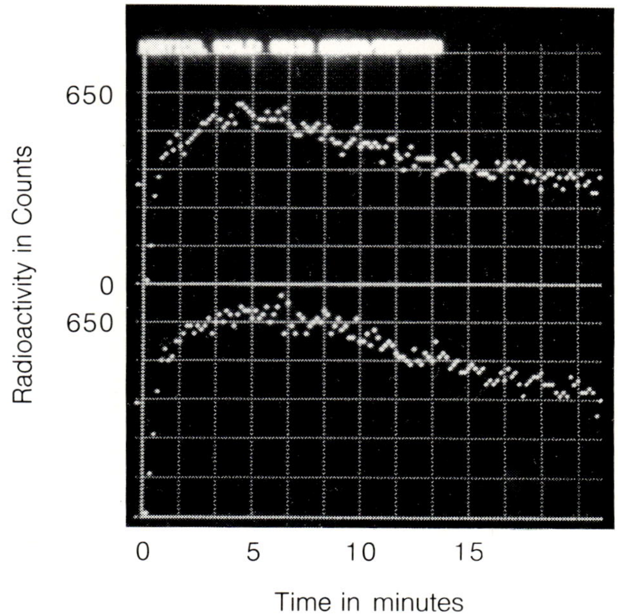


E Renogram

**FIG. 13. HYPERTENSION AND ASSOCIATED CHRONIC RENAL DISEASE IN A 16-YEAR-OLD GIRL. A.** Blood flow studies performed with Tc-99m DTPA shows evidence of arterial perfusion to both kidneys. However, the computerized analysis (**B**) shows somewhat flattened tracings, which are similar for both the right and left sides. **C.** Static renal imaging with Tc-99m DTPA shows no evidence of obstructive uropathy, but there is reduced clearance of the radioactive material from the blood as evidenced by the relatively elevated blood radioactivity. These findings suggest reduced glomerular filtration. **D. I-131 Hippuran Imaging.** Although there is renal visualization during the interval 2 to 4 minutes, there is a persistence in renal radioactivity consistent with the reduced excretion. **E. Renogram.** The curves from both kidneys reflect the findings seen on I-131 Hippuran imaging. Transit time is prolonged to 5 minutes, and excretion is markedly reduced to a similar degree bilaterally. That no disparity appears between the right and left renograms points toward the absence of unilateral renal ischemia. Thus, the Hippuran studies in this patient helped determine that renal angiography for the purpose of discovering unilateral renal artery stenosis should not be performed.

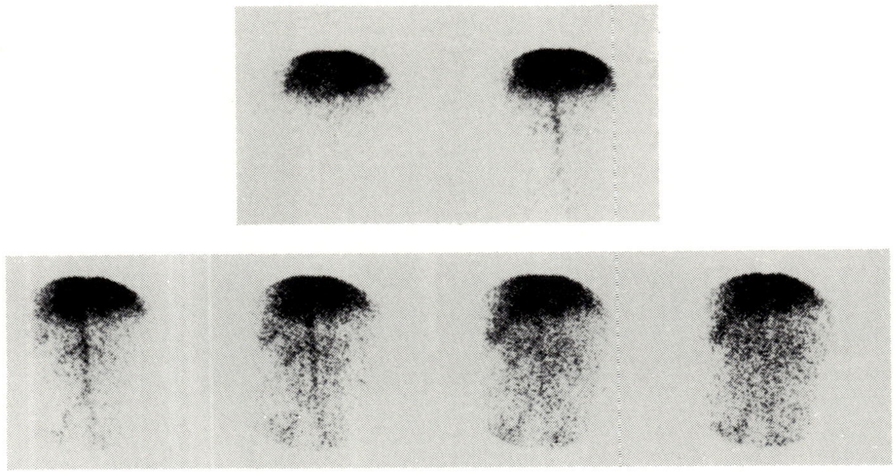

A Posterior Blood Flow

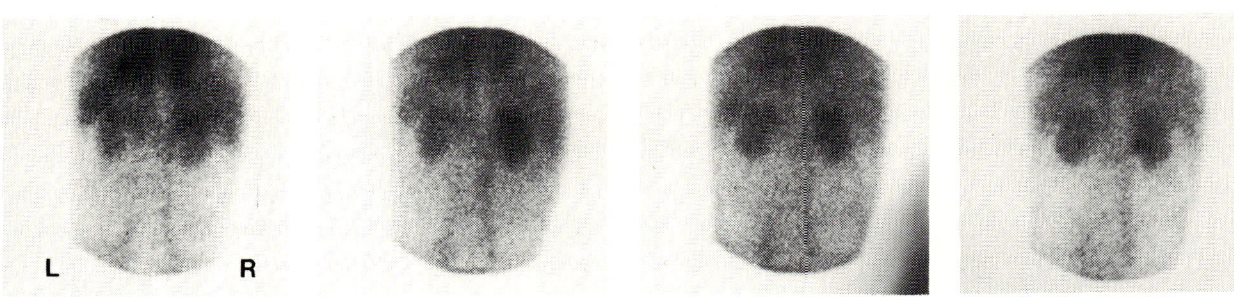

B 2 minutes 5 minutes 15 minutes 30 minutes

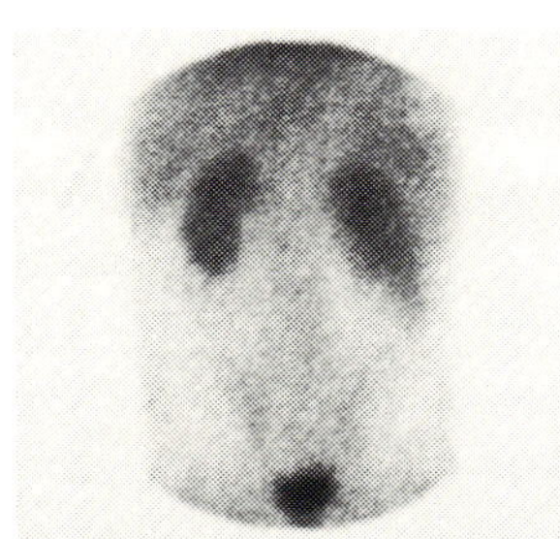

24 hours

Static DTPA Imaging

**FIG. 14. A, B.** (See legend page 410)

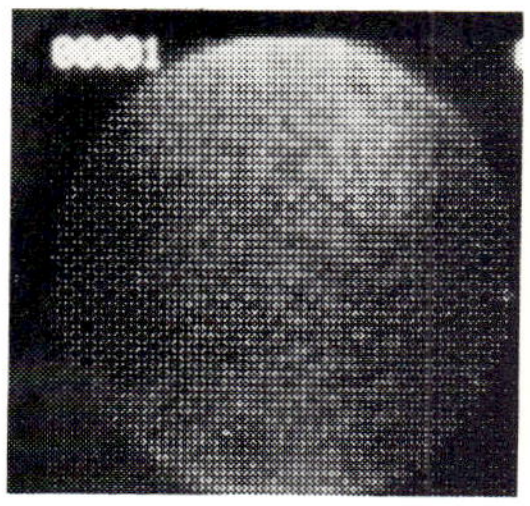

C 0 to 2 minutes

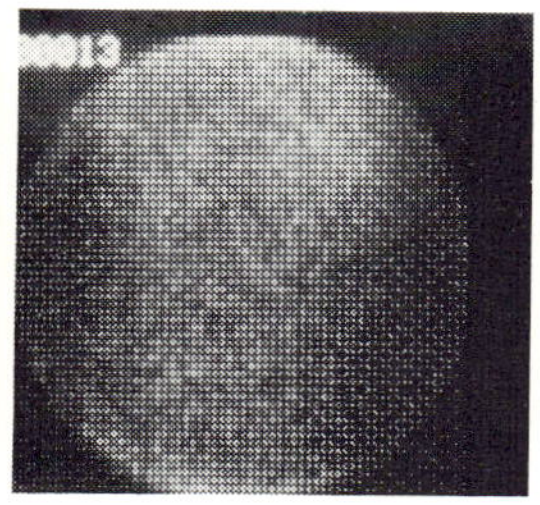

2 to 4 minutes

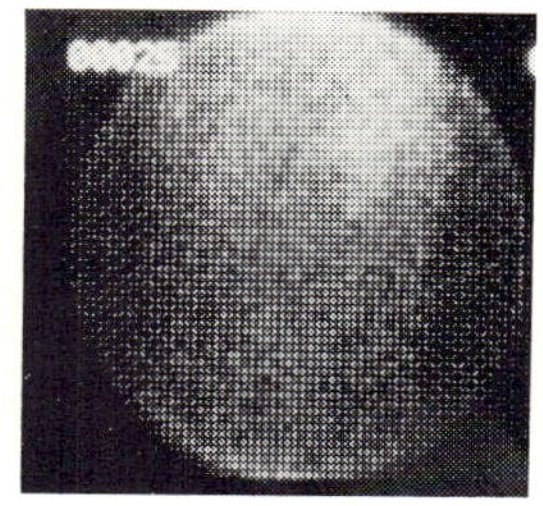

4 to 6 minutes

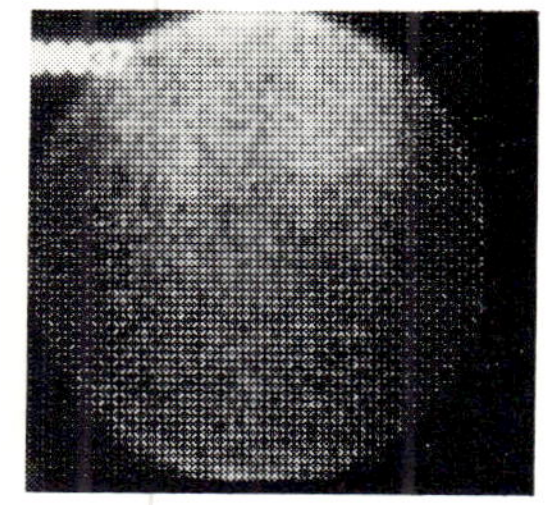

6 to 8 minutes

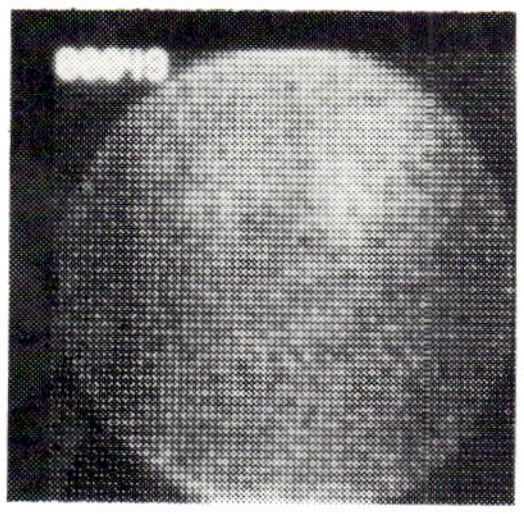

8 to 10 minutes

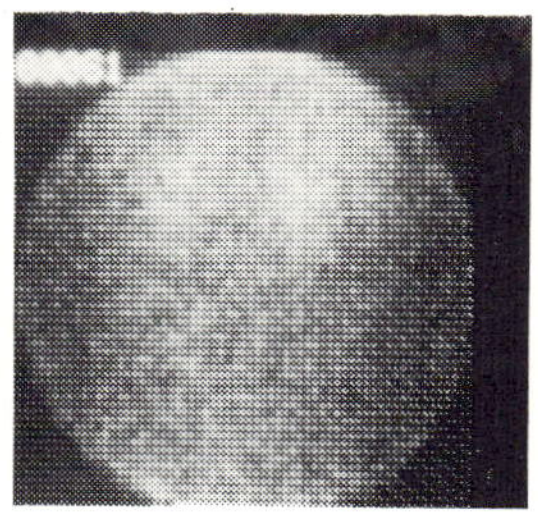

10 to 12 minutes

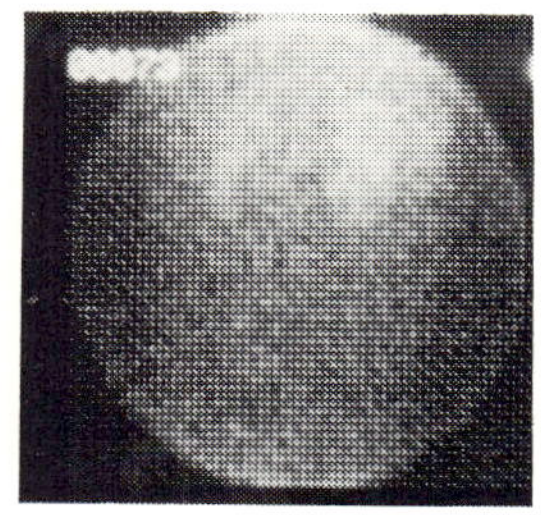

12 to 14 minutes

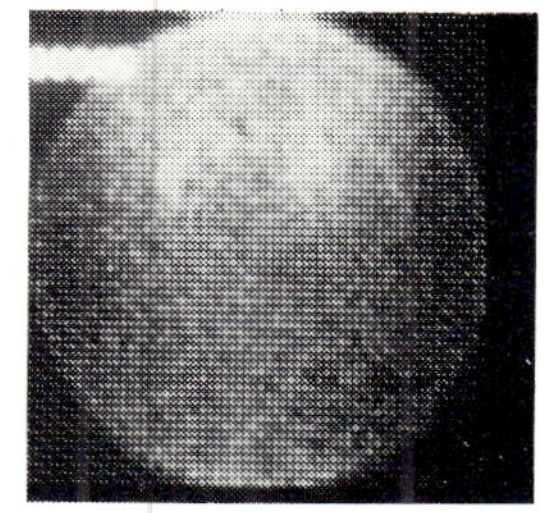

14 to 16 minutes

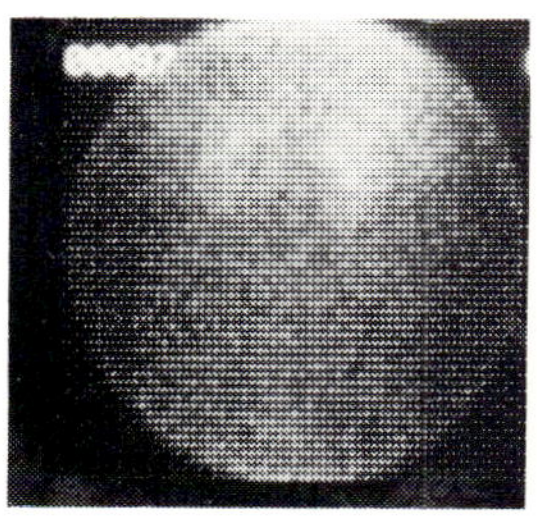

16 to 18 minutes

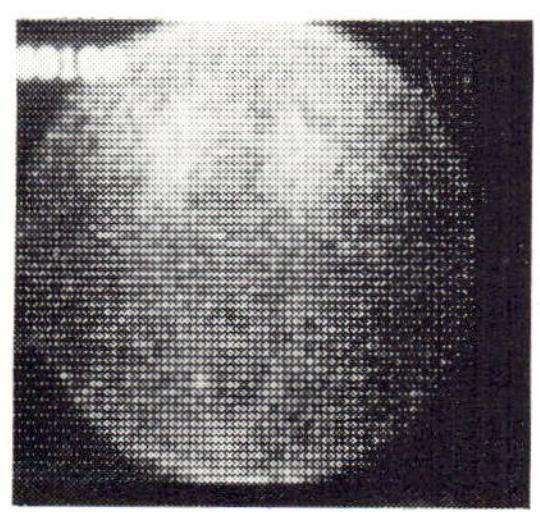

18 to 20 minutes

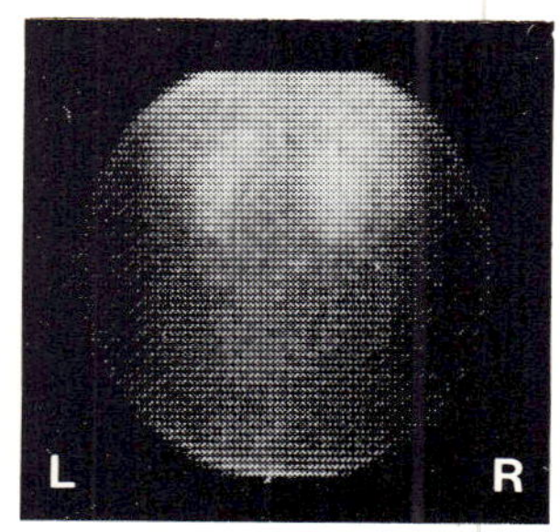


D Composite Hippuran Image

I-131 Hippuran Imaging

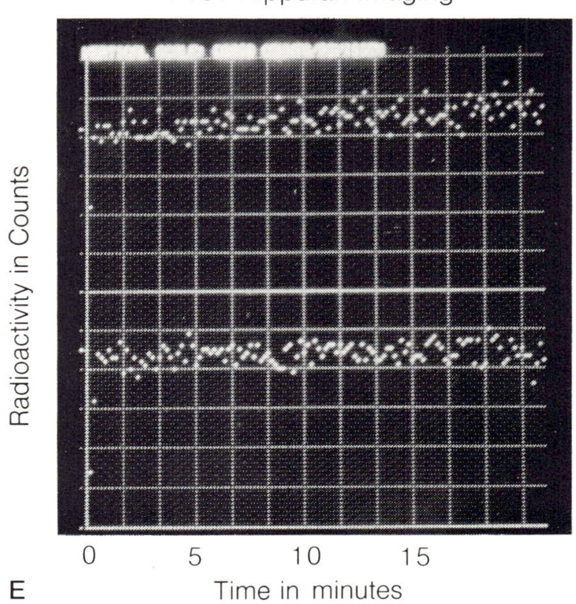


Renogram

E

**FIG. 14. C, E.** (See legend next page)

**FIG. 14.** **CHRONIC GLOMERULONEPHRITIS AND MARKEDLY IMPAIRED RENAL FUNCTION BILATERALLY.** Evidence of the extensive involvement is seen in the studies of this 12-year-old boy. **A.** Blood flow studies do not sharply identify the kidneys during the arterial phase (Tc-99m DTPA). **B.** Static Tc-99m DTPA imaging reflects the slow blood clearance of the radioactive material due to the marked reduction in glomerular filtration. **C.** Identification of both kidneys appears late (8 to 10 minutes) on the serial I-131 Hippuran imaging. **D.** The composite Hippuran image shows how faintly the kidneys are visualized in association with reduced tubular uptake of the radioactive material. **E.** Renogram shows somewhat flattened curves, which are characteristic of chronic, severe parenchymal disease. Both uptake and excretion of radionuclide show marked impairment.

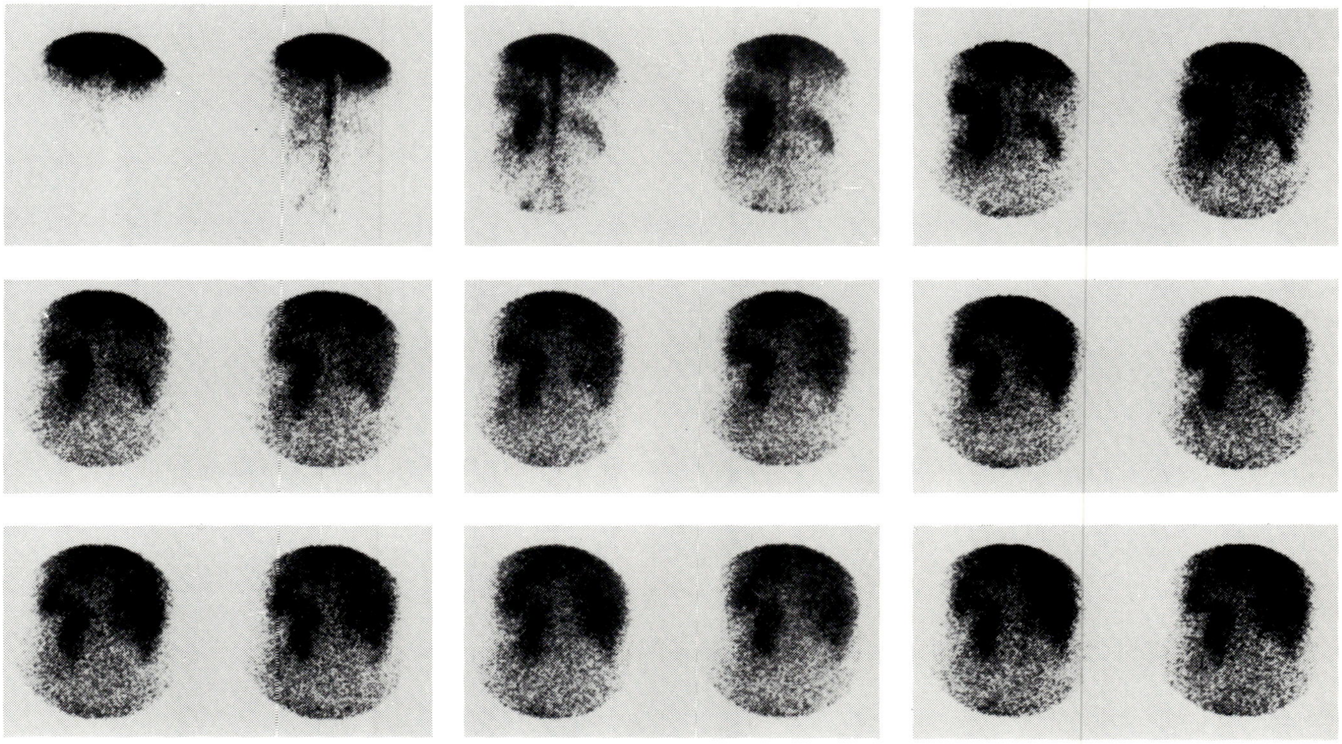

A Posterior Blood Flow

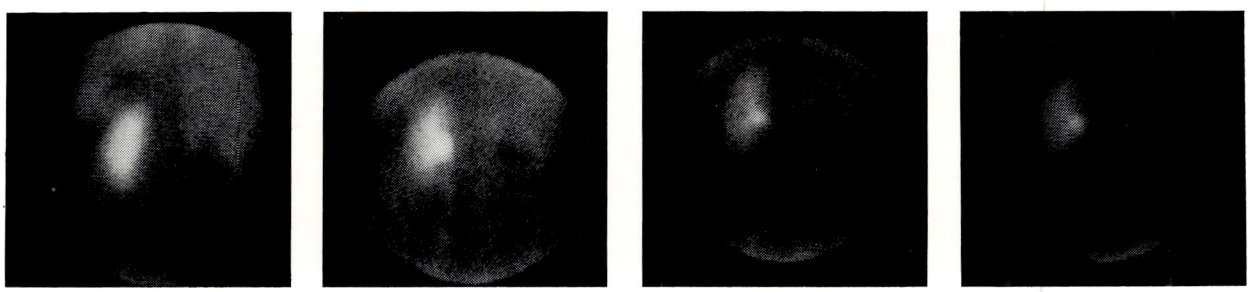

B 2 minutes 5 minutes 15 minutes 30 minutes

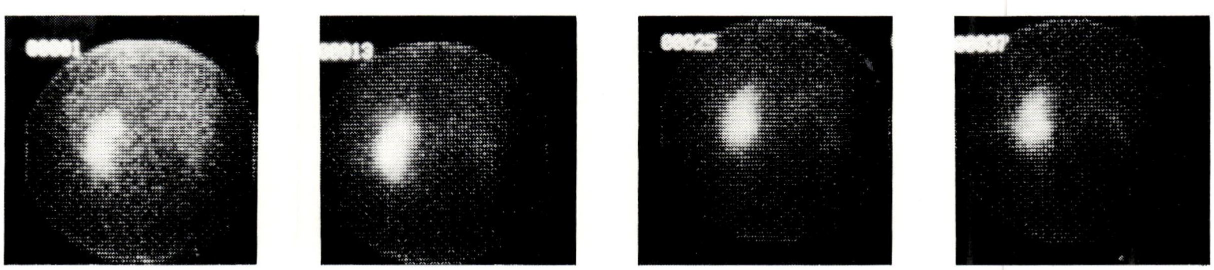

C 0 to 2 minutes 2 to 4 minutes 4 to 6 minutes 6 to 8 minutes

**FIG. 15. A, B, C.** (See legend next page)

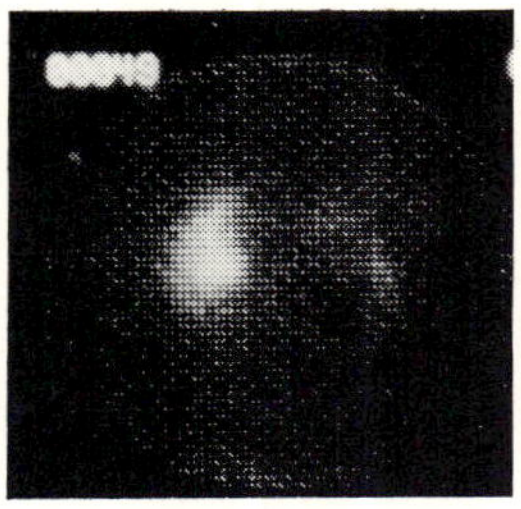

C 8 to 10 minutes

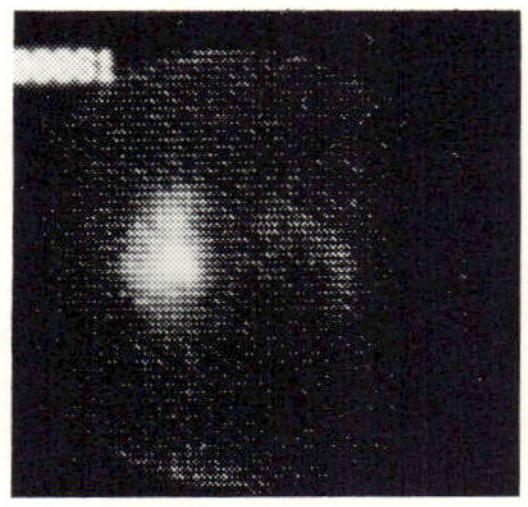

10 to 12 minutes

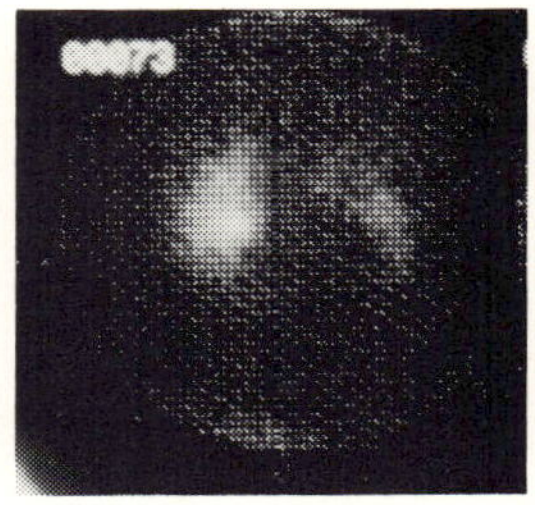

12 to 14 minutes

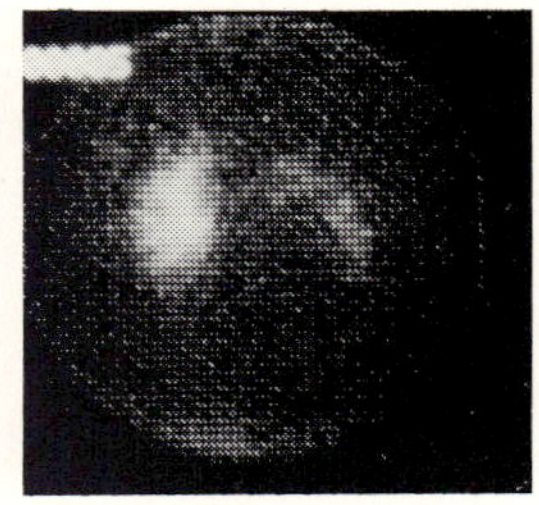

14 to 16 minutes

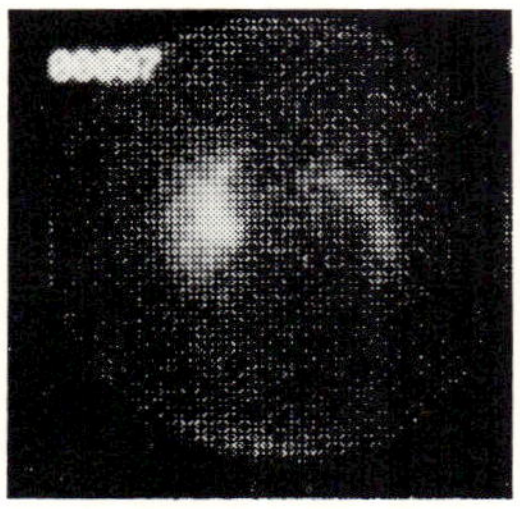

16 to 18 minutes

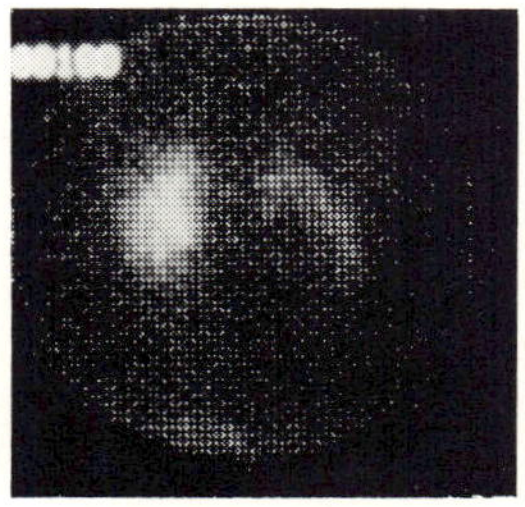

18 to 20 minutes

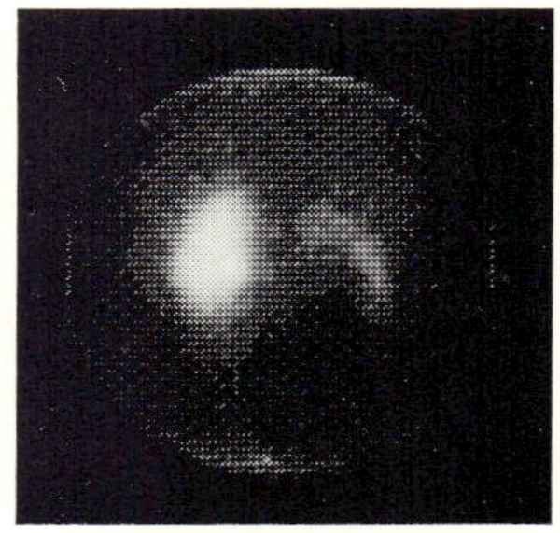

D Composite Image

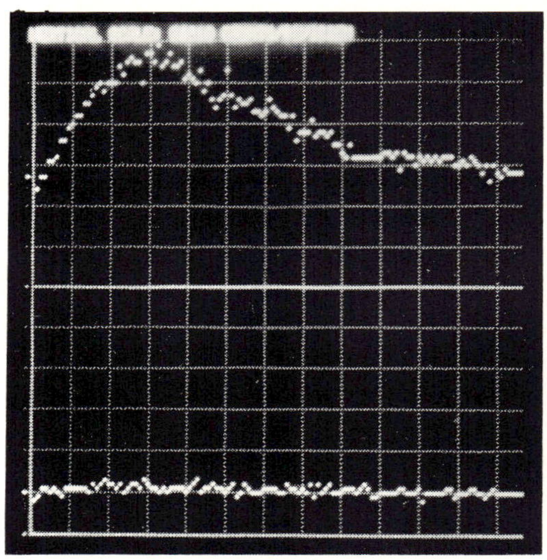


E Renogram

**FIG. 15. NONFUNCTIONING KIDNEY RESULTING FROM OBSTRUCTIVE UROPATHY SECONDARY TO NEOPLASM. A.** Blood flow studies performed in the posterior position show evidence of arterial perfusion to both kidneys. However, radioactivity in the right kidney was not persistent and indicated the absence of sufficient glomerular filtration to enable renal visualization (Tc-99m DTPA). **B.** Static Tc-99m DTPA imaging shows a normal left-sided sequence of early cortical visualization followed by excretion. The right side shows only faint cortical activity with no suggestion of excretion. **C.** Serial I-131 Hippuran imaging shows evidence of normal uptake and excretion in the left kidney but only cortical accumulation in the right kidney. **D.** The composite I-131 Hippuran image indicates that the radionuclide is present only in a shell of cortical tissue. **E.** The I-131 Hippuran renogram shows evidence of a nonfunctioning right kidney. The patient was found to have chronic obstruction secondary to extension from carcinoma of the cervix.

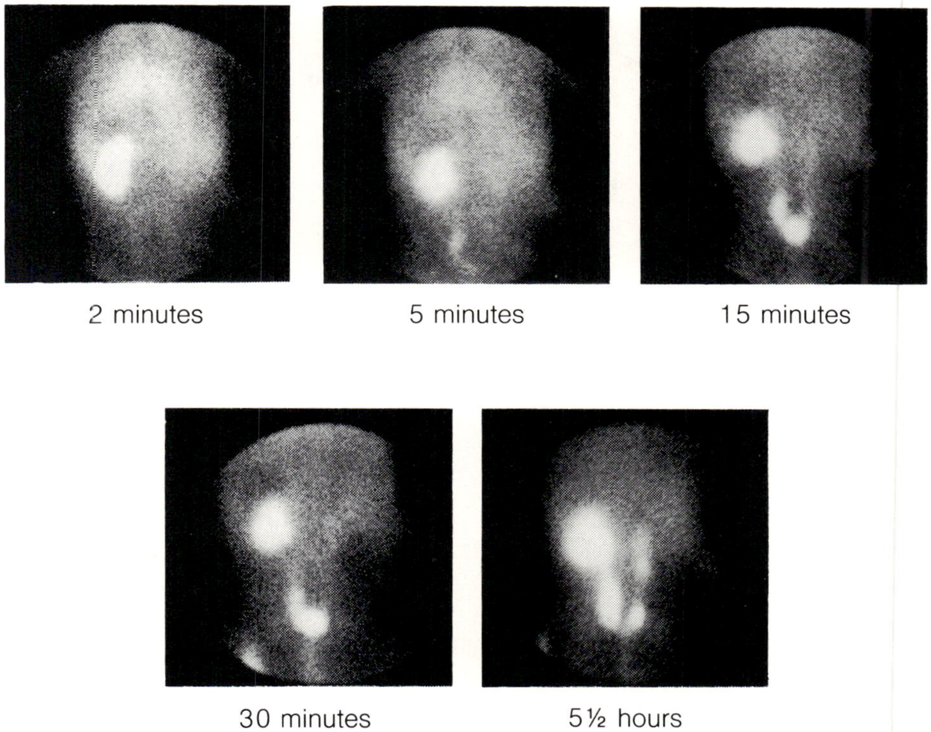



**FIG. 16. BILATERAL REFLUX SEEN ON Tc-99m DTPA IMAGING.** Observations on Tc-99m DTPA imaging may be misleading without associated, specific roentgenologic diagnostic studies. Persistent ureteral visualization may be due to reflux, as well as obstruction. In this patient with a nonfunctioning right kidney, Tc-99m DTPA imaging shows continued visualization of the distal left ureter. However, a contrast voiding cystourethrogram showed evidence of bilateral reflux. The DTPA study shows ureteral reflux on the right side and reflux to the ureter and renal pelvis on the left. If there is a question of reflux, it is often helpful to perform the imaging procedure in *both* the sitting and recumbent positions.

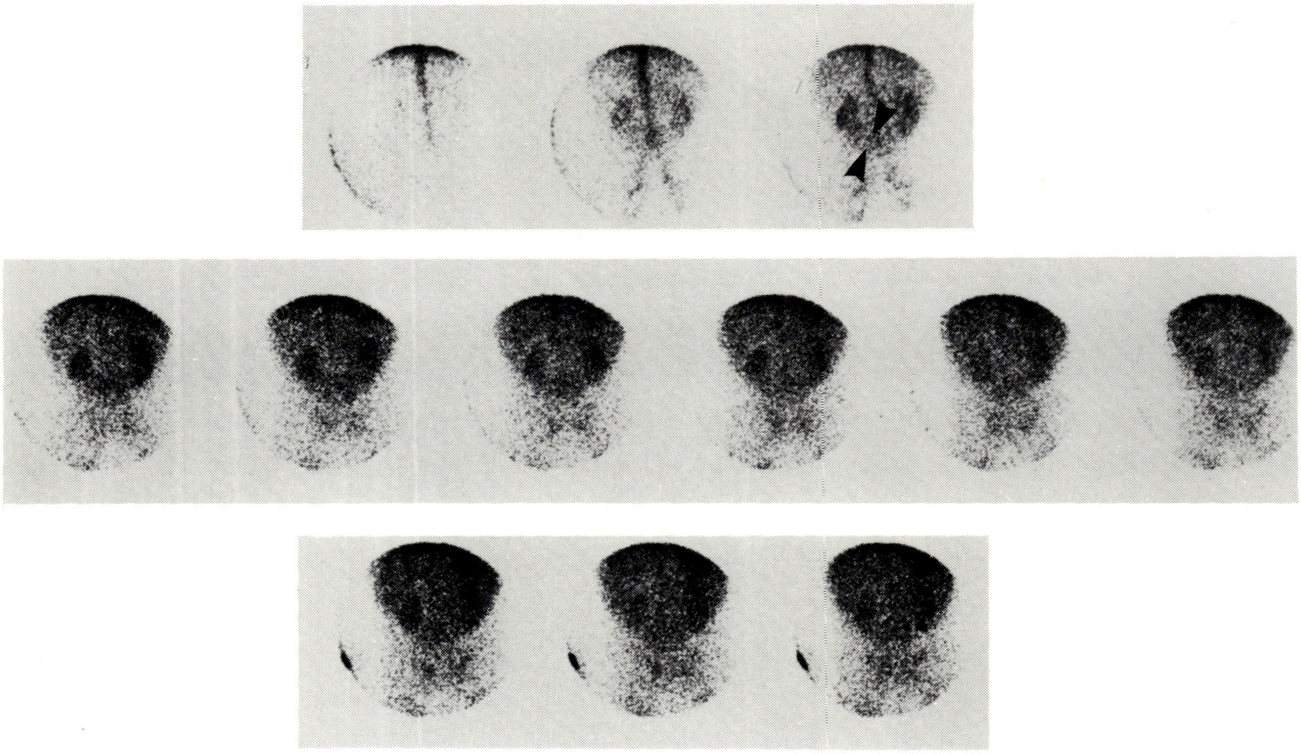

A Posterior Blood Flow

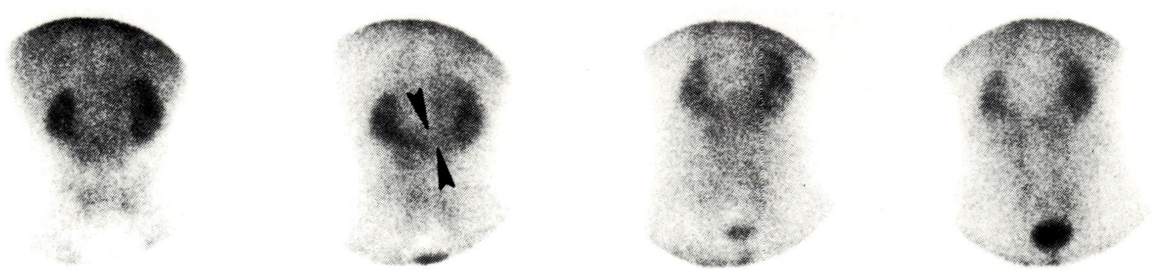

B 2 minutes 5 minutes 15 minutes 30 minutes

**FIG. 17. HORSESHOE KIDNEY.** The site of fusion (arrows) can be identified on both the blood flow study (**A**) and static imaging (**B**).

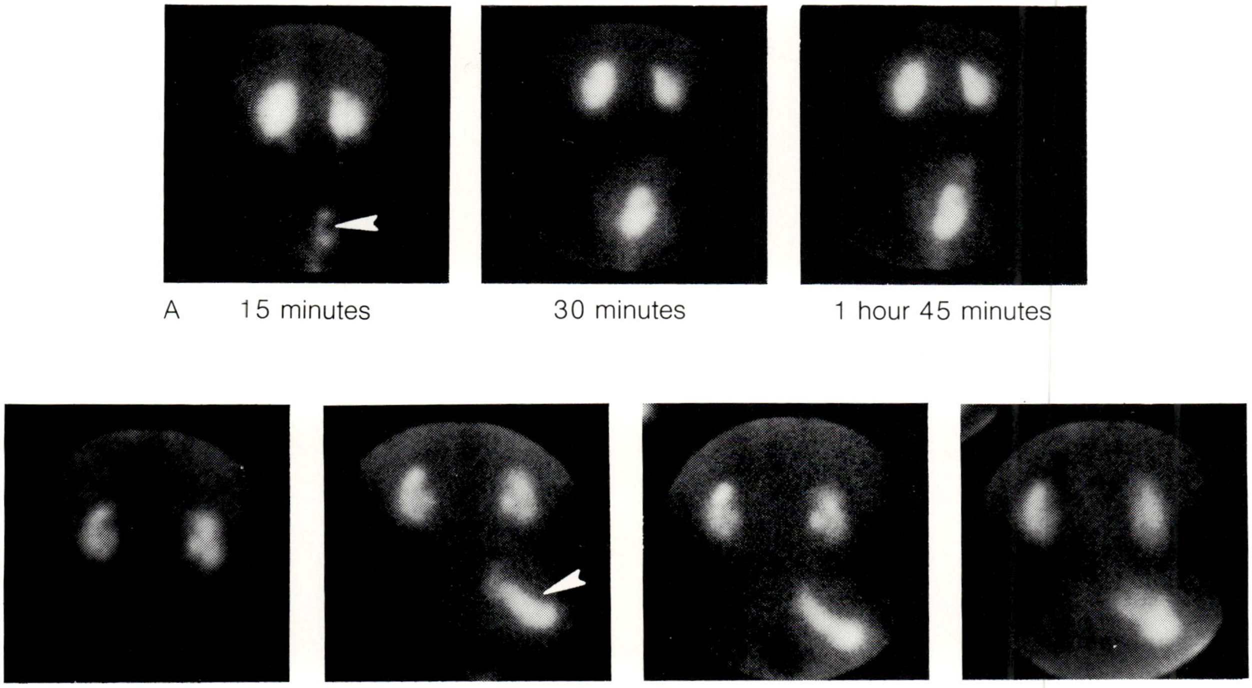

A 15 minutes 30 minutes 1 hour 45 minutes

B 5 minutes 15 minutes 45 minutes 2½ hours

**FIG. 18.** ILEAL CONDUIT. **A.** The site of the ileal bladder (arrow) appears to be related to the usual position of the urinary bladder as seen on selected static images. **B.** Eccentrically situated ileal conduit (arrow) in a patient (Tc-99m DTPA).

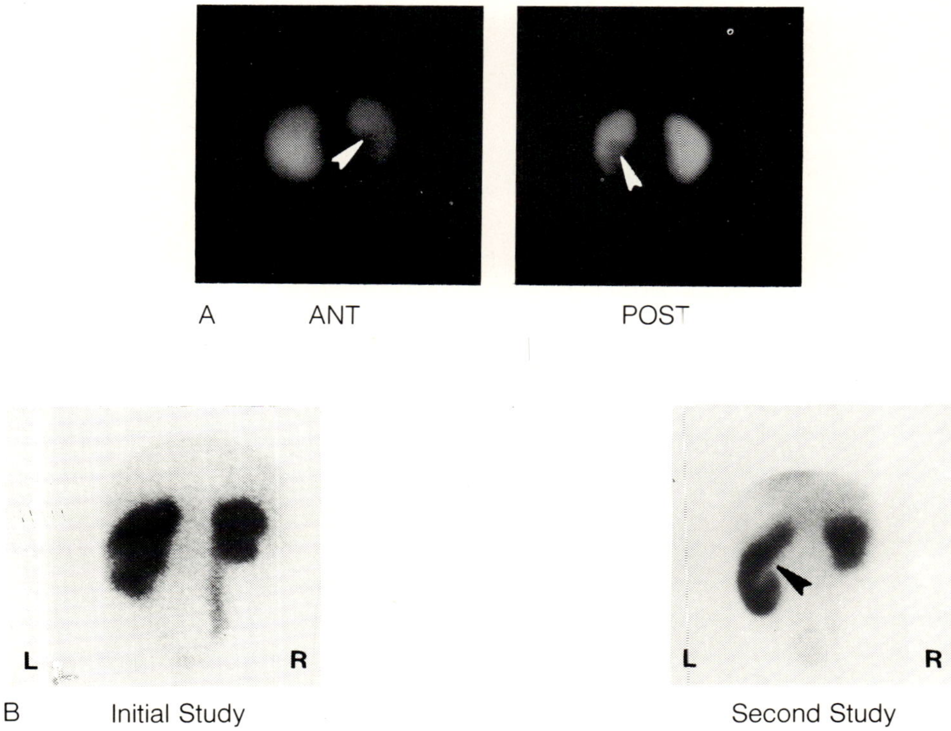


**FIG. 19.** **Tc-99m DMSA IMAGING.** Since the radionuclide becomes localized in the proximal tubules, renal images represent functioning cortical tissue. Imaging was performed 2 hours following injection. **A.** The right renal image is normal. This patient has left-sided pyelonephritis associated with reflux on that side. The involvement in the lower half of the left kidney has resulted in loss of cortical tissue (arrow) in this region. **B.** Progressive changes in a child with hydronephrosis and pyelonephritis. The relatively thin shell of cortical tissue in the left kidney (arrow) in the second study, associated with marked hydronephrosis, is indicative of progressive destruction and replacement of renal cortical tissue. Compare this to the initial study, which was performed 2 years earlier.

## Renal Transplantation

Nuclear medicine studies are relied on heavily in the evaluation of patients with a transplanted kidney. Among the studies most commonly employed are Tc-99m DTPA blood flow and static imaging, Tc-99m glucoheptonate blood flow and static imaging, and I-131 Hippuran imaging and renogram generation.

It is often most convenient for such procedures to be carried out at the bedside during the early postoperative period. Such studies are greatly facilitated by a portable scintillation camera with computer capabilities—either an on-board computer or a remote terminal connected to a stationary computer.

The patency of the arterial supply to the transplanted kidney can be easily determined from a radionuclide blood flow study using Tc-99m DTPA. Static imaging may also be performed with the same radionuclide to help determine the functional status of the kidney. Given the sites at which kidneys are transplanted, imaging should usually be performed in the anterior position.

Specific information in regard to whether or not a rejection reaction might have occurred can be obtained from I-131 Hippuran imaging and renogram generation. Such studies may be performed at intervals of 3 or 4 days if a rejection reaction is suspected.

As pointed out earlier in this chapter, the renal image is most sharply identified three to five minutes following I-131 Hippuran injection. Thereafter, renal radioactivity decreases as the I-131 Hippuran is excreted into the bladder. Care must be exercised in the identification of both the renal and bladder images, since they are often in very close anatomic relation in the patient with a renal transplant. Such normal radioactive Hippuran imaging will be associated with a renogram curve of normal configuration in which the three segments are clearly recognized.

Failure of the kidney to be visualized on I-131 Hippuran imaging during the first 10 minutes may be seen with interference with the arterial supply to the kidney. On the other hand, increased renal radioactivity 10 or 15 minutes after radionuclide administration, with little or no bladder activity visible, may herald the onset of a rejection phenomenon. Identical imaging findings may also be seen with mechanical obstruction and acute tubular necrosis. However, an initial increase in renal radioactivity up to, for example, 10 minutes, that is followed by a gradual increase in bladder activity, is usually a sign of only temporary renal tubular impairment.

As expected, renogram tracings parallel the findings of I-131 Hippuran imaging. However, distinctive findings related to whether or not a rejection reaction is occurring may be more clearly identified from the inspection and analysis of the renogram curve that is generated.

The onset of a rejection phenomenon may be indicated by a renogram showing an obstructive pattern (of the intrarenal type). These findings are in part associated with ischemic changes in the renal tubules secondary to the rejection reaction affecting the peritubular capillaries. Subsequent renograms 3 or 4 days later may show curves with a pattern of nonfunction (no accumulation phase) in the patient having a hyperacute or accelerated rejection reaction.

It is important to remember that a renogram curve with an "obstructive" pattern in a transplanted kidney may also be associated with mechanical obstruction, cortical necrosis, acute tubular necrosis, and arterial occlusion. If the last is suspected, arterial patency may be determined with radionuclide angiography. (The images presented in this section on transplantation were supplied by Dr. Eva V. Dubosky, Veterans Administration Medical Center, Birmingham, Alabama.)

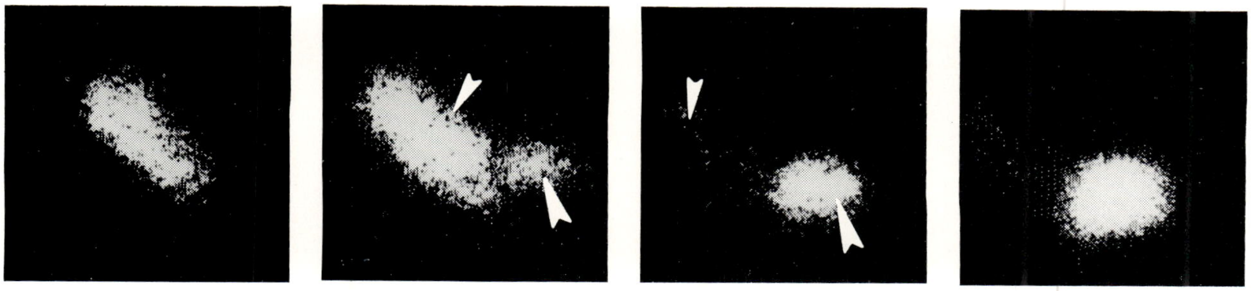

A 0 to 3 minutes 3 to 6 minutes 11 to 14 minutes 21 to 24 minutes

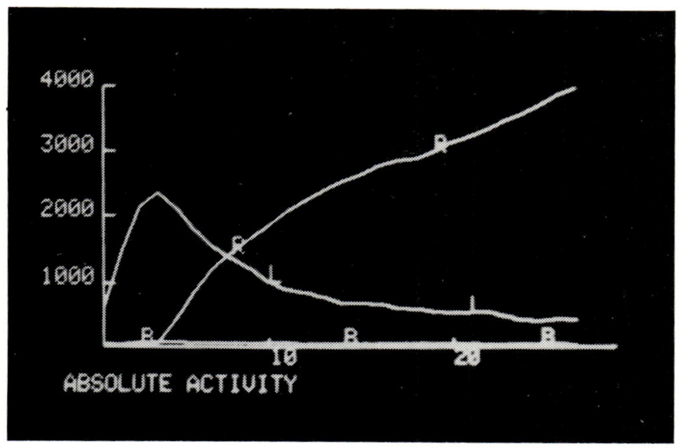


B

**FIG. 20.** NORMAL I-131 HIPPURAN IMAGING AND RENOGRAM GENERATION. **A.** Selected frames following injection of 150 $\mu$Ci of I-131 Hippuran show evidence of normal tubular uptake during the first 2 frames with radioactive material starting to appear in the bladder ( larger arrows) during the 3- to 6-minute interval. Excretion of the radioactive material from the renal transplant (small arrows)is almost complete, as seen on the images at 11 to 14 minutes and 21 to 24 minutes. **B.** The computerized renogram curve (L), generated through region of interest studies of the transplanted kidney, is normal (see Fig. 11). Note the gradual ascending bladder curve (R) which reflects its increasing activity as the radioactive material is excreted from the kidney into the bladder. (Courtesy of Dr. Eva V. Dubovsky, Veterans Administration Medical Center, Birmingham, Alabama)

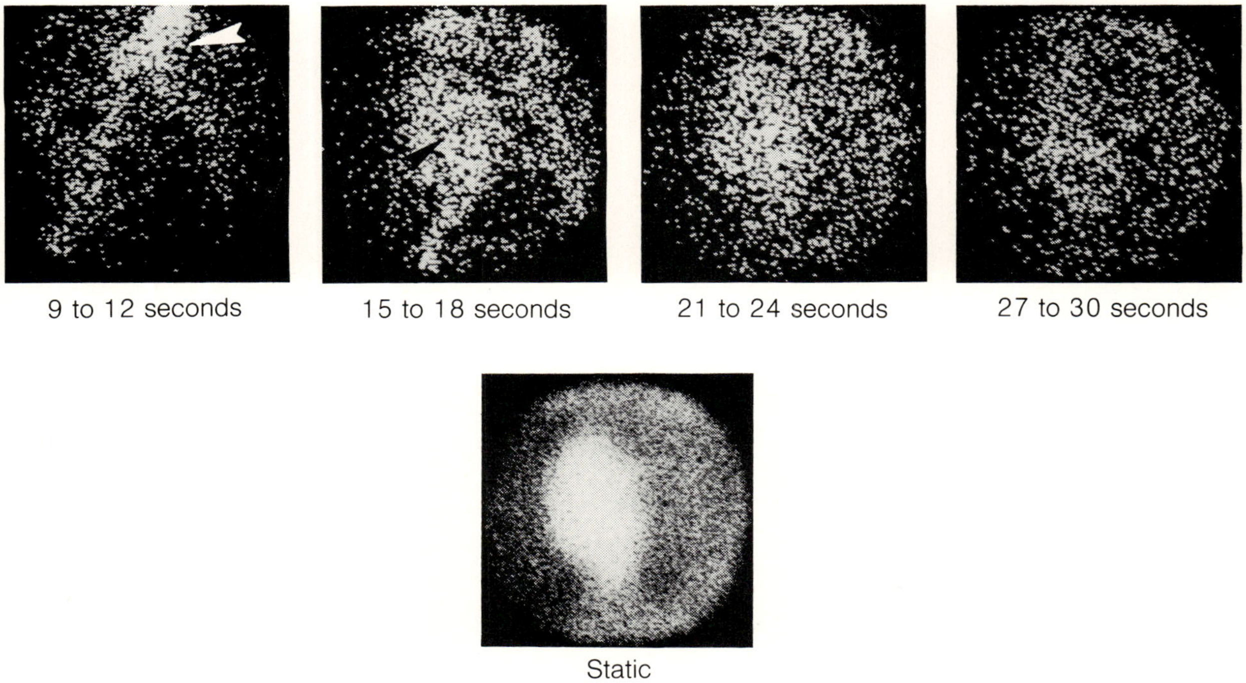


**FIG. 21.** NORMAL BLOOD FLOW STUDY. Imaging during the arterial phase demonstrates the distal abdominal aorta (larger arrow) and, 3 seconds later, the transplanted kidney (small arrow) is seen. Note the rapid transit of the Tc-99m DTPA through the kidney so that there is a barely visible renal impression as the arterial phase ends (27 to 30 second image). The transplanted kidney is again identified on static imaging immediately following the blood flow study. (Courtesy of Dr. Eva V. Dubovsky, Veterans Administration Medical Center, Birmingham, Alabama)

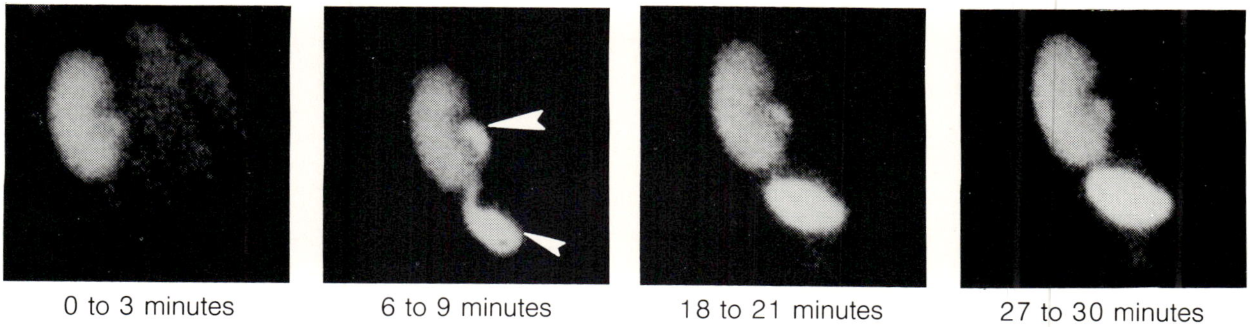


**FIG. 22. NORMAL STATIC IMAGING WITH TC-99M-GLUCOHEPTONATE.** Imaging during the 0–3 minute interval following tracer administration demonstrates the functioning cortex of the renal transplant. During the 6- to 9-minute interval, there is excretion, with demonstration of the renal pelvis (larger arrow) and bladder (small arrow). Since the Tc-99m-glucoheptonate is also a cortical imaging agent, radioactive material continues to remain in the kidney although there is continued excretion as seen by the bladder image. (Courtesy of Dr. Eva V. Dubovsky, Veterans Administration Medical Center, Birmingham, Alabama)

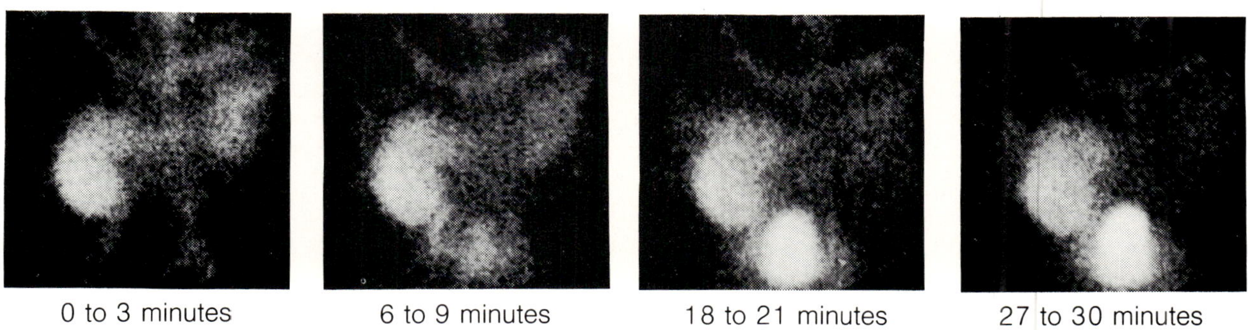


**FIG. 23. ACUTE REJECTION.** Although there is evidence of renal function and excretion, the elevated background radioactivity and persistence of radioactivity in the vascular structures are findings that may characterize an acute rejection reaction. During the 27- to 30-minute interval, there is still considerable radionuclide present that has not been handled by the transplanted kidney (Tc-99m glucoheptonate). (Courtesy of Dr. Eva V. Dubovsky, Veterans Administration Medical Center, Birmingham, Alabama)

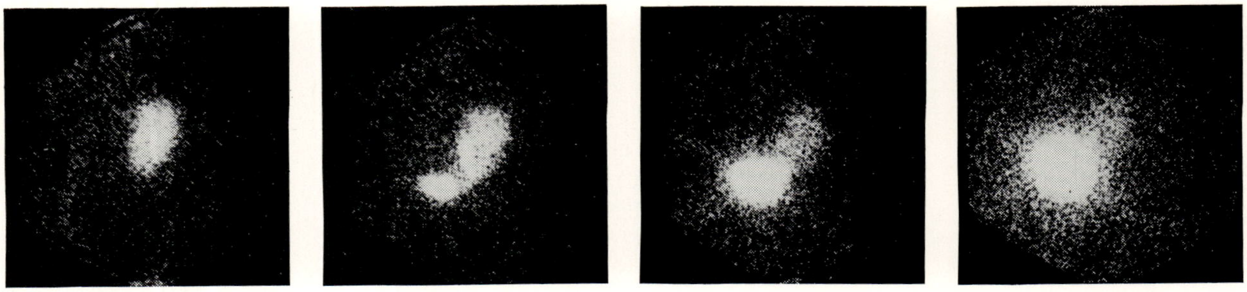

A 0 to 3 minutes 3 to 6 minutes 12 to 15 minutes 24 to 27 minutes

I-131 Hippuran Imaging

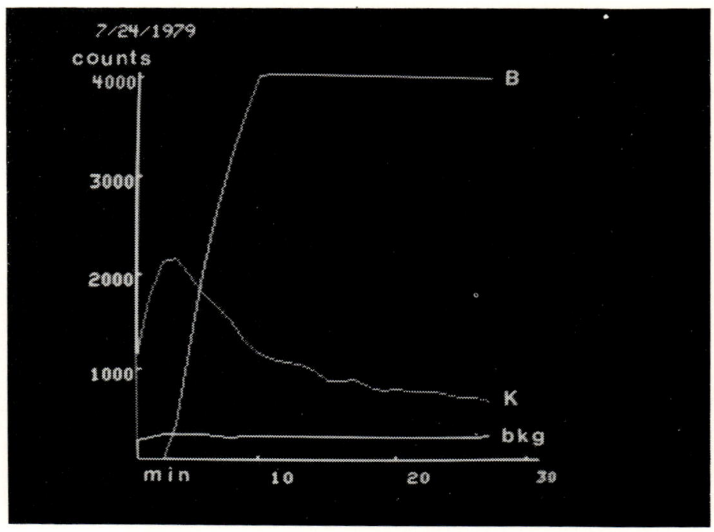


Renogram

**FIG. 24. A.** (See legend on page 425)

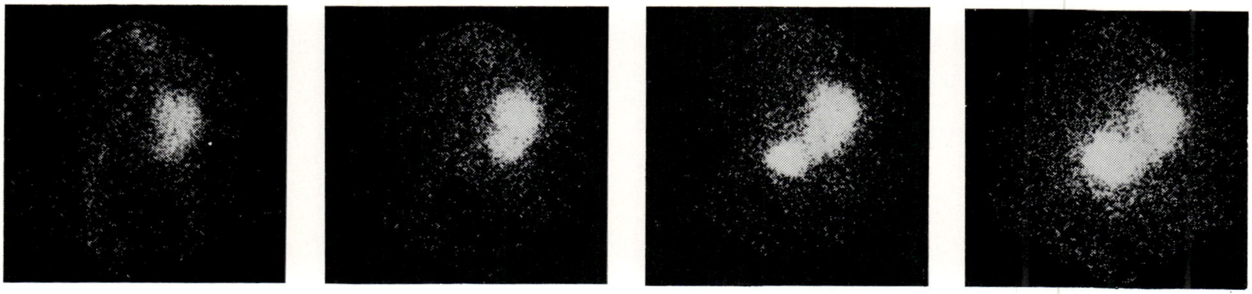

B 0 to 3 minutes 3 to 6 minutes 12 to 15 minutes 24 to 27 minutes

I-131 Hippuran Imaging

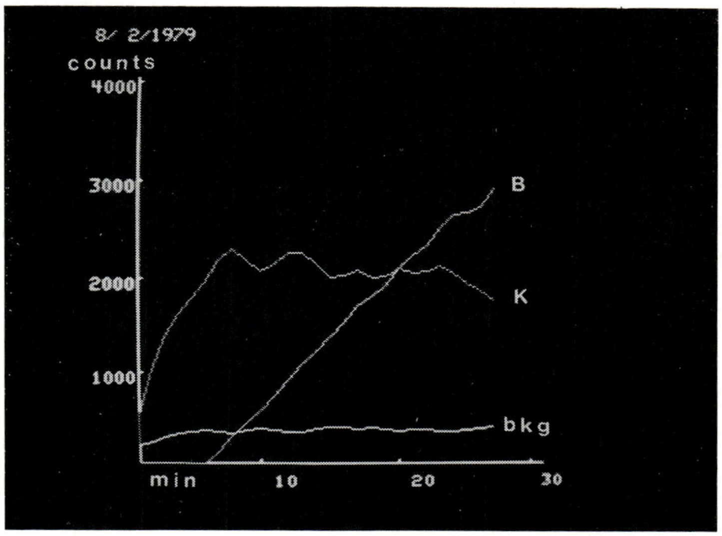


Renogram

**FIG. 24. B.** (See legend on page 425)

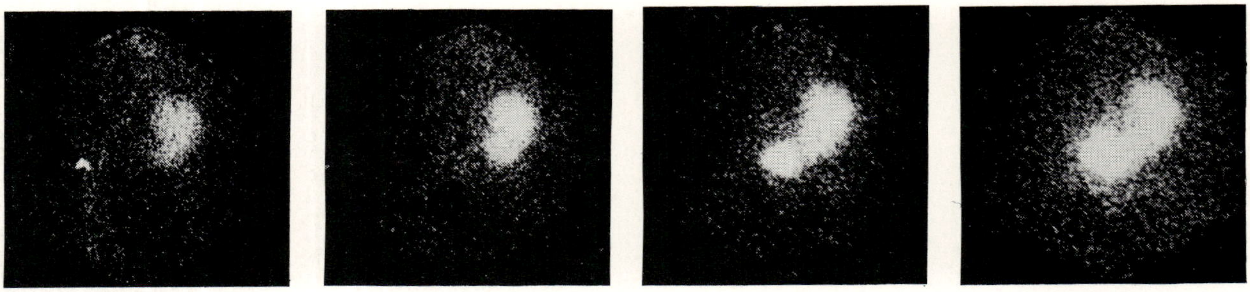

C 0 to 3 minutes | 3 to 6 minutes | 12 to 15 minutes | 24 to 27 minutes

I-131 Hippuran Imaging

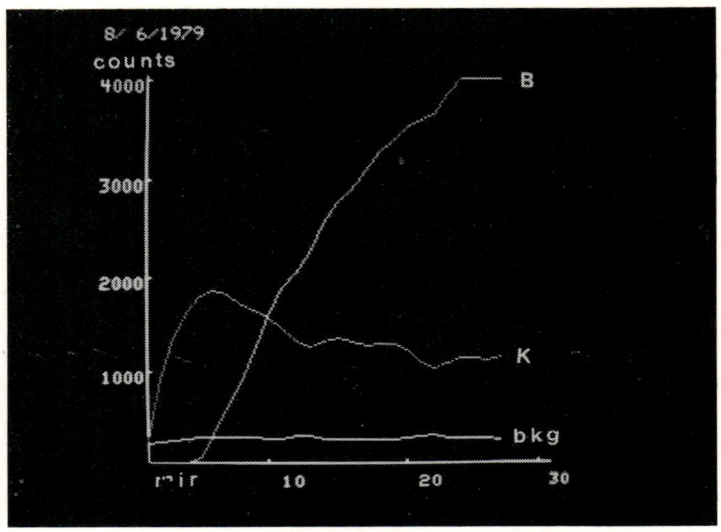


Renogram

**FIG. 24. C.** (See legend page 425)

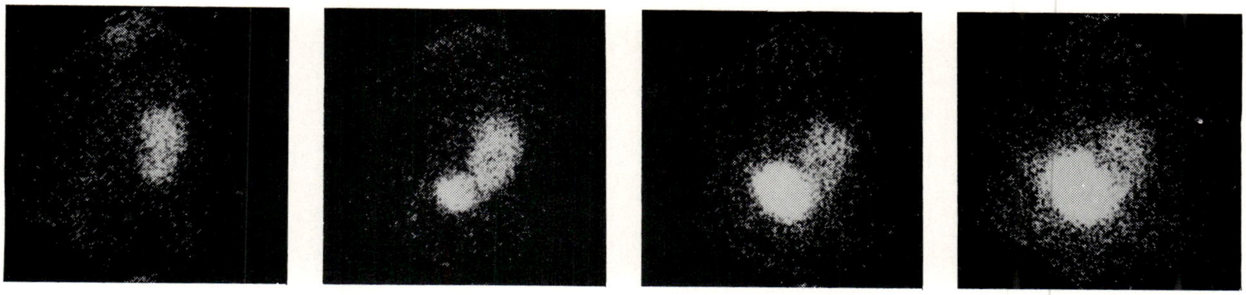

D 0 to 3 minutes | 3 to 6 minutes | 12 to 15 minutes | 24 to 27 minutes

I-131 Hippuran Imaging

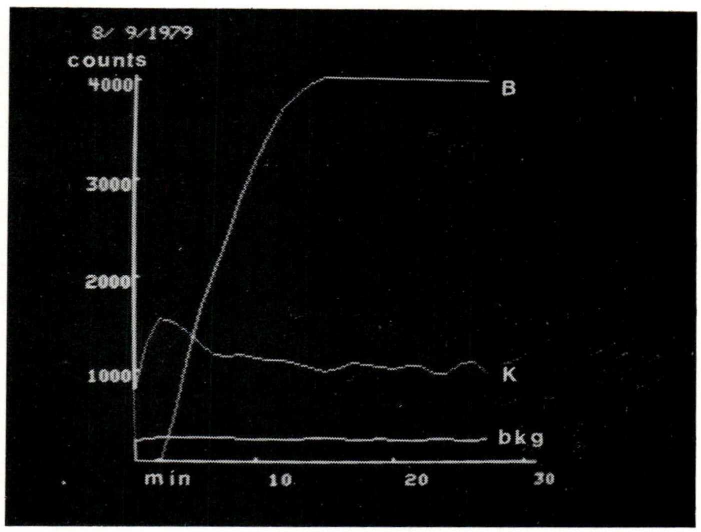


Renogram

**FIG. 24. I-131 HIPPURAN IMAGING AND RENOGRAM GENERATION IN ACUTE REJECTION.** Moderately acute rejection is characterized by an initial decline in excretory function, which is followed by a decrease in the effective renal plasma flow. With improvement, the excretory function increases first. Serial studies of a patient with a moderately acute rejection reflect these findings. **A.** Initial sequential I-131 Hippuran imaging performed 5 weeks following transplantation shows no evidence of impaired excretion. **B.** At 9 days, there is a marked reduction in excretion and this is especially well seen on the renogram. **C.** At 13 days the excretory impairment, although still present, is less marked. **D.** At 16 days, excretion has practically returned to normal and this coincides with the patient's clinical improvement. (Courtesy of Dr. Eva V. Dubovsky, Veterans Administration Medical Center, Birmingham, Alabama)

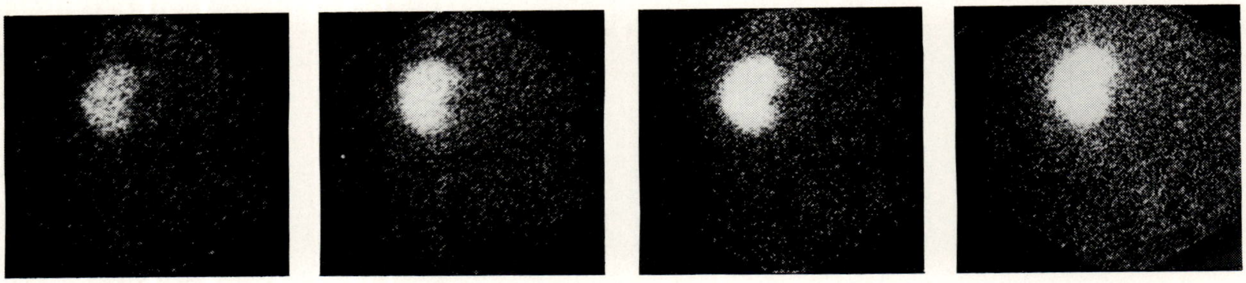

A 0 to 3 minutes | 3 to 6 minutes | 12 to 15 minutes | 24 to 27 minutes

I-131 Hippuran Imaging

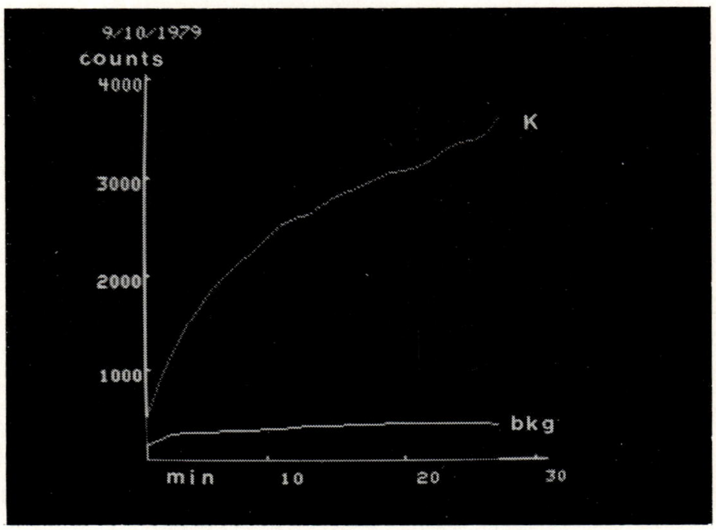


Renogram

**FIG. 25. A.** (See legend page 428)

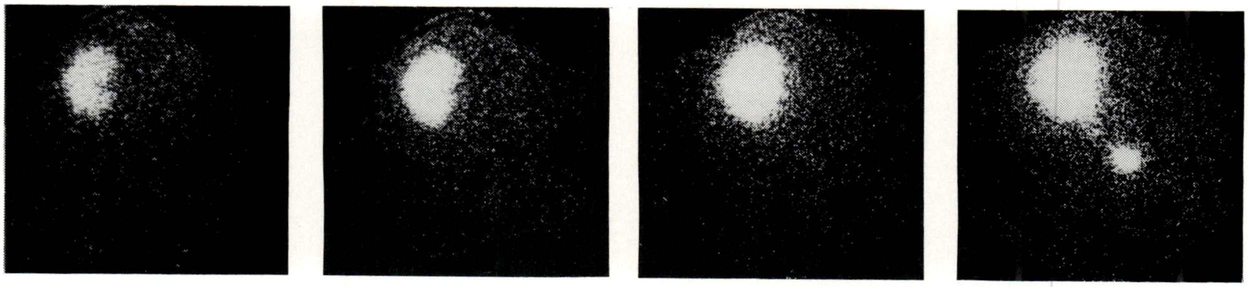

B 0 to 3 minutes　　3 to 6 minutes　　12 to 15 minutes　　24 to 27 minutes

I-131 Hippuran Imaging

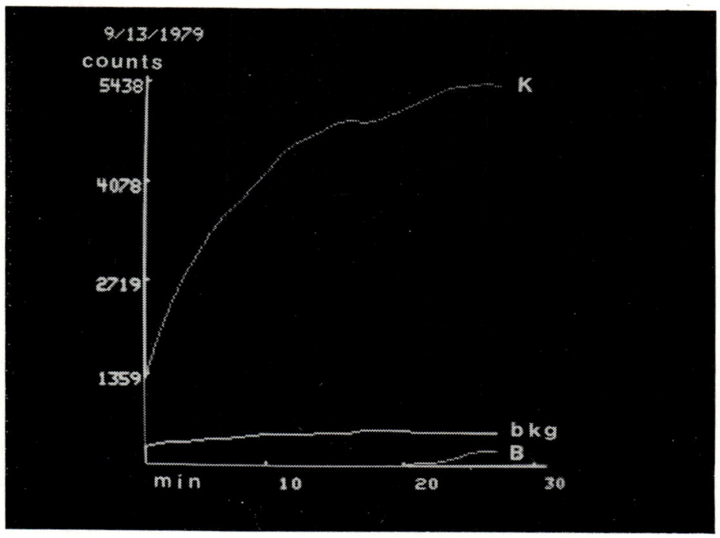


Renogram

**FIG. 25. B.** (See legend next page)

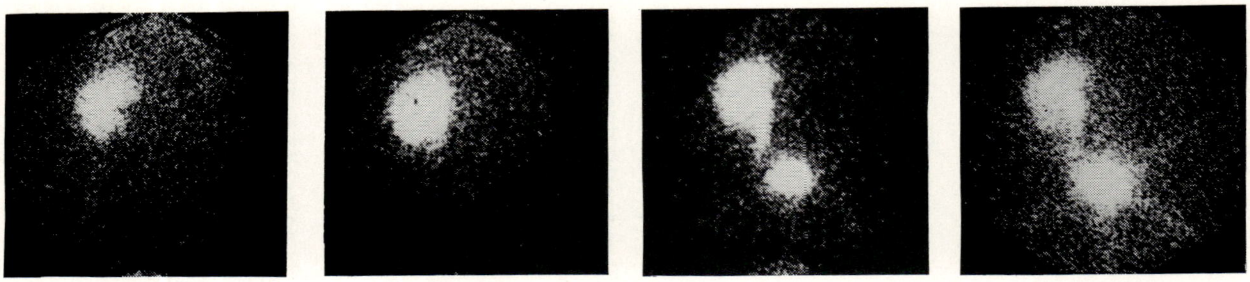

C 0 to 3 minutes | 3 to 6 minutes | 12 to 15 minutes | 24 to 27 minutes

I-131 Hippuran Imaging

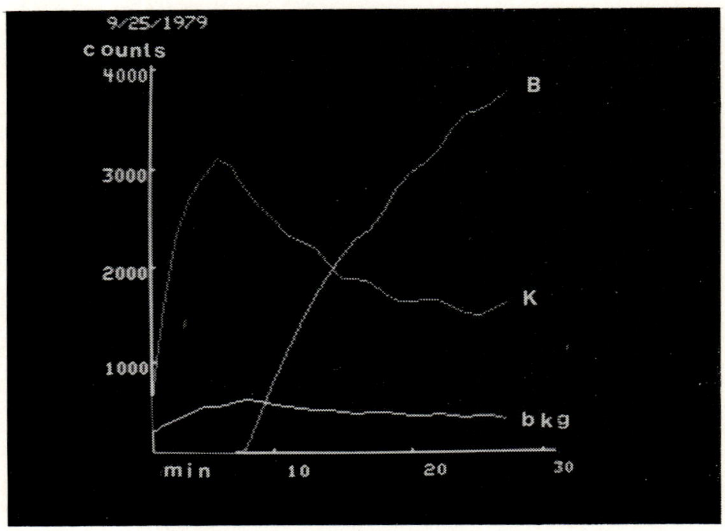


Renogram

**FIG. 25. I-131 HIPPURAN IMAGING AND RENOGRAM GENERATION IN ACUTE TUBULAR NECROSIS.** The nuclear medicine studies in a typical course of uncomplicated acute tubular necrosis are characterized initially by little or no excretion. **A.** In this patient, who received a kidney transplant, the I-131 Hippuran studies 3 days later showed no evidence of excretion. Imaging showed accumulating radioactivity in the transplanted kidney with no evidence of bladder visualization. The accompanying renogram showed a continual rise in the accumulation phase with no hint of an excretory fall. **B.** At 6 days after transplantation, imaging shows some evidence of I-131 Hippuran excretion. There is some reflection of this on the tracing, as there appears to be the start of an excretory curve and bladder activity can now be monitored. **C.** At 12 days, the renogram tracing exhibits its characteristic 3 segments. The transit time is normal and excretion is only slightly reduced. A completely normal study is common by the end of the third week. A return to normal occurs more rapidly in moderate or mild cases of acute tubular necrosis. (Courtesy of Dr. Eva V. Dubovsky, Veterans Administration Medical Center, Birmingham, Alabama)

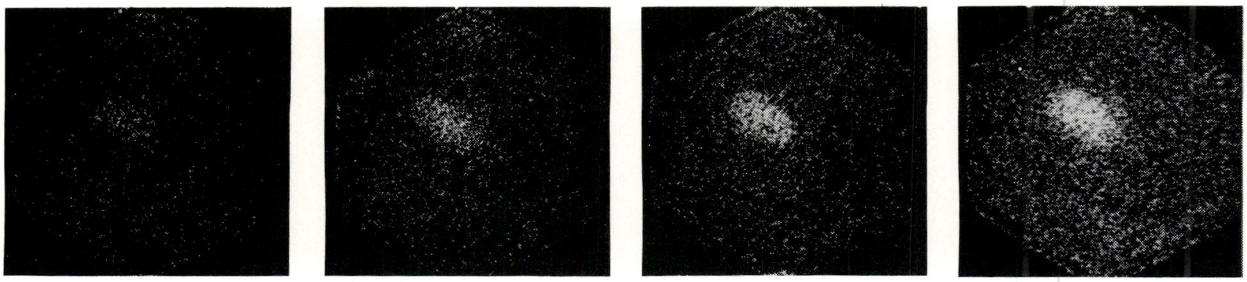

A 0 to 3 minutes 3 to 6 minutes 12 to 15 minutes 24 to 27 minutes

I-131 Hippuran Imaging

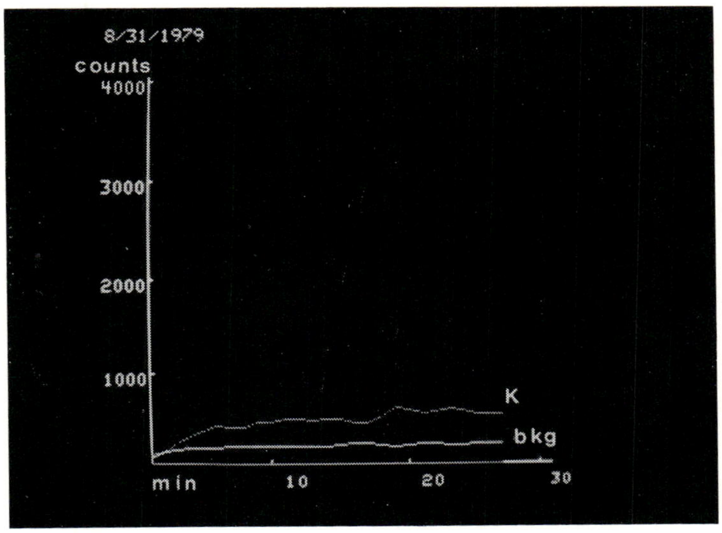


Renogram
One-Day Post-Transplantations

**FIG. 26. A.** (See legend on page 434)

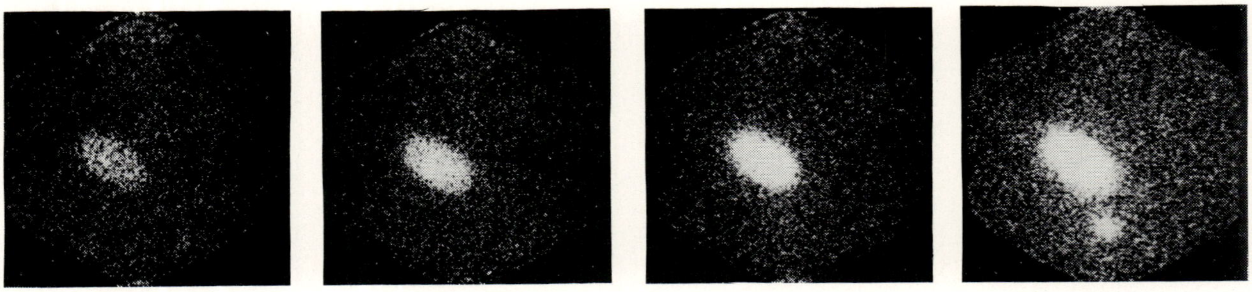

B 0 to 3 minutes | 3 to 6 minutes | 12 to 15 minutes | 24 to 27 minutes

I-131 Hippuran Imaging

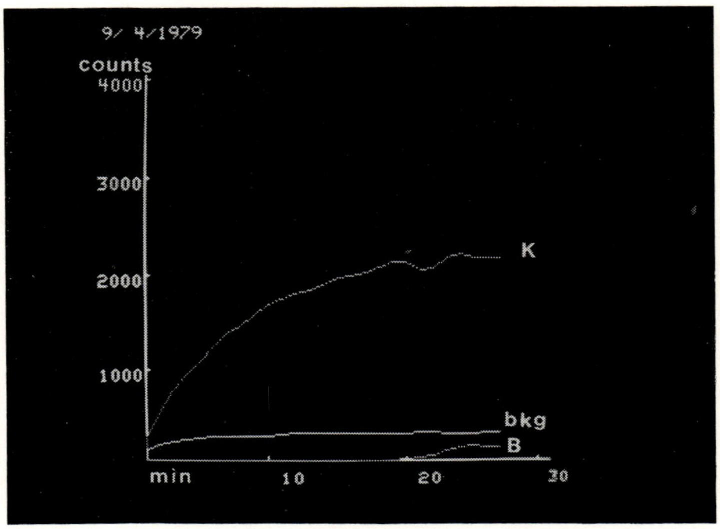


Renogram

Six Days Post-Transplantation

**FIG. 26. B.** (See legend on page 434)

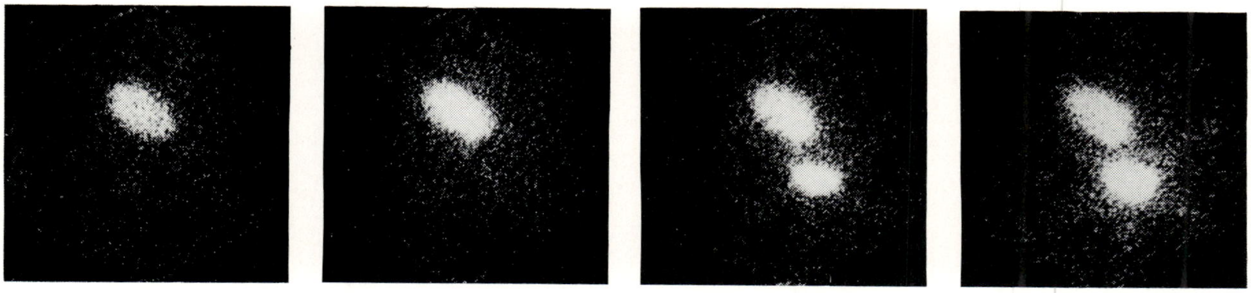

C 0 to 3 minutes 3 to 6 minutes 12 to 15 minutes 24 to 27 minutes

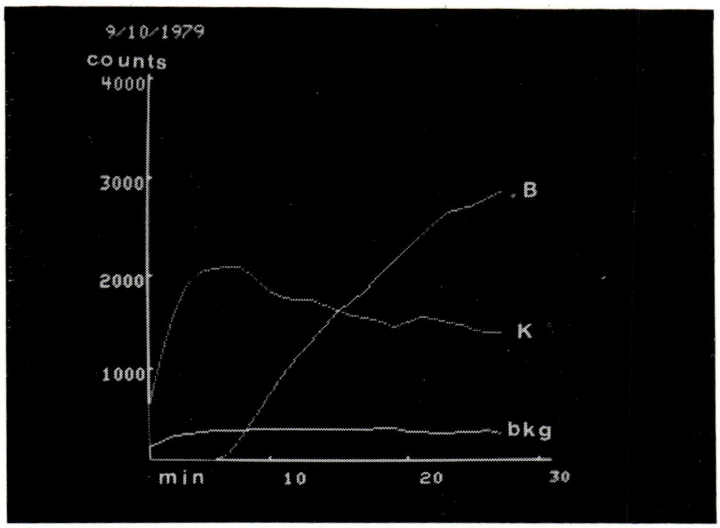


Renogram

Twelve Days Post-Transplantation

**FIG. 26. C.** (See legend page 434)

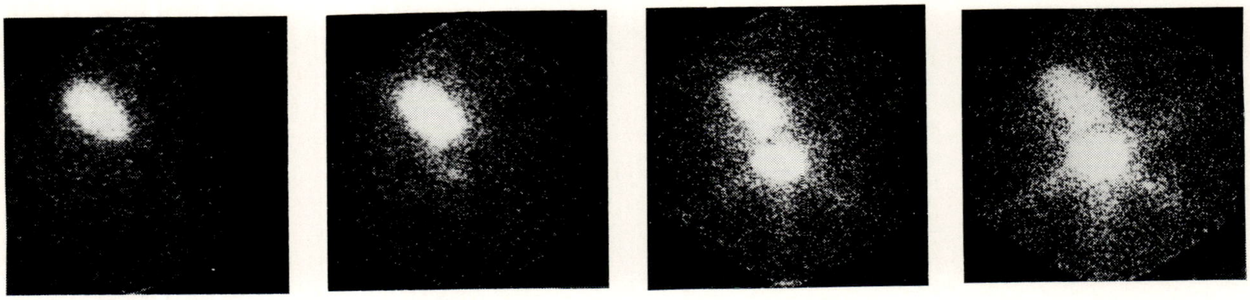

D 0 to 3 minutes — 3 to 6 minutes — 12 to 15 minutes — 24 to 27 minutes

I-131 Hippuran Imaging

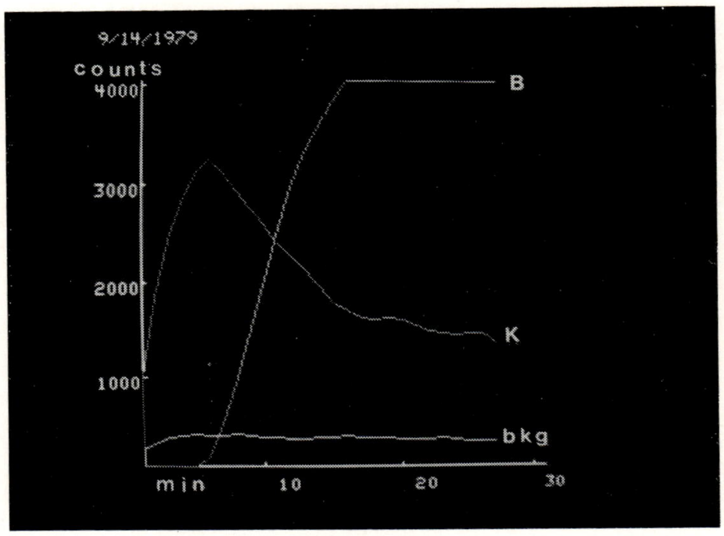


Renogram
Sixteen Days Post-Transplantation

**FIG. 26. D.** (See legend page 434)

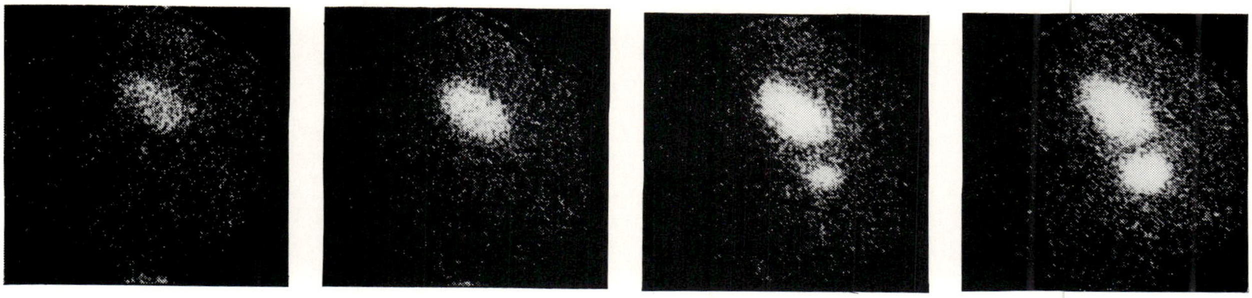

E 0 to 3 minutes 3 to 6 minutes 12 to 15 minutes 24 to 27 minutes

I-131 Hippuran Imaging

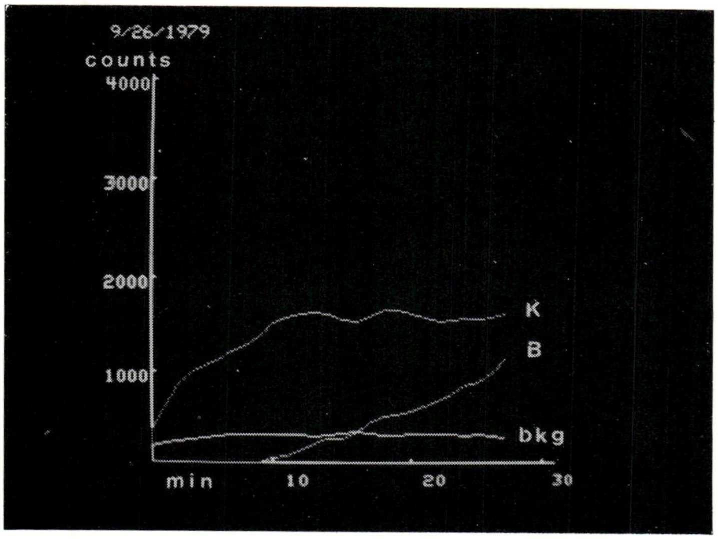


Renogram
Four Weeks Post-Transplantation

**FIG. 26. E.** (See legend next page)

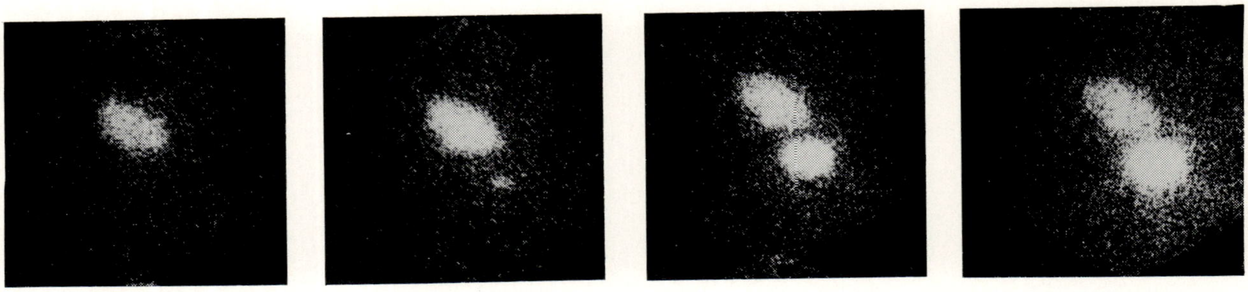

F 0 to 3 minutes 3 to 6 minutes 12 to 15 minutes 24 to 27 minutes

I-131 Hippuran Imaging

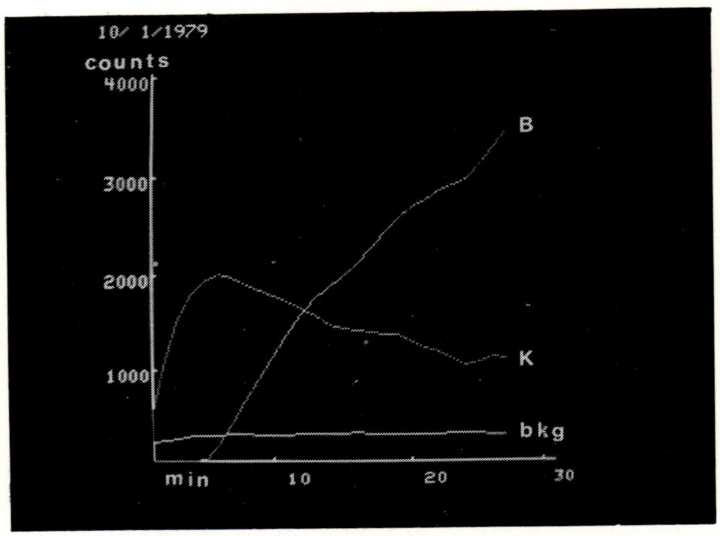


Renogram

Thirty-three Days Post-Transplantation

**FIG. 26.** **I-131 HIPPURAN IMAGING AND RENOGRAM GENERATION IN ACUTE TUBULAR NECROSIS COMPLICATED BY ACUTE REJECTION. A.** Studies performed one day following transplantation show no evidence of excretion. These findings may be indicative of acute tubular necrosis. The accumulation of the radioactive material is less than what would be expected. **B.** Six days after transplantation excretory function is still markedly impaired but there is faint evidence of excretion at about 25 minutes. **C.** The improvement from the acute tubular necrosis is not apparent 12 days after transplantation. Excretion is noted and the renogram configuration now exhibits 3 distinct segments. **D.** Further improvement is noted 16 days following transplantation. Note the bladder imaging as early as the 3- to 6-minute interval. **E.** At 4 weeks after transplantation, there is an unanticipated reduction in excretory function, heralding the onset of a rejection reaction. However, at 33 days (**F**) the rejection phenomenon is subsiding and this is indicated by the rapid improvement in excretion. (Courtesy of Dr. Eva V. Dubovsky, Veterans Administration Medical Center, Birmingham, Alabama)

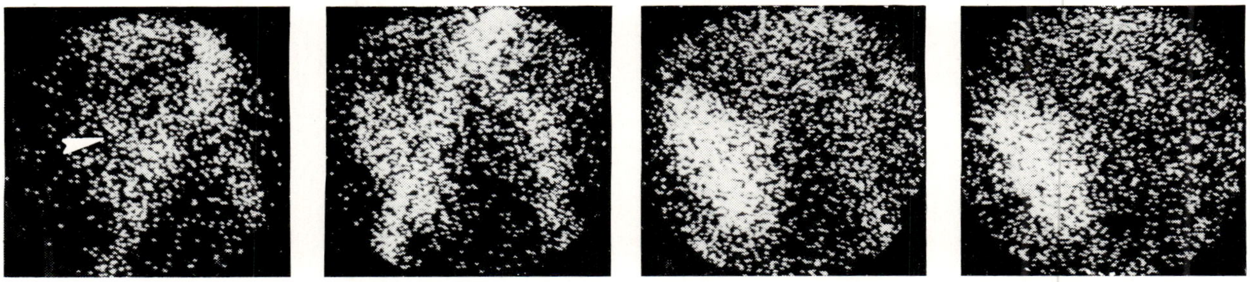

9 to 12 seconds | 15 to 18 seconds | 21 to 24 seconds | 27 to 30 seconds

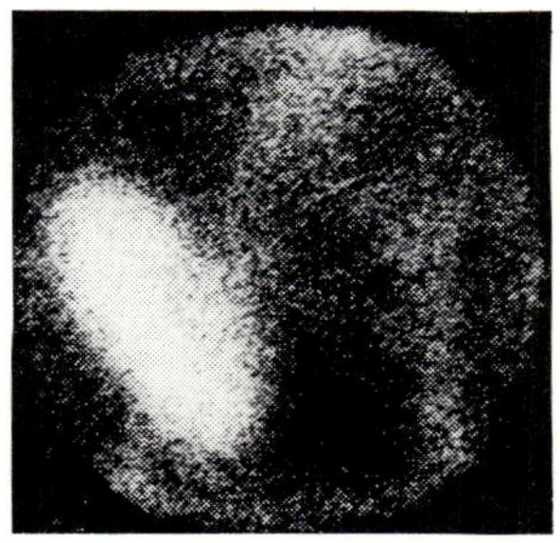

Static

**FIG. 27. BLOOD FLOW IMAGING IN CHRONIC REJECTION.** That there is arterial perfusion to the transplanted kidney is evidenced by the beginning renal visualization (arrow) during the arterial phase (9- to 12-second interval). Instead of a normal rapid transit through the kidney, the transit of the Tc-99m DTPA is prolonged, resulting in a well-defined renal image toward the end of the blood flow study (see Fig. 19). The static image taken immediately following the blood flow study further illustrates the clearly defined renal image. *Continued visualization of the renal image during the blood flow study may be a sign of chronic rejection.* (Courtesy of Dr. Eva V. Dubovsky, Veterans Administration Medical Center, Birmingham, Alabama)

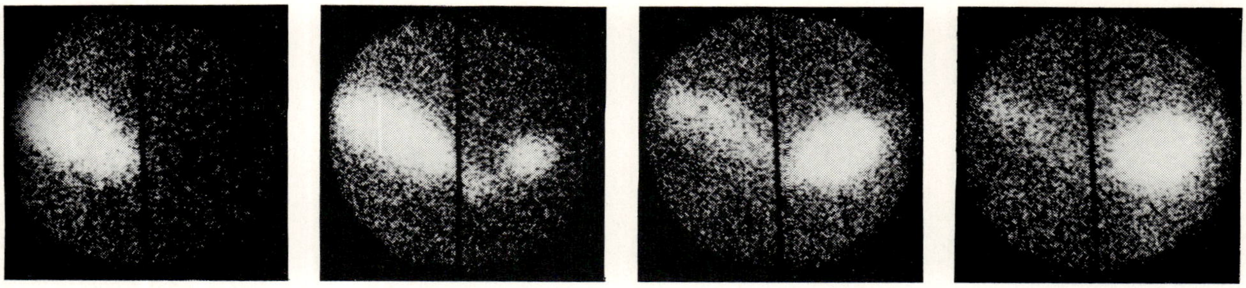

A 0 to 3 minutes 3 to 6 minutes 12 to 15 minutes 24 to 27 minutes

I-131 Hippuran Imaging

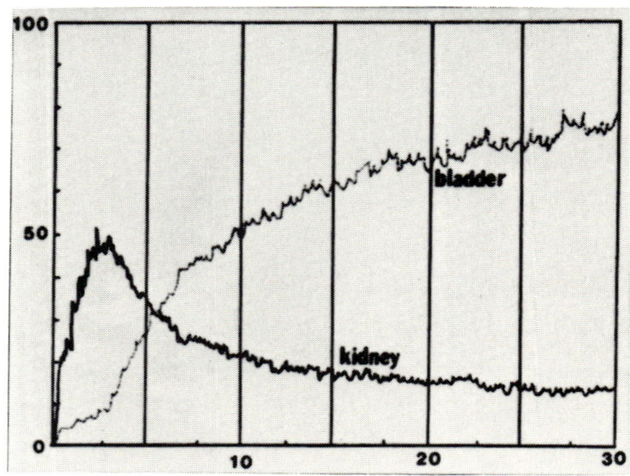


Renogram
One Year After Transplant

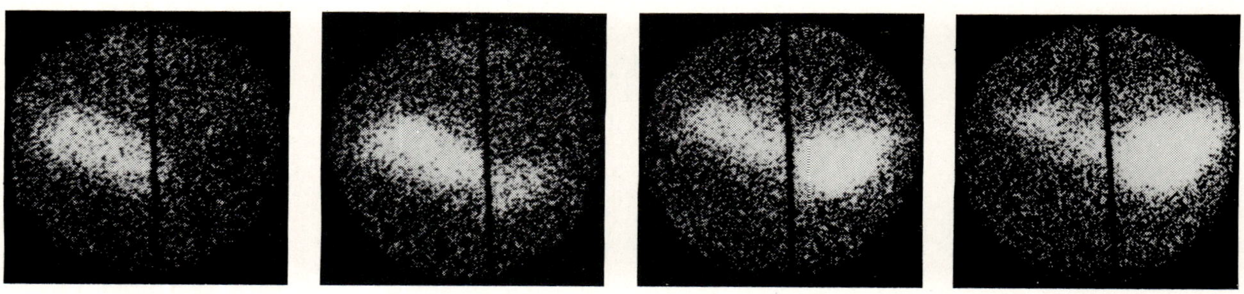

B 0 to 3 minutes 3 to 6 minutes 12 to 15 minutes 24 to 27 minutes

I-131 Hippuran Imaging

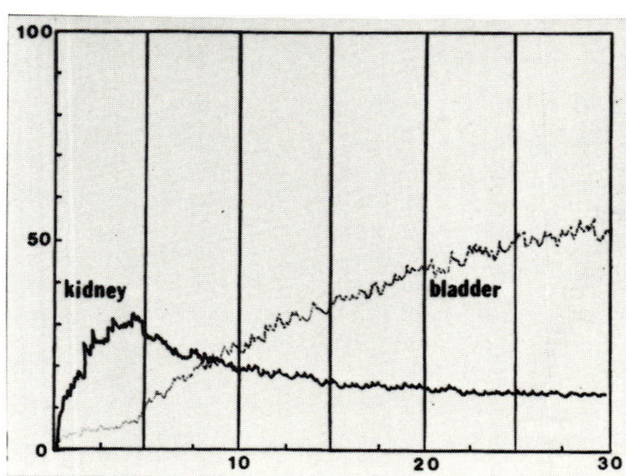


Renogram
Three Years After Transplant

**FIG. 28. A, B.**
(See legend next page)

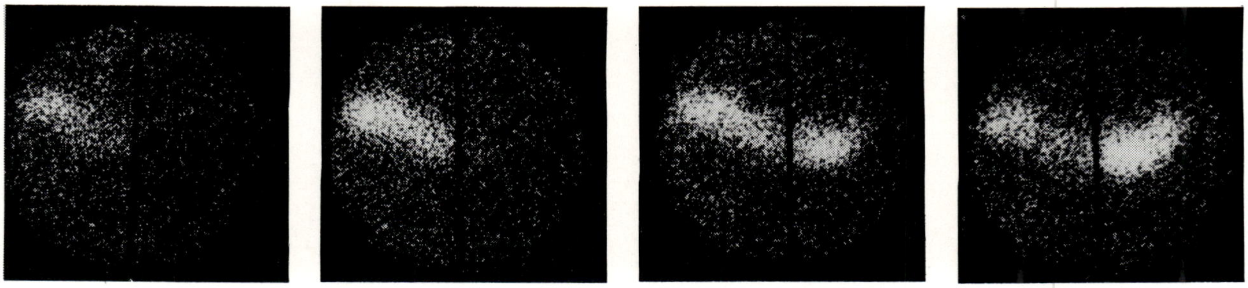

C 0 to 3 minutes 3 to 6 minutes 12 to 15 minutes 24 to 27 minutes

I-131 Hippuran Imaging

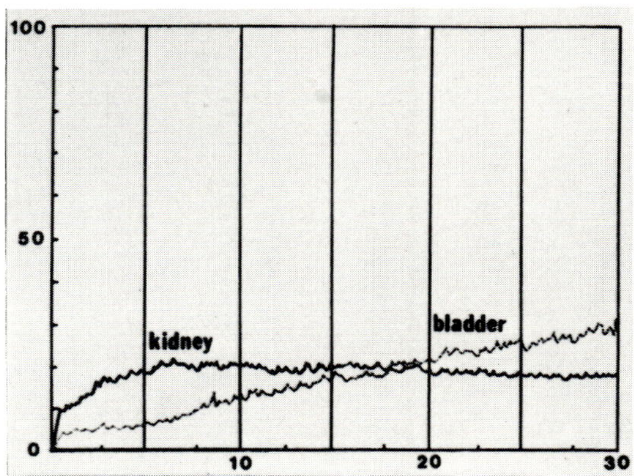


Renogram
Five Years After Transplant

**FIG. 28. I-131 HIPPURAN IMAGING AND RENOGRAM GENERATION IN CHRONIC REJECTION.** This patient received a renal transplant in 1971 and initially had no problems related to renal function. **A.** Examinations performed in 1972 showed normal I-131 Hippuran studies. **B.** The effective renal plasma flow started to diminish in 1974, 3 years after transplantation, indicating the gradual onset of chronic rejection. It can be seen that excretion is reduced when compared to the 1972 study. **C.** The patient continued to exhibit further impairment in renal excretion and these findings are reflected in the renal imaging and renogram performed in 1976, 5 years after transplantation. The patient's renal impairment was progressive and a graft nephrectomy was done in 1977. (Courtesy of Dr. Eva V. Dubovsky, Veterans Administration Medical Center, Birmingham, Alabama)

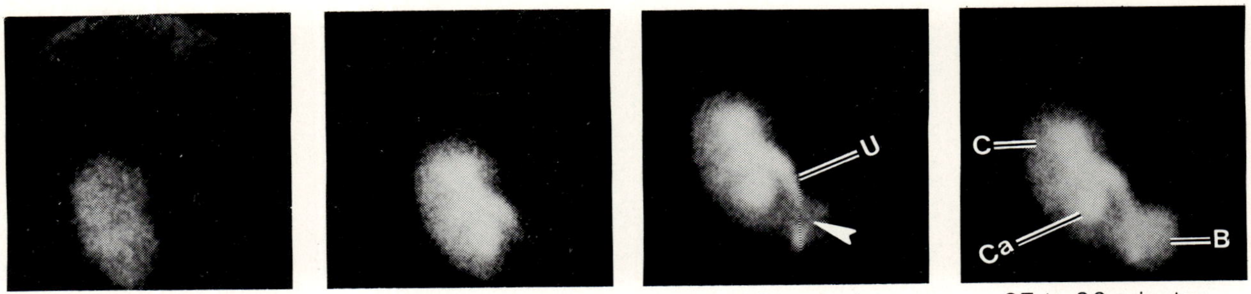


0 to 3 minutes | 6 to 9 minutes | 18 to 21 minutes | 27 to 30 minutes

## MECHANICAL COMPLICATIONS IN RENAL TRANSPLANTATION

**FIG. 29. OBSTRUCTION AT URETERO-VESICAL JUNCTION DUE TO POST-SURGICAL EDEMA.** Sequential static images show evidence of partial obstruction at the uretero-vesical junction (arrow), causing some retention of radioactive material in the renal transplant. There is evidence of partial obstruction in the image performed during the 18- to 21-minute interval. Note the sharp image of the ureter (U), the diminishing activity in the renal cortex (C), the greatly increased radioactivity in the calyces (Ca) and the indistinct imaging of the bladder (B). Since the obstruction is incomplete, continued imaging will show gradually increasing bladder activity (Tc-99m glucoheptonate). (Courtesy of Dr. Eva V. Dubovsky, Veterans Administration Medical Center, Birmingham, Alabama)

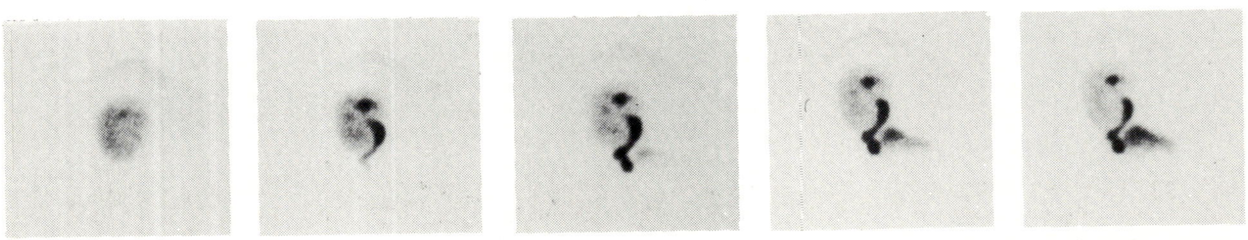

0 to 3 minutes | 3 to 6 minutes | 6 to 9 minutes | 9 to 12 minutes | 12 to 15 minutes

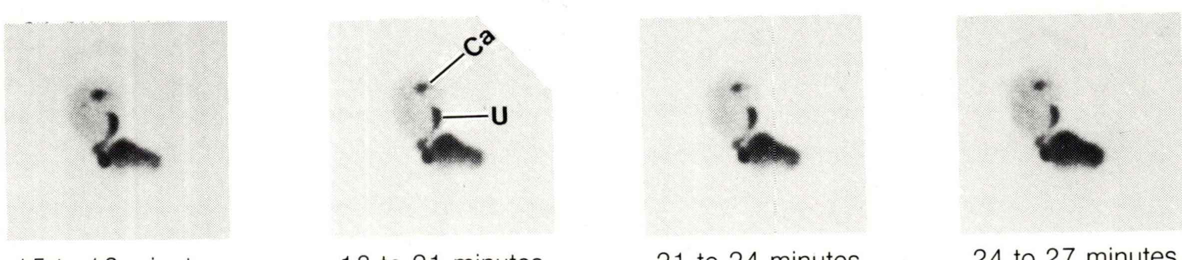


15 to 18 minutes | 18 to 21 minutes | 21 to 24 minutes | 24 to 27 minutes

**FIG. 30. INCOMPLETE OBSTRUCTION AT URETERO-VESICAL JUNCTION DUE TO POST-SURGICAL EDEMA.** In this case, the problem is less severe than that seen in Fig. 27. Note the persistent identification of the ureter (U) throughout, a finding suggesting at least partial obstruction in this case. Abundant bladder activity is not seen until the 15- to 18-minute interval. Calycyeal (Ca) retention is noted throughout (Tc-99m glucoheptonate). (Courtesy of Dr. Eva V. Dubovsky, Veterans Administration Medical Center, Birmingham, Alabama)

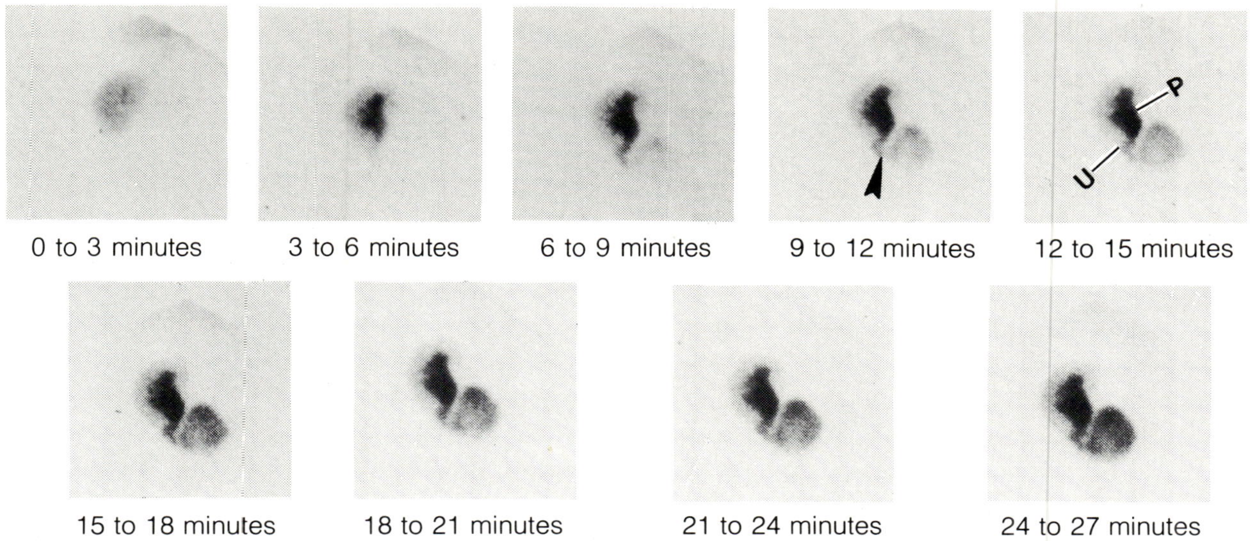


**FIG. 31. OBSTRUCTION AT URETERO-VESICAL JUNCTION DUE TO STRICTURE AT THAT SITE.** Note the persistence of radioactivity in the renal pelvis (P) and ureter (U), findings which are hallmarks of obstruction. Although there is some bladder activity, indicating that the obstruction is not total, the continued accumulation of radioactivity in the renal pelvis and ureter point to the severity of the situation. The site of obstruction (arrow) is easily identified. (Tc-99m glucoheptonate). (Courtesy of Dr. Eva V. Dubovsky, Veterans Administration Medical Center, Birmingham, Alabama)

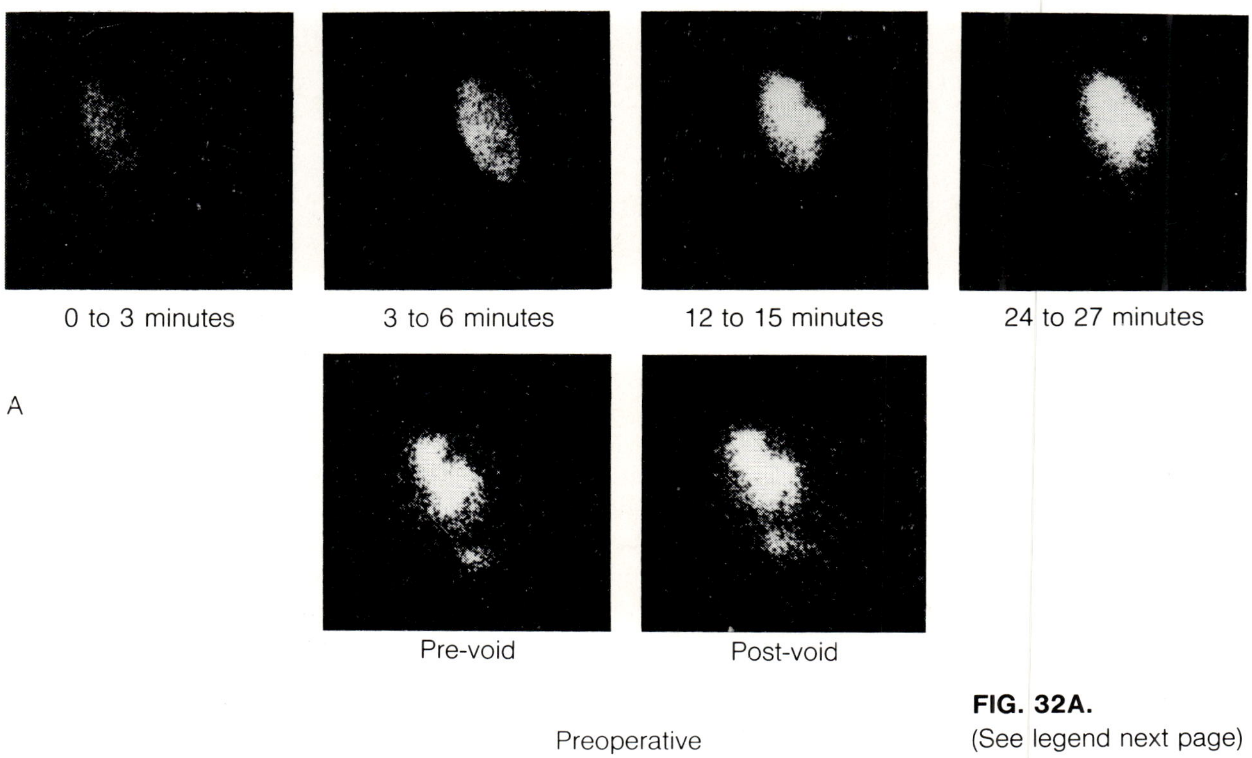


**FIG. 32A.**
(See legend next page)

0 to 3 minutes 3 to 6 minutes 12 to 15 minutes 24 to 27 minutes

B

Pre-void Post-void

Postoperative

**FIG. 32. I-131 HIPPURAN RENAL IMAGING IN URETERO-PELVIC JUNCTION OBSTRUCTION. A.** Evidence of obstructive uropathy is seen on imaging 8 months following transplantation. There is barely any evidence of radioactive material reaching the bladder. At surgery performed 2 weeks later, it was found that the obstruction was caused by adhesions around the middle third of the ureter; the obstruction was relieved with lysis of the adhesions. **B.** Imaging performed one week following surgery shows no evidence of obstructive uropathy any longer. Note the pre- and post-voiding images before and after surgery. (Courtesy of Dr. Eva V. Dubovsky, Veterans Administration Medical Center, Birmingham, Alabama)

## ANATOMIC CHANGES

### Renal Tissue Replacement or Destruction

Although a localized area of absent radioactivity on renal imaging may be easily visualized, the precise identification of the etiology of such an abnormality is often made with great difficulty or is beyond the reliability of proper interpretation. Thus, a number of space-occupying lesions may have a similar appearance on static imaging. It is not unusual for lesions such as cysts, tumors, and abscesses to have a similar appearance on imaging.

A number of refinements have been introduced to more clearly define an abnormality seen on radionuclide renal imaging. It is well known, for example, that a simple cyst of the kidney may be identified on a blood flow study as an avascular area, while a neoplasm, such as a hypernephroma, will usually show increased radioactivity on blood flow imaging. Despite the ability to differentiate between two types of lesions in certain selected situations, in the majority of cases it is far more difficult to suggest a diagnosis.

A large body of nuclear medicine physicians prefer that emphasis not be placed on renal imaging for the precise identification of renal space occupying lesions. Considering the possible diagnostic precision that may be possible from ultrasound, computed tomography, and roentgenologic studies of the urinary system, they feel that attention in such cases should be directed to diagnostic screening procedures employing these methods rather than to radionuclide imaging. This is the point of view held by the authors of this Atlas as is reflected in the brief treatment of this subject. To be sure, this opinion is not shared by all nuclear medicine physicians.

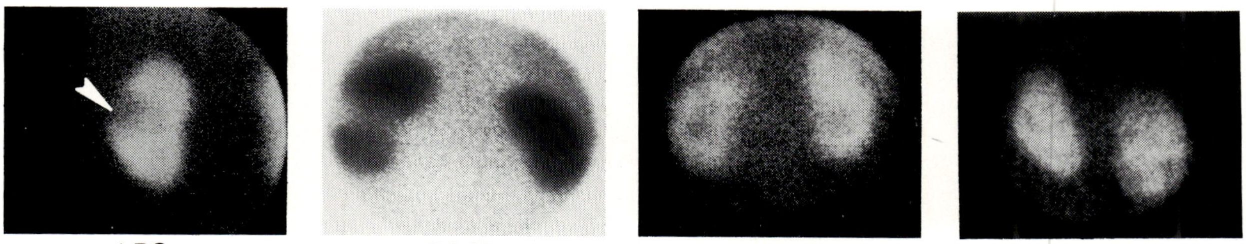

A LPO Cortical Cyst

B POST Intrarenal Cyst

C POST Bilateral Intrarenal Cysts

D POST Polycystic Disease

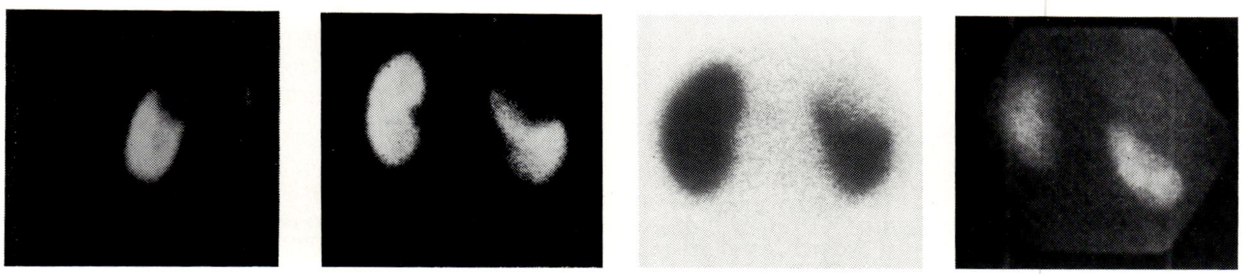

E POST Hypernephroma

F POST Hypernephroma

G POST Hypernephroma

H LPO Renal Corbuncle

**FIG. 33. SPACE OCCUPYING LESIONS.** It is often possible to correctly identify the etiology of a space-occupying lesion from renal imaging alone. However, renal imaging is usually not a precise method for determination of whether or not, for example, an abnormality is cystic or due to neoplasm. **Renal cysts. A.** Solitary cortical cyst (arrow) which has a somewhat rounded appearance. **B.** Large, solitary intrarenal cyst which appears to bisect the left kidney. **C.** Bilateral intrarenal cysts. **D.** Polycystic disease. The visualization of multiple, small, rounded areas of absent radioactivity bilaterally suggests that polycystic disease is indeed present. **Neoplasm.** Unfortunately, there are no characteristic features on static imaging to establish a diagnosis of neoplasm. In **E** and **F**, the site of the upper pole hypernephroma in each of 2 patients shows the area of tumor replacement and remaining, functioning renal tissue to be sharply and smoothly demarcated. Although visible, the tumor–kidney interface is less clearly defined in **G. Inflammatory lesion.** Although a renal abscess can be identified with Ga-67 imaging, such demonstration may also be seen with renal imaging agents. **H.** Renal carbuncle seen as poorly defined area of reduced activity (arrow) at right lower pole. (**B** and **G** courtesy of Dr. L. Silver, Queens Hospital Center, Jamaica, NY; **D** courtesy of Dr. M. Friedlander, Polyclinic Medical Center, Harrisburg, PA; **H** courtesy of Dr. J. Rockett, Baptist Memorial Hospital, Memphis, TN)

## Suggested Reading

Ball, JD, Maynard CD: Nuclear imaging in urology. Urol Clin North Am 6:321–342, 1979

Bingham JB, Maisey MN: An evaluation of the use of $^{99m}$Tc-dimercaptosuccinic acid (DMSA) as a static renal imaging agent. Br J Radiol 51:599–607, 1978

Bueschen AJ, Witten DM: Radionuclide evaluation of renal function. Urol Clin North Am 6:307–320, 1979

Diethelm AG, Dubovsky EV, Whelchel JD, et al. Diagnosis of impaired renal function after kidney transplantation using renal scintigraphy, renal plasma flow and urinary excretion of hippurate. Ann Surg. 191:604–616, 1980.

Dubovsky EV, Diethelm AG, Tauxe WN. Differentiation of cell-mediated and humoral rejection by orthoiodohippurate kinetics. Arch Intern Med 137:738–742, 1977

Holten I, Storm HH: Kidney scintigraphy with $^{99m}$Tc-DMSA and 131 I-hippurate. Scand J Urol Nephrol 13:275–281, 1979

Kawamura J, Hosokawa S, Yoshida O: Renal function studies using $^{99m}$Tc-dimercaptosuccinic acid. Clin Nucl Med 4:39–45, 1979

Kirchner PT, Ed: *Nuclear Medicine Review Syllabus.* New York, Society of Nuclear Medicine, 1980, pp 323–384

Lome LG, Pinsky S, Levy L: Dynamic renal scan in the nonvisualizing kidney. J Urol 121:148–152, 1979

McAfee JG: Radionuclide imaging in the assessment of primary chronic pyelonephritis. Radiology 133:203–206, 1979

Mogensen P: *Strategy in Clinical Renography.* Copenhagen, Laegeforeningens Forlag, 1979

Ormrod D, Miller T, Stewart E: Technetium-99m sulfur colloid localization in renal infection: experimental evaluation. Invest Urol 16:23–26, 1978

Preston DF, Luke RG: Radionuclide evaluation of renal transplants. J Nucl Med 20:1095–1096, 1979

Steyn JH, MacDonald AF, Keyes WI, et al: An assessment of computerised isotopic renal section scanning. Br J Urol 50:437–441, 1978

# Index